REMOVABLE ORTHODONTIC APPLIANCES

T. M. GRABER, D.M.D., M.S.D., Ph.D.

Professor, Pediatrics and Anthropology,
Zoller Dental Clinic;
Chairman, Orthodontics, University of Chicago;
Kenilworth Dental Research Foundation
Kenilworth, Illinois

BEDRICH NEUMANN, M.D.

Former Chief Orthodontist
Regional Hospital
Ostrava, Czechoslovakia

W. B. SAUNDERS COMPANY • PHILADELPHIA • LONDON • TORONTO

W. B. Saunders Company: West Washington Square
Philadelphia, PA   19105

1 St. Anne's Road
Eastbourne, East Sussex BN21 3UN. England

1 Goldthorne Avenue
Toronto, Ontario M8Z 5T9, Canada

Library of Congress Cataloging in Publication Data

Main entry under title:

Removable orthodontic appliances.

Previous ed. (1966) by A. M. Schwarz and M. Gratzinger.

Includes index.

1. Orthodontic appliances.   I. Graber, Touro M.
II. Neumann, Bedrich.   III. Schwarz, Artur Martin,
Removable orthodontic appliances. [DNLM: 1. Ortho-
dontic appliances, Removable. WU400 R389]

RK527.S46 1977   617.6'43'0028   76-14681

ISBN 0-7216-4190-3

Removable Orthodontic Appliances   ISBN   0-7216-4190-3

Last digit is the print number: 9   8   7   6   5

Dedication

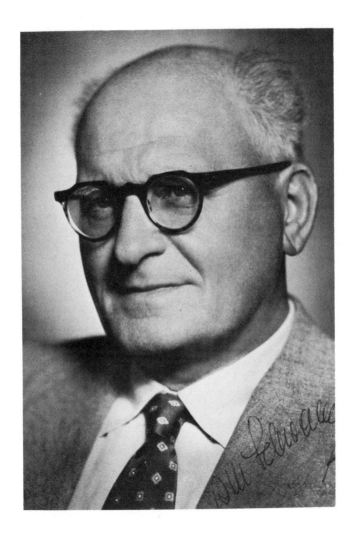

To Martin Schwarz, Scientist, Biologist, Clinician, and Teacher

Preface

The genesis of this book may be traced to Martin Schwarz. As General Chairman of the 1960 American Association of Orthodontists' meeting in Washington D.C., I had the pleasure of inviting him to take part in one of the first truly international meetings held under the aegis of the AAO. With VIPs like Hotz, Häupl, Korkhaus, Begg, and Lager, Schwarz was in his element. A major surgical operation right before the meeting would surely have sidelined most men, but Schwarz, with an indomitable will, literally got out of bed to attend the meeting because he had made the commitment. A great biologist and scientist, a consumate cephalometrician, a superb clinician, and a great teacher with boundless enthusiasm, his *Lehrgang der Gebissregulung* was the orthodontic bible of Europe. He had taken the myriad of appliances that were used and had organized them into an orderly system, which was treatment objective oriented.

A. M. Schwarz (May 16, 1887–June 15, 1963) had graduated as an M.D. in 1913. After military service in World War I, he returned to Vienna and was employed in various departments of the University Hospital in Vienna (otorhinolaryngology, surgery, and pathology). But his first love, finally, was dentistry. Albin Oppenheim was his teacher in orthodontics. Dr. Schwarz soon started to publish a number of valuable reports on treatment procedures and on his research in the development of occlusion and the prevention of malocclusion. He became associated in practice with Professor Bernhard Gottlieb, regarded as one of the foremost periodontists of his time. Gottlieb headed a group of specialists who devoted themselves to histologic studies. There Martin Schwarz found the help he needed for his own investigations on tissue changes incident to orthodontic tooth movement (Intern. J. Orthod., *18*:331, 1932).

In 1933, Schwarz was appointed to the medical faculty of the University of Vienna, and became professor and chairman of his department in 1951. In 1939, he took over the small orthodontic department of the Vienna Municipal Health Service. At that time about 100 children were receiving orthodontic treatment there. Under his guidance, the number was expanded to 3000. Forty dentists made up the staff and received orthodontic training by working in the clinic three half days a week without pay.

Most important for the further work of Schwarz was the close cooperation established with Alfred Kantorowicz and Gustav Korkhaus of Bonn, Germany. Kantorowicz had developed an economically feasible and systematic school dental care program. His special endeavor was to extend that service to include ortho-dontics. Based on the extensive research work of Korkhaus, the two men tried to clarify the etiology of malocclusion, thus making preventive and interceptive orthodontic procedures possible. At that time, however, the potential for prac-tical application of their research was limited, preventing extension of ortho-dontics to larger segments of the public. Schwarz, with his further development of the active plate, and Andresen and Häupl, with their activator, became the catalysts, making the treatment of large numbers of children possible.

The apparent but deceptive simplicity of these removable orthodontic appliances encouraged many dentists to employ orthodontic treatment in their practices. Since there were no adequate training facilities, nor sufficient appro-priate postgraduate instruction possibilities, Schwarz tried to fill the gap by writing textbooks giving detailed information on diagnosis and treatment. The step-by-step presentation of diagnostic and therapeutic procedures and deci-sions provided lucid and systematic guidance for dentists. In the final edition, the textbook appeared in two volumes, with 1600 pages, 1200 figures, and 4300 single illustrations.

Like most American orthodontists at the time of our 1960 AAO meeting, I was literally a "doubting Thomas" about removable appliances. I had just finished an extensive survey of AAO membership the previous year on what the future developments were likely to be (*Orthodontics in 1969*) and there had, in-deed, been the prediction by our membership that we all would be using more removable appliances in the next ten years. But I took a rather dim view of this, as a step backwards into proliferating mediocrity, performing a little bit for a lot of patients, not the best possible for each individual. Removable appliances were those gadgets used by non-specialists, both in Europe and America, when they had not been trained in the mastery of the more sophisticated fixed appliances. At the time, most of the claims of successful treatment seemed more like prop-aganda than anything else. Since they couldn't use fixed appliances, proponents of removable appliances had to talk a good game and show carefully selected cases.

In 1961, I attended the European Orthodontic Society meeting in Bologna. Martin Schwarz came down from Vienna with some of his confreres. He asked me to come up to his room and see representative cases treated with removable appliances. I well remember my accepting reluctantly, with an indulgent smile and, inwardly, a condescending, "Come now, do you really expect me to believe that what you will show me is in the same league as fixed appliance results?" I had just driven down from Zurich with Rudi and Margi Hotz. Before we left, I spent an afternoon in the prestigious orthodontic department headed by Professor Hotz at the University of Zurich. Twenty-six patients, one right after another, had been called in, each showing superb correction of a Class II, Division 1 malocclusion. All had been treated with a monobloc, the propulsor, designed by Mühlemann and modified by Hotz. Very impressive, but I was so thoroughly imbued with the idea that only fixed appliances could routinely do the job that the true impact had not sunk in as yet. I reasoned that these cases were probably due to the outstanding clinical ability and genius of Rudi Hotz, but I doubted that others could do the same.

I went across town in a ridiculously small taxi, with all four of us squeezed in, to Schwarz's hotel. Spread out on the bed, which occupied most of his hotel room, were the contents of two large valises. I found out later, with some degree of flattery, that the material had been brought specially just to show to me. In the hour and a half we spent going over every conceivable kind of malocclusion, I really learned the potential of removable appliances. No doubt about it, *in the right hands, with the proper case selection*, a great deal could be done—often more easily, with less potential damage, and sometimes even more rapidly. The Hotz cases were not unique, but only part of the story—a most important part, of course, but here were cases of every type of malocclusion. I remember Martin Schwarz asking me, with a rather triumphant smile on his face, after we were finished, "Well now, what do you think of it? Do you really have to do everything the hard way, with every tooth banded?"

Martin Schwarz was a meticulous orthodontist, with each case subjected to total diagnostic scrutiny. His cephalometric analysis (roentgenostatics) was more sophisticated and pertinent than most of the so-called analyses making the rounds in America as "cephalometrics." When I got back home, I helped translate and get his material published in the AJO. And when Max Gratzinger, a distinguished disciple of Schwarz and a leader in his own right, wanted help on the English translation and publication of *Der Lehrgang*, I stepped in with real interest, because I saw something for the American orthodontist which could help many more people.

Professor Schwarz did not live to see the English edited version, *Removable Orthodontic Appliances*, published in 1966. The book was successful, however, and very probably was an opening wedge in the stainless steel fortress built and defended by American orthodontists.

Many advances have occurred in removable appliances in the last 10 to 15 years. When Saunders asked me to revise and update the 1966 Schwarz-Gratzinger book, I knew this would be a major undertaking. I consulted with Bedrich Neumann of Czechoslovakia, who has seen more of European orthodontics in toto, and has been associated with more leaders, than anyone else. His "elder statesman" status and avid interest in current developments made unique qualifications. He pointed out that the Schwarz-Gratzinger book was based on a book written years before and that there was a new generation of leaders and of appliances. The laborious efforts to make the necessary changes soon made it apparent that it was impractical to do a second edition of the Schwarz-Gratzinger book, as fine as it was. We agreed to form a team and to work together on the major task of culling European orthodontic techniques for those with the greatest potential for American orthodontic specialists and for American children.

A new book incorporating "the latest and best" in removable appliances has been written. Many have lent a helping hand. In particular, eminent orthodontic statesmen like Ascher, Bimler, Fränkel, Herren, Hotz, Karwetzky, Klammt, Mills, Schmuth, Slagsvold, Stockfisch, Taatz, and Woodside have made important contributions. And Schwarz is still there, too—with his ingenious active plates, both single and double, and his detailed instructions on activator fabrication— still right up to date.

We have tried to give the most complete information possible within the limitations imposed by the book. To accomplish this, it was necessary not only to get the cooperation of the authors involved, but also to give them an opportunity to state their case. In the writing and editing we have tried hard to unify the book and create a logical "flow." This has been possible only to a limited degree. Disagreement in the views of the different authors could not be eliminated without distorting their opinions. Some contradictions in the various chapters exist. But this is no different than in multiauthored texts by American authors (*Current Orthodontic Concepts and Techniques,* for example), and should stimulate the critical and interested reader to resolve these differences in his own mind.

We now have over a quarter of a century of National Health Scheme orthodontics by Britain, using mostly removable appliances, to serve as a basis of assessment of the good and the bad. Hans Eirew, an eminent British orthodontist, has recently studied European orthodontics under the aegis of the World Health Organization. He visited various orthodontic centers in Europe and then made a comparision of British and European procedures. As an active clinician on the British scene, a leader in British orthodontic society affairs, and a disciple of Rolf Fränkel, he is well qualified to make this appraisal. He writes, "In suitable cases—and here, case selection is important—functional treatment, particularly by the modern devices, has a great deal to offer. It can successfully be employed at an earlier age than other methods. . . . Both the amount and burden of treatment may be reduced. In the following clinical situations, functional appliances appear to score over the removable plates and fixed appliances commonly used in Britain:

1. Where there is need for mandibular advance.
2. Where there is need for bite opening.
3. Where there is need for increased lower face height.
4. Where there is need for arch widening.
5. For early treatment of Class III.
6. In Class II, Division 2.
7. In open bite cases.

Eirew lists the following contraindications for functional appliances like the activator, Bionator, Fränkel function corrector, Stockfisch Kinetor, and Bimler Oral Adaptor.

1. Single arch treatment.
2. Movement of single teeth or small localized adjustments.
3. Rotations.
4. Severe crowding.
5. Angle Class II, with normal mandibular development and prenormal (protrusive) middle third.
6. Angle Class II with prominence of the bony chin.
7. Patients of questionable cooperation.
8. Patients unable to tolerate bulky removable appliances.
9. Patients with allergic reaction to appliance materials.
10. Patients lacking appliance control owing to other physical or mental handicaps.

Eirew points to the evident predominance in the use of simple removable plates in Britain, of functional appliances in central Europe, and of sophisticated multibanded appliances in the United States and Australia. He writes, "It is my belief that this exclusiveness is irrational, uneconomic in many cases and often conducive to bad results." He is critical of the low level of British accomplishment, with the lack of proper training of British dentists to do anything but simple plates and extractions. He makes a plea for more emphasis on diagnosis (cephalometrics in particular), on patient education, on the long-term effects of treatment such as they are providing British children, and on the elimination of orthodontic wastage—the large number of uncompleted cases, owing to the delegation of work to semitrained operators and the lack of patient education.

Eirew stresses the universal European criticism of British orthodontics because of overemphasis of simple treatment, preoccupation with undergraduate orthodontics, and the disunity among British orthodontists. He quotes one Dutch academic as saying, "We pay five times as much as you for our orthodontics, but we get fifty times the value. That is good economics!" And again, with reference to the semitrained practitioner, "A patient seeking professional advice, be it from a surgeon, physician, dentist or orthodontist, has the right to expect that this man is fully trained."

It must be obvious even to the uninitiated that potentially analogous problems exist on this side of the Atlantic, and that it is relatively easy to extrapolate from the British to the American scene. Eirew, in his report, stresses the theme of this book—that better all round treatment would doubtless result if a larger proportion of orthodontists had all three systems—simple plates, functional appliances, and multibanded fixed appliances—at their command, and were able to employ them selectively. Based on his experience, he suggests the following categories for each:

1. Mild irregularities, upper canine retraction, simple incisor retraction, movement of tooth in crossbite—the use of a simple removable plate with a spring, screw, or elastic.
2. Severe rotations or crowding, major movement of individual teeth or tooth groups—fixed appliances.
3. Bite opening or closure—dynamic functional appliances.
4. Bimaxillary protrusion—extraction of first premolars and fixed multibanded appliances.
5. Class II, Division 1 malocclusion.
   a. True maxillary protrusion with normal mandibular development and posture—upper arch extractions predominating, upper canine and incisor retraction by removable plates or fixed appliances, headgear.
   b. Mixed maldevelopment affecting both jaws—intermaxillary traction, fixed or removable or simple functional appliances.
   c. Marked mandibular retrusion, reduced lower face height—dynamic functional appliances.
6. Class II, Division 2 (Deckbiss)—function corrector, extractions in molar regions only.
7. Class III Malocclusion.
   a. Early treatment—dynamic functional appliances.
   b. Late treatment—fixed multibanded techniques.

Most American orthodontists would take exception to one or more of these suggested corrective approaches. But there can be no question that a wider use of removable appliances will enlarge the orthodontic armamentarium, make some things easier, serve more patients, and permit the orthodontic specialist to meet any practice challenge from third party enlargement of service. We must learn from the lessons of the British National Health Scheme. A real message seems to be that we do not emulate their mistakes. If we are to believe the critics of British orthodontics, the public has not been served well, by and large, mostly because the system was thrust on them before they had time for preparation. In defense of our British confreres, they really had no choice at that time. Very few orthodontically trained dentists existed in England, and they had to "make do" the best that they could. The blame lies with the proliferating governmental bureaucracy which has imposed its dictates on both the dental profession and the public.

Subsequent preoccupation with training dental students and technicians in the mechanical aspects of appliance manipulation in England has resulted in needless mass extractions and familiarity with only the simpler removable appliances. In the final analysis, only the orthodontic specialist or fully trained professional has the specialized biological background, the intensive training in diagnostic procedures, and the ability to use the broadened armamentarium properly. And to do the job right, it has to be a broad-based multi-appliance facility. Treatment must be patient problem oriented, not appliance system dictated.

There is a certain degree of urgency now for the orthodontic specialty to inform itself of the potentials and pitfalls of all types of removable appliances, so that stop-gap procedures will not be necessary and so that dentistry is not forced to render a substandard service to the public because of unwise politico-social decisions.

T. M. GRABER

BEDRICH NEUMANN

Acknowledgments

This book is a team effort. Some chapters are totally the effort of the authors listed. Others have been rewritten. A liberal amount of editing has been done in most instances. Particular credit is given to Olav Slagsvold, Professor and Head of the Orthodontic Department at the University of Oslo, for Chapter 7; to Donald Woodside, Professor and Head of the Orthodontic Department, University of Toronto, for Chapter 12; and to Dr. H. P. Bimler, who has lectured at a number of universities and is currently in private orthodontic practice in Wiesbaden, Germany, for Chapter 13.

Others who have contributed heavily to the final versions of various chapters are Rudi Hotz, former Professor and Head of the Department of Orthodontics, University of Zurich; Robert Shaye, Associate Professor of Orthodontics at the University of Louisiana, for Chapter 5; Professor Felix Ascher of Munich for Chapter 9; H. Metzelder of the German Democratic Republic for Chapter 10; G. Klammt of Görlitz, Germany, for Chapter 11; Hugo Stockfisch of Stuttgart, Germany, for Chapter 14; Rolf Fränkel of Zwickau, German Democratic Republic, for Chapter 15; Herbert Margolis of Boston, Mario Tenebaum of Buenos Aires, J. R. E. Mills of London, J. P. Pfeiffer and D. Grobety of Lausanne and Vevey, Switzerland, and Hugo Stockfisch of Stuttgart for Chapter 16. Equally important are contributions to Chapter 8 by Paul Herren of Berne, G. P. F., Schmuth of Bonn, and R. Karwetzky of the German Democratic Republic. I am grateful for the editorial assistance provided by Geraldine Udell.

Of course, the book would not even exist without the guiding light of Martin Schwarz, whose presence is very much felt in Chapters 2, 3, and 8, and even in other parts of the book. His *Lehrgang der Gebissregelung* was the original inspiration. Schwarz and Max Gratzinger fathered *Removable Orthodontic Appliances*, first published in 1966 by W. B. Saunders Company. This book was taken from the *Lehrgang*. Though both eminent elder statesmen of orthodontics are no longer living, it is only fitting that we and all those who have contributed acknowledge our debt in orthodontics to them.

T. M. Graber

B. Neumann

Contents

Chapter 1
SOCIOECONOMIC, HISTORICAL, AND
BIOPHYSICAL CONSIDERATIONS............................... 1

    Socioeconomic Considerations...................................... 1
    Historical and Biophysical Development........................ 5

Chapter 2
THE ACTIVE PLATE...................... 12

Chapter 3
SCHWARZ DOUBLE PLATE........................... 51

Chapter 4
THE UTILIZATION OF MUSCLE FORCES BY
SIMPLE APPLIANCES 63

Chapter 5
THE GUIDE PLANE PLATE AND PROPULSOR
IN THE TREATMENT OF CLASS II,
DIVISION 1 MALOCCLUSION...................................... 93

Chapter 6
FUNCTIONAL JAW ORTHOPEDICS: THE
CHANGES OF A CONCEPT... 118

Chapter 7
ACTIVATOR DEVELOPMENT AND PHILOSOPHY......... 133
    by Olav Slagsvold

Chapter 8

THE ACTIVATOR: USE AND MODIFICATIONS............ 183

Chapter 9

THE BIONATOR... 229

Chapter 10

CUTOUT OR PALATE-FREE ACTIVATOR.................... 247

Chapter 11

THE ELASTIC OPEN ACTIVATOR................................ 253

Chapter 12

THE ACTIVATOR... 269

by Donald G. Woodside

Chapter 13

THE BIMLER APPLIANCE... 337

by H. P. Bimler, M.D., D.D.S.

Chapter 14

THE KINETOR... 501

Chapter 15

THE FRÄNKEL APPLIANCE (THE FUNCTION CORRECTOR)... 526

Chapter 16

REMOVABLE APPLIANCES WITH EXTRAORAL FORCE 567

Chapter 17

EPILOGUE: A PHILOSOPHICAL PERSPECTIVE.. 597

INDEX.. 603

CHAPTER 1

Socioeconomic, Historical, and Biophysical Considerations

SOCIOECONOMIC CONSIDERATIONS

This book is meant to show the therapeutic value of removable appliances. Although the variety and kinds of appliances discussed may seem excessive to the neophyte, a careful reading of all sections, together with experience with each appliance, will make it abundantly clear why they have been chosen. It will then be possible to recognize the common denominators of all appliances and to correlate special appliance features more precisely with the results attained. The greatest emphasis is placed on an exhaustive diagnostic regimen prior to appliance selection, for important information is usually gained here on the kind of malocclusion most likely to respond favorably with a specific type of removable appliance. Such diagnostic acumen is likely to be forthcoming only from those who have had orthodontic specialty training and prior experience with fixed appliances.[1] The maximum benefit possible will, perhaps, be a combination of parts of the different appliances described herein, or removable appliances used in conjunction with multibanded techniques (see Chapter 5). Woodside demonstrates the importance of adequate diagnosis and the limitations imposed by morphogenetic pattern and specific appliance design on the ultimate treatment results. There is no "cook-book" for removable any more than there is for fixed appliances, and cult-oriented dogmas and "systems" in removable appliance techniques can create as much operator anxiety and frustration as their counterparts in multibanded techniques.

A number of orthodontic leaders are addressing themselves to a study of the future of orthodontics these days, and with good reason. It is here, perhaps, that removable appliances may play a significant role, used alone as preventive, interceptive, or corrective devices, or in conjunction with fixed appliances. "Changing Times" is more than the name of a business magazine—it is a way of life. Reference, of course, is made to the socioeconomic flux and the mushrooming role of third-party involvement in medical and dental care.

Despite the fact that the birth rate is slowing down, there are still millions of children who have not had and cannot obtain the benefits of orthodontic treatment. Schulman estimates that the 4.5 million children in the age group who need orthodontic treatment today will not be expected to be more than 3.5 million in ten years.[2] But only 2 to 3 per cent of these potential patients are at present receiving orthodontic treatment. Various studies indicate that 50 per cent of children could benefit from orthodontics. Simple mathematics demonstrates a large, untapped pool of patients, with demand for services directly related to just how much of the financial investment will be made by third-party agencies, private or governmental or both.

Wilbur Johnston, president of the American Association of Orthodontists (1977–1978), recently outlined the healthy growth of third-party involvement in dentistry.[3] In 1968, 6.9 million people had dental coverage. By 1970, the number had jumped to 12 million. By 1972, it had surpassed 17 million. Five million more were added by 1974, as 22 million people, including spouses and children, were receiving dental coverage through more than 11,000 employee group insurance plans across the country. By the end of 1977, the total expected is 35 million. The projection for 1980 is 60 million people in the U.S.A. enrolled in dental prepayment plans. Today, nearly one of five persons who sees his dentist once a year has some degree of third-party help. With at least a dozen National Health Insurance bills before Congress now, stressing dental care for children, another 30 to 40 million could be added to the total number of persons in prepayment plans.

Very clearly, the current status of orthodontists with less than full practices could change drastically overnight. What would happen? Is there any precedent elsewhere to give us some inkling? Even granting the differences in socioeconomic conditions, as well as in training and psychological attitudes of dentists in other countries, it may be worthwhile to review some of the recent studies of the British system, based on their experiences for a quarter of a century.

The need for orthodontic treatment has been assessed by T. D. Foster and A. J. Walpole Day, in children aged 11 to 12 years.[4] No orthodontic treatment was found necessary in 40.1 per cent of the sample. Treatment by planned or guided extraction was deemed sufficient in 22 per cent. Active tooth movement with appliances, with or without extraction, was indicated in 37.9 per cent.

In another study, S. Haynes examined 566 boys and 619 girls in the same age group.[5] Only 30.7 per cent were thought not to need treatment. Selective extraction procedures without appliances seemed indicated in 24.2 per cent; extractions and removable appliances in 30.0 per cent. Use of fixed appliances and extractions was projected in only 2.5 per cent! An analysis of these data indicates extractions were needed in 59.7 per cent. Without extraction, 7.8 per cent should be treated with removable appliances and only 1.7 per cent with fixed appliances.

The clinical assessment concerning serial extraction and choice of appliances would undoubtedly be different for orthodontists who are trained in and use only multibanded appliances. Yet the use of removable appliances may provide at least a partial solution to the problem. It has been demonstrated that the results achieved with these devices, even if they fall short of complete correction (and such is not always possible with fixed appliances, either), will be stable and quite satisfactory to most patients whose obvious malocclusion has been reduced by effecting a significant cosmetic and psychological improvement. Reitan points up the reduced iatrogenic potential of removable appliances with less likelihood of root resorption and alveolar crest damage.[6]

In England and Wales, orthodontic treatment is actually provided for 25 per cent of the child population.[7] This figure is based on the number of children annually accepted for treatment, at present about 200,000, and the average number of children in each age group from 5 to 15 years. With the continuity of treatment from year to year, treatment at that rate is thus provided for all children. There are, however, considerable regional variations. Demand is not met where there are too few dentists or, as in sparsely settled rural areas, where dentists are not readily accessible. In some urban sections, 50 per cent of the children receive orthodontic care.

The methods of orthodontic treatment used most of the time in Great Britain are simple and the objectives limited. In the hands of a highly competent specialist, they may yield impressive results; however, some clarification and additional information would seem desirable. Malocclusions requiring treatment should be more exactly defined. Treatment recommendations are necessarily subjective. It is interesting to note, however, that whereas Haynes recommended therapy by extractions only in 24.2 per cent using no appliances,[5] Rose limited such procedures to only 1.4 per cent of his treated cases.[8] Such a discrepancy indicates significant differences in treatment philosophy and objectives. It would be very interesting to compare children in a region where maximum therapy had been provided for a number of years with a similar group where only a few children had received treatment. What would the malocclusion index be? The potential dental health status? Enough American orthodontists have now made the trek to Great Britain to study the British system to consider their results seriously. Initial skepticism and criticism of the early years have given way to thoughtful analysis and an earnest desire to know more about how they have met and solved their problems. The chances that we will face the same problems in the next decade are very real now, if we watch political and social trends. The astute American orthodontist will plan ahead—he has the chance to do what his British confrere could not do and thus he may learn the best ways to serve society well.

To the best of our knowledge, this is the first book on orthodontic therapy with removable appliances that has been written specifically for the orthodontic specialist, already trained in multibanded fixed appliances. Such extensive information covering the various appliances from active plates to the various functional devices has never before been provided in one volume. Yet we are mindful of the limitations of any form of therapy. It is our hope that this book will dispel a number of half-truths and myths, too often propounded by nonspecialists, who have not "traveled the orthodontic specialty road." Unsubstantiated claims include the following:

1. Removable appliances require less training.
2. Removable appliances are always easier to adjust.
3. Removable appliances, since they are ostensibly easier to use and supposedly require less training, are part of the province of pedodontics and general dental practice.
4. Removable appliances eliminate the need for extraction.
5. Removable appliances eliminate the need for fixed appliances.
6. Removable appliances can do things that fixed appliances cannot do, such as stimulating condylar and dental arch growth.

If we have been successful in attaining our objectives, selective validity for the following claims may be demonstrated.

1. A larger patient load may be carried.
2. Auxiliary personnel, under the direct and continual control of the orthodontic specialist, can help the orthodontist serve more children and maintain a first class level of practice.
3. Removable appliances may be used for certain preventive and intercep-

tive tasks in the deciduous and mixed dentitions. Carefully diagnosed and selected malocclusions may be treated completely, using removable appliances alone.

4. Total investment of the orthodontic specialists' chair time and materia technica is reduced.

5. Removable appliances, by virtue of longer treatment guidance, have more potential for control of growth and development.

6. A higher level of patient cooperation is often required with removable appliances. Special help and training in motivational techniques may be necessary for the orthodontist and his staff.

7. Removable appliances, properly handled and used in conjunction with fixed appliances, will help meet the increased demand from society.

Certain specific limitations of removable appliances are recognized. Stahl of Heidelberg, Germany, lists several treatment tasks in which fixed appliances are superior.[9]

1. Rotation of teeth.
2. Uprighting of tipped teeth.
3. Paralleling movement of teeth in the dental arch.
4. Treatment of supra- or infraocclusion of one or several teeth.
5. Buccal or lingual bodily movement of teeth.
6. Torque.
7. Obtaining the precise interdigitation.

The immediate or ultimate need of tooth movement requiring the use of the multibanded techniques is not recognized or foreseen without expert diagnosis and treatment planning. Frequently, it will become apparent only during the course of treatment. By the same token, the reader will recognize that removable appliances have also become much too sophisticated to use without similar diagnostic and therapeutic planning. Successful treatment by the pedodontist or general practitioner who has not had orthodontic training is unlikely.

Before and after World War II, when the development of modern removable appliances was just beginning, the number of trained orthodontists in Europe was negligible. Active plates and activators, introduced mainly in the German-speaking parts of the continent, were very simple devices. Since for socioeconomic reasons there had been no way to treat an appreciable portion of the child population, the new possibilities aroused great enthusiasm and the results achieved were grossly overestimated and judged prematurely. Since it took American orthodontists some 40 years to recognize the futility of promiscuous expansion of the dental arches, they should not look too condescendingly on Europeans who learned the lesson somewhat later.

In Great Britain, the sudden expansion of the responsibilities of the Dental Health Service, which included orthodontic treatment, necessitated that it be done by the rank and file of the profession. Quite understandably, the results of these activities on both sides of the English Channel did not appeal to American orthodontists. The opinion became firmly entrenched that removable appliances are vastly inferior and not worth studying at all. Second rate service with removable appliances in the hands of orthodontically unqualified dentists in the United States and Canada strongly supported this prejudgment.

Yet conditions in Europe have changed and continue to change. There is no need to minimize honest differences of opinion and attitudes due to tradition and socioeconomic conditions. There is, however, an orthodontic specialty

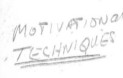
MOTIVATIONAL TECHNIQUES

in existence on the other side of the Atlantic which can be justly proud of its achievements. We are thoroughly convinced that it is not only advisable but necessary for the American orthodontist to study the methods developed in other countries and to use them to the advantage of both the patient and the orthodontist.

Some may fear that the publication of this book will aid and abet the undesirable activities of dentists attempting the treatment of malocclusion without the necessary training and knowledge to do so. Unfortunately, such moral intransigence and malpractice have not been impeded in the past by lack of information. However, such activities will not be enhanced materially by the objective presentation of new material, most of which is unsuited for the pedodontist and general practitioner. Quite the contrary, if there is a "market" for removable appliances, is it not better to appeal to the orthodontist who has mastered all the techniques necessary to bring the treatment to a successful conclusion? Can the 7500 orthodontists in the United States and Canada afford to ignore the whole development of removable appliances?

Whether 70, 50, or 25 per cent of our children could benefit from orthodontic treatment is not the issue for discussion. It is a fact that at present only 2 to 3 per cent are receiving orthodontic care in the United States. With proper indoctrination, significantly more children could be helped by the orthodontist, using some removable appliances. Recent surveys indicate that most orthodontic practices are not full. The growing cadre of orthodontists is capable of expanding its services. Removable appliances are made by technicians, so chairside time is greatly reduced. By the time these devices have become an established part of American orthodontics, there is every indication that they will be very much needed, considering the current development of third-party involvement.

The techniques thought worthwhile are described in this book. The chapter on the activator by Woodside shows how much such appliances may benefit from exact diagnosis and indications for treatment, based on research and complete records. Harvold's recent book on activators demonstrates the same thing. In a similar manner, other American orthodontists will certainly add much to the knowledge contained in this book. The description of the various methods will make the book useful. It may, however, become even more important as a starting point for future development.

HISTORICAL AND BIOPHYSICAL DEVELOPMENT

The biomechanical principles of orthodontic tooth movement are essentially the same, whether fixed or removable appliances are used. The reader may, therefore, be referred to recently published textbooks.[6, 10] However, some knowledge of the history and a short discussion of some problems specifically related to the subject of this book will be interesting to the reader.*[11]

In the earlier writings, there was a diversity of views concerning the nature of orthodontic tooth movement. Harris (1863)[12] saw it as a result of bone resorption on one side and bone deposition on the other side of the root. This view was supported by Talbot (1888),[13] Guilford (1898),[14] and others. Kingsley (1877),[15] later supported by Farrar (1888),[16] claimed that a bending of the alveolar bone would take place during orthodontic tooth movement. These surprisingly contemporaneous theories were based on clinical observation and macroscopic studies. Recent concepts might well have negotiated a compromise between these opposing views. It is suggested that the remodeling of bone occurring with tooth movement is subsequent to the bending of the alveolar bone.[17]

The first histological study of the problem was published by Sandstedt.[18,][19] The importance of some of his observations, such as hyalinization and undermining resorption, was appreciated only some tens of years later. For the development of orthodontic thinking, the investigations of Oppenheim (1911), proved to be most important.[20] Oppenheim was a disciple of E. H. Angle and very well known on both sides of the Atlantic. He interpreted his findings as a refutation of Walkhoff's pressure theory.[21] Following earlier advocates of the concept of the correction of malocclusion by bending the alveolus. Walkhoff's theory fostered the concept of overcoming the tension of the bone by strong pressure for a very short time. The permanency of the result was to be achieved by prolonged retention. Whatever the merits of Oppenheim's interpretation of his findings, it served well as a scientific foundation for Angle's empirically developed methods of treatment. Later, the results of Oppenheim's investigations, together with Angle's appliances, won recognition throughout the whole world. From then on, orthodontic treatment was regarded as tantamount to an artificially effected resorption and deposition of bone.

It is interesting that, with the swinging of the pendulum, the application of strong forces has been revived for palate splitting.[22-26] Using different methods, heavy "orthopedic" forces have proved their worth for the treatment of malocclusion,[27, 28] and have shown their efficiency by experimental investigation.[29]

The immense practical importance of tissue reaction to orthodontic treatment was brought to the attention of the profession by Ketcham's observations on root resorption, subsequent to treatment with orthodontic appliances.[30, 31] For obvious socioeconomic reasons, German-speaking and American orthodontists reacted differently to these findings. It led to a parting of the ways. In the United States, the pathologic effects inherent in orthodontic therapy were recognized. Heavy, rigid appliances, apparently responsible for the largest share of root resorption, were abandoned in favor of more resilient and efficient devices, such as the Angle edgewise appliance.[32] This may be considered the beginning of the modern multibanded technique, capable of utilizing gentle force application.

Further research revealed that root resorption and flattening of the alveolar crests can occur regularly without orthodontic treatment.[33-35] The indi-

---

*A detailed historical review is to be found in Reitan's fundamental study,[11] from which the references 12 to 16, 18, 19 and 21 are quoted.

vidual reaction of each patient was a major concern, to be observed carefully during actual appliance manipulation, regardless of the appliance being used.

In the beginning, the impact of multibanded technique was minimal in Britain and on the continent. Few specialists were adequately trained in the exacting details of appliance fabrication and manipulation. Only the most affluent could afford the greater cost of treatment, as compared to the cost when removable appliances were used. Korkhaus made an effort to improve the situation with his book on *Modern Orthodontic Therapy* in 1928.[36] This excellent text, based on the use of the Mershon lingual appliance, and also elements from the Lourie high labial arch technique, elaborated the possibilities of fixed appliances in the correction of most malocclusions. The first report by Ketcham was cited as supportive evidence for the relative innocuousness of these appliances.[30]

The claim of "biological superiority" of removable appliances was reinforced, however, after the pioneering clinical work of Andresen and Nord. The active plate of Schwarz, with his supplemental confirming tissue research, and the Häupl modification and development of the Andresen activator, also supported by definitive research, proved much more attractive to European orthodontists, however. The substantiating tissue reaction research and minimal iatrogenic tissue response claims literally "won the day."

Schwarz recognized the intimate relationship of force magnitude and tissue response and classified orthodontic forces into four degrees of biologic efficiency.[37]

First Degree of Efficiency.   These are forces below the threshold of stimulation to activate orthodontic tooth movement: (a) they are of too short duration, as, for example, a few minutes of thumbsucking by children before going to sleep; (b) they are balanced by compensatory forces such as the pressure of lip and cheeks from the outside and the tongue from the inside of the dental arch; (c) the forces of mastication are not artificially reinforced; (d) they are too weak to provoke tooth movement. Even the smallest force, however, may be effective if permitted to exert its influence long enough. It should be noted that according to Schwarz's definition, the Frankel appliance would effect tooth movement by forces of the first degree of biologic efficiency.

Second Degree of Efficiency.   These forces were regarded by Schwarz as the most favorable to achieve continuous tooth movement without root resorption. Resorption of alveolar bone in the pressure zone will happen at the same rate as deposition in the area of tension. Such forces are still weaker than the blood pressure in the capillary blood vessels, that is, 15 to 20 grams per square centimeter of the compressed periodontal membrane. They will be effective if permanent or exerted frequently in the same direction. Forces of a magnitude many times that pressure may nevertheless belong to the second degree of efficiency. The condition here is that the pressure is effective only over the distance of 0.1 mm. That is half the thickness of the periodontal membrane Schwarz assumed to measure 0.2 mm.* For that reason, the strong pressure of the jack screw will be innocuous.

Third Degree of Efficiency.   These forces interrupt the blood circulation

---

* There are variations in the width of the periodontal membrane, depending on the teeth, the area of the root, and the age of the patient. In the narrowest and potentially most endangered areas, it measures only 0.1 mm., on the average.

in the periodontal membrane. They are of medium strength, 20 to 50 grams per square centimeter. The tissues are not yet crushed. They will recover if circulation is restored before permanent damage is done. Under these circumstances, the repeated application of medium strong forces, interrupted in time, is conducive to resorption and deposition of alveolar bone. If, however, the pressure continues, it will cause necrosis of the periodontal membrane with subsequent damage to the surface of the alveolar socket and the cementum of the tooth. This is the most frequent cause of root resorption.

Fourth Degree of Efficiency. These forces are of such magnitude that the periodontal membrane is crushed between the root and the alveolar bone in the areas of greatest pressure. If continuous, the consequence is extensive necrosis of the alveolar bone and root resorption. Irreparable damage may be caused to the tissues involved.

The classification proposed by Schwarz is based on the assumption that the magnitude and duration of force are closely and regularly connected with the histologic reaction to the force. Schwarz probably underrated the frequency and extent of spontaneous root resorption. This, however, is a highly variable phenomenon. Furthermore, he did not take into consideration the hyalinization and posthyalinization periods seen by Reitan and others. Schwarz himself had called attention to that phenomenon as first described by Sandstedt, yet he did not appreciate its importance. Reitan[38] regards the division of force into four degrees of severity as too theoretical. "No such gradations are observed in histologic sections. The force effect is related more to the anatomical environment and the time factor than to anything else. In recent experiments in the rat, molars were moved labially or lingually with continuous force. A force of 4 grams produces hyalinized zones quite similar to those produced by 100 grams force." According to Schwarz, however, the gradation of force served well, especially because it called attention to the damaging effects of excessive force, such as those of the third and fourth degree.

Häupl was the other outstanding personality forming the European orthodontic, or as it has now been called, "jaw-orthopedic," thinking. He based his working hypothesis on the writings of Roux, whose theory on bone formation ascribed the greatest importance to trophic stimuli. These would "shake the bone substance" and increase cell activity of the osteoblasts, leading to the deposition of bone. Häupl claimed that the activator would provide such stimuli, leading to primary bone formation on the pressure side. That newly formed bone would move the tooth.[39] Häupl and Eschler experimented on three dogs. Muscular activity of the jaws was completely prevented by cutting of nerves. Then applied pressure by a fixed appliance did not lead to osteoblastic activity within two days. When, however, the teeth of the third experimental animal were tapped with a wooden stick, such bone formation activity was observed. These observations led Häupl to reject the theory of Flourens, who had stated that pressure would lead to the resorption of bone.[40]

According to the theory of tissue reaction evolved by Häupl, pressure would only narrow the periodontal space. When that happens, the tissue is made sensitive to functional stimuli providing the essential "shaking of the bone molecules." Then and there, bone deposition and resorption would occur. The most favorable way to achieve it would be by the use of "passive" appliances, not permanently narrowing the periodontal space. Although these teachings were soon disputed and rather convincing objections were made by

Reitan and others, they had an enormous impact on contemporary orthodontics in parts of Europe. Enthusiastic followers condemned all active, fixed, or removable appliances and limited themselves to the exclusive use of the activator. Others accepted active plates too; yet they were unanimous in rejecting fixed appliances about which they knew nothing. These were not practical, anyway, for economic reasons at that time.

The adherents of the use of plates and activators could quite correctly comment on the possible unfavorable sequelae of treatment with fixed appliances, dubbed "inimical to tissues." Yet there was no recognition of the fact that important tooth movement most likely to cause damage is beyond the possibilities of removable appliances. There was no awareness of the frequency and extent of root resorption in untreated dentitions.[34-36, 41] Without changing his views, Häupl conceded in 1955 that it is difficult to discern by histologic research the differences in the tissue changes brought about by the various appliances, whether they are passive, active, fixed, or removable.[42]

The fixed appliances, however, re-entered the European scene triumphantly, as soon as economic conditions made the use of multibanded techniques in parts of Europe possible. The recriminations against their use were not revoked. Like the old soldiers of the military song, they faded away. Notwithstanding the historical cycles, outstanding clinicians have, over the years, succeeded in extending the possibilities of removable appliances. The following chapters will bear testimony to their achievements. The concepts of tissue reaction evolved by Schwarz and Häupl have been superseded by more perfect knowledge. That knowledge will again be modified in due course by the progress of science. Yet these great men and others of their stature have opened the door and shown the way.

American orthodontists may have been right when likening the stand against fixed appliances to that of the fox who was sure the grapes were sour. They found removable appliances clumsy, erratic in performance, and seldom capable of achieving complete correction. The opinion expressed in 1959,[43] predicting only slightly to moderately increased use in the United States by 1969, was even too optimistic. It would, however, be rash to foresee the same for 1979.

Objectively considered, there is some truth in the criticism leveled against fixed appliances. The perfect alignment of the dentition is achieved at a price. Without very great care, that price may be high.[44] Even competent treatment will not prevent significant root resorption.[45-47] Not all facial contours appear to be improved after the extraction of four premolars, an essential part of all too many treatment plans.

Although our knowledge is incomplete, we may rightly assume, from clinical experience, that removable appliances generally will do little harm to periodontal tissues. A slight loosening of the teeth, regarded as conducive to successful tooth movement when multiband techniques are used, would quite rightly very much alarm the orthodontist using removable devices. Yet these appliances, too, may cause damage in some cases. A labial bow pressing on a protruding incisor may damage the pulp of the tooth. A canine rotated by a whip spring may be loosened excessively.

Such risks are increased by improper handling of the appliance. Far greater, however, is the danger of faulty treatment by lack of proper diagnosis and misguided planning. Even the trained orthodontist may go wrong when disregarding the differences in the philosophies of the two systems. The relative innocuousness and simple technique of making some of these appliances do not provide a license for their misuse by the insufficiently trained and educated.

Properly used, removable appliances will correct many malocclusions. They will considerably improve and lessen the challenge of others. Treatment undertaken in the mixed dentition will not delay or complicate further treatment in the permanent dentition, if it is needed. Rather, it can make such therapy considerably simpler and more successful. The potential and very useful combination of fixed and removable appliances, and of the use of extraoral force with removable appliances, has hardly been explored yet.[48] Once the profession has grasped the potential and the possibilities, the lingering doubts about the usefulness of removable appliances will soon be dispelled. A prophetic editorial recently appeared in the American Journal of Orthodontics,[49] and it would seem pertinent. "There may be honest differences, but other nationals have shown a greater interest in learning, for example, our methods with fixed appliances, than we have in learning their methods with removable appliances. It won't be long till they are better men for it if Americans fail to learn what is being accomplished in other countries."

References

1. Ackerman, J., and Proffit, W. R.: Diagnosis and planning treatment in orthodontics. *In* Graber, T. M., and Swain, B. F. (Eds.): Current Orthodontic Concepts and Techniques, 2nd ed. Philadelphia, W. B. Saunders Company, 1975.
2. Schulman, M. L.: The future of orthodontics. J. Clin. Orthod., *9*:435–436, 1975.
3. Johnston, W. D.: The evaluation of health care systems and the contribution dentistry must make to preserve the best of private practice and the highest level of dental care. Lester Burket Alumni Lecture, Philadelphia, May 16, 1975.
4. Foster, T. D., and Walpole Day, A. J.: A survey of malocclusion and the need for orthodontic treatment in a Shropshire school population. Br. J. Orthod., *1*:73–78, 1974.
5. Haynes, S.: Orthodontic treatment needs in English children, age 11–12 years. Br. J. Orthod., *1*:9–12, 1973.
6. Reitan, K.: Biomechanical principles and reactions. *In* Graber, T. M., and Swain, B. F. (Eds.): Current Orthodontic Concepts and Techniques, 2nd ed. Philadelphia, W. B. Saunders Company, 1975.
7. Stephens, C. D., and Bass, T. P.: Regional variations in the provision of orthodontic treatment in England and Wales. Br. J. Orthod., *1*:13–17, 1973.
8. Rose, J. S.: A thousand consecutively treated orthodontic cases—a survey. Br. J. Orthod., *1*:45–54, 1974.
9. Stahl, A., and Paul, C. L.: Über die Indikation abnehmbarer Apparate im Rahmen der vorwiegend mit der Multibandtechnik durchgeführten Kieferorthopädischen Behandlung. Osterr. Z. Stomatol., *66*:334–337, 1969.
10. Graber, T. M.: Orthodontics: Principles and Practice. 3rd ed. Philadelphia. W. B. Saunders Company, 1972.
11. Reitan, K.: The initial tissue reaction incident to orthodontic tooth movement. Acta Odontol. Scand., Suppl. 6, 1951.
12. Harris, C. A.: The Principles and Practice of Dental Surgery. Philadelphia, Lindsay and Blakiston, 1863.
13. Talbot, E. S.: Irregularities of the Teeth and their Treatment. Philadelphia, Blakiston Company, 1888.
14. Guilford, G. M.: Orthodontia or Malposition of the Human Teeth, Its Prevention and Remedy. Philadelphia, Davis and Sons, 1898.
15. Kingsley, N. W.: An experiment with artificial palates. Dent. Cosmos, *19*:231, 1877.
16. Farrar, J. N.: A Treatise on the Irregularities of the Teeth and Their Correction. New York, International News Company, 1888.
17. Baumrind, S.: A reconsideration of the propriety of the "pressure-tension" hypothesis. Am. J. Orthod., *55*:12–21, 1969.
18. Sandstedt, C.: Nägra bidrag til tandregleringens teori. Stockholm, 1901.
19. Sandstedt, C.: Einige Beiträge zur Theorie der Zahnregulierung. Nord. Tandl. Tidskr., *5*:236, 1904; *6*:1, 1905.

20. Oppenheim, A.: Die Veränderungen der Gewebe insbesondere der Knochen bie Verschiebung der Zähne. Oester. Ung. Vjschr. Zhk., *27*:302, 1911.
21. Walkhoff, O.: Beitrag zur Lehre von den Kieferveränderungen beim Richten der Zähne. Corresp. Bl. Zahnärzte, *29*:193, 1900.
22. Graber, T. M.: An appraisal of the developmental deformities in cleft palate and cleft lip individuals. Q. Bull., Northwestern Univ. Med. School, *23*:153, 1949.
23. Graber, T. M.: Changing philosophies in cleft palate management. J. Pediatr., *37*:400, 1950.
24. Derichsweiler, H.: Die Gaumennahtsprengung. Fortschr. Kieferorthop., *14*:234, 1953.
25. Isaacson, R. J., Wood, J. L., and Ingram, A. H.: Forces produced by rapid maxillary expansion. Angle Orthod., *34*:256, 1964.
26. Haas, A. J.: The treatment of maxillary deficiency by opening the midpalatal suture. Angle Orthod., *35*:200, 1965.
27. Graber, T. M., Chung, D. B., and Aoba, J. T.: Dentofacial orthopedics versus orthodontics. J. Am. Dent. Assoc., *75*:1145, 1967.
28. Graber, T. M.: Dentofacial orthopedics. *In* Graber, T. M., and Swain B. F. (Eds.): Current Orthodontic Concepts and Techniques, 2nd ed. Philadelphia, W. B. Saunders Company, 1975.
29. Droschl, H.: The effect of heavy orthopedic forces on the maxilla in the growing Saimiri sciureus (squirrel monkey). Am. J. Orthod., *63*:449–461, 1973.
30. Ketcham, A. H.: A preliminary report of an investigation of apical root resorption of permanent teeth. Int. J. Orthod., *13*:97, 1927.
31. Ketcham, A. H.: A progress report of an investigation of apical root resorption of vital permanent teeth. Int. J. Orthod., *15*:310–325, 1928.
32. Angle, E. H.: The latest and best in orthodontic mechanism. Dent. Cosmos, *70*:1143–1158, 1928; *71*:164–174, 260–270, 409–421, 1929.
33. Henry, J. L., and Weinmann, J. P.: Pattern of root resorption and repair of human cementum. J. Am. Dent. Assoc., *42*:270, 1951.
34. Massler, M., and Malone, A. J.: Root resorption in human permanent teeth. Am. J. Orthod., *40*:364–372, 1954.
35. Massler, M., and Perreault, J. S.: Root resorption in the permanent teeth of young adults. J. Dent. Child., *21*:158–164, 1954.
36. Korkhaus, G.: Moderne orthodontische Therapie. Berlin, Herrmann Meusser, 1928.
37. Schwarz, A. M.: Lehrgang der Gebissregelung, 2nd ed., Vol. 2. Vienna, Urban and Schwarzenberg, 1956.
38. Reitan, K.: Quoted in Schwarz, A. M., and Gratzinger, M.: Removable Orthodontic Appliances. Philadelphia, W. B. Saunders Company, 1966.
39. Häupl, K.: Gewebsumbau und Zahnverdrängung in der Funktionskieferorthopädie. Leipzig, J. A. Barth, 1938.
40. Eschler, J., and Häupl, K.: Die Drucktheorie Flourens vor dem Forum tierexperimenteller Untersuchungen. Z. Stomatol., *38*:423–453, 1940.
41. Hotz, R.: Wurzelresorptionen an bleibenden Zähnen. Fortschr. Kieferorthop., *28*:217–224, 1967.
42. Häupl, K.: Die Gewebsveränderungen unter dem Einfluss Kieferorthopädischer Apparate. *In* Die Zahn-Mund und Kieferheilkunde, Vol. 5. München-Berlin, Urban and Schwarzenberg, 1955.
43. Graber, T. M., and Chung, D. B.: Orthodontics in 1969. Am. J. Orthod., *45*:655–681, 1959.
44. Graber, T. M.: Postmortems in post-treatment adjustment. Am. J. Orthod., *52*:331–352, 1966.
45. Rudolph, C. E.: An evaluation of root resorption occurring during orthodontic treatment. J. Dent. Res., *19*:367–371, 1940.
46. Phillips, J. R.: Apical root resorption under orthodontic therapy. Angle Orthod., *25*:1–22, 1955.
47. De Shields, R. W.: A study of root resorption in treated Class II, Division 1 malocclusion. Angle Orthod., *39*:231–245, 1969.
48. Van der Linden, F. P. G. M.: The application of removable orthodontic appliances in multiband techniques. Angle Orthod., *39*:114–117, 1969.
49. Dewel, B. F.: International relations, personal conduct and the London Congress. Am. J. Orthod., *64*:95, 1973.

CHAPTER 2

The Active Plate

THE CONSTRUCTION OF THE ACTIVE PLATE

The removable appliances used at present were developed before World War II. At that time, there were two distinctly different devices, the active plate and the activator, the first using forces from within the appliance, the other utilizing muscular forces. Further development and diversification have led to the construction of appliances that combine the use of extrinsic and intrinsic forces. Nevertheless, the division into "active" and "functional" appliances is still possible and useful.

HISTORICAL BACKGROUND

Soon after the invention of vulcanite, it was introduced as material for dentures; also, it was soon used for "regulating devices." Of historical importance is the Coffin plate (1881), with the spring that is still part of present appliances. It was then made of piano wire. N. W. Kingsley first described his plate for "jumping the bite" in 1880. It was the forerunner of modern functional appliances.[1] Pierre Robin in 1902 constructed the first split plate with an incorporated screw that he had designed. The plate also had a hinge in the posterior end of the split for eccentric expansion. He had not found this type of appliance reported in the literature, in spite of his "most careful bibliographic research." It was used to gain "the immense distance of 4 mm.," as he wrote, to align a crowded upper central incisor.[2] In England, J. H. Badcock in 1911 described an expansion plate with an efficient screw that he had designed.[3] But in the next three decades these plates were eclipsed by Edward H. Angle's fixed appliances, which dominated the orthodontic world. Only the Hawley retainer came to stay.

In 1929, at the meeting of the European Orthodontic Society in Heidelberg, C. F. L. Nord presented very simple screw split plates meant for the treatment of the masses.[4] The orthodontists who were present apparently were not impressed.[5] His paper, however, triggered further development. At the Ninth International Dental Congress in Vienna (1936), M. Tischler demonstrated quite sophisticated active plates.[5] Two years later, A. M. Schwarz published a textbook entirely devoted to treatment with plates. There the designs of different split plates with various screws were shown.[6] These plates, with some modifications and improvements, are still in use.

The active plate contains a number of basic components:

1. The baseplate
2. The clasps

3. Active elements
    a. Labial wire
    b. Springs
    c. Screws
    d. Elastics

In addition to these, extraoral traction, infrequently used with the original designs of the active plate, is becoming more important.

The operator will select a combination of all these elements to construct the device for the particular treatment. The choice is made according to the requirements of the case at hand, the mechanical possibilities offered by the different parts, and last, but not least, the preference of the orthodontist.

The Baseplate

The baseplate usually is made of acrylic and its main purpose is threefold: (1) as a base of operations to carry all working parts; (2) to serve as anchorage; and (3) to be an active part of the appliance itself as indicated by the specific orthodontic problem.

As a Base of Operation. The maxillary plate is in contact with the palatal aspects of all teeth, except where the plate is cut away for a special purpose. It should extend to a point just distal to the last erupted molar. That will help prevent rocking and the displacement in an anteroposterior direction. The

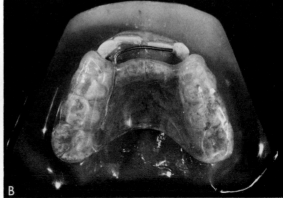

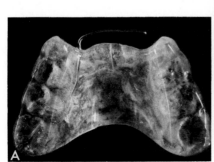

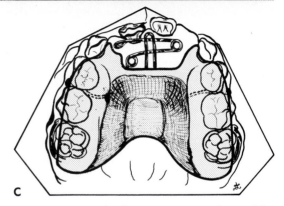

Figure 2–1. *A,* Palatal view. Simple plate blocking open the bite to move lingually locked incisor labially. *B,* Appliance on model. (After George M. Anderson.) *C,* Modified removable palatal appliance to move central incisor labially. Finger spring is deeply anchored in acrylic and recurves twice by forming helical coil loops before it engages the malposed central incisor. In this manner, a light but continuous force is exerted on the tooth. A "spring guard" protects the spring from functional stress and prevents the spring from creeping incisally. Added retention is given to the palatal portion with circumferential clasps on the first permanent molars and by carrying the acrylic up over the occlusal. Anterior cross-bite may be corrected with this type of appliance. (From Graber, T. M.: Orthodontics: Principles and Practice, 3rd ed. Philadelphia, W. B. Saunders Company, 1972.)

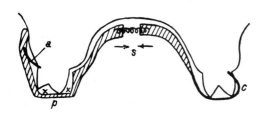

Figure 2–2. Drawing of maxillary plate to show buccal flange extension. The method for reducing the arch width, using a pull screw, *S*, on the plate. Schematic cross section. *Left*, Plate covering the buccal teeth to block the bite; *p*, bite block; *a*, covered arrow; *x*, free spaces to permit the lingual tipping of the tooth, which is moved by the screw and by the arrow, *a*. (From Schwarz, A. M., and Gratzinger, M.: Removable Orthodontic Appliances. Philadelphia, W. B. Saunders Company, 1966.)

placement of screws for different treatment objectives or the need for stabilization usually will make it necessary to cover the whole palate. However, a plate cut out in the midline to expose a large part of the palate is more comfortable to wear. With a screw in the midline, a plate covering the entire palate may even cause difficulties in the course of expansion.[7] On the other hand, a screw placed anteriorly may necessitate an undesirable thickening of the plate in the sensitive area. These construction details are discussed later in this chapter.

To serve a special purpose, the plate may be extended to cover the buccal teeth, forming bite blocks. The opening of the bite thus achieved will make it easy to align incisors locked in lingual occlusion. In the early mixed dentition, such simple appliances may not even need to be retained by clasps (Fig. 2–1).[8] Occasionally, if deemed necessary, the plate may also cover parts of the buccal aspect of the alveolus (Fig. 2–2), or the tuberosities (see Fig. 2–34).

The limits of the mandibular plate are determined by the height of the alveolar process. This is not as critical as it would be with a complete or partial denture. Retention depends on clasps and the appurtenances of the orthodontic appliance itself. The plate should be made thicker in the lower alveolar region. A plate modeled into the undercut in this region might be impossible to insert or painful to the gingival tissues. A sufficiently thick peripheral portion will make it possible to remove the appropriate part of the acrylic (Fig. 2–3).

As an Anchorage Unit and Working Part. The baseplate provides resistance against active forces. Its contact with the teeth and the palate will augment decisively the anchorage obtained from the clasps and labial bow. An example of a simple and effective use of a plate is shown in Figure 2–1. (See also Figure 2–4.)

Plates divided by screws will provide anchorage in addition to serving as working parts. An expansion plate, split in the midline, is an excellent example of a reciprocal anchorage appliance. In other designs, shown later in this chapter, the plate is split so as to use as much as possible for anchorage, leaving smaller parts to effect tooth movement.

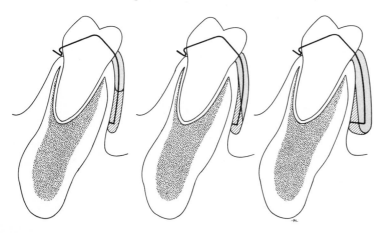

Figure 2–3. Fashioning of baseplate for removable lower appliance. Lower molar region usually requires relieving to allow insertion. Hence, periphery should be made thicker to permit removal of acrylic from tissue contacting surface. (After Adams, C. P.: Removable Orthodontic Appliances. Third edition. Bristol, John Wright & Sons, 1964, Figure 22.)

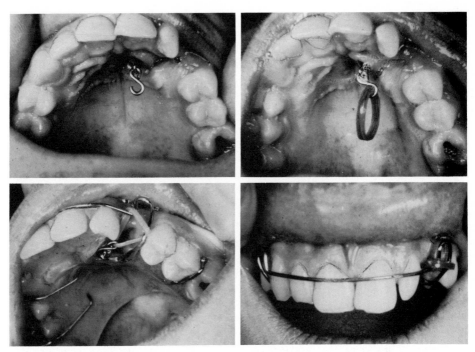

Figure 2-4. Versatile use of removable palatal appliance. Maxillary left canine is uncovered for a 14-year-old girl. There is adequate space in the arch. *Top,* A hook is cemented on the exposed canine crown, and an elastic is attached. *Bottom,* A plain Hawley type appliance is worn, with a cut-out portion for the impacted canine. The elastic is stretched from the hook to the labial bow and loop of the appliance. As the canine moves toward its correct position, a spur may be soldered on the labial bow loop to maintain tension on the elastic and to ensure proper direction of pull. Elastic is changed every day by the patient. (From Graber, T. M.: Orthodontics: Principles and Practice, 3rd ed. Philadelphia, W. B. Saunders Company, 1972.)

Another working part of the plate may be a bite plane, built in to level the bite. The bite plane may be inclined to form a guide plane intended to bring the mandible forward or retain it in its forward position. The maxillary bite plane is a very useful tool in the treatment of temporomandibular joint disturbances, periodontal disease, bruxism, excessive overbite, and so on. This subject, however, has been dealt with sufficiently in orthodontic textbooks.[9]

The margins of the baseplate can be fabricated in different ways (Fig. 2-5).

Figure 2-5. *A,* The buccal papilla is shaved to an extent of 1 to 2 mm. before the arrow clasp is bent (x); thus the arrow will fit exactly. *B,* If the margin of the plate touches the tooth gingivally of the arrow, a bodily movement may occur during expansion; in this case, the lingual margin of the gingiva, instead of the buccal papilla, may be shaved a little (x). *C,* If the margin of the plate is broad, covering nearly the whole lingual surface of the tooth, the clasp (K) prevents the growth in height, pressing the tooth into the broad and concave margin of the plate. *D,* The arrow (K) is situated gingivally of the greatest circumference of the buccal surface (x); therefore it does not prevent the growth in height of the tooth, but stimulates it, provided the margin (r) of the plate (p) is thin. (From Schwarz, A. M., and Gratzinger, M.: Removable Orthodontic Appliances. Philadelphia, W. B. Saunders Company, 1966.)

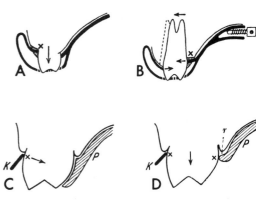

The Clasps

To perform all its functions, the baseplate must be maintained securely in place. Tissue apposition and adhesion and the extension of the acrylic between the teeth or below the region of their greatest convexity enhance the anchorage, but will rarely be sufficient. Nearly all plates, therefore, are attached to the teeth by clasps, a great variety of which have been designed. The oldest and, for a considerable time, most generally used is the arrow clasp of A. M. Schwarz.[10] It is made of a single piece of stainless steel wire, usually 0.024 in. (approximately 0.7 mm.) in diameter. The construction and design are illustrated and described in Figures 2–5, 2–6, and 2–29D. The special pliers shown, however, are not regarded as necessary by most technicians. After the first three steps have been made, the tip is bent gingivally (Fig. 2–6). The operator must take care that the vestibular part of the clasp is carefully bent to stay within the limits of the attached mucosa at a distance of about 1 mm. to avoid contact with the soft tissue.

The anterior arm of the clasp, which is inserted into the plate, crosses over the mesial contact point of a premolar or deciduous molar. From there, the clasp forms two or three arrows with the tips fitted into the interproximal areas. The posterior arm runs distal to the last fully erupted tooth and inserts again into the plate. The clasp is thus one continuous wire with both ends anchored in the acrylic. The tip of the arrow lies just gingival to the greatest circumference of the crown. As shown in Figure 2–5, the inter-relationship of the tip and the margin of the baseplate may be varied in different ways so as to enhance the working of the appliance. If the buccal papilla is scraped slightly on the cast, the tip will slightly impinge on it in the interproximal area. Additional bending of the tip in an apical direction may serve the same purpose. This step may be necessary in some instances to increase the hold of the clasp

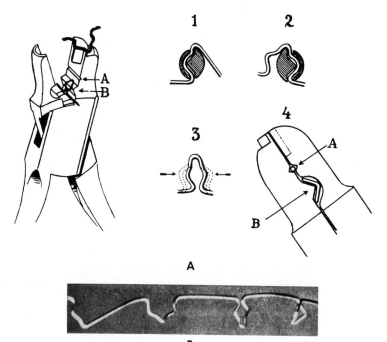

Figure 2–6. Bending the arrows using the arrow-forming pliers of A. M. Schwarz.* The material used is stainless, highly elastic steel, usually 0.7 mm. *A,* Four steps of the procedure: *1* and *2,* bending the first and second half of the clasp using the working top of the pliers; *3,* reducing the width, using the small groove A; and *4,* bending the arrow using the part B. *B,* The four steps, shown in one piece of wire. (From Schwarz, A. M., and Gratzinger, M.: Removable Orthodontic Appliances. Philadelphia, W. B. Saunders Company, 1966.)

*Manufactured by R. Thurriegl, Medical Instruments, Vienna IX, Schwarzspanierstrasse 15. Similar arrow clasp-forming pliers are available in other countries.

Figure 2–7. If the teeth are very short in a mixed dentition, the clasp cannot find sufficient retention. In such a case shallow grooves ground into the enamel of the deciduous teeth are useful to get insertion for the arrows. Horizontal grooves, parallel to and near the bucco-gingival margin, are made with flame-shaped and knife-edged diamond stones. *A* and *B,* The position of the stones and of the arrows shown in their relation to the surface of the teeth. *C,* Buccal view of the arrow in situ. *D,* The stones used. (From Schwarz, A. M., and Gratzinger, M.: Removable Orthodontic Appliances. Philadelphia, W. B. Saunders Company, 1966.)

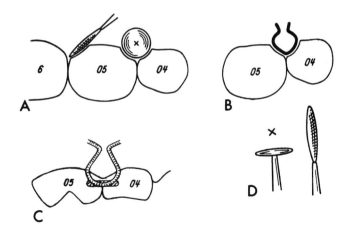

on the teeth. The contact of the tip with the papilla must remain within safe limits, however. Excessive pressure has to be avoided.

The expanse of wire between the arrows makes the arrow clasp of Schwarz more elastic than others, enhancing its effectiveness. Another advantage is the possibility of adjusting the arrows slightly in an anterior or posterior direction. This step may prove useful if, for example, a deciduous second molar is shed during treatment. Bending the arrows slightly against the first premolar and first molar will increase the hold on the teeth. Bending the tips against the teeth to further their movement, for example, in a posterior direction, is only of marginal importance. The many bends of the Schwarz clasp demand great care in its formation. It must not be bent around a sharp edge. This could damage the wire internally, and breakage will occur at a stressed and weakened point. The distance from the acrylic will, however, make repair by soldering feasible. (See section on repairs later.)

If the deciduous teeth used for retention of the plate are short and conical, the grinding of a shallow groove into the teeth has been recommended (Fig. 2–7). This should be done if the finished plate will not be retained by the clasp and the teeth in question will be shed soon. If such a contingency develops, however, providing sufficient anchorage by cemented bands with buccal lugs seems preferable.

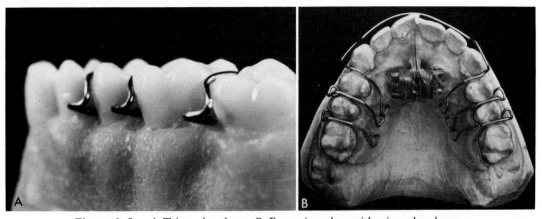

Figure 2–8. *A,* Triangular clasps. *B,* Expansion plate with triangular clasps.

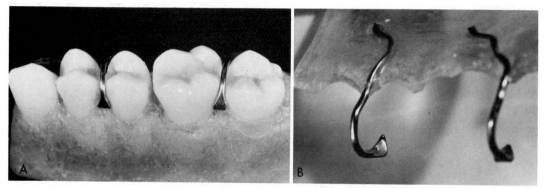

Figure 2-9.   *A* and *B,* The arrow pin clasp.

The use of the continuous clasp is convenient in combination with lateral bite blocks, as crossing the occlusion under the acrylic can be avoided. It also is recommended to facilitate further eruption of the buccal teeth. The continuous eyelet clasp, which will be shown later, is superior for such purposes (see Fig. 2–10).

In recent years, preference has often been given to other designs or clasps. Among these, the triangular clasp is most popular. Essentially, it is a single arrow on a wire crossing the contact point (Fig. 2–8). Excellent retention is provided without any irritation of the gingival tissues. It is easily formed and replaced with a minimal effort when broken. A prefabricated clasp is available,

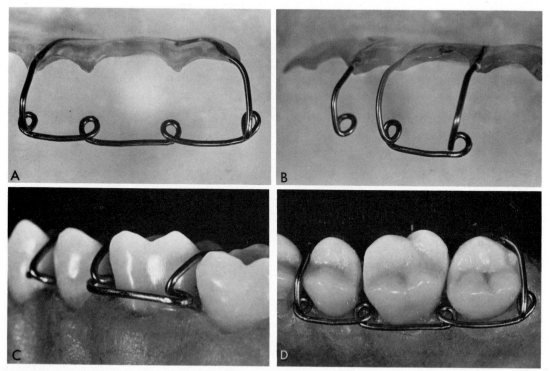

Figure 2-10.   *A* and *B,* The simple and the double eyelet clasp. In contradistinction to the use of the Adams clasp, the hold of the double eyelet clasp may be increased by bending the bridge slightly away from the tooth. *C* and *D,* The continuous eyelet clasp.

or it can be made in advance by the technician and stored. Special pliers to form triangular clasps are available but are not really necessary.

Similar in action are two manufactured clasps, the well-known ball clasp (Fig. 2–4) and the arrow pin clasp (Fig. 2–9). The latter is a solid arrow bent to penetrate into the interdental space. It provides a firm grip on the teeth. The patient cannot easily dislodge it by a tug on the clasp itself, only by pulling on another appurtenance of the plate, such as the labial wire. It is a device worth considering in special cases.

The eyelet clasp is similar to the triangular clasp. Heideborn and Burgert[11] have shown how to use it to embrace a single tooth; it is usually used as a continuous clasp (Fig. 2–10). Since it is formed without sharp bends, springy hard wire may be used and breakage is unlikely. Being well away from the gingival tissue, a deformed wire usually does not injure the mucosa. The eyelet clasp for a single tooth does not have the firm grip of the Adams clasp, but it is easier to make. The continuous eyelet clasp has many advantages, however. Embracing three teeth, it offers four eyelets against the two arrows of other designs. The first and last eyelets are placed below the greatest circumference of the tooth. As mentioned above, it is somewhat more convenient under lateral bite blocks and will not impede further eruption of teeth.

The orthodontist will soon find reasons for the selection of a particular clasp to serve a specific purpose. An eyelet clasp, for example, is rather long when embracing four teeth. In such a case, triangular clasps are preferable. These will also penetrate deeper into the interdental space and will be chosen for the distal movement of teeth with a Y-plate. In this instance, a clasp-like wire must be placed before the most anterior tooth to be shifted to ensure its participation in the movement.

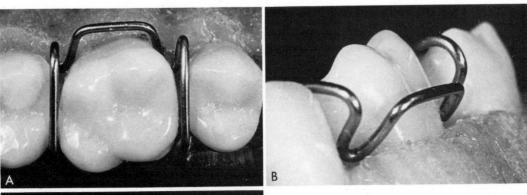

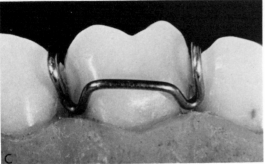

Figure 2–11. The Adams clasp. *A,* The arrows must not contact the adjoining teeth. The arrows should not be too short and the bridge between them should be straight. *B,* The bridge between the arrows is kept well away from the buccal surface of the tooth and from the gingival tissues. The clasp is brought into close contact with the tooth by bending the tags. Bending the bridge for this purpose should be avoided. *C,* An often neglected detail is to tilt the arrows to make them correspond to the slope of the gingival margins.

Certainly the clasp preferred by the greatest number of orthodontists is the Adams clasp (Fig. 2–11). It is the most versatile and provides the strongest anchorage for the plate.[12] The clasp is made of 0.7 mm. hard stainless steel wire; for canines, 0.6 mm. wire is preferred. The first step is to form the arrows. These should be at a distance in accordance with the size of the tooth clasped, so that the bridge between the arrows remains straight. All bends are made with the fingers over the pliers, firmly gripping the wire. The arrows should be reasonably long so as to keep the bridge between them at a proper distance from the tooth as well as from the gingival tissues. Clasps preformed to that stage are available in different sizes. The next step, often neglected, is to tilt the arrows buccally to make them correspond to the slope of the gingival margins. Then the arrows are slightly squeezed to narrow them appropriately, after which the tags are bent over the contact points. They must lie snugly between the teeth in order not to disturb the occlusion. The tips of the arrows should be placed below the widest circumference of the teeth. If the tooth is not fully erupted, the plaster below the gingival margin must be slightly trimmed to reach a part of the tooth still covered by the gingiva. When inserted, the arrow will then depress the gingiva slightly. Conversely, with fully erupted teeth with a large undercut visible, the arrow must not be placed too

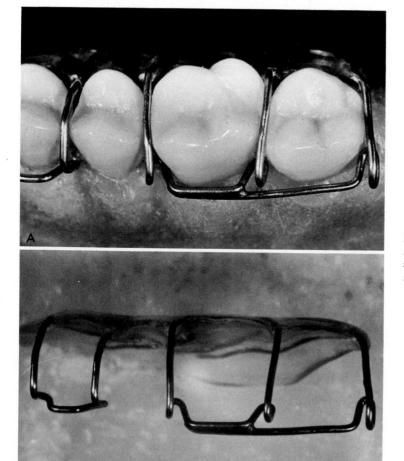

Figure 2–12. *A* and *B*, The Adams clasp with an accessory arrow clasp on the second molar.

far beyond the widest circumference. The finished clasp will be brought into close contact with the tooth it grips by bending the tags at the angle between the occlusal and buccal part of the wire. To increase the hold by bending the bridge and narrowing the distance between the arrows will lessen the efficiency of the construction.

Among the variations of the Adams clasp, two are of special importance. The addition of an accessory arrow to the clasp will provide maximum anchorage in the molar region. Thus, especially after bilateral extraction of premolars, planned movement of buccal and subsequently of anterior teeth is facilitated (Fig. 2–12).

If extraoral traction is required, a tube may be soldered to the bridge of the clasp (see Chapter 16).

In spite of the superior qualities of the Adams clasp, its exclusive use should not be encouraged. There may be instances in which a tooth strongly gripped by the clasp will be less easy to move. Too tight a grip may elongate the tooth. Also the use of simpler constructions may save time in the laboratory.

Occasionally, a simple circumferential clasp may be used to provide additional retention. After premature loss or shedding of deciduous molars, for example, a clasp on the deciduous canine in conjunction with an efficient clasp on the molar will provide retention and stabilization of the plate in the anterior region.

A simple clasp design is the Duyzings clasp (Fig. 2–13). It is made by two wires emerging from the plate to cross the occlusion over the anterior and posterior contact point of the tooth clasped. Each wire then goes above the greatest circumference of the tooth to the middle of the tooth and back again below, using the undercut. It is also possible to use only half of that clasp or a half extended to the anterior or posterior part of the tooth.[13]

If retention of a clasp is doubtful, or if an especially strong hold must be secured, a crown or a band with a buccal lug or a piece of wire welded to it may be cemented on the molar, occasionally also on a premolar. A circumferential clasp engaging these appurtenances will enhance retention (Fig. 2–14).

Active Elements

Labial Wire. The labial wire or labial bow may have two functions. One, exemplified by the Hawley retainer, is to hold the plate in place and to retain the teeth, a passive function. The other is to serve as an active element for the movement of teeth. However, in this capacity it will also serve simultaneously to stabilize the appliance. Most of the time it will play a dual role, with some parts of the wire retaining teeth and other parts moving teeth. The purpose of the

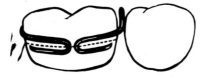
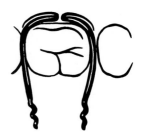

Figure 2–13. The Duyzings clasp. (From Duyzings, J.A.C.: Orthodontic Applicances. Leiden, Stafleu and Tholen, 1969.)

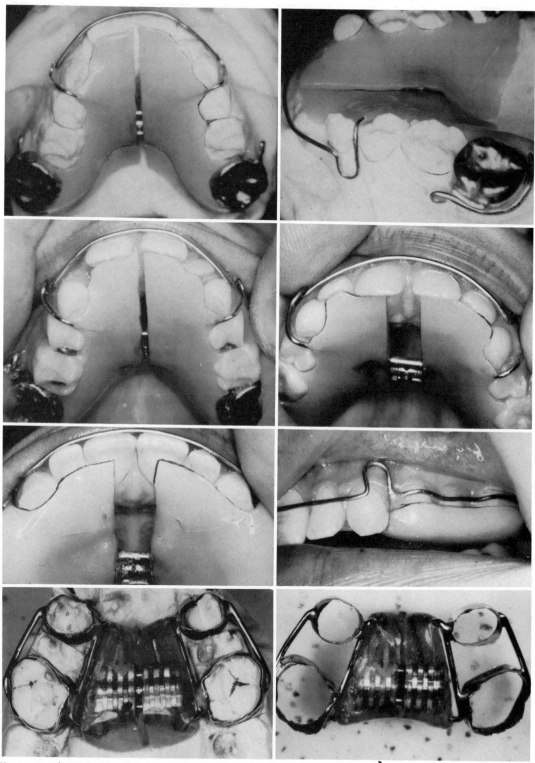

Figure 2–14. Palatal expansion appliance is held in place with full-coverage metal crowns and buccal lugs, to which circumferential clasps hook. The buccal arms of the clasps snap over the lugs, preventing dislodgment when the jackscrew is turned periodically. Bands with lugs may be used instead of crowns. Bottom row is a rapid palatal expansion appliance, which is cemented to molars and premolars. (From Graber, T. M.: Orthodontics: Principles and Practice, 3rd ed. Philadelphia, W. B. Saunders Company, 1972.)

labial wire will determine its dimension. It varies from 0.6 to 0.9 mm. Every labial wire, even the smaller gauge, is capable of exerting considerable pressure, enough to cause damage to the pulp and the periapical region. The operator must be conscious of that fact and bear in mind that the labial wire is the part of the generally innocuous removable appliance most likely to do irreparable harm.

For retention, the labial bow will generally follow the design of the Hawley retainer, embracing the six anterior teeth with the arms joining the acrylic of the plate between the canine and first premolar. The bow may, however, be restricted to the four incisors or any part of the anterior region, or it may extend as far distally as the second premolar or even the first molar. Such may be necessary in extraction cases so as not to impede the movement of the teeth in a posterior direction.

When used to effect tooth movement, the arms as well as the labial arc of the bow may be activated (Figs. 2–15 and 2–16). These wire configurations are effective in a number of cases. Despite the use in conjunction with expansion, some technical details are shown that may prove to be useful. After extractions, however, the labial wire is often omitted altogether during the first phase, when canines and the first premolars are moved distally. When these tooth movements have been achieved, incisors and canines are aligned by a labial bow which will also reduce the overjet (Fig. 2–17). The possibility of using a longer labial wire has been mentioned already.

A variation of the labial bow is the high labial arch combined with different designs of the "apron spring"[14] (Fig. 2–18). It is an attractive and effective device; however, these constructions are not quite so simple to make. Some seem vulnerable to dislodgment and deformation and may even be potentially harmful if not used by a well-trained specialist.

Springs. The auxiliary springs used for tooth movement are of two types: (1) closed or continuous loop springs; (2) free-end springs. Free-end or cantilever springs may have a helical coil incorporated, and these are used most

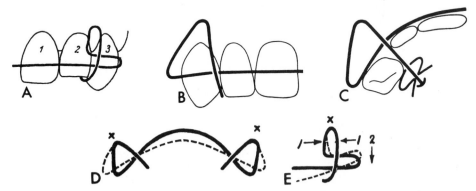

Figure 2–15. The loop of the labial bow of the canine. *A* and *B,* Commonly used shapes in front view. *C,* The shape of 1 in *A,* as seen from below, to show the rotation of the canine; gingival to the prolonged arm of the labial bow a lingual spring turns the mesial ridge of the canine labially, while the labial bow turns its distal ridge lingually; the little arrowhead at the end of the arm of the labial bow marks the point where the wire emerged from the plastic material of the plate. *D* and *E,* Activation of the labial bow at the loop; *D,* opening the bend x; *E,* compressing at first the bend x (arrows 1) and bending down the horizontal loop (arrow 2). To be activated lingually, the loop is bent against the canine. (From Schwarz, A. M., and Gratzinger, M.: Removable Orthodontic Appliances. Philadelphia, W. B. Saunders Company, 1966.)

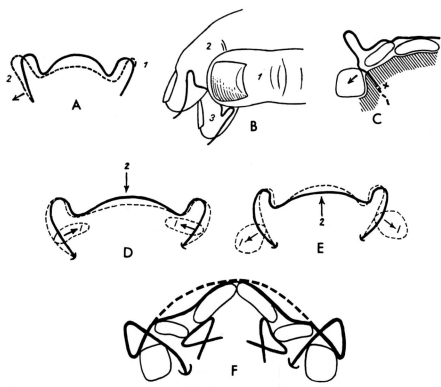

Figure 2–16. Activation of the labial bow. *A,* The bow is flattened and the loops carefully reduced (as in *1*), either with pliers or *(B)* with the fingers. *C,* In order to touch a definite point on the tooth, little "noses" may be bent; the arm is bent to move the canine distally (arrow), as shown in *A. D* and *E,* Both arms are used to move teeth mesially or distally. The distance between the arms is reduced (mesial movement) or increased (distal movement), but the secondary effect imparted to the bow in this way is different. *D,* To move the lateral incisors mesially (arrows 1), the bow is activated, reducing the distance between both arms (solid line). When the plate is inserted, the bow snaps in, gliding along the distal surfaces of the teeth (dotted line), the distance between the arms being enlarged. In this way also, the bow itself is automatically activated (arrow 2). Therefore, combined retrusion and mesial movement are accomplished. *E,* To move the canines distally (arrows 1), the bow is activated, increasing the distance between the arms (solid line). When the plate is inserted, this distance is reduced (dotted line) and so the bow itself automatically is released (arrow 2). In this case, if we intend to combine retrusion and distal movement, one or the other movement may fail. *F,* It is a common mistake to fit the labial bow, in a case of rotated teeth, following their initial position (solid line). The correct initial shape in this case is indicated by the dotted line. The bow is formed from the beginning in the nearly final shape of the corrected arch, touching in this way all prominent margins of the teeth and providing the space for the other aspects, which have to be moved labially. (From Schwarz, A. M., and Gratzinger, M.: Removable Orthodontic Appliances. Philadelphia, W. B. Saunders Company, 1966.)

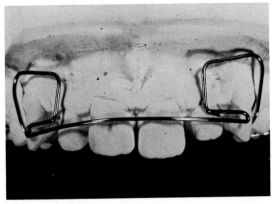

Figure 2–17. Labial bow to align anterior teeth and to reduce overjet. (From Neumann, B.: Removable appliances. *In* Graber, T. M., and Swain, B. F. (Eds.): Current Orthodontic Concepts and Techniques, 2nd ed. Philadelphia, W. B. Saunders Company, 1975. Courtesy of Dr. J. R. E. Mills, London, England.)

frequently. To exert the necessary pressure on the tooth or teeth to be moved, the spring has to be activated. The manner in which this is done is shown in Figure 2–19 for free springs and in Figure 2–20 for closed or continuous loop springs. Used only occasionally, but very effective, is another design described by Schwarz. He called this the "paddle spring" (Fig. 2–21).

Helical coil springs are most effective for the distal movement of canines and premolars into a postextraction space (Fig. 2–22). The spring is "boxed in." Thus the acrylic protects it occlusally. The wire forming the spring is anchored in the acrylic and then turns to cross the spring, thus preventing it from being dislodged gingivally. If, for hygienic reasons or to allow better control of the spring, the plate is cut back, the guide wire will be overlying the spring or a double guide wire will be made (Fig. 2–23). Similar in construction is the two-looped safety pin spring for the labial movement of upper incisors (Fig. 2–24). The coil should be wound so that when the spring acts, the coil tends to unwind (Fig. 2–25). Protected palatal or lingual springs are generally of 0.5 to

Text continued on page 29

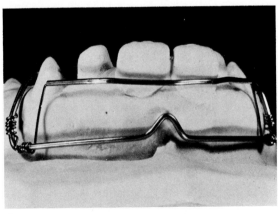

A

Figure 2–18. High labial bow with different designs of apron springs. (*A*, from Neumann, B.: Removable appliances. *In* Graber, T. M., and Swain, B. F. (Eds.): Current Orthodontic Concepts and Techniques, 2nd ed. Philadelphia, W. B. Saunders Company, 1975. Courtesy of Dr. J. R. E. Mills, London, England. *B, C,* and *D* from Tulley, W. J., and Campbell, A. C.: A Manual of Practical Orthodontics. Bristol, John Wright and Sons, Ltd., 1960.)

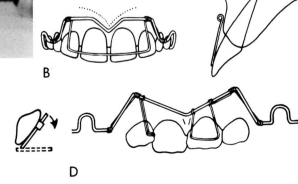

B

C

D

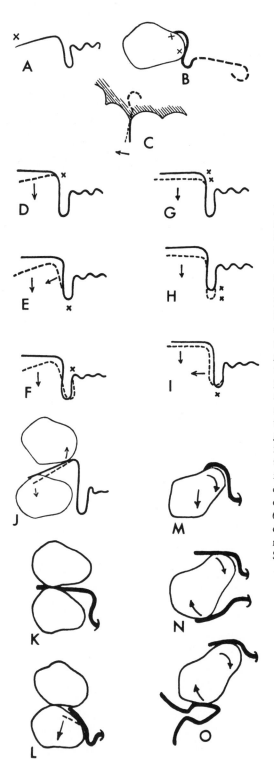

Figure 2–19. The finger spring. *A,* Typical shape made of 0.6 to 0.7 mm. wire; the undulated part is for insertion in the plastic material. *B,* Usually a hook at the end (interrupted line) is sufficient to anchor the wire in place. *C,* The simple finger spring, used to make small movements; its activation is in the direction of the arrow (dotted line). *D* to *I,* Activation of the typical finger spring. The bends at points x in *D, E, G,* and *H* intend mesio-distal movements only; in *E* and *I,* mesiodistal and buccal movements combined. The bending shown in *G* elongates the free end, which must be gradually shortened. *J,* A common error when bending the spring as shown in *D* to *F.* The bend prevents the proximal tooth from following the moved one; a space results. *K,* Another common error: the end of the finger spring is too long to snap in short of the contact point; the correct place for the spring is at the gingival margin. *L,* The correctly situated spring. *M* to *O,* Simple finger springs can be used to effect minor rotations of the upper premolars, the crowns of which make such movements possible: *M,* rotation combined with mesiodistal movement; *N,* rotation using two springs: the contact for the buccally working spring must be free; *O,* rotation, using a lingual spring and the arrow of a clasp. (From Schwarz, A. M., and Gratzinger, M.: Removable Orthodontic Appliances. Philadelphia, W. B. Saunders Company, 1966.)

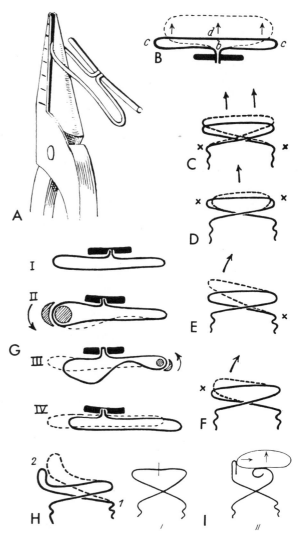

Figure 2–20. Activation of the loop spring. *A,* Pliers for gradually opening a loop.* With every mark on the pliers the diameter of the male part of the pliers increases by 1 mm. *B,* Symmetrical bending (arrows); with every activation a widening of only 1 mm. must be made. *C,* Activation lifting the spring at points x. *D,* Same method as shown in *B.* *E* and *F,* Asymmetrical activation. *G,* Changing the stage of the spring (*I* to *IV*): *II,* The pliers are turned (arrow) until the shape shown in III results. *III,* The other bend is turned (arrow) and the first larger bend compressed to form the shape shown in *IV*. This transformation of lingually placed anterior springs sometimes becomes necessary in cases in which one of their points of application is lost due to the expansion of the plate. *H,* The pliers are turned at bend 2, and the spring lifted around 1. The spring is activated to move the tooth mesiodistally also. *I,* The loop spring is converted into two fingers, which move or retain the tooth (incisor) in the direction of the arrows, after the loop spring has done its work. (From Schwarz, A. M., and Gratzinger, M.: Removable Orthodontic Appliances. Philadelphia, W. B. Saunders Company, 1966.)

---

*The loop spring for fixed appliances was introduced by A. M. Schwarz in 1925 (Mershon's lingual arch). The spring shown here is soldered to an arch wire.

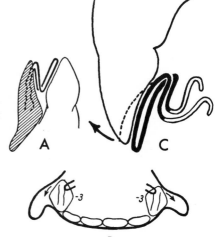

Figure 2–21. The paddle spring. Its shape is that of a hairpin, formed of 0.5 mm. wire, and it is bent to form a paddle. It is activated by bending it toward the tooth. *A* and *B,* Turning a lower canine (arrow) combined with the labial arch. *C,* Tipping lingually retruded upper central incisor labially. A hook spring is used as shown here. (From Schwarz, A. M., and Gratzinger, M.: Removable Orthodontic Appliances. Philadelphia, W. B. Saunders Company, 1966.)

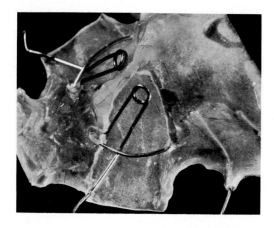

Figure 2–22. Boxed-in helical coil spring for retracting upper canines into extraction spaces. (From Neumann, B.: Removable appliances. *In* Graber, T. M., and Swain, B. F. (Eds.): Current Orthodontic Concepts and Techniques, 2nd ed. Philadelphia, W. B. Saunders Company, 1975. Courtesy of Dr. J. R. E. Mills, London, England.)

Figure 2–23. Helical coil springs protected against distortion by guide wires with plates cut back. *A,* Guide wire overlying the spring. *B,* Spring placed between double guide wires.

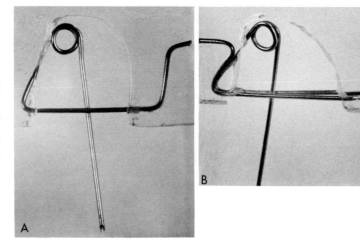

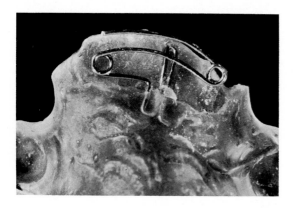

Figure 2–24. Boxed-in two-looped safety pin spring to move upper incisors forward with centrally placed guide wire to prevent distortion. This spring is used mostly in conjunction with lateral bite blocks. (From Neumann, B.: Removable appliances. *In* Graber, T. M., and Swain, B. F. (Eds.): Current Orthodontic Concepts and Techniques, 2nd ed. Philadelphia, W. B. Saunders Company, 1975. Courtesy of Dr. J. R. E. Mills, London, England.)

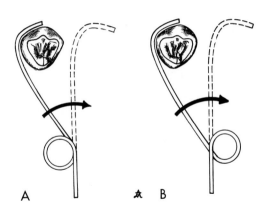

Figure 2–25. Correct (*A*) and incorrect (*B*) methods of winding helical coil finger spring for use in removable palatal appliance. To activate spring, helical coil should always be closed—never opened—for optimal efficiency. The coil tends to unwind when acting. (From Graber, T. M.: Orthodontics: Principles and Practice, 3rd ed. Philadelphia, W. B. Saunders Company, 1972.)

A   A   B

0.6 mm. diameter wire; unprotected buccal springs are illustrated in Figure 2–26 and are of 0.7 mm. wire. They are used for the distal movement of more buccally displaced canines. For apparent technical reasons, the coil must be opened when the spring is activated. With the stronger wire the spring will, however, work equally well. The coil must not be placed distally. That will make activating the spring difficult, because the anterior part of the spring will slide down and become ineffective. The same configuration with the end turned to lie flat on the buccal surface of a premolar will move the tooth in a palatal direction. For limited movements of single teeth, small springs have proved useful. They need only a little space and will effect more precise movements, such as rotating an incisor against the labial wire. They are formed as closed loops, double loops or, using double wire with a small coil, straight or S shaped; 0.4 or 0.5 mm. wire is used (Fig. 2–27).

The rotation of a canine is rather difficult with a removable appliance, but it can be achieved by the "whip" appliance.[15] A 0.35 mm. wire is attached to a bracket on the canine band. The flexible spring is hooked under the labial bow and produces a very gentle rotating force (Fig. 2–28).

Springs of larger dimensions (1.1 to 1.25 mm. diameter) may be used as Coffin springs for expansion, instead of screws. One or two such springs may be incorporated into a maxillary plate. A circular lingual wire below the buccal segment acrylic parts, joining them at the distal end, is used for a similar mandibular appliance. A very careful activation is needed so as not to dislodge the clasps from the teeth. It is probably easier to see the difficulty of using this device than the advantage of using it.

Screws. Except for the rather infrequent use of Coffin springs mentioned

Figure 2–26. Unsupported canine retracting spring to move the tooth into the space left by the extraction of the first premolar. (From Neumann, B.: Removable appliances. *In* Graber, T. M., and Swain, B. F. (Eds.): Current Orthodontic Concepts and Techniques, 2nd ed. Philadelphia, W. B. Saunders Company, 1975. Courtesy of Dr. J. R. E. Mills, London, England.)

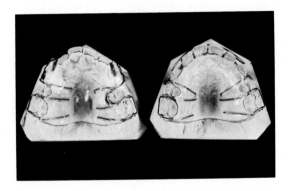

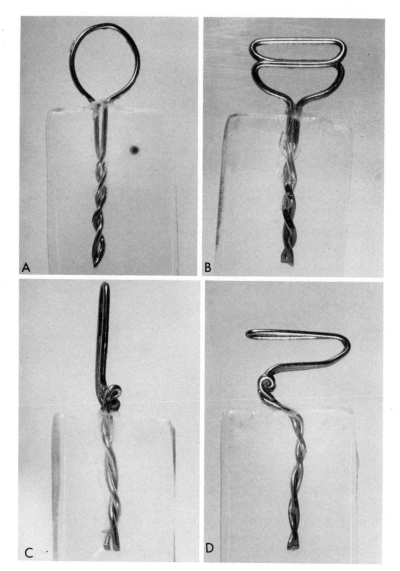

Figure 2-27. Small springs for the movement of single teeth. *A,* Loop spring. *B,* Double loop spring. *C,* Spring for mesial or distal movement. *D,* Spring for rotation, generally in conjunction with a labial bow. These springs are made mostly of 0.4 mm. wire; *A* and *B,* when used with the activator, also of 0.5 mm. wire. Twisting the wire of the tags facilitates placement in the wax. With springs *A* and *B* the portion emerging from the acrylic is left straight to prevent breakage. The small coils with *C* and *D* increase the elasticity.

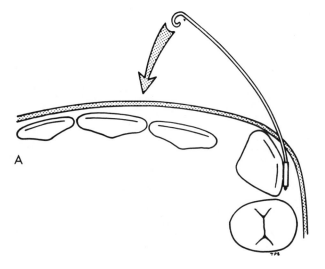

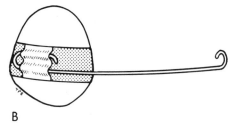

Figure 2-28. The whip appliance. (From Tulley, W. J., and Cryer, B. S.: Orthodontic Treatment for the Adult. Bristol, John Wright and Sons, Ltd., 1969.)

above, the baseplate when used as a working part is divided and driven apart by screws. An equal division of the plate will create a reciprocal anchorage for both parts. By dividing the plate into larger and smaller parts, the larger will provide added anchorage for the movements of the smaller part or parts. Different designs applying these principles are shown with the description of how to use the active plate.

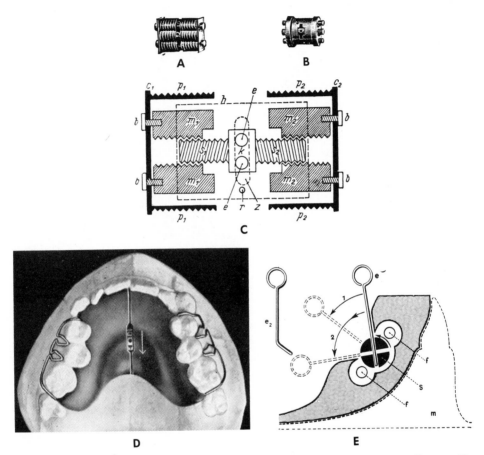

Figure 2–29. Orthodontic screws. *A*, Normal type A (in natural size). *B*, Smaller type B. *C*, Cross section through type A. The screw is opened to half its maximal expansions. (S_1S_2, the screw; *k*, head of the screw with holes for the key, *e*; m_1m_2, the nuts (guiding female parts of the screw); *b*, (dotted line), case with slot, *z*, and mark, *r*, which indicates the direction in which the screw is to be turned; p_1p_2, casing attached with the tiny screws, *b*). *D*, An upper expansion plate showing an arrow in the small groove near the opening of the screw, indicating the direction in which to turn; another mark above the screw indicates the point at which the dentist makes periodic measurements to ascertain that the widening is progressing according to schedule. *E*, Schematic sagittal section through the anterior part of an upper expansion plate on the model (*S*, the screw with the two holes for the key; *f*, the guiding rods; *e*, the key put in one hole which is situated near the anterior border of the slot *z* shown in *C*); arrow 1 shows a turn of 45 degrees, which is called a "half turn", arrow 2 indicates a turn of 90 degrees, until the key is stopped by the posterior borders of the slot, called a "whole turn." With this movement the next of the four holes appears at the anterior part of the slot. The patient or his parents must be explicitly instructed in the use of the screw. If the screw is placed at the side of the plate, the bent key, e_2, is used. (From Schwarz, A. M., and Gratzinger, M.: Removable Orthodontic Appliances. Philadelphia, W. B. Saunders Company, 1966.)

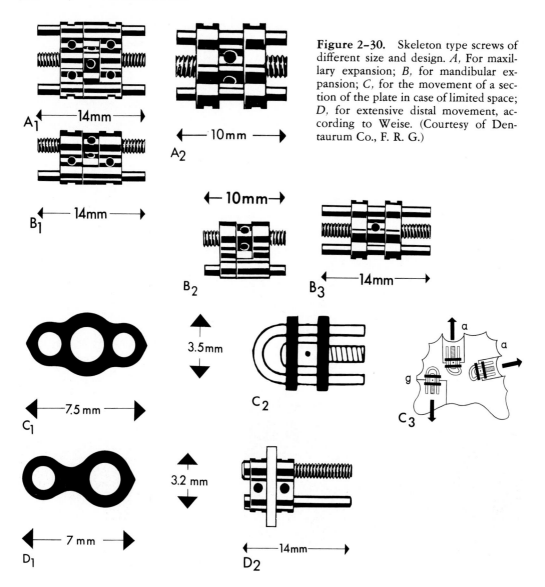

Figure 2-30. Skeleton type screws of different size and design. *A,* For maxillary expansion; *B,* for mandibular expansion; *C,* for the movement of a section of the plate in case of limited space; *D,* for extensive distal movement, according to Weise. (Courtesy of Dentaurum Co., F. R. G.)

The screw, when turned 90 degrees, will drive the parts of the plate apart 0.2 mm. That should mean narrowing the periodontal membrane 0.1 mm. on each side. It has been argued that such a mild reduction of space would not interrupt the circulation of blood, thus creating the ideal orthodontic conditions for the transformation of bone. There is clinical evidence that the movement of teeth is thus brought about in a harmless and effective way. There are other factors still to be considered, however.[16]

Screws and their construction and working mechanism are shown in Figure 2–29. Over the years since Schwarz first introduced these in his plates, an abundance of screws has come into being. In a recent attempt to collect the various types of screws currently used in Europe, no less than 254 were found.[17, 18] Some of these were identical products of different manufacturers. Others, although fundamentally similar, are yet different in one small way or another. So it is safe to say that 200 screws of different types are still in existence.[19]

In practice, only a very limited selection is used by most orthodontists. There is, however, an advantage in selecting the proper size and design of screw for the particular action of the plate.

The encased expansion screws shown in Figure 2–29 are sturdy and resist stress. The spiral part, however, may sometimes turn back. The skeleton type of screws with part of the spiral embedded in the acrylic is superior in this respect and therefore generally preferred now. Such screws are available in various sizes, broader for maxillary, narrower for mandibular plates. The smaller size also is effective for the distal movement of teeth (Fig. 2–30*A* and *B*). When space for the screw is limited for a distal movement, the construction is facilitated by unequally divided special screws with the entire spiral on one side (Fig. 2–30*C*). A screw of this type, making possible a distal movement of up to 8 mm., was designed by Weise. It can be used to advantage for the distal movement of both premolars after the extraction of the upper first molar unilaterally or bilaterally (Fig. 2–30*D*).

In some instances the use of the pull screw may seem desirable. In such cases, an expanded encased screw is inserted and subsequently closed to effect the desired tooth movement (see Fig. 2–34). A skeleton type screw cannot be used the same way. When the screw is expanded the spiral is pulled out of the acrylic. The closing of such a screw inserted in the expanded state will break the acrylic. A way to avoid such a contingency will be shown later. Special pull screws are, however, available (Fig. 2–31*A*), making improvisation unnecessary.

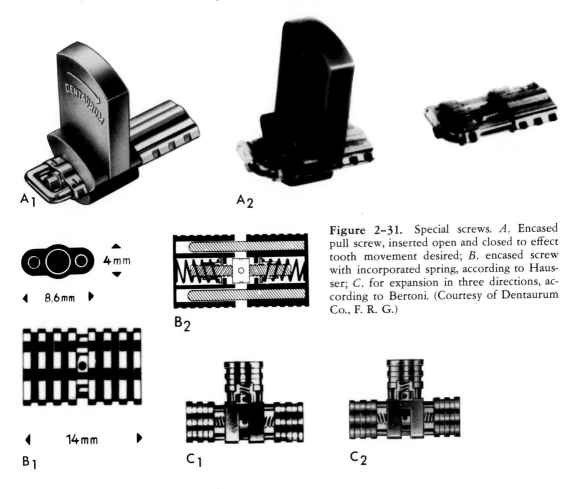

Figure 2–31. Special screws. *A*, Encased pull screw, inserted open and closed to effect tooth movement desired; *B*, encased screw with incorporated spring, according to Hausser; *C*, for expansion in three directions, according to Bertoni. (Courtesy of Dentaurum Co., F. R. G.)

A screw activating a limited spring action has been designed by Hausser (Fig. 2–31C). A complete turn of this screw will expand it 0.7 mm.; that means a quarter turn, divided for both sides, is less than 0.1 mm. on each side. By incorporating a spring, this limited pressure will be kept constant. The screw of Bertoni (Fig. 2–31C) provides the possibility of a forceful expansion in three directions.

The usual maxillary split plate can be adapted for symmetrical expansion by the incorporation of a piece of wire at the distal end of the split palate. When the screw is opened, the two parts of the plate are kept together at the posterior end. The screw permits some freedom, so the plate will open fanwise anteriorly about 4 mm. With a special screw constructed for this purpose, an opening of 8 mm. can be achieved. The screw is made of two parts, a hinge and a special screw permitting a slight rotation inside the disk (Fig. 2–32A). Anoth-

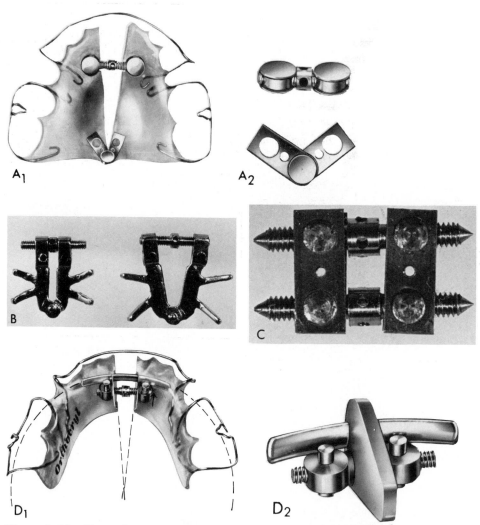

Figure 2–32. Eccentric screws. *A,* For fanwise maxillary expansion; *B,* Wipla expansion screw, length 8.2 or 7.2 mm., width 18.0 or 15.0 mm. *C,* for making possible anterior and posterior fanwise expansion up to 4 mm.; *D,* for eccentric mandibular expansion. (Courtesy of Dentaurum Co., F. R. G.)

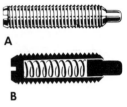

Figure 2–33. Screw with incorporated spring for the movement of single teeth. (Courtesy of Dentaurum Co., F. R. G.)

er construction incorporates the hinge with the screw in one piece (Fig. 2–32*C*). The latter is more stable and the laboratory procedure is easier. It is recommended for the maxillary expansion of operated palate cases. A screw designed for anterior and posterior expansion is shown in Figure 2–32*C*.

For eccentric mandibular expansion, a screw designed by G. Müller is available (Fig. 2–32*D*). However, the expansion has a slight sagittal component. This will lead to a tendency to unseat the clasps, which will have to be adapted accordingly.

Small screws are made which are able to exert precise limited pressure on single teeth. An example of these, with a spring incorporated, is shown in Figure 2–33. These screws are available in different lengths. Thus, after the first small screw is used, it may be exchanged for a longer one if its range of action is spent and further tooth movement is required.

Elastics. Elastics in conjunction with removable appliances are used for the movement of single teeth and groups of teeth, and for intermaxillary traction. An excellent use of an elastic is shown in Figure 2–4. An exposed impacted canine is moved to its proper position. The possibility of varying the construction in order to give the pull of the elastic any desired direction makes this simple appliance very effective indeed. Springs and screws may still be preferred to the use of elastics, depending on the task, as shown in Figure 2–34.

An elastic between two hooks in the canine labial region may replace the labial wire for the retrusion or retroinclination of spaced incisors. The upper plate must be cut away behind the incisors to make the movement possible. The curvature of the upper arch will not favor that procedure in some cases. A mandibular plate to serve the same purpose should have its buccal parts joined anteriorly by a lingual bar. The acrylic in this area would impede the retrusion of the teeth. The use of such techniques is generally limited to adult orthodontics, in conjunction with periodontal treatment, as a preliminary measure to splinting and similar therapy.

Intermaxillary elastics with removable plates are shown in Figure 2–35. Many conventional plates are often used in this way. In the treatment of Class II, Division 1 malocclusion, the elastics are slipped over the U bend of the labial bow. From there, they extend obliquely down and back to a hook extended into the buccal vestibule from the lower plate. Variations of clasps to accomodate elastics have also been designed. Part of the original Schwarz technique with active plates and elastics has never really had widespread use. Lately there has been a revival in their use, however, with quite clever variations by some clinicians to solve specific problems. Fixed appliances, or combined fixed and removable appliances, may be easier and more effective to use in most instances. Nevertheless, the reasons cited by Hotz for using intermaxillary elastics from a guide plane to molar bands connected by a lingual arch are valid. There are further interesting possibilities for the use of intermaxillary elastics in conjunction with extraoral traction.

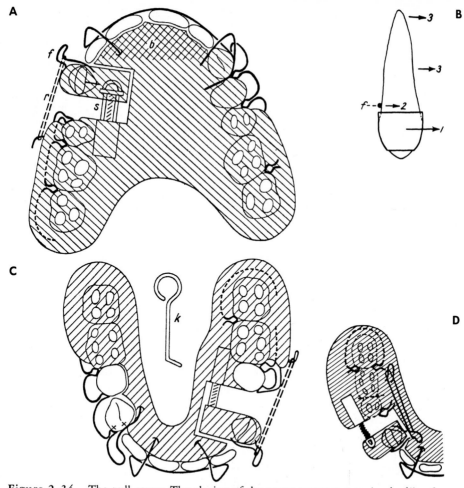

Figure 2–34. The pull screw. The closing of the screw removes a canine bodily after extraction of p_1 (or a p_1 after extraction of p_2). *A,* The usual construction of an upper plate for moving the right canine. The canine is embraced by a band, which becomes part of an acrylic block; the block is attached to the anterior part of the open screw (Fig. 2–29*A*). If the plate is inserted, the band covers the canine like a thimble. *f* is a finger spring touching the tooth close to the mesiogingival margin of the band. It is activated by an elastic, *r.* (The purpose of this arrangement is explained in *B.*) Other details of the plate: tuberosities included as anchorage, p_2, m_1, m_2, covered by acrylic as bodily anchorage (the cusps eventually are exposed); an anterior bite plane; if the jaws are closed the plate is kept in place by the lower teeth (or by a lower plate) anteriorly and in both molar areas (three point contacts as intermaxillary anchorage); covered arrows buccally situated between M_1 and M_2; the labial bow (0.7 mm. wire) serving as anchorage only touches the incisors and the left canine near the incisal edges (bodily resistance); its right arm crosses the arch between the right lateral and central incisors without touching the teeth; hence the movement of the right lateral and medial incisor, which occurs to a greater or lesser degree simultaneously with the distal movement of the right canine, is not prevented. *B,* The finger spring, *f,* rests mesiogingivally below the margin of the band. This part of the band is overhanging, since it does not exactly fit the bell-shaped crown. Therefore the finger spring is placed there to act in the direction of arrow 2, advancing the bodily movement (arrows 3). Arrow 1 is the force of the screw. *C,* The same plate for bodily distal movement of the left lower canine. Covered arrow is seen on the lingual side between M_1 and M_2; the same details for stationary anchorage as in the upper jaw except, of course, tuberosity anchorage. In both jaws the extraction of both first premolars is planned. In the upper jaw, *A,* the treatment is depicted as beginning at the right side after extraction of right p_1. The left half of the jaw serves as anchorage. In the lower jaw the second phase of the treatment is initiated. The right p_1 was extracted and the canine already moved close to the p_2. A remaining distance of about 1 mm. must be corrected by activating the anterior arm x and arrow x of the clasp. This corrected right half of the jaw serves now as anchorage. *D,* If there is lack of space in a narrow jaw, the pull screw is attached buccally. (From Schwarz, A. M., and Gratzinger, M.: Removable Orthodontic Appliances. Philadelphia, W. B. Saunders Company, 1966.)

Figure 2–35. Intermaxillary elastics for correction of Class III malocclusion (true prognathism inferior). Both arches and the palate are covered with acrylic, which retains the teeth bodily ("horseshoe appliances"). Clasps may be added. Vertical hooks for the elastics (100 grams force) attached in the area of the lower canines provide traction in the most favorable direction for the forward movement of the upper arch, even if the jaws are moderately opened. This appliance may be worn during the night and also several hours during the day. The chincap also should be worn during the night. (From Schwarz, A. M., and Gratzinger M.: Removable Orthodontic Appliances. Philadelphia, W. B. Saunders Company, 1966.)

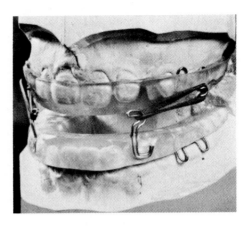

Fabrication and Repairs of Active Plates

The fabrication of a simple Hawley type appliance is shown in Figure 2–36. Curing under pressure is more desirable, however, for active plates. More complicated constructions should be waxed, flasked, and boiled out for greater precision. Wires and screws have to be kept securely in place in different ways, according to the manner in which the plate is made.

For repairs, endothermic acrylic is generally used. A broken labial wire can be repaired by soldering or preferably by electrowelding (Fig. 2–37). The same procedure is possible with the Schwarz continuous arrow clasp or with an Adams clasp. Other clasps are easily replaced when broken. Some are fabricated for just that reason (for example, the Stockfisch and Bimler appliances).

If an extension screw has been opened to its maximum adjustment, the midsagittal crevice created in the plate is filled with baseplate wax. The softened wax is adapted to the palate. Plaster is poured under the plate. After hardening, the wax is removed. The screw is cut out, turned back, and the space between the halves of the plate and around the newly inserted screw is filled with endothermic acrylic. The plate is cut appropriately, finished, and polished. If the screw has moved only a section of the plate, it will be sufficient to cut out the acrylic only around the half of the screw in the section. Otherwise the procedure is the same as described above.

If a skeleton type screw has to be used as a pull screw, the spiral parts and guide wires emerging from the screw are covered with a small amount of cold-curing acrylic. After the hardening of the acrylic, the screw may be opened and placed as desired. The space for the threaded section, now withdrawn into the female portion, will thus be left open.

The laboratory technician should be provided with a sketch showing the situation of the wires, clasps, and screws and how the plate is cut into sections. The drawings need not be elaborate works of art, but must show clearly the essential details. Written directions should be added if there could be any doubt about the work to be done.

For further construction details, fine texts like that of Philip Adams are available.[12] Careful selection of a well-trained technician is important. Most large metropolitan areas now have laboratories capable of fabricating excellent removable orthodontic appliances, to the prescription of the orthodontist.

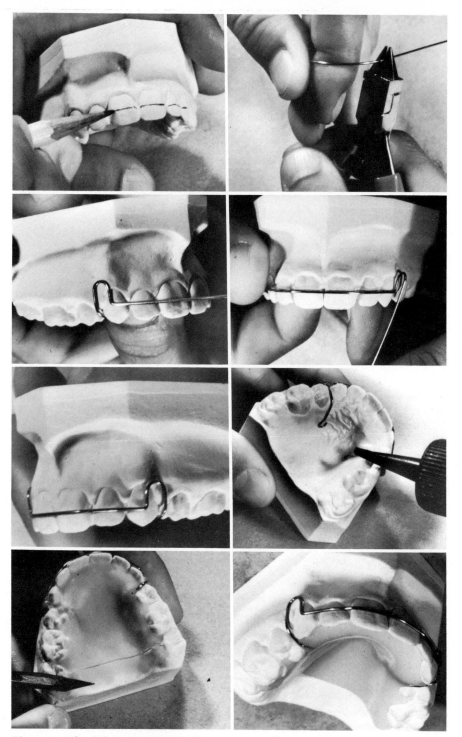

Figure 2-36. Fabrication of Hawley-type removable appliance. Pencilled line (upper top left) shows level of labial wire placement. No. 139 pliers (upper right) are used to make the bends and loops in the shaped 0.030 inch nichrome or stainless steel wire bow. Drawing the wire between the thumb and forefinger gently will make the approximate anterior arch curvature. After the bow is bent to the desired shape and is passive, it is placed on the model and the acrylic portion is fabricated. Usually this is done by the "cold-cure technique" of adding acrylic powder and monomer alternately. Conventional waxing and flask or pressure curing is also possible. Polishing is the same as for a denture. (From Graber, T. M.: Orthodontics: Principles and Practice, 3rd ed. Philadelphia, W. B. Saunders Company, 1972. Courtesy of J. A. McNamara, Jr.)

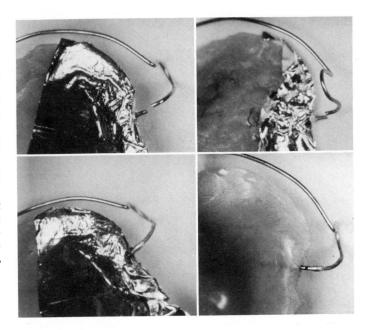

Figure 2–37. Broken labial wire, being repaired on a removable upper orthodontic appliance. Acrylic has been cut back at wire exit from acrylic and covered with aluminum foil. Only the broken end protrudes (top). Lower left shows soldered labial wire, with foil still in place. Foil is then removed and acrylic and wire cleaned and polished. Electric soldering using a welder attachment is even better, if available. (From Graber, T. M.: Orthodontics: Principles and Practice, 3rd ed. Philadelphia, W. B. Saunders Company, 1972.)

THE USE OF THE ACTIVE PLATE

The orthodontist, confronted with an almost overwhelming abundance of elements to choose from for the construction of the active plate, will have to make up his mind how to use it. The task for the appliance is the application of force to effect the planned movement of teeth. For that the device must be well contrived mechanically, technically precisely executed with respect for the biological preconditions for the success of the therapy. Yet, whether fixed or removable appliances are used, orthodontic treatment is no simple biomechanical problem. The attainment of the result and especially its stability are dependent also on morphogenetic pattern, muscular function, simultaneous growth and development, and other factors. Some of these contributing factors still need clarification and further investigation.[20] Also when using removable appliances, clinical judgment and the skill of the operator and his ability to attend to minute details will ultimately determine the level of possible achievement.

With active plates, the direction and the amount of the forced applied are under complete control, and secure anchorage is provided. These are the advantages the operator should know and use to the fullest extent. But if he is not equally well aware of the limitations imposed by these methods, it will be very much to his and his patient's disadvantage.

There are many uses for the removable plate. Some are not "active" at all, such as those used as a periodontal splint or a "dental crutch." Others are used as retainers or with a built-in bite plane to open the bite. Such are described in Graber's textbook.[9] Active plates are used to assist in solving other dental problems, for instance, as a preliminary measure before placing bridges and castings. The pulling down of an impacted canine is shown in Figure 2–4. Other minor irregularities amenable to simple correction have to be treated with some circumspection. The alignment of very slightly crowded maxillary incisors with a Hawley type upper plate after stripping the contacts with a lightning strip will usually necessitate grinding of the incisal margins of the opposing incisors to remove occlusal interference to the retraction. A lip or finger habit may cause the malposition of a single upper central incisor. With occlusion permitting, and with adequate space for the tooth, the gentle pressure of the labial wire will bring the incisor into alignment and in due course may also stop the habit. The appliance may be modified to intercept both finger and tongue habits.

A divergent midline diastema (narrower at the gingival than the incisal margin) may be corrected with finger springs emerging from the plate, moving the incisors together. The permanency of the result will depend partly on the mesial movement of the erupting canines absorbing the surplus space. There is, however, the danger of tipping the incisors mesially. For this reason, most orthodontists using plates will often prefer a small fixed appliance with bands and appropriate attachments, assuring a parallel movement of the incisors. The tendency to relapse seems to be considerable. The same is true for the alignment of slightly rotated incisors with adequate space in the arch. If the rotation was primarily due to crowding, the alignment of the incisors after the creation of the necessary space can be quick and permanent. Gentle pressure of the labial wire, combined with the action of a finger spring from the palatal side, effectively eliminates incisor rotations (Fig. 2–16F). A "free" rotation which requires apical movement and paralleling is better corrected with a fixed appliance, however.

The treatment of anterior crossbite is simple and rewarding. If the plate with a lateral bite plate or bite block is worn continuously, including during meals, there will be a strong tendency for the autonomous correction of the incisor locked in lingual occlusion. Any kind of spring will bring it quickly into line. If the labial movement of more than one tooth is required, a safety pin spring (Fig. 2–24) is a good choice. Selective pressure on each tooth to be moved may be exerted by small loop springs of 0.4 or at most 0.5 mm. diameter wire.

For the treatment of these conditions, there is the choice between maxillary plates with springs and lateral bite blocks or appliances incorporating an inclined bite plane seated on the mandibular dentition. Preference usually is given to the former, judged by patient convenience. The lower inclined plane will open the bite. This is beneficial if there is a deep bite, but if the original overbite is shallow, there will be less retention for the tooth moved and relapse may follow. If the overbite is very small or nil, the tipping of the incisors will remove the possibility of retention. The palatal appliance then is preferable, since it also serves as a retainer, or a functional appliance such as the Bionator should be used. Obviously, a correct diagnosis is imperative. The operator should not attempt correction of a basal Class III malocclusion by either of the appliances just described for local crossbite conditions. If the differential diagnosis is a pronounced Class III tendency, a Frankel appliance (FR III) is recommended (see Chapter 15). Treatment with a functional appliance may also be instituted if the result of the treatment with an active plate does not seem to be stable (see Chapters 8 to 14).

The overwhelming majority of active plates are used for the treatment of crowding, excessive overjet, or a combination of these conditions in patients with a Class I or mild Class II skeletal pattern. The best results will be achieved when there is no need for treatment of the mandibular dentition and the correction of the maxillary malocclusion is sufficient (one arch treatment). Extraction in both arches will give acceptable results also when there will be autonomous correction or the necessity of only minor mechanical interference in the lower dentition, with appliances again used mainly in the maxillary arch. A third, more controversial possibility is to content oneself with the correction of the conspicuous maxillary malocclusion and the continued existence of minor irregularities or residual postextraction spaces in the lower dentition. Such a solution may be satisfactory to many patients and the achievable optimum even where the multibanded technique is an alternative treatment means.

The preponderant use of appliances for the maxillary dentition only is shown by a survey of one thousand consecutive treated orthodontic cases, published recently by one of the most competent English orthodontists.[21] About three quarters of the patients had maxillary teeth extracted and 42 per cent had teeth removed from the mandible. In 92.7 per cent, appliance treatment for the upper arch only was used; in 1.5 per cent it was confined to the lower arch; 2.6 per cent had therapy applied to both arches. Thus only 4.1 per cent had active treatment in the lower arch, less than 10 per cent of the extraction cases. It should be mentioned that only 0.8 per cent of the patients treated had fixed appliances and 0.5 per cent myofunctional therapy. Looking back over some cases, which were all started seven or eight years ago, the author states that "today one might actively treat more of the lower arches. Certainly more of them would have had extractions from the mandible, in order to lessen the risk of late incisor crowding."[21]

There is no intention to enter here into the controversy regarding complete correction versus compromise treatment. The emphasis is on careful diagnosis, prognosis, and appliance limitations. The operator who disregards these prerequisites and who is not aware of the limitations imposed by therapy with active plates may find himself in the uncomfortable position of having started a treatment he is unable to complete satisfactorily.

The design of plates using springs as active parts is comparatively simple. The baseplate is held in place to serve as a secure base of operation. Springs of the desired form are fitted in to effect the planned tooth movement. Number and action of the springs are limited to the quantity not affecting the stability of the plate. Beware of trying to do too many things at once with active plates.

If screws are used, the baseplate then serves also as a working part. It is divided into sections driven apart by one or more screws. The tasks undertaken vary from simply moving a first molar to create space for the second premolar or moving a tooth into alignment for which space has been provided, to expanding the dental arch in a sagittal or transverse direction, or both.

"Lateral expansion of both upper and lower arches for the relief of crowding places teeth in an unstable relationship to their muscular environment and they will inevitably relapse."[14] That dictum will meet with approval of English-speaking orthodontists on both sides of the Atlantic. Nevertheless, under certain conditions mentioned later, lateral expansion may be indicated and appliances to effect it are shown also in English textbooks.[21]

After World War II, when the wave of extractionism reached the shores of the continent from the United States, the reaction was to emphasize apparently successful expansion of the dental arches and seeming stability of the results obtained, showing impressive isolated examples. Hotz begged to differ and later took the lead in having post-treatment results examined. Reports of 250 cases from his clinic were published.[22, 23] Others followed so that now a more cautious attitude prevails.[24-30] Yet in none of the textbooks published in German from 1968 to 1973 is the possibility of successful expansion within limits denied.[31-37] According to Schmuth,[37] transversal expansion by plates will be stable only to the extent of 3 to 4 mm. and will in most cases relapse if this amount is exceeded. These are only average values; in some cases, expansions of 8 to 10 mm. remained totally or largely permanent.[37]

Investigations by Skieller,[38] using the Björk implant method, and by Lebret[39] have shown that some widening of the palatal vault is stimulated by the active plates with screws. This research seems to support the permanency of moderate expansion.

In a more recent study using measurements from exact scale photographs, C. W. Schwarze[40] has shown that the benefits of transverse expansion are further reduced by the subsequent mesial drifting of the posterior teeth. Among the 110 patients investigated, 75.4 per cent had a follow-up examination 9 to 13 years after the beginning of treatment. Although the average expansion during treatment had been only 3.65 mm., there was an average relapse of 2 mm., leaving as the long-range result a widening of only 1.65 mm. The size of the relapse was correlated with the size of the preceding expansion and independent of the duration of retention.

Less controversial and more stable are the results of sagittal (anteroposterior) retraction. It is facilitated by the absence of maxillary third molars and may be greatly helped by extraoral traction. Even without this, 3 to 4 mm. may be gained to align a canine or, as is frequently desirable, a second premolar. There is little probability of relapse.

Cases with minimum overbite have to be watched closely during any kind of expansion treatment with active plates. Treatment has to be abandoned or altered instantly if the bite begins to open. The open bite thus artificially produced often has a tendency to remain. The alternative is the use of vertical pull head-gear with the intraoral appliance, either fixed or removable. The Milwaukee brace-like effect of these intermittent extraoral head-cap appliances has been demonstrated conclusively by Graber.[42]

In spite of these uncertainties, there are indications for lateral expansion of the dental arch. Unilateral and bilateral crossbite may be corrected, although rapid expansion may possibly be contemplated for the latter in rare cases. The often-present lingual inclination of the buccal teeth will facilitate a greater expansion. A comparatively small space gained by transverse expansion will permit the alignment of a slightly crowded upper incisor locked in lingual occlusion. The correction will improve the function, leading to further au-

Text continued on page 46

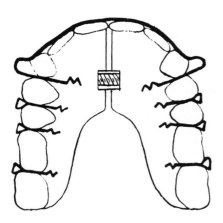

Figure 2–38. The plate, showing a split along the midline, is used for the treatment of bilateral crossbite and minor crowding of the incisors. In this, as in most other figures, triangular clasps are shown. They are the simplest to form and are indicated in all these cases, although in some cases other clasps may serve equally well or even better.

Figure 2-39. Plate for unilateral crossbite. The larger part of the plate forms a block to serve as anchorage for the movement of the smaller part. The anchorage may be reinforced by the base plate covering the palatal aspects of the buccal teeth on the side of the correct occlusion. Adams clasps may be used to advantage here. The plate is thin on the side to be moved. Bite blocks may also support the correction (see Fig. 2-52).

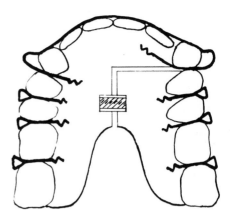

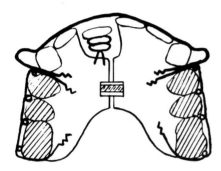

Figure 2-40. Slightly crowded upper central incisor locked in lingual occlusion is tipped forward by a double loop spring after space is provided by moderate expansion. Lateral bite blocks are used. The plate is held in place by continuous eyelet clasps (see Fig. 2-1 for a similar construction).

Figure 2-41. Expansion of the maxillary arch and subsequent labial tipping of slightly crowded upper central incisors in Class II, Division 2 malocclusion. The double loop springs can be adapted sagittally and mesially to remain in proper contact with the teeth moved. The closed bite is to be opened by a bite plate. The springs may be boxed in (see Fig. 2-1). Such plates are recommended for preliminary treatment before the insertion of functional appliances such as the Bionator.

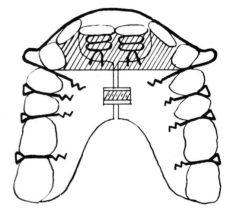

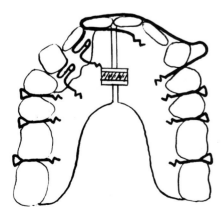

Figure 2-42. Expansion plate for the alignment of crowded upper right canine and lateral incisor. The right central incisor has moved over the midline and is brought back by the labial arch fastened with both ends inserted in the left side of the plate. Small helical springs exert pressure on canine and lateral incisor. 0.5 mm. or double 0.4 mm. wire is used for the springs. The double wire enhances resistance to dislocation without loss of elasticity.

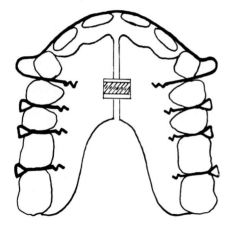

Figure 2–43. Expansion and reduction of overjet as a preliminary treatment in Class II, Division 1 malocclusion.

Figure 2–44. Y-plates. The original Y-plate of A. M. Schwarz used for the alignment of crowded canines by sagittal and lateral expansion. Lateral expansion is less if the screws are directed more sagittally.

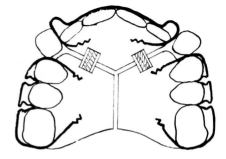

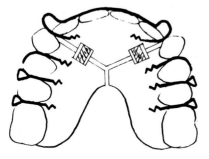

Figure 2–45. Y-plates. The modernized Y-plate. A large part of the palate is left uncovered. Triangular clasps are used in place of the Schwarz arrow clasp. Small clasps anterior to the first premolars are necessary to make these teeth participate in the movement.

Figure 2–46. Y-plate. The insertion of the tags of the labial wire into the lateral parts of the plate exerts a slight pressure in a posterior direction on the anterior part of the plate when the screws are turned. This serves to stabilize the anterior portion of the plate. The loops of the labial wire are small, permitting contact of the labial wire with the canines to guide them into the space provided by the expansion.

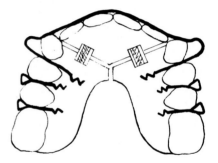

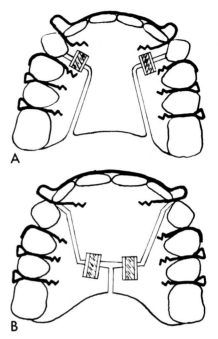

Figure 2-47. *A* and *B*, These two designs stabilize the anterior part of the plate by extending it over a large part of the palate. The screws act nearly entirely in a posterior direction. This will produce only a minimum of lateral expansion to compensate for the movement of teeth into a wider diameter of the dental arch.

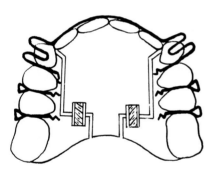

Figure 2-48. A very effective variation of the Y-plate. Insertion of the labial wire into the lateral parts is combined with coverage of the largest possible part of the palate by the anterior part of the plate. U loops of the labial wire exert a slight pressure on the canines and are simultaneously activated by the turning of the screws. Anchorage with all Y-plates may be reinforced by turning the screws on one side only alternately each week. A case treated with this appliance is shown in Figure 2-53.

Figure 2-49. Y-plate for the movement of teeth on one side only.

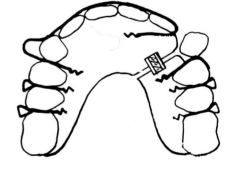

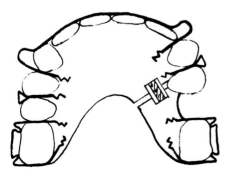

Figure 2-50. Plate for opening the space for upper second premolar. The same plate may be used with screws on both sides for bilateral action. Similar constructions are made to serve the same purpose in the mandibular arch.

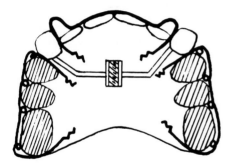

Figure 2–51.   Plate for labial movement of all incisors. Lateral bite blocks are added for increased anchorage or for incisors in lingual occlusion.

tonomous improvement. Lingually inclined and slightly crowded maxillary central incisors in Class II, Division 2 malocclusion may be freed by a very small gain of space and tipped labially. Functional retrusion can be relieved and the correction of the Class II condition facilitated. In many instances minor expansion will make further treatment much easier, particularly with elimination of abnormal perioral muscle function.

As mentioned before, some expansion plates are designed so that the part of the plate serving as anchorage is made as large as feasible to enhance its sta-

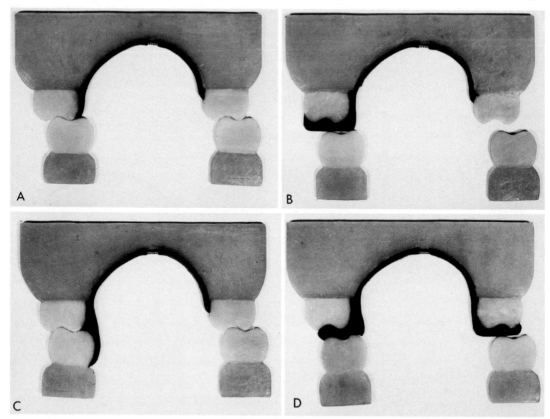

Figure 2–52.   Cross sections of plates designed for the treatment of cross bite. Anchorage is increased in different ways. *A*, The margin is extended on one side, short on the side to be moved. *B*, Unilateral blocking of the bite. *C*, Extending the plate to contact the antagonists (according to A. M. Schwarz). *D*, Bilateral blocking of the bite with imprints of the antagonists left on one side; a flat surface on the side to be moved.

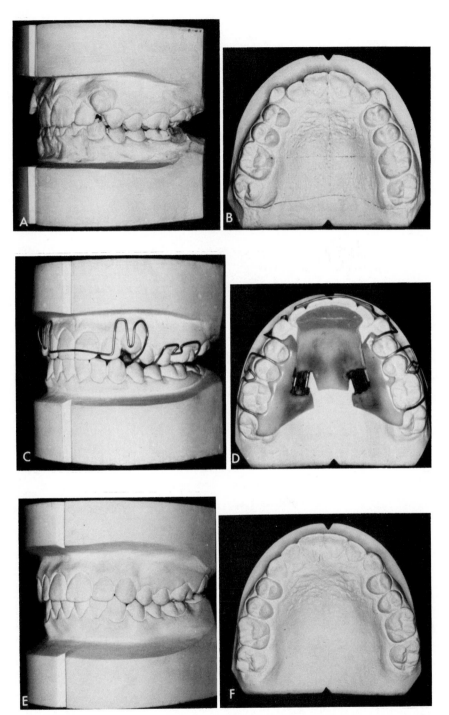

Figure 2-53. Case treated with Y-plate shown in Figure 2-48. Loss of space for upper canines erupting labially. *A* and *B*, Before treatment. *C*, After six months of treatment, with appliance inserted. *D*, Appliance used. The screws are parallel to the buccal teeth. To improve the deep overbite, to facilitate tooth movement, and to correct the distal occlusal relationship, an inclined guide plane was added. Progress must be checked closely so as not to open the bite excessively. *E* and *F*, The finished case. (From Reichenbach-Brückl-Taatz Kieferorthopädische Klinik und Terapie, 7th ed. Leipzig, J. A. Barth, 1971. Courtesy of Dr. H. Taatz and J. A. Barth Verlag, Leipzig, G. D. R.)

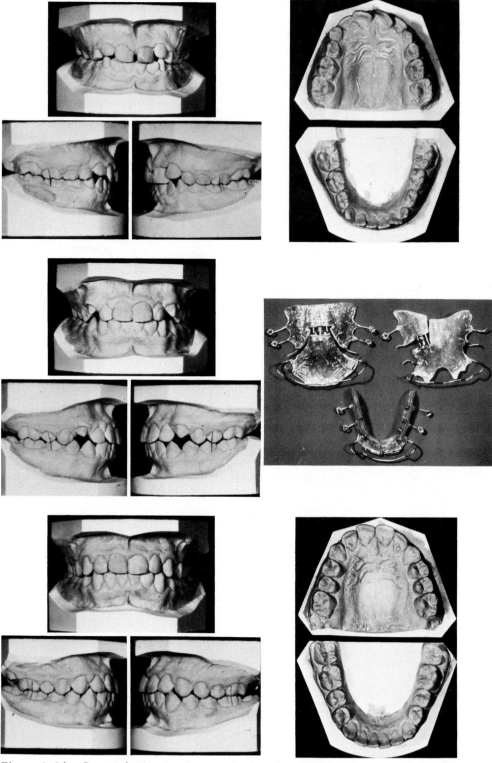

Figure 2-54. Case study showing the use of active plates in the guidance of a developing dentition over a five-year period. Casts on top are original malocclusion, a Class 1 problem, with rotated incisors and a mild arch length deficiency. Removable upper and lower appliances were placed to correct rotations, to move lingually inclined maxillary incisors to the labial, and to distalize the maxillary right molar segment. Screws and springs were the major appurtenances employed (see appliances, middle figure). The casts on the bottom are of the completed correction (courtesy of P. Herren).

48

bility and to facilitate the movement of smaller parts of the plate. In other cases, reciprocal anchorage is used to move both parts of the plate, not always necessarily to the same extent. The kind of clasp used, the form of the labial wire, the direction of the screws, together with the unequal division of the plate are combined to effect the desired change in the form of the dental arch. The practical application of these principles is shown by the designs of different plates (Figs. 2–38 to 2–52). A case treated to relieve the crowding of the canines is shown in Figure 2–53.

Active plates are the most versatile of the removable appliances. Even when constructed in the simplest manner, they may serve a variety of purposes as splints and retainers, and for uncomplicated tooth movements. British orthodontists have proved that combined with extractions, active plates provide a possibility of treating great numbers of patients in an economical and (within the given limits) very effective manner. A number of orthodontic problems can be solved partly or totally by the judicious use of screws.

There are more difficult cases requiring a sequence of appliances, with the plan of treatment repeatedly adjusted according to development and the result achieved at each stage. In such a continuous diagnostic and decisional process, as Graber termed it,[41] active plates play an important role.

Intermaxillary elastics extended from upper to lower plates may correct Class II or Class III conditions. Other possibilities shown later in the book are the double plate of A. M. Schwarz and the guide plane of R. Hotz. The usefulness of plates is greatly increased by extraoral traction. The considerable experience already gained with this combination may be only the beginning of a promising development.

The spectacular achievements of functional appliances seem to be able to steal the limelight (activators; Bimler, Stockfisch, and Fränkel appliances: Bionator; etc.). Yet active plates certainly will remain an essential part of treatment with removable appliances.

References

1. Kingsley, N. W.: A Treatise on Oral Deformity with Appropriate Preventive and Remedial Treatment. New York, Appleton & Co., 1880.
2. Robin, P.: Observation sur un nouvel appareil de redressement. Rev. Stomatol., 9:423–432, 1902.
3. Badcock, J. H.: The screw expansion plate. Trans. Br. Soc. Orthod., May–Dec., 1911, pp. 3–8.
4. Nord, C. F. L.: Loose appliances in orthodontia. Trans. Eur. Orthod. Soc., 1929.
5. Neumann, B.: Personal recollections.
6. Schwarz, A. M.: Gebissregelung mit Platten. Vienna, Urban & Schwarzenberg, 1938.
7. Schmuth, G. P. F.: Difficulties and failures experienced with active plates. Trans. Eur. Orthod. Soc., 1967, pp. 63–70.
8. Anderson, G. M.: Treatment procedures of simple form which have proved their worth. Am. J. Orthod., 37:181–187, 1951.
9. Graber, T. M.: Orthodontics, Principles and Practice, 3rd ed. Philadelphia, W. B. Saunders Company, 1972.
10. Schwarz, A. M. and Gratzinger, M.: Removable Orthodontic Appliances. Philadelphia, W. B. Saunders Company, 1966.
11. Heideborn, M. O., and Burgert, R.: Oesenklammern-Neuartige Halteelemente für aktive Platten. Zahnärztl. Welt/Reform., 80:387–390, 1971.
12. Adams, C. P.: The Design and Construction of Removable Orthodontic Appliances, 4th ed. Bristol, John Wright & Sons, Ltd., 1970.
13. Duyzings, J. A. C.: Orthodontic Appliances. Leiden, Stafleu & Tholen N. V., 1969.
14. Tulley, W. J., and Campbell, A. C.: A Manual of Practical Orthodontics. Bristol, John Wright & Sons, Ltd., 1960.
15. Tulley, W. J., and Cryer, B. S.: Orthodontic Treatment for the Adult. Bristol, John Wright & Sons, Ltd., 1969.

16. Reitan, K.: Biomechanical principles and reactions. *In* Graber, T. M., and Swain, B. F. (Eds.): Current Orthodontic Concepts and Techniques, 2nd ed., Philadelphia, W. B. Saunders Company, 1975.
17. Dausch-Neumann, D., and Khawari, A.: Die in der Kieferorthopädie gebräuchlichen Schrauben. Fortschr. Kieferorthop., *30*:413–421, 1969.
18. Khawari, A.: Schrauben im Dienst der Kieferorthopädie für abnehmbare Apparate. Med. Dissertation, Tübingen, 1968.
19. Dausch-Neumann, D.: Personal communication, February 15, 1972.
20. Moorrees, C. F. A., Burstone, C. J., Christiansen, R. L., Hixon, E. H., and Weinstein, S.: Research related to malocclusion. Am. J. Orthod., *59*:1–18, 1971.
21. Rose, J. S.: A thousand consecutive treated orthodontic cases—a survey. Br. J. Orthod., *1*:45–54, 1974.
22. Hotz, R.: Versuch einer Klassifizierung von Erfolg und Misserfolg. Fortschr. Kieferorthop., *23*:338–344, 1962.
23. Bamert, S.: Ergebnisse von Nachuntersuchungen kieferorthopädisch behandelter Fälle. Med. Dissertation, Zürich, 1961.
24. Brückl, H., and Reimann, G.: Nachuntersuchung behandelter Schmalkiefer. Fortschr. Kieferorthop., *23*:355–365, 1962.
25. Schmuth, G. P. F.: Ueberprüfung kieferorthopädischer Behandlungsergebnisse. Dtsch. Zahnärztl. Z., *17*:981–986, 1962.
26. Costa del Rio, D.: Untersuchungen über das Rezidiv der transversalen Expansion. Fortschr. Kieferorthop., *23*:395–400, 1962.
27. Land, I.: Nachuntersuchungen von abgeschlossenen und abgebrochenen kieferorthopädischen Behandlungsfällen. Med. Dissertation, Köln, 1965.
28. Schmuth, G. P. F.: Behandlungszeit–Retentionszeit–Rezidive. Fortschr. Kieferorthop., *27*:22–31, 1966.
29. Brückl, H., and Otto, G.: Weitere Nachuntersuchungen behandelter Schmalkiefer. Fortschr. Kieferorthop., *28*:377–388, 1967.
30. Schumacher, H.-A.: Befunderhebungen an kieferorthopädisch behandelten Gebissen. Probleme und Ergebnisse bei fünf- und mehrjähriger Nachuntersuchungsfrist. Med. Dissertation, Bonn, 1970.
31. Ascher, F.: Praktische Kieferorthopädie. München, Urban & Schwarzenberg, 1968.
32. Reichenbach, E.: Kieferorthopädie in Hofer-Reichenbach-Spreter von Kreudenstein-Wannemacher: Lehrbuch der klinischen Zahn-Mund- und Kieferheilkunde, 4th ed. Vol. 2. Leipzig, J. A. Barth, 1968.
33. Weise, W.: Die Behandlung. *In* Haunfelder, D., Hupfauf, H., Ketterl, W., and Schmuth, G.: Kieferorthopädie, Praxis der Zahnheilkunde, vol. IV, München, Urban & Schwarzenberg, 1969.
34. Hotz, R.: Orthodontic in der täglichen Praxis. Bern, Hans Huber, 1970.
35. Reichenbach E., Brückl, H., and Taatz, H.: Kieferorthopädische Klinik und Therapie. Leipzig, J. A. Barth, 1971.
36. Eschler, J., Rakosi, T., and Witt, E.: Kieferorthopädie für den praktischen Zahnarzt. München-Gräfelfing, Werk. Edmund Banaschewski, 1971.
37. Schmuth, G. P. F.: Kieferorthopädie, Grundzüge und Probleme. Stuttgart, Georg Thieme Verlag, 1973.
38. Skieller, V.: Expansion of the midpalatal suture by removable plates analyzed by the implant method. Trans. Eur. Orthod. Soc., 1964, pp. 143–158.
39. Lebret, L. M. L.: Changes in the palatal vault resulting from expansion. Angle Orthodont., *35*:97–105, 1965.
40. Schwarze, C. W.: Expansion and relapse in long follow-up studies. Trans. Eur. Orthod. Soc., 1972, pp. 263–274.
41. Graber, T. M.: Serial extraction: A continuous diagnostic and decisional process. Am. J. Orthod., *60*:541–575, 1971.
42. Graber, T. M., and Swain, B. F. (Eds): Current Orthodontic Concepts and Techniques, 2nd ed. Philadelphia, W. B Saunders Company, 1975.
43. Herren, P.: Indikationen und Kontraindikationen für abnehmbare und festsitzende kiefer orthopädische Apparate. Schweiz. Monatsschr. Zahnheilkd., *85*:291–308, 1975.

CHAPTER 3

Schwarz Double Plate

The so-called double plate of Martin Schwarz attempted to combine the advantages of the activator and the active plate.[1] For the treatment of Class II, Division 1 malocclusion, the maxillary appliance was modified by extending flanges into the lower dental arch, usually in the anterior region (Fig. 3–1*A* to *C*). The extensions were originally made of acrylic (Fig. 3–1*D* to *F*), but wire elements were added and incorporated later (Fig. 3–1*H* and *I*). At present, instead of the design shown in Figure 3–1*H*, two independent loops are generally made.[2] The relation of the lower part of the appliance to the upper is determined by the construction bite, as it is described in the chapter dealing with the activator. The forward positioning of the mandible should be limited routinely to 5 mm., or at the most 7 mm. This limit should not be exceeded, even in patients with a larger overjet. Disregarding this rule may create difficulties in the closing movement of the mandible, bringing the two parts of the appliance together. The closing maneuver also must not be impeded by an improper inclination of the extended flanges.

A gradual increase of the forward positioning of the mandible may be achieved by bending the metallic guiding elements (Fig. 3–1*I*). If there is improvement in the distoclusion, however, which makes it desirable, the same effect can be achieved by first coating the lower plate with petroleum jelly and then adding endothermic acrylic to the anterior surface of the upper extension. The mandible is then guided into a more anterior position during the closing maneuver. If it is not possible to adapt the wire elements to a more advanced anterior positioning, the available space should make it possible to add acrylic onto the wires to achieve the guiding effect.

One advantage of the double plate is the possibility of independently expanding either the upper or the lower dentition, or both at the same time. With a Class II, Division 1 malocclusion, maxillary expansion usually is necessary. As a consequence, the upper extension will become wider also. In the case of a routine forward positioning, the necessary space for the lower plate can be provided when the appliance is fabricated. With the double plate, the possibility of lateral mandibular movements also makes the wearing of the appliance more comfortable, and may even provide some functional stimuli. If, however, the appliance is meant to correct a lateral mandibular deviation, such shifting is not permissible and an angular shape of the extension should be chosen (Fig. 3–1*F*).

An alternate construction of the double plate employs lateral flanges (Fig. 3–2). It is based on similar designs introduced by Pedro Planas (Madrid) and Charles Nord (Amsterdam).[2] As developed originally by Schwarz, only the an-

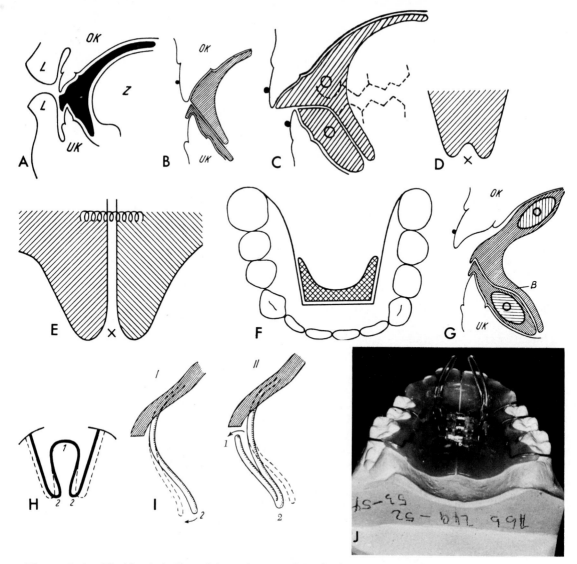

Figure 3–1. The identical effect of the activator and the double plate in jumping the bite. *A*, Cross section through the anterior part of the jaws with an activator (black) in place (*L*, lips; *OK*, upper jaw; *UK*, lower jaw; *Z*, tongue) *B*, The principle of the double plate: the activator (shown in *A*) is divided obliquely and, with clasps, the two separated parts are attached as plates to the teeth. *C*, The usual construction of the double plate with anterior guiding flange made of plastic. The anterior parts of the plates touch each other; the lower incisors are kept in place (no intrusion occurs); the lateral teeth are apart, but the margins of the plates are designed to prevent the growth of the teeth in height, and in addition the tongue is interposed. *D* and *E*, The lower end of the guiding flange (view from behind) (*E*, if an expansion screw is used; *x*, free space for the lingual frenum). *F*, Angular-shaped upper anterior guiding flange, fitting into the angular-shaped lingual surface of the lower plate, for exact positioning of the lower jaw. *G*, The double plates with expansion screws and the anterior guiding element, *B*, made of 1.5 mm. wire. *H*, The shape of the metallic guiding element. Note how it can be adapted for the expansion by flattening loops 1 and 2. *I*, Activation of the plate to move the lower jaw successively forward: *I*, bending the end (arrow 2); *II*, bending the loop (arrow 1). The guiding element made of wire is indicated if the dentist prefers to move the lower jaw forward step by step. *J*, The now preferred design with two independent loops. Courtesy of Professor H. Taatz, Halle, GDR. (From Schwarz, A. M., and Gratzinger, M.: Removable Orthodontic Appliances. Philadelphia, W. B. Saunders Company, 1966.)

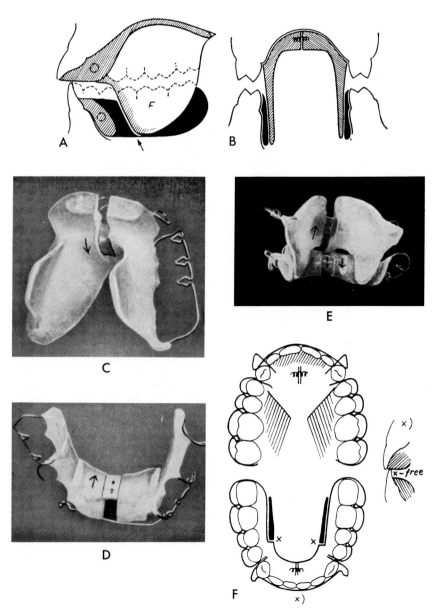

Figure 3-2. The double plate with lateral guiding wings. *A,* Sagittal cross section to show the double plates in the mouth; the black area represents the lingual surface of the lower plate with the inclined guiding groove (arrow), the lateral wing of the upper plate, F, sliding along the groove; the inclination of the guiding groove and the corresponding anterior guiding surface of the wing is 60 to 70 degrees in relation to the occlusal plane. Note that the lower plate, being low, leaves a free space with the anterior bite plate of the upper plate. Thus the lower incisors bite against the bite plate, which tends to intrude them. Between the buccal teeth (dotted line) there is also open space to permit their eruption. *B,* Diagram of a transverse cross section; the lateral wings of the upper plate touch the lingual surface of the lower (black). Note the free space between the posterior teeth so that they can erupt. *C to E,* Used double plates. Expansion (open screws) and forward positioning of the mandible were achieved. *E,* The plates assembled, view from the lingual aspect. *F,* Sketch of a pair of double plates with screws for simultaneous expansion. Note the supplementary sketch (right), which is the instruction for the technician to keep the lower plate low. In this manner (by intruding the lower incisors), the deep bite will be partly corrected. (From Schwarz, A. M., and Gratzinger, M.: Removable Orthodontic Appliances. Philadelphia, W. B. Saunders Company, 1966.)

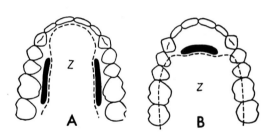

Figure 3-3. The relation of the double plates to the tongue and their effect on the tongue. *A,* The upper plate with lateral guiding wings (black). The tongue, *Z,* prevented by the wings from lying between the posterior teeth, is laterally compressed; its tip is free. Speech is not impaired. *B,* The upper plate with the anterior guiding flange (black). *Z* (dotted line), the tongue, which spreads laterally because its tip is pushed back by the plate. Its lateral margins rest between the posterior teeth, thus preventing their eruption. Speech is impaired, but tongue thrust is prevented. (From Schwarz, A. M., and Gratzinger, M.: Removable Orthodontic Appliances. Philadelphia, W. B. Saunders Company, 1966.)

terior margin of the wings is used as an exact guide. The mandibular plate is kept low in its anterior portion (Fig. 3–2*A*). The mandibular incisors contact the maxillary bite plane and thus receive an intrusive force. The teeth in the upper and lower buccal segments are kept apart. The wings also serve to keep the tongue out of the interocclusal space. Thus, the posterior teeth are free to erupt (Figs. 3–2*B* and 3–3*A*). Eruption is facilitated by the lateral bite opening, because of the forward positioning of the mandible in the established construction bite, as well as the contact of the lower incisors with the bite plate, immediately behind the maxillary incisors. The precise guidance of the inferiorly extending flanges prevents the lower jaw from moving laterally into an occluding position. The inferior margin of the wings must be rounded and smoothed to prevent irritation. The inclination of the guiding surfaces and the length of the wings must be shaped in such a manner that the mandibular arch is automatically guided into the intended protrusive relationship with each closing movement. The rounded ends of the wings are important in helping to establish this guidance. If the angulation is improper, too short or too steep, the mandible is

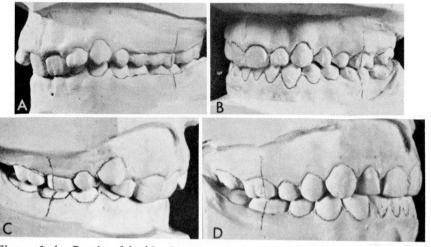

Figure 3-4. Results of double plates (see Fig. 3–2). *A* and *B,* Result of one pair of double plates. *A,* Class II, Division 2 malocclusion in a 14-year-old girl. *B,* The effect of the plates, worn during the night only, after 14 months. The lingual retrusion of the central incisors is not yet completely corrected (spaces appear between the upper and lower incisors) because the large apical base of this typical "Class II, Division 2 jaw" would need larger teeth. *C* and *D,* Result of two pairs of double plates. *C,* Class II, Division 2 malocclusion in an 11-year-old boy; *D,* after two years. (From Schwarz, A. M., and Gratzinger, M.: Removable Orthodontic Appliances. Philadelphia, W. B. Saunders Company, 1966.)

prevented from assuming the desired position, because the wings strike against the lower plate and block the bite. In addition, if the mouth is kept open during sleep, because the lower plate hits against the wings of the upper plate, the initial retruded position of the mandible is accentuated rather than reduced.

Clinical experience has shown that with a properly designed appliance, the patient usually requires only a few nights to learn to maintain the mandible in the moderate protrusion relationship that has been established. The process of accommodation is helped by wearing the appliance as much as possible during the day in the initial phase of adjustment. Then the plates can be worn mainly

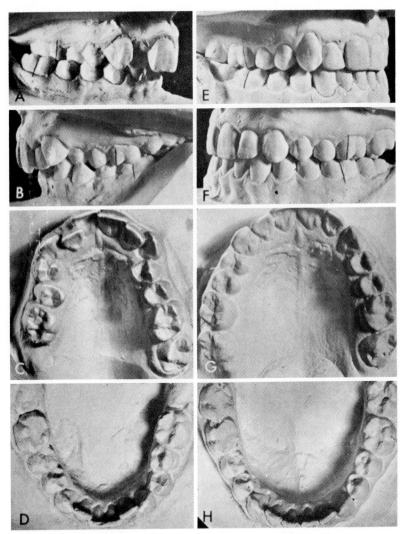

Figure 3–5. Result of treatment using two pairs of double plates. Cases best suited to treatment with double plates are cases in which, in addition to correction of the abnormal intermaxillary relationship, individual repositioning of some teeth and transformation of the arch form must be performed, and cases of Class II, Division 2 malocclusion. *A to D,* Class II, Division 2 malocclusion in a 12-year-old boy; note the anterior crowding, the cross-bite of the right p_1 and M_1 and the left p_1. *E to H,* Effect of two pairs of plates worn for two years, each pair used one year. (From Schwarz, A. M., and Gratzinger, M.: Removable Orthodontic Appliances. Philadelphia, W. B. Saunders Company, 1966.)

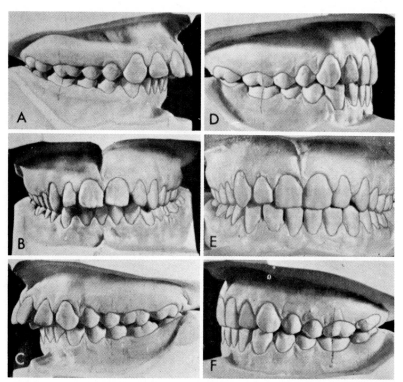

Figure 3-6. Result of treatment with one pair of double plates. Such cases of a typical Class II, Division 1 malocclusion are most suitable to be treated with the activator, because all that is necessary is expansion, retrusion of the upper incisors, raising the bite, and developing the lower jaw to obtain the normal occlusion. Movement of individual teeth is not necessary. In the case presented here, however, a 13-year-old girl lost the activator after several weeks and the parents, instead of cooperating with the doctor, refused the appliance "because it hindered sound sleep." Therefore double plates were made. *A* to *C,* Before treatment; *D* to *F,* effect of the plates after nine months. (From Schwarz, A. M., and Gratzinger, M.: Removable Orthodontic Appliances. Philadelphia, W. B. Saunders Company, 1966.)

at night. Inserting them for two to three hours during the day, however, is essential for rapid progress. Sometimes even the success or failure of treatment depends on this added time. If the patient tends to hold his mouth open, or breathe through the mouth, the effectiveness of the double plate is greatly reduced. The same, of course, holds true for the activator under similar conditions. The widening of the maxillary arch without appreciable similar modification in the mandibular arch should be planned for in the initial stages of therapy. Thicker wings can then be made and their accommodation by grinding the lateral surfaces is possible. Thin wings may be reinforced by the addition of cold-curing acrylic on the lingual aspect.

The two types of double plates described differ not only in their construction, but particularly in their relation to the tongue and their effect on the tongue. The upper plate with lateral guiding wings will prevent the tongue from lying between the posterior teeth (Fig. 3–3*A*). The tip of the tongue is free. Speech is not impaired and wearing during the day is facilitated. The deep overbite that is generally associated with Class II, Division 1 malocclusion will be corrected by the stimulated eruption of the posterior teeth. The leveling of the bite should be further helped by the intrusion of the mandibular incisors which contact the maxillary bite plate, as mentioned previously. The upper plate with the anterior guiding flange (Fig. 3–3*B*) tends to force the tongue back. The lateral margins of the tongue will then tend to insert between the upper and lower posterior teeth, preventing their eruption. Consequently, this type of double plate is indicated in cases of slight overbite or open bite, where interocclusal space is minimal or inadequate. The interposition of the tongue thus re-establishes a normal "freeway space," which is lacking in most open-bite malocclusions. As mentioned later, the double plate may also serve to advantage in the final phase of orthodontic therapy, and as a retention device which can restore overbite that has been overcorrected during prior mechanotherapy.

Impressive results have been achieved with the use of the double plate (Figs. 3–4 to 3–7). It is apparent that the appliance construction tends to combine the advantages of the active plate with those of the activator. Thus, there is simultaneous correction of different malocclusion characteristics. The construction enhances the seating of the appliance, by virtue of mutual contact; this assists in retention and provides additional anchorage. The effective use of such possibilities is again shown in the treatment of the case presented in Figures 3–8 to 3–10. The plates with the design shown in Figure 3–9 could not have been inserted singly. The retention provided by the clasps would have been insufficient. The arrow clasp on the right upper posterior teeth is activated to provide a slight distal movement of these teeth, assisted by small

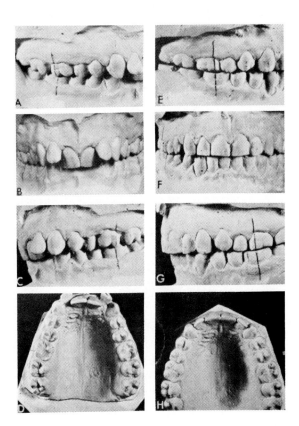

Figure 3–7. Class II, Division 2 malocclusion in a 24-year-old woman with "rest position anterior to occluding position." *A* to *D*, Before treatment. Note in *B* the visualized side tangents converging downward. *E* to *H*, After treatment (three years later). Double plates were used, worn during the night only. (From Schwarz, A. M., and Gratzinger, M.: Removable Orthodontic Appliances. Philadelphia, W. B. Saunders Company, 1966.)

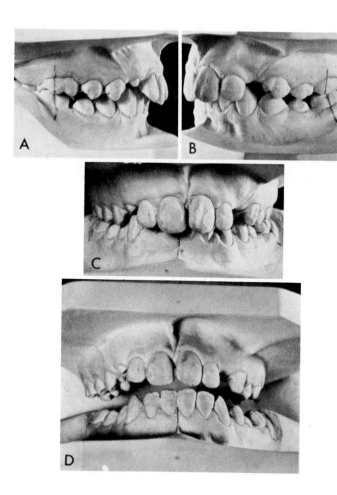

Figure 3–8. How to use the construction bite in a case of unilateral retro-occlusion. *A* to *C,* Right side Class II malocclusion in an 11-year-old child. Examination of the model reveals that the upper and lower incisor midline coincides with the true midline of the jaws. Therefore the deviation of the lower incisor midline to the right *(C)* indicates the displacement of the lower jaw as a whole to the right. The upper arch is sagittally symmetrical; gnathic Class II malocclusion. The purpose of the construction bite is to correct or even to overcompensate for this unilateral malocclusion, moving the lower midline to coincide with the upper, or even a little to the left. The upper and lower incisors do not occlude in edge-to-edge bite, 1.5 to 2 mm. apart, as shown in *D. D,* A wax bite is taken and the models are mounted in a fixator (see Fig. 3–11), showing clearly which secondary malpositions of the arches (alveolar symptoms) are present. The lower right lateral teeth and the left upper lateral teeth must be moved buccally. These movements will be combined with the intermaxillary correction by using double plates; an additional distal movement of the upper right lateral teeth to an extent of 1 to 2 mm. will facilitate the treatment. (From Schwarz, A. M., and Gratzinger, M.: Removable Orthodontic Appliances. Philadelphia, W. B. Saunders Company, 1966.)

springs on the lingual. Such springs tend to lessen the retention of the clasp, however, and have been made obsolete by the use of extraoral traction. However, the reciprocal pressures keep the plates in place, and this enhances the different simultaneous spring actions. Concurrently, the distocclusion and any midline deviation are corrected. This type of combined action is especially favorable in the treatment of Class II, Division 2 malocclusions.

In spite of the advantageous features of the double plates and excellent results shown in the literature, the appliances have met with rather limited acceptance. One of the reasons may be that the appliances are more complicated to fabricate and adjust. Also, the claim is made that they are less comfortable to wear than other competing appliances. The double plate appliance is meant to expand the dental arches and to correct the distal relationship at the same time. Yet expansion has often been only partially successful at best, and the creation of a Class I jaw relationship may be done more effectively by the newer functional appliances. Schwarz contended that the patient will swallow twelve to eighteen hundred times a day and each time will move the mandible forward to make the plates efficient. However, recent research on deglutition indicates that

Figure 3-9. Sketch of the appliances used to treat the malocclusion shown in Figure 3-8. Since the lower jaw must be moved to the left, with the lower midline 1 mm. to the left in relation to the upper for overcompensation of the present position, the right lateral wing is used for guidance. The left upper lateral teeth must be moved buccally (springs); to keep the plate in place the right canine is used (Adams clasp). The bite must be blocked and the deep bite removed by the upper anterior bite plane, and by the lower plate (additional front sketch), permitting the growth in height of the posterior teeth. In addition, the growth in height of the upper right posterior teeth is also guided distally 1 to 2 mm. to advance the normal occlusion. In similar cases, other necessary individual corrections, such as alignment of the anterior teeth or expansion, may be provided. (From Schwarz, A. M., and Gratzinger, M.: Removable Orthodontic Appliances. Philadelphia, W. B. Saunders Company, 1966.)

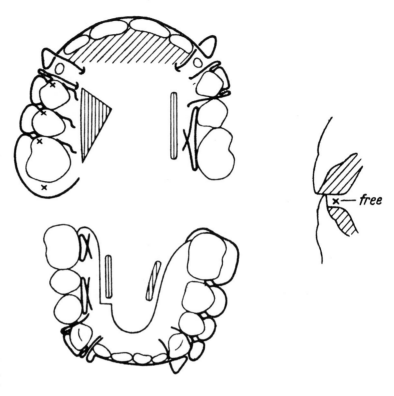

Figure 3-10. The case shown in Figure 3-8, three years after beginning of treatment. The plate shown in Figure 3-9 was used for two years, after which an activator was worn for retention. The patient uses this appliance from time to time for retention. (From Schwarz, A. M., and Gratzinger, M.: Removable Orthodontic Appliances. Philadelphia, W. B. Saunders Company, 1966.)

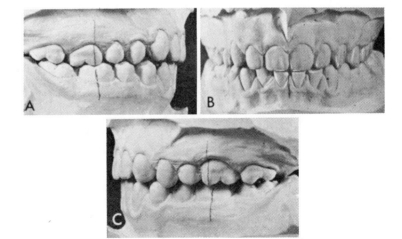

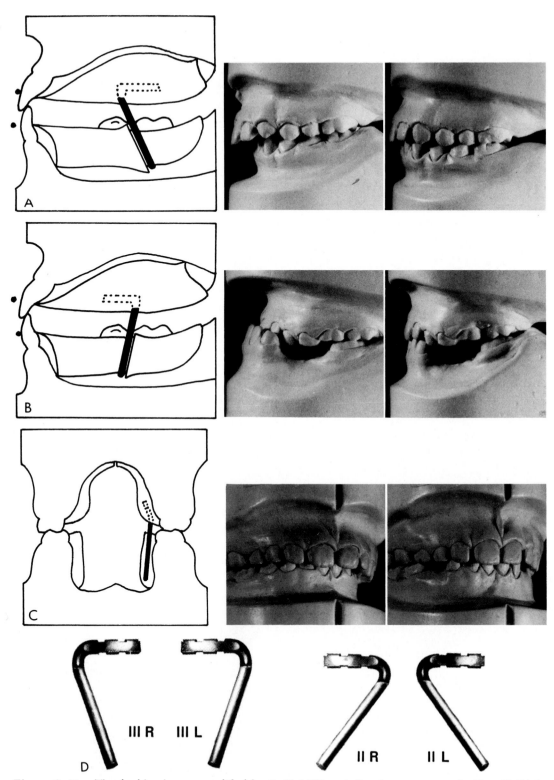

Figure 3-11. The double plates as modified by G. H. Müller. *A,* For the treatment of a Class II, Division 1 malocclusion, corrected by the appliance in one and a half years. *B,* For the treatment of Class III malocclusion; case shown was corrected in three months. *C,* For treatment of lateral deviations of the mandible, wire placed unilaterally. Case shown was corrected in one year. *D,* The wires used for the plates. (Courtesy of Professor G. H. Müller, Göttingen, FRG.)

children from five to twelve years old have a lower frequency of swallowing—800 to 1200 times every 24 hours.[3] The range for adolescents and adults as indicated by Lear and co-workers[4] is 233 to 1008, with a mean of 585 swallows every 24 hours. During sleep, the frequency is reduced to an overall mean of 7.5 hourly swallows.[4] The importance of the reduced swallowing frequency at night and the effect on the appliance have not been determined.

Notwithstanding these reservations, the double plate may be helpful to attain limited objectives. Adolescents and young adults, unable or unwilling to wear fixed appliances, may be treated if the malocclusion is not too extensive. Schmuth often uses the double plate after accomplishing most of his objectives with other appliances.[5] The double plate is thus used for the final stage of active therapy and for retention. The appliance may help to improve the nearly normal intermaxillary relations and to correct minor residual deviations. A similar technique for the correction of Class III conditions by means of extension of the mandibular plate into the maxillary area was also devised by Schwarz. The appliance has not proved effective, however. A widely recommended modification of the double plate has been introduced by G. H. Müller.[6-8] The lateral wings are replaced by wires of 2.0 mm. diameter. These are incorporated into the maxillary plate, bilaterally for the treatment of Class II, Division 1 or Class III malocclusions (Fig. 3–11*A* and *B*). The unilateral construction for lateral deviations of the mandible is shown in Figure 3–11*C*. For Class II, Division 1 malocclusion, the wires form an angle of about 70 degrees opening posteriorly. For Class III malocclusions, the angle opens about 85 degrees anteriorly. The wires must be placed parallel to each other in the anteroposterior as well as the vertical direction. A slight vertical convergence, however, is permitted. The upper and lower plates are fabricated in wax to allow for the placing of the wires. Inclined planes cut into the lower plate for guiding the wires. They cross the upper margin of these plates between the second premolar and first molar. The wires are fixed temporarily in position and the bent parts providing anchorage are inserted into the heated upper plate. The wires are placed as far laterally as possible, so as not to impede the tongue. If only maxillary expansion is planned, some excess space is left for the wires in the construction of the inclined planes of the mandibular plate. Further space is provided by grinding the lower plate and by bending the wires appropriately with strong plier beaks. Any necessary adaptations for an anteroposterior change are made by the removal or the addition of acrylic. The wires are available in the prefabricated state, or they may be fashioned from a 2.0 mm diameter wire. The heavy single wire has been found to be superior to the use of two smaller gauge wires.

The forces created by the mutual contact of the plates may press the clasps between the teeth. This should be prevented by the addition of occlusal rests, as is done for a prosthetic appliance. The treatment time of the cases shown in Figure 3–11 was one and a half years for case A, three months for case B, and one year for case C. In this case, an expansion screw was inserted into the mandibular plate. The laterally placed wires do not impede speech. The patient had little difficulty wearing the appliances day and night after a short adjustment period. Treatment of young adults is especially facilitated by this appliance.

While double plates are more complicated than some of the other appliances, it is felt that the skilled and experienced operator will find them most useful, sometimes extending the possibilities of the active plate in selected cases.

References

1. Schwarz, A. M.: Lehrgang der Gebissregelung, 2nd ed., Vol. 1. Vienna, Urban & Schwarzenberg, 1956.
2. Schwarz, A. M., and Gratzinger, M.: Removable Orthodontic Appliances. Philadelphia, W. B. Saunders Company, 1966.
3. Graber, T. M.: Orthodontics, Principles and Practice. Philadelphia, W. B. Saunders Company, 1972.
4. Lear, C. S. C., Flanagan, J. B., Jr., and Moorrees, C. F. A.: The frequency of deglutition in man. Arch. Oral Biol., *10*:83–99, 1965.
5. Schmuth, G. P. F.: Kieferorthopädie—Grundzüge und Probleme. Stuttgart, Georg Thieme Verlag, 1973.
6. Müller, G. H.: Die Doppelplatte mit Oberkiefer-Spornführung. Fortschr. Kieferorthop., *23*:243–50, 1962.
7. Müller, G. H.: Die Abkehr von der kieferorthopädischen Monotherapie. Studieweek, 1965.
8. Müller, G. H.: Personal communications, 1972, 1973.

CHAPTER 4

The Utilization of Muscle Forces by Simple Appliances

Conventional active plates as well as appliances using extraoral traction rely on the use of intrinsic force. This is because the source of the force exerted on the teeth and other structures is partly within the appliance itself. The bimaxillary active plates, working by moving the mandible either forward or backward from its centric occlusion, make additional use of muscle forces. The appliances described in the following pages are primarily effective because of the exclusive use of muscle forces. They have only an occasional minor treatment objective allocated to active intrinsic moving parts. It is with historical deference to the men who first devised this type of "muscle mechanics" treatment, using appliances that were to be effective in their own right and yet serve as forerunners for functional jaw orthopedic appliances, that we write this chapter.

Inclined planes, oral screens, and lip bumpers transmit force directly to the teeth. Certain other simple appliances that are closely related to this first group are the guide plane plate (Vorbissplatte) of Hotz and the propulsor of Mühlemann and Hotz. They are discussed in Chapter 5, since they represent a stage of development between the oral screens or inclined planes and the more sophisticated functional jaw orthopedic appliances.

The second group of appliances consists of the activator and the various modifications. The changing concepts of such functional appliances, the historical development, and the use and modifications of the classical activator are covered in Chapter 6 through 14. This group is distinguished primarily by the fact that the appliance moves the mandible downward and forward (except in Class III malocclusion), activating the muscles attached to it and to the surrounding structures. The resultant force that is created is transmitted not only to the teeth but to other structures as well. The third group is the Fränkel appliance, the function corrector or function regulator (FR), which owes its effect primarily to the bone and tooth position changes created by changing muscle balance and forces working on these tissues and on the periosteum. While there are mandibular positional changes produced by the FR appliance, similiar to those of the activator, the major thrust is to work through appliance effects in the oral vestibule, on the outside of the dental arches, by the use of oral screenlike shields. Hence, the third group could logically be considered a development of both the first and second groups and is discussed in Chapter 15.

INCLINED PLANE

The inclined plane was introduced by Catalan more than 150 years ago.[1] The plane was fashioned from various materials and placed on the mandibular incisors. Now, using endothermic acrylic, it may be formed directly on the mandibular incisors (Fig. 4–1). However, this is usually less desirable than the indirect technique of making the guide plane on a plaster model, saving chair time and insuring a better product. Various textbooks describe the details of fabrication and use; thus, the appliance will not be described here. It should be stressed, however, that a fixed inclined plane should be limited to the simplest cases. In crossbite cases where patient cooperation is in question for removable appliances, the cemented guide plane is particularly effective.

A modification of the simple inclined plane is the Oppenheim splint.[10] When it was first indroduced, it was made from vulcanite, with a little gold

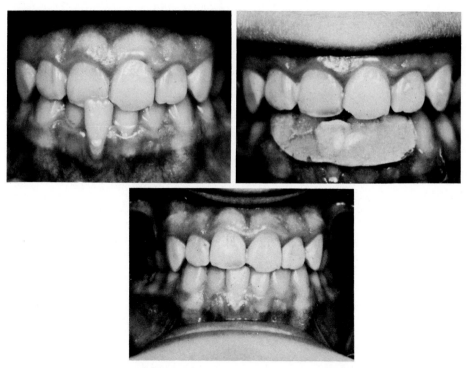

Figure 4–1. Correction of lingual crossbite of maxillary central incisor by endothermic inclined plane formed directly on lower incisors. Oblong mass of setting acrylic was forced over lower incisors, adapted with fingers to approximate contour desired, and removed when it started getting hard and warm. After setting completely and cooling off, it was trimmed to proper size, polished, checked in the mouth for correct inclination and coverage, and cemented. The plane was worn for only six days and removed. The remaining adjustment was due to the forces of occlusion after the incisor had been brought across labially. This type of fabrication is less desirable than the indirect technique of making the inclined plane on a plaster model, however. (From Graber, T. M.: Orthodontics: Principles and Practice, 3rd ed. Philadelphia, W. B. Saunders Company, 1972.)

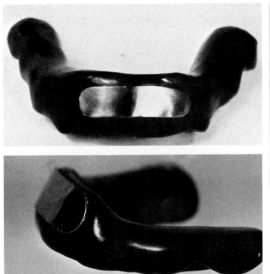

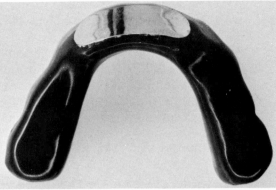

Figure 4-2. The original Oppenheim splint. Polished metal incline is imbedded in vulcanite, which covers mandibular teeth. It is now made of acrylic without the metal incline. Acrylic covering posterior teeth is ground away 1 mm. at a time, so only maxillary incisors in lingual crossbite engage metal incline. This is done periodically, so that force is minimal and yet prevents unwanted eruption of mandibular buccal segments. Appliance must be worn at all times, including meals.

inclined plane incorporated to engage the displaced incisors (Fig. 4–2). The splint is fashioned with the premolars and molars occluding on the splint also. The appliance is activated by grinding the occlusal surfaces approximately 1 mm. so that the only teeth that touch are the displaced incisors engaging the inclined plane. The rest of the splint is out of occlusion. With the incisor movement, the posterior teeth occlude again and acrylic must be ground off to restore inclined plane force for the teeth in crossbite. In this instance, the force is minimal and desirable particularly for teeth with the roots not fully developed (Fig. 4–3).

A frequently used inclined plane adjunct is made merely by adding an inclined plane to a mandibular Hawley type retaining appliance. Occlusal rests are used on the molars for stabilization. A variety of clasps, described in various texts, may be used. Clasps are not so important, however, since the labial arch

Figure 4-3. Drawing of splint action shown in Figure 4-2. Hatch-marked area is ground away on superior surface, out of contact with maxillary buccal teeth by about 1 mm. each time. (From Graber, T. M., and Swain, B. F. (Eds.): Current Orthodontic Concepts and Techniques, 2nd ed. Philadelphia, W. B. Saunders Company, 1975.)

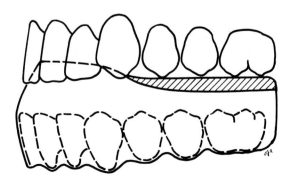

and the acrylic offer quite adequate retention (Fig. 4–4). This appliance has the advantage that the labial bow can be used to retract labially malposed incisors back into alignment (Fig. 4–5). It is also possible to add acrylic to the occlusal surfaces of the posterior teeth to make lateral bite blocks and then use the appliance in the same manner as the Oppenheim splint.

It should be emphasized that in the construction of the inclined plane, great care must be taken to insure that only the tooth or teeth in crossbite are in contact with the acrylic. The resultant force is the by-product of a combined depressing and anterior vector (Fig. 4–6). The steeper the plane, the greater the anterior vector will be. But even with a steep plane, there is a depressing force on the incisor. All inclined planes have the characteristic of opening the bite by allowing the posterior teeth to erupt. Thus, the inclined plane is contra-indicated unless there is an appreciable amount of overbite. Otherwise, even a slight opening of the bite will eliminate the stabilization of the orthodontic correction by the occlusion itself.

The cemented simple inclined plane is best suited in deep bite cases because it takes advantage of a larger than normal interocclusal clearance and helps to correct the deep bite while eliminating the crossbite. If the bite is not so deep, the Oppenheim splint is a safer appliance. Even if the appliance is checked infrequently, no harm can happen, because the bite blocks prevent further eruption of posterior teeth. If the overbite is shallow, and the use of an

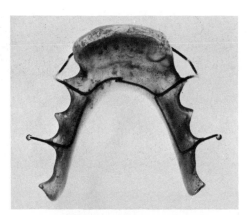

Figure 4-4. Inclined plane added to mandibular Hawley-type retainer, Labial bow can still retract lower incisors, while inclined plane stimulates forward movement of tooth in crossbite. Muscle forces provide sufficient force for maxillary incisor movement, but intrinsic appliance force is used in the lower arch.

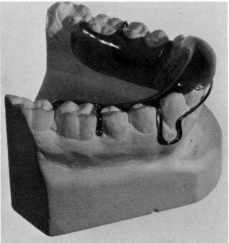
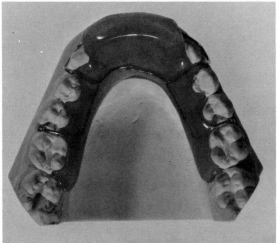

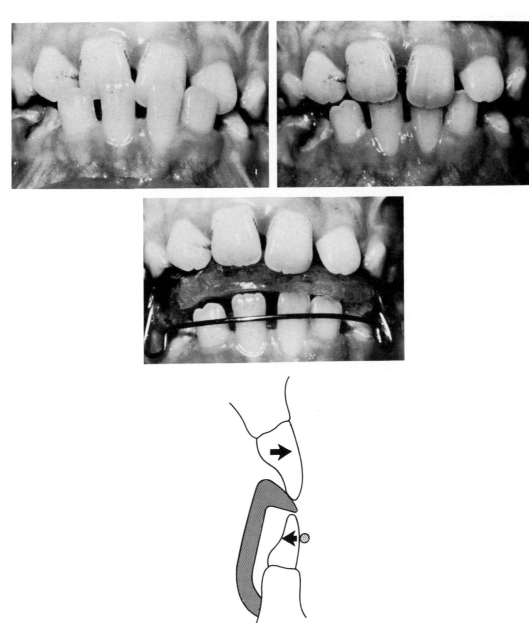

Figure 4–5. Pseudo Class III malocclusion, with mesial displacement of mandibular incisors. Mandibular removable appliance provides inclined plane to guide maxillary incisors labially. Acrylic is cut away on lingual of mandibular incisors and labial arch exerts a retrusive force to upright incisors, close spaces, and correct crossbite. Diagram shows force vectors. (From Hotz, R.: Orthodontics in Daily Practice. Baltimore, Williams and Wilkins, 1974.)

inclined plane is contraindicated, a maxillary plate with bite blocks on posterior teeth and springs behind the displaced maxillary incisors can be used to correct the anterior crossbite (see Chapter 2). It is not so important in the use of the upper plate that reciprocal forces are being exerted on the lower, labially

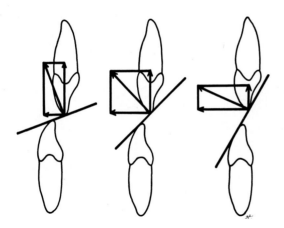

Figure 4–6. Force vectors of the inclined plane, with different angulations. The steeper the plane, the greater the forward pressure on the maxillary incisor. (After Lundström, A.: Introduction to Orthodontics. Stockholm, Ivar Haeggströms Boktryckeri AB, 1960.)

displaced incisors. Usually, as soon as the crossbite is eliminated, there is a speedy autonomous correction of the displaced mandibular incisors, under the combined forces of the occlusion and the lip. In deep bite cases, the use of the maxillary active plate is, however, not recommended, because buccal bite-opening blocks would have to be too high and thus would be uncomfortable for the patient. They would tend to perpetuate the abnormally deep bite.

Regardless of the construction, all inclined plane appliances or any removable appliances designed to correct a crossbite must be worn continuously. If the appliance is removed during eating, this will generally force the tooth back toward the original malposition. The repeated jiggling may damage the tooth and loosen it. Contact sports or even horseback riding and skiing, because they cause undue momentary pressures, may make the wearing of a splint undesirable. Actual fracture of an incisor might be possible by a sudden hard blow. Despite the apparently cumbersome construction, children seem to adapt well in two to three days. When used properly, the inclined plane, enlisting functional forces, can achieve the correction in a few days. Seldom does it take any longer than six weeks. Sometimes, after correction, it is advisable for the child to wear the removable inclined plane during sleeping hours as a guard against the tendency to move the mandible forward and to bring the corrected incisor lingually again . If the inclined plane fails to achieve more than an end-to-end incisal relationship, an active plate with lingual spring should be used, or possibly, an activator.

VESTIBULAR AND ORAL SCREENS

The vestibular screen was introduced by Newell in 1912 and it was used quite regularly in England before World War II.[1] The foremost German proponent was Körbitz (Fig. 4–7). Most recently, the vestibular oral screen has been widely advocated by Nord,[4,5] Hotz,[6] Kraus,[7,8] and Fingeroth and Fingeroth.[9]

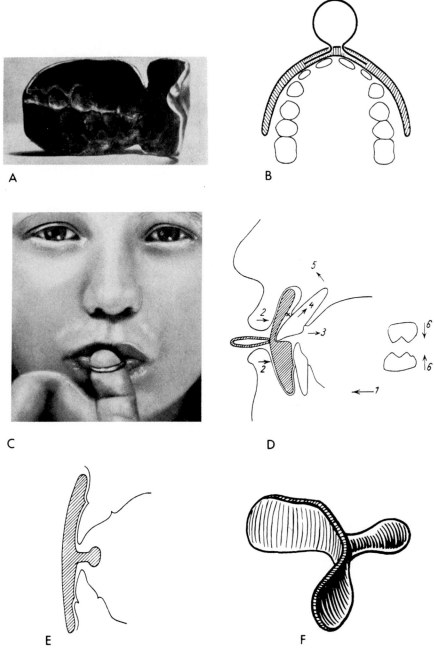

Figure 4–7. The vestibular screen or "lip molder" (Newell; A Korbitz). *A,* Original form, view from inside. *B,* Modification of Hotz. The plate, bucally broader than the arches, keeps off the pressure of the cheeks and directs the pressure of the lips to the labially inclined anterior teeth. *C,* The ring on the plastic is used for lip exercises (Hotz). *D,* Additional effects. Arrow 1: the lower jaw is moved forward; arrow 2: the hypotonic lips are induced to work; arrows 3, 4, and 5: if the incisal edges of the upper incisors are caught, they are retruded (arrow 3) and intruded (arrow 4) and since the apex is moved facially (arrow 5), growth in length of the maxillary apical base is stimulated. A free space *(x)* permits these changes: if the screen is constructed in rest position the posterior teeth grow occlusally, raising the bite (arrow 6). *E,* In cases of open bite the tongue is kept away by a projection made of acrylic or wire (Hotz). *F,* Modification of Rehak. The screen combined with a nipple, which protrudes but is retained by the lips. Thus the natural sucking movements are used to enhance the effect of the screen. Some children prefer this appliance to the Nuk exerciser. (From Schwarz, A. M., and Gratzinger, M.: Removable Orthodontic Appliances. Philadelphia, W. B. Saunders Company, 1966.)

69

The vestibular screen has turned out to be a versatile and certainly a most simple appliance in the early treatment of dental arch deformities when they are caused or aggravated by faulty muscle function.

The oral screen can be used for the correction of the following conditions: (1) thumb-sucking, lip biting and tongue thrust; (2) mouth breathing when airways are open; (3) mild distoclusions with premaxillary protrusion and open bites in deciduous and mixed dentition; and (4) flaccid orofacial musculature.

The simple form of vestibular screen or shield is a commercially manufactured polyamide or thermoplastic appliance (Fig. 4–8). It is particularly valuable in the early deciduous dentition. The appliance can be used to intercept mouth-breathing, thumb-sucking, or lip-sucking habits and to correct developing alveolar protrusions or open bites. The lips exert pressure through the plastic against the anterior part of the dentition and its alveolar support, while the buccal part of the screen is wide enough to keep the pressure of the cheeks off the posterior teeth (2 to 3 mm. clearance on each side in the first deciduous molar area), letting the tongue mold and expand the narrowed dental arches.

The deciduous dentition is a particularly valuable stage in which to use the vestibular screen. Treatment kits are available with six rubber molds to permit pouring of plaster models in different sizes and shapes to fit the particular patient. Plaster molds may be altered to better match the patient's arch form. A clear or opaque thermoplastic blank of the correct size is then chosen. It is heated gently over a Bunsen flame (Fig. 4–9), and then formed on the right size plaster model, using a moist towel. The notched border fits the maxillary cast. If there is a low frenum, an acrylic bur can be used to deepen the midline notch. Breathing holes may be enlarged if desired. The vestibular screen is then tried on the plaster study models of the patient and modified by adding on the margins or by cutting away and polishing. Minor shape changes may be made by reheating, to insure that the screen contacts the incisors, but stands 2 to 3 mm. away in the buccal segments. Figure 4–10 shows a transparent screen in place on the study models of a patient in the early mixed dentition stage. Note the plastic extension, particularly in the maxillary vestibular fornix.

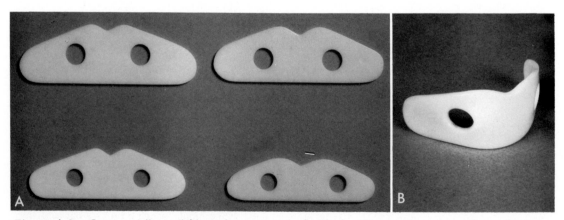

Figure 4–8. Commercially available oral screen or mask. Blanks *(A)* come in various sizes, and may be formed by heating gently with a Bunsen burner to the approximate shape of the dental arches *(B)*. (Courtesy of Rocky Mountain Orthodontics.)

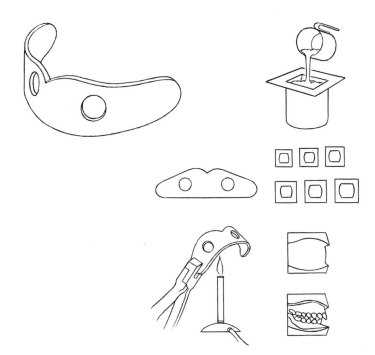

Figure 4-9. Steps in oral screen fabrication. Proper sized rubber mold is chosen, and poured up in plaster, allowed to set and separated. Six sizes of molds are available. The plaster model is modified by adding or subtracting plaster to conform more nearly to the shape of the arches of the particular patient. The correct size thermoplastic oral screen blank is chosen, heated gently over the Bunsen flame, and formed over the plaster model with a moist towel. It is then taken to the study models of the patient and modified further as needed, as to shape and peripheral extension. Care is taken to polish the margins, preventing irritation. (Courtesy of Rocky Mountain Orthodontics.)

For an older patient it is preferable to use a vestibular screen fabricated especially for the particular patient. The appliance may be made out of endothermic acrylic, although thermoplastic blanks are usually used, by applying heat and pressure and making the material conform to the area desired, directly on the articulated plaster casts.

The plaster casts for the appliance construction must include the complete vestibular fornix. In the case of a developing distoclusion, the appliance is made with the jaws in a nearly normal sagittal relationship. The working bite or construction bite is taken in the patient's mouth. The mandible is moved forward to Class I relationship and the bite is opened 2 to 3 mm. If the sagittal

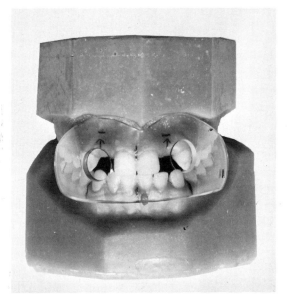

Figure 4-10. Transparent oral screen in place on study models. Plastic contacts protruding central incisors in maxillary arch but stands away from other areas, particularly in the buccal segments. (Courtesy of Rocky Mountain Orthodontics.)

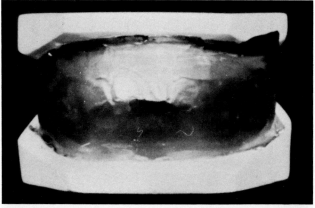

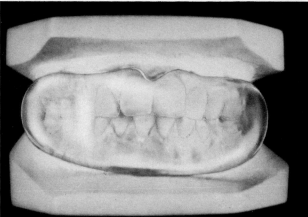

Figure 4–11. Vestibular screen construction by waxing up. (The screen may also be made with a construction bite.) Casts are waxed together with sticky wax, and labial and buccal surfaces are foiled after undercuts are filled with wax (top). Oral screen is then waxed up and constructed of acrylic (bottom). (From Graber, T. M., and Swain, B. F. (Eds.): Current Orthodontic Concepts and Techniques, 2nd ed. Philadelphia, W. B. Saunders Company, 1975.)

relationship is normal to start with, there is no need to change it for the construction bite. If the overbite is normal or if there is an open bite, the bite should not be opened for the appliance. The plaster casts with the correct construction bite are then fixed on a simple articulator.

Depending on the nature of the dental arch deformation and the effect desired, the vestibular screen is constructed so that the teeth and alveolar structures either receive or are relieved of muscular pressure. In the case of an open bite, there is often no need to expand the buccal segments and the appliance is allowed to rest on the tissues, whereas in the usual premaxillary protrusion, the dental arches are narrowed and the screen is constructed so that only the intraoral forces act on the canine premolar parts of the arches. The buccal aspects of the teeth and alveolar portions are therefore covered with a thin layer of wax where the appliance should stay away from the soft and hard tissues (Fig. 4–11). For instance, in a Class II, Division 1 malocclusion, with protruding upper incisors, the wax covers other parts except the lower half of the labial surfaces of the upper incisors. The buccal surfaces of the teeth and the alveolar processes are then covered with two layers of wax which extend to the mesial aspects of the first molars. This wax matrix is invested and processed in acrylic. When worn, the appliance contacts only the maxillary incisors, while holding the cheeks away from the buccal segments. This is the standard type of vestibular screen and the one used most frequently. The appliance can, however, be varied and several modifications can be made.

Finger Sucking

The sequelae of finger sucking are well known. Narrow maxillary arch, unilateral crossbite, anterior open bite, hyperactive mentalis and hypoactive upper lip muscles, together with the tendency for the lower lip to cushion to the lingual of the maxillary incisors, are self-perpetuating entities, when joined by compensatory and adaptive forward tongue posture and retained infantile deglutitional thrusting patterns. The early placement of a vestibular screen will not only intercept the worsening situation but actually correct an existing

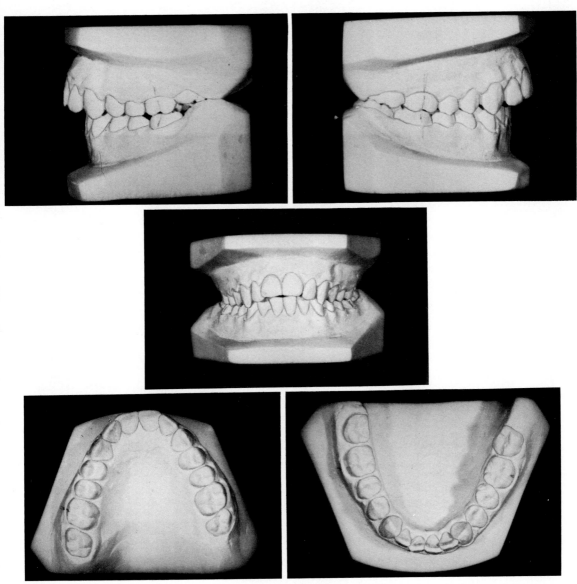

Figure 4–12. Class II, Division 1 malocclusion with history of fingersucking from birth. Oral screen (Fig. 4–11) was inserted and maxillary right and left premolars extracted. (From Graber, T. M., and Swain, B. F. (Eds.): Current Orthodontic Concepts and Techniques, 2nd ed. Philadelphia, W. B. Saunders Company, 1975.)

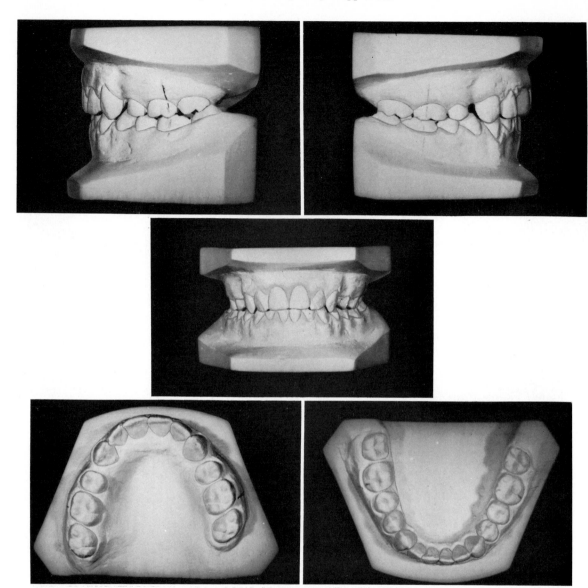

Figure 4-13. The same patient as in Figure 4-12, one year later. Habit has stopped, spaces have almost closed in extraction sites, and overjet and overbite are now normal. Oral screen was worn on a gradually reduced basis for 14 months longer. No change was made in the appliance at any time. Result was stable. Note autonomous improvement in mandibular incisor segment. (From Graber, T. M., and Swain, B. F. (Eds.): Current Orthodontic Concepts and Techniques, 2nd ed. Philadelphia, W. B. Saunders Company, 1975.)

malocclusion and Class II condition (Figs. 4-12 and 4-13).[5] The best time from a patient compliance standpoint is 3½ to 4 years of age, preferably in the spring or early summer. Three to six months of intensive use may be all that is necessary.

Mouth Breathing

To increase the usefulness of the appliance as a muscle training apparatus, Hotz recommends the addition of a wire loop to the front part of the screen.[6]

Figure 4-14. To prevent breathing difficulties, Kraus has recommended the use of breathing holes (top). Breathing difficulties are more psychological than real, however. When oral screen is used as an exerciser to develop tonicity of perioral musculature, Hotz recommends use of an embedded metal ring for insertion and withdrawal (bottom). Instead of a wire "pull ring," a small hole may be made in the center of the screen, through which a string with a button on the end is pulled flat against the lingual. Tension exerted is transmitted to the screen and requires increased lip tonicity to maintain the oral screen in place. (From Graber, T. M., and Swain, B. F. (Eds.): Current Orthodontic Concepts and Techniques, 2nd ed. Philadelphia, W. B. Saunders Company, 1975.)

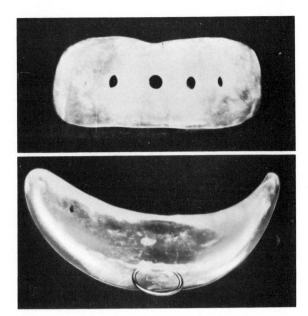

The patient pulls the appliance forward from the loop while at the same time trying to resist the force with the lip muscles (Fig. 4-14). Actual rubber exercisers may also be used (Fig. 4-15). These exercises have also proved useful in improving the mobility of scar tissue structures around the mouth, particularly in cleft lip patients. Fingeroth and Fingeroth place "breathing holes" in the labial aspect of the screen. They then use a button and string, inserting the button on the lingual and instructing the patient to perform exercises for at least half an hour a day, pulling on the string and resisting the forward pull on the screen with the lips.[9] Garliner has recommended similar exercises, using large convex plastic buttons on string.[10] Lip seal exercises also form an important part of the Fränkel appliance routine.[11]

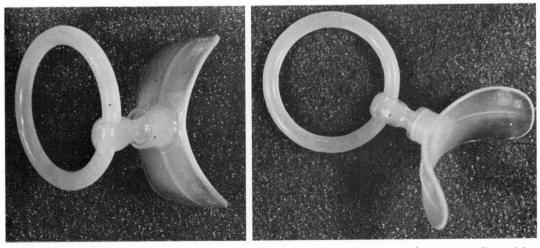

Figure 4-15. Rubber exerciser, simulating a small oral screen, which is also used to improve lip tonicity and oral seal through daily usage during such activities as watching television. An actual improvement in excessive overjet and spacing is possible.

Mixed dentition Class II, Division 1 type malocclusions with mouth breathing are often associated with excessive epipharyngeal lymphoid tissue. A vestibular screen may prove to be a psychological hazard in those cases. As nasal breathing seems difficult, small holes may be made in the screen, as recommended by Kraus. The upper half of Figure 4–14, shows how the holes may be placed.[4] These are cut in the appliance when it is first given to the patient, and then the holes may be gradually reduced in size with acrylic as the patient becomes accustomed to the wearing of the appliance. Kraus has claimed that the reduction of the mouth breathing actually helps eliminate some of the excessive adenoid tissue bulk. His clinical observations were confirmed in a study done at the Children's Nose and Throat Clinic in Prague.[12] When a tonsillectomy and adenoidectomy have been performed, the screen may also be used to reduce or eliminate postoperative mouth breathing and to enhance nasal breathing, since the passages are free postoperatively. Harvold and Linder-Aronson have shown the etiologic aspect of mouth breathing and the need to eliminate the habit.[13, 14] Figures 4–16 and 4–17 show an example of vestibular screen therapy during the mixed dentition.

As might be expected in the use of functional appliances, there has been

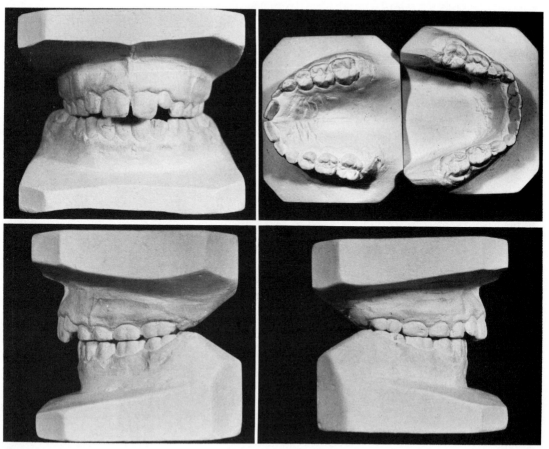

Figure 4–16.   Female patient, aged seven years, two months, with poor lip tonicity, unilateral Class II malocclusion, and excessive overjet. Vestibular screen was made with the construction bite restoring normal interdigitation.

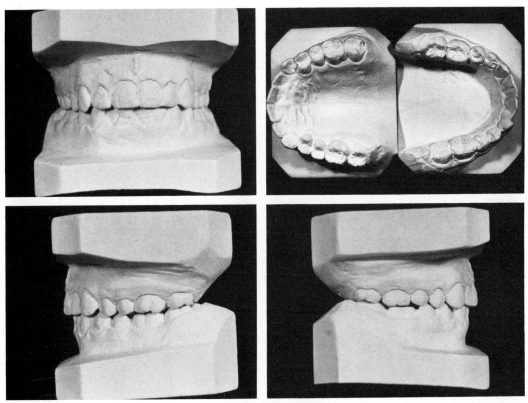

Figure 4–17. Same patient as Figure 4–16, at 12 years of age. Overjet was reduced in one year from 6.5 mm. to 3.6 mm. and the distance between maxillary first deciduous molars increased from 33.0 mm. to 35.7 mm. First molar increase was from 39.3 mm. to 42.9 mm. A new vestibular screen was placed and worn by the patient until eruption of premolars and canines. The first premolar dimension increased to 36.4 mm. and the first molar dimension increased to 44.7 mm., with the overjet staying at 3.0 mm.

some semantic confusion over the use of descriptive terms by different clinicians. While some have made no differentiation between the terms oral and vestibular screen, Kraus limited the term "oral screen" to those appliances with the primary objective of controlling tongue function (Fig. 4–18). Kraus developed the theoretical concept that by inhibiting faulty muscle function, normal development could be achieved and malocclusions could be intercepted without the appliance actually touching the teeth. In his version of the vestibular screen, the material extended into the vestibule in contact with the alveolar process but did not touch the teeth at all.

Other variations of Kraus combine oral and vestibular screens to make a "double oral screen" (Fig. 4–20).[5] A smaller lingual screen is attached to the vestibular screen with two 0.036 inch wires which run through the bite in the lateral incisor area. Such construction can be useful in tongue thrust–open bite cases. This appliance has the potential of simultaneously eliminating mouth breathing, tongue thrusting, and dental protrusion. Figure 4–21 illustrates other double screen variations of Kraus. Figure 4–22 shows models of a result that can be achieved with the double oral screen. Selmer-Olsen has recommended a similar construction for the "double screen" and writes in support of the theoretical basis of action.[15]

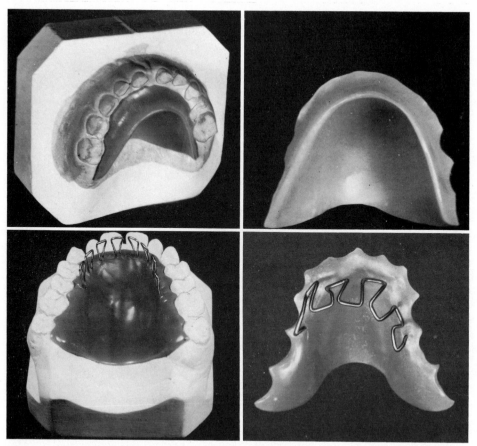

Figure 4-18. Oral screen appliances. These appliances may be made solely of acrylic (upper pictures) or of acrylic combined with wire loops (lower pictures). Their primary objective is to control tongue function. Ball clasps may be added in the molar area to increase the retention of the appliance and reduce the tendency for the posterior end to drop when the tongue thrusts forward. (From Graber, T. M.: Orthodontic Principles and Practice, 3rd ed. Philadelphia, W. B. Saunders Company, 1972.)

1. The appliance prevents mouth breathing, and the respiration is forced through the nose and past the swollen lymphatic tissues, reducing the "exudative diathesis" or nasal secretions which clog the nose. The column of air thus stimulates nasal breathing.

2. The increased nasal air activity stimulates nasal tissues, sinuses, and paranasal circulation and may have a favorable influence on growth of contiguous osseous structures.

3. Since nasal breathing is more difficult and requires more work than mouth breathing, the oral screen induces a more intensive exercise of muscles of respiration in general. (Small holes are made in the screen in the beginning for breathing, but are gradually closed as the patient adapts.)

4. The double screen automatically keeps off the deforming lip and tongue pressure from the upper and lower front teeth.

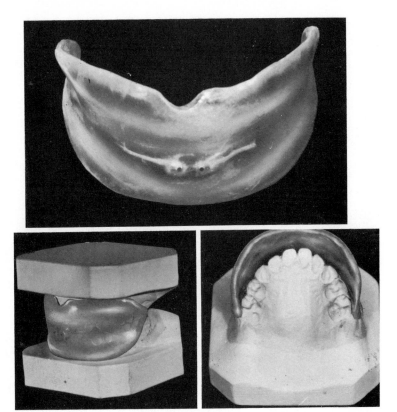

Figure 4–19. Vestibular screen of Kraus, carried well into the sulci, in contact with the basal alveolar process, but not touching the teeth at all. The primary effect would be expansion, but with little lingualizing potential on the maxillary incisors, if excessive overjet was present. (Courtesy of Frantisek Kraus. From Graber, T. M.: Orthodontics: Principles and Practice, 3rd ed. Philadelphia, W. B. Saunders Company, 1972.)

5. The appliance discourages both thumb-sucking and tongue thrusting, as well as abnormal postural position of tongue and lips.

6. The appliance stimulates muscle exercise, much like chewing gum, enhancing the tonicity and serving also as a tension release as the patient works against the appliance.

7. The lingual pressures of the oral screen portion can retrude maxillary incisors and upright them, closing spaces at the same time. Adding gutta percha to the lingual aspect, or additional acrylic or finger springs may enhance favorable incisor positioning.

The vestibular or oral screen should be worn by the patient every night and also during the day whenever possible. For instance, a good time is while doing school work or watching television. The patient is also instructed to perform lip exercises several times a day for a few minutes at a time, or at least 30 to 45 minutes in a 24-hour period. The lips should be kept in contact all the time to enhance the effect of the appliance and to improve the lip seal.

There is no need to check the patient in the office more often than every six to eight weeks, once the patient has adjusted to the appliance and there is an assurance that the appliance is being worn.

When some progress has been achieved with the use of the oral screen, it is advisable to reactivate it by adding acrylic on that portion of the appliance that is contiguous to the labial surface of the maxillary incisors. If this is not done, the screen may contact the border area of the mucosa and vestibule, reducing the effect on the teeth and the immediate supporting alveolar bone.

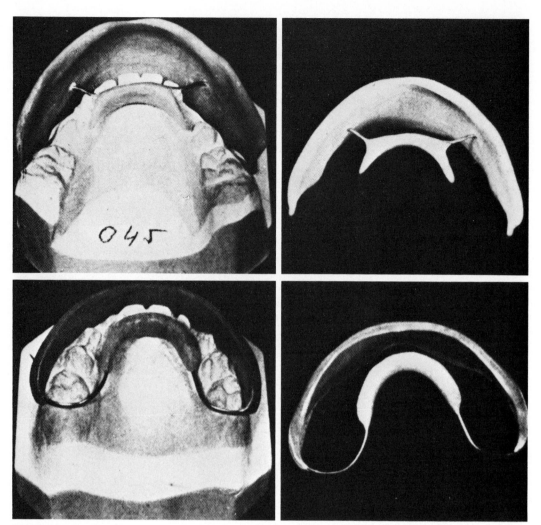

Figure 4–20. Double oral screen of Kraus. In top pictures, 0.036 inch wires run through to lingual side at distal of lateral incisors, to support an acrylic anti–tongue thrusting screen. Major control is for lips and tongue. In bottom pictures, double screen designs, lips, cheeks, and tongue are controlled. (Courtesy of Frantisek Kraus.)

As with all appliances, there are limitations. Seldom is the vestibular or oral screen the total mechanotherapy. Rather, it should be thought of in terms of an initial assault on the orthodontic problem. The screen is especially suitable in the treatment of developing malocclusions which are associated with an aberrant muscular pattern. The beneficial effect of the screen manifests itself in es-

Figure 4–22. Narrow maxillary arch and anterior open bite, corrected by double oral screen (buccal shields and lingual oral screen). The patient's own muscle forces have been channeled to correct the malocclusion. (Courtesy of Frantisek Kraus. From Graber, T. M.: Orthodontics: Principles and Practice, 3rd ed. Philadelphia, W. B. Saunders Company, 1972.)

Illustration on opposite page

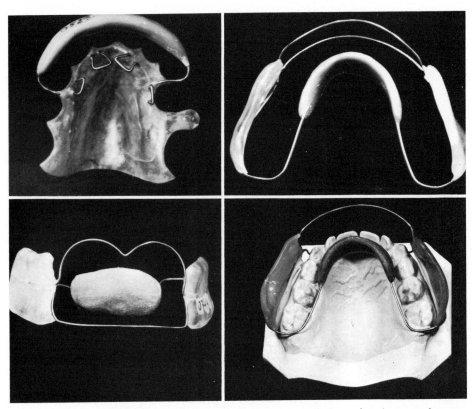

Figure 4-21. The Kraus "double screen," combining vestibular and oral screen elements for tongue, lip and cheek muscle control. Upper left appliance controls lip and tongue muscles, remaining views illustrate appliances designed to control excessive buccinator contraction and anterior tongue thrust. For a lateral tongue thrust, the oral screen portion would be modified and extended posteriorly. (Courtesy of Frantisek Kraus. From Graber, T. M.: Orthodontics: Principles and Practice, 3rd ed. Philadelphia, W. B. Saunders Company, 1972.)

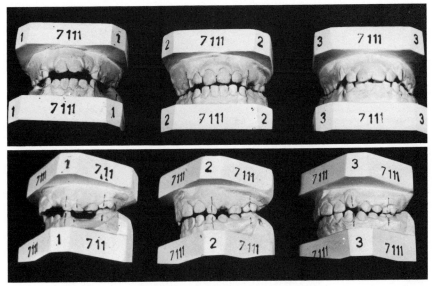

Figure 4-22. *See opposite page for legend.*

tablishing a better muscle balance between the tongue and the buccinator mechanism. As the mandible assumes a more mesial position with the guidance of the screen, the tongue follows it, filling up the oral cavity. At the same time, the vestibular screen helps correct the faulty relationship of the upper and lower lips to each other, and a normal lip seal becomes possible. In developing distoclusions, the constructed forward position of the mandible is also assumed to have an effect on the protractor and retractor muscles that are responsible for the mandibular position in the sagittal plane. In the new habitual position, the protractor muscles are shortened, while the retractor muscles are lengthened. This, together with the other favorable changes, e.g., widening of the maxillary arch, rounding off the protruding maxillary incisors, and strengthening of the perioral muscles, contributes to the development of a proper functioning occlusion.

Where there is a buccal crossbite condition already present, the vestibular screen usually improves the maxillary intercanine width, but it may not correct the buccolingual relationship completely. In such instances, other types of re-

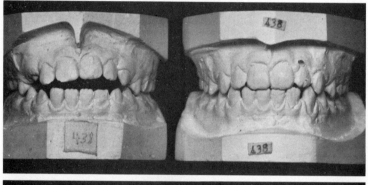

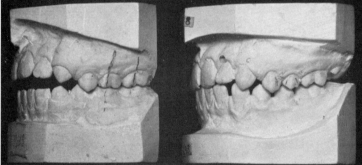

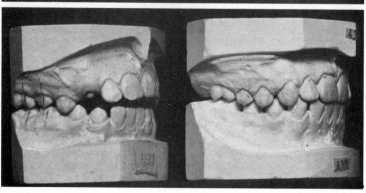

Figure 4–23. Open bite malocclusion and bimaxillary protrusion, corrected with four months' wearing of vestibular screen (mask). (Courtesy of A. I. Fingeroth.)

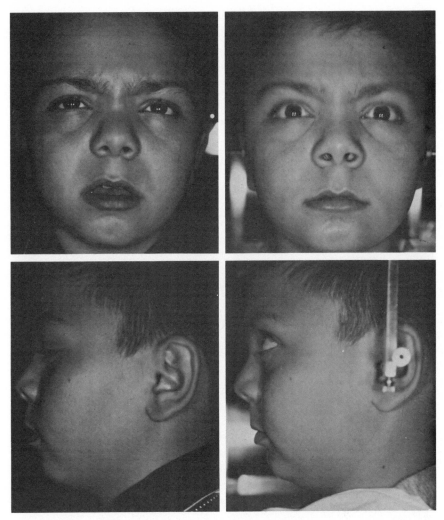

Figure 4-24. Before (left) and after (right) facial views of patient in Figure 4-23. (Courtesy of A. I. Fingeroth.)

movable appliances may be required, such as a split-palate appliance with an expansion screw in the center and acrylic over the maxillary occlusal surfaces. The double screen prevents anterior tongue thrust and should eliminate the prolonged infantile deglutitional pattern so often seen in mouth-breathing, thumb-sucking children. The tongue drops back and moves superiorly in the oral cavity, widening the maxillary intercanine dimension. Many of the oral malformations are the result of combined tongue and lip activity, with the lip, particularly, exacerbating the overjet, proclining the maxillary incisors, and retroclining and crowding the mandibular incisors. The vestibular screen is an effective mechanism for reducing or eliminating hyperactive mentalis muscle activity by itself. But to improve upper lip hypotonicity, an exercise discipline must be established and maintained. Figures 4–23 to 4–27 illustrate the effectiveness of oral screens in reducing malocclusions.

It is estimated that about 50 per cent of developing dentitions demonstrate a flush terminal plane relationship, with the upper and lower buccal segments

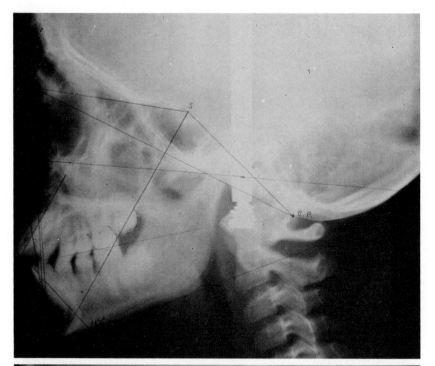

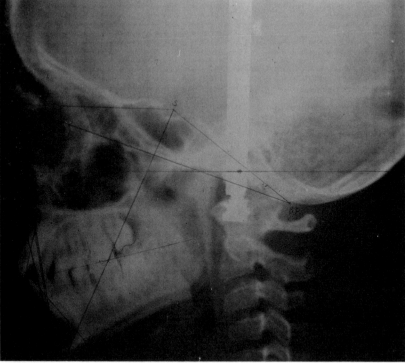

Figure 4-25. Before (above) and after (below) lateral cephalograms. The mandibular plane angle and facial angle remained the same at 25 and 82 degrees, respectively. Apical base difference remained the same, with a slight reduction in angle of facial convexity. The main changes are in the interincisal angle (107 to 125 degrees), the lower incisor to the occlusal plane angle (32 to 30 degrees), the lower incisor to mandibular plane angle (113 to 107 degrees), and the upper incisor to the NP plane (10.5 mm. to 8.5 mm.).

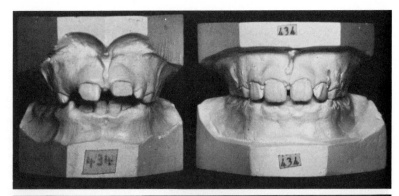

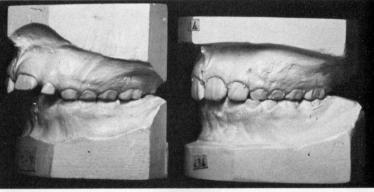

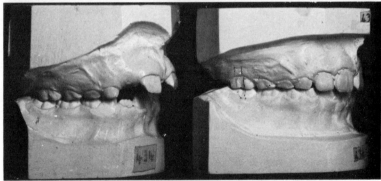

Figure 4–26. Class II, Division 1 malocclusion, with confirmed lower lip habit. Vestibular screen wear for one year. Overbite is still excessive, but interdigitation and overjet have been improved. Hyperactive mentalis muscle activity was eliminated. (Courtesy of A. I. Fingeroth.)

in an end-to-end relationship in the mixed dentition (Fig. 4–28). With the loss of the deciduous molars, the differential mesial drift of the first permanent molars, using the larger leeway space in the lower arch and the greater second deciduous molar width, allows the establishment of proper interdigitation. Abnormal lip and tongue activity can convert a flush terminal plane relationship into a full-fledged Class II, Division 1 malocclusion. This is why it is so important to intercept such cases in the deciduous or early mixed dentition periods, using simple devices like the vestibular screen or oral mask, as it is called by Fingeroth and Fingeroth.[9] In the event that a full Class II malocclusion has already been established, the wearing of an oral screen, even though it has been made with a construction bite that has positioned the mandible forward, may not correct the anteroposterior malrelationship. In such cases, the orthodontist may turn to a functional appliance such as the propulsor (Chapter 5), activator (Chapter 8), or perhaps a Fränkel appliance (Chapter 15).[16] There should be

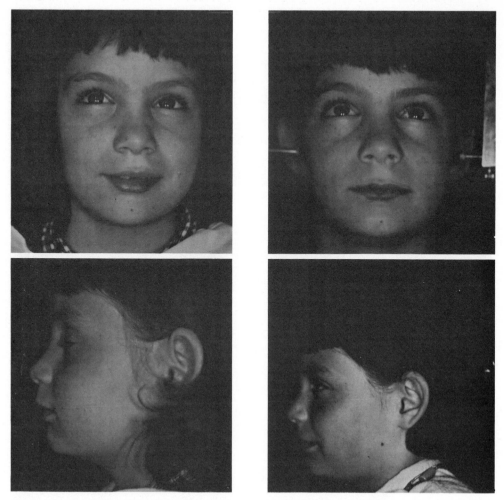

Figure 4–27. Before (left) and after (right) facial views of patient in Figure 4–26. (Courtesy of A. I. Fingeroth.)

no hesitancy to change appliances if the need is there. Vestibular and oral screens are best suited to work with abnormal lip and cheek activity. However, they may be used in conjunction with extraoral force appliances, which will reduce the basal discrepancy, allowing the oral screen to achieve its maximum potential of restoring lip tone and posture (Figs. 4–29 and 4–30). A fuller discussion of extraoral and removable appliances is presented in Chapter 16.

THE LIP BUMPER

Occasionally, when the problem is primarily a lower lip habit which flattens and crowds the lower anterior segment while leaving the maxillary arch relatively normal, a lower vestibular screen may be used, as the diagrams in Figure 4–31 show. Hyperactivity of the mentalis muscle can be eliminated, in a manner similar to that of the lip shields of the Fränkel appliance (see Chapter 15).

Another modification of the simple vestibular screen is the combined fixed and removable appliance called the lip bumper (or plumper, in some quarters).

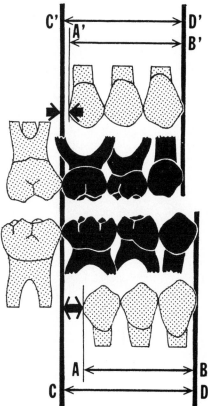

Figure 4–28. "Flush terminal plane" relationship of maxillary and mandibular buccal segments. The larger "leeway space" in the lower arch (averaging 2.7 mm.) permits greater anterior drift of the first permanent molars when the second deciduous molars are lost, eliminating the Class II molar relationship tendency. (From Graber, T. M.: Orthodontics: Principles and Practice, 3rd ed. Philadelphia, W. B. Saunders Company, 1972.)

Since it is the lower lip, by virtue of the hyperactive mentalis muscle, which does the most damage, the lip bumper is usually made for the mandibular arch. First permanent (or second deciduous) molar bands or crowns are made, with 0.040 inch horizontal buccal tubes soldered to receive the wire and acrylic

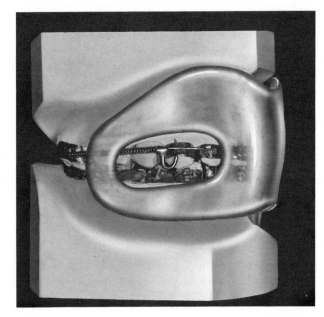

Figure 4–29. Vestibular screen, modified to fit over multibanded appliance, with opening to receive extraoral force "J" arms. (Courtesy of Rocky Mountain Orthodontics.)

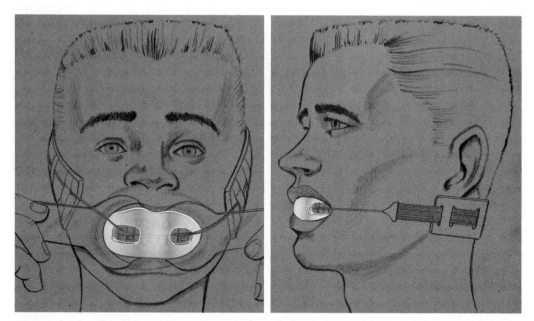

Figure 4-30.   Drawings to illustrate use of vestibular screens with extraoral force and fixed orthodontic appliances. (Courtesy of Rocky Mountain Orthodontics.)

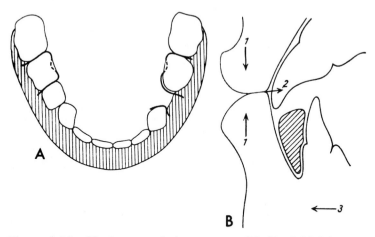

Figure 4-31.   The lower vestibular screen, modified by A. M. Schwarz. *A,* Modification to enhance stability, with clasps snapping into a little groove on the lingual of a deciduous molar, or by using lingual arrow clasps at strategic interproximal areas. *B,* The purpose is to prevent hyperactive mentalis and orbicularis oris muscle activity, and the tendency to cushion to the lingual of the maxillary incisors during deglutition. The result is normal lip closure and lingual pressure on the protruding maxillary incisors (see arrows). There is a tendency to posture the mandible forward in these problems (arrow 3), which is beneficial. (From Schwarz, A. M., and Gratzinger, M.: Removable Orthodontic Appliances. Philadelphia, W. B. Saunders Company, 1966.)

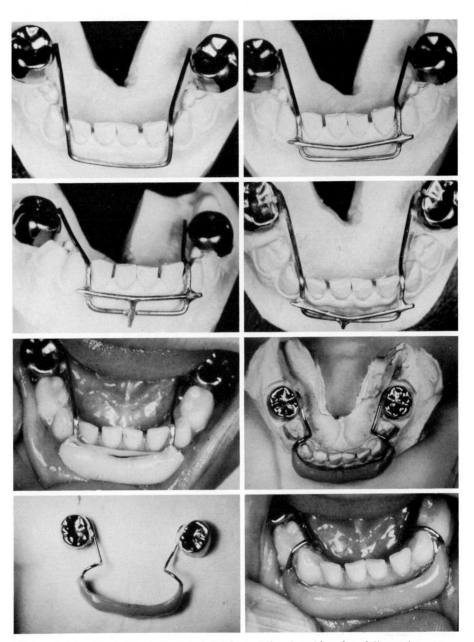

Figure 4-32. Lip habit appliance. A 0.040 inch bar is soldered to full metal crowns on second deciduous or first permanent molars. Bar may cross from lingual to labial either mesial or distal to canine, depending on occlusion and anterior spacing. The operator should be sure that labial assemblage is 2 to 3 mm. anterior to the labial aspect of lower incisors. Model is foiled first before endothermic acrylic is adapted to wire framework. Appliance is cemented in place for a period of three to six months, depending on severity of lip habit and amount of overjet. (From Graber, T. M.: The "three M's:" muscles, malformation, and malocclusion. Am. J. Orthod., 49:418–450, 1963.)

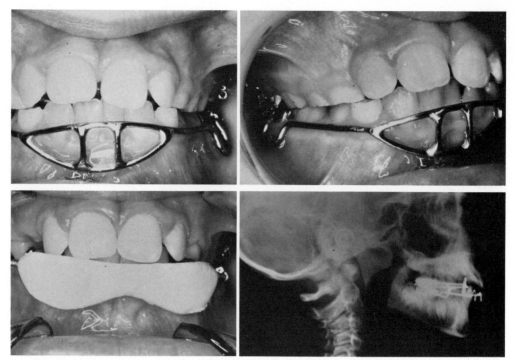

Figure 4–33. Metal lip shield (above) tied into 0.040 inch buccal tubes. Acrylic lip shield is also tied in, with open coil spring element mesial to tube to keep shield away from lower incisors and to transmit distalizing force to first permanent molars. Lateral cephalogram (lower right) shows same patient, but with the addition of a lingual tongue thrust crib attached to the maxillary molar bands. Both lip and tongue are then controlled to eliminate excessive overjet.

assembly or with wire and acrylic portion soldered to metal crowns (Fig. 4–32 and 4–33).[17] The wire may be tied into the tubes and worn continuously, or removed by the patient and worn as directed by the orthodontist. The anterior and removable portion can be a wire skeleton only or an acrylic shield (Fig. 4–33), both serving to keep the lip away from the lower incisors, preventing its cushioning to the lingual of the maxillary incisors during posture and function.

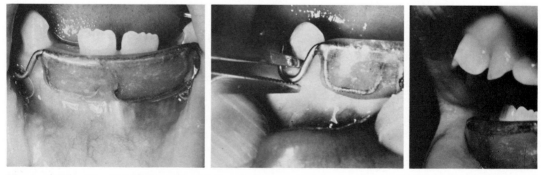

Figure 4–34. Lip shield being adjusted directly in the mouth by opening vertical loops in wire framework, to move the acrylic portion away from the teeth, as the tongue moves the lower incisors forward. Mentalis muscle activity is greatly reduced or eliminated during deglutition with the lip bumper in place.

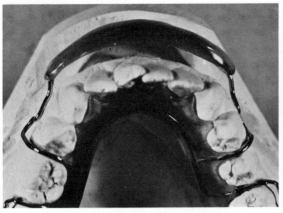
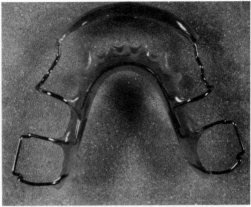
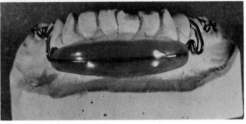

Figure 4-35. Modified lower Hawley-type removable appliance, with lip shield away from lower incisors. Mentalis muscle hyperactivity is discouraged, while lower incisors may move forward under tongue pressure.

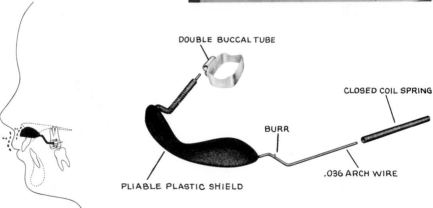

DOUBLE BUCCAL TUBE

CLOSED COIL SPRING

BURR

PLIABLE PLASTIC SHIELD

.036 ARCH WIRE

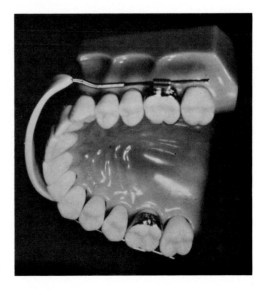

Figure 4-36. *Above* and *right,* Denholtz muscle anchorage appliance in use in maxillary arch. Coil spring exerts a distalizing effect on the banded first permanent molars with upper lip contraction and exercises. (Courtesy of Rocky Mountain Orthodontics.)

The tongue will then tip the lower incisors labially, increasing arch length and reducing crowding and excessive overjet. This type of muscle anchorage may actually be used to upright mandibular molars in conventional orthodontic therapy or to restore space that has been lost through premature loss and mesial drift of molar teeth. Coil spring elements may be used instead of loops or stops at the molar tubes, providing a gentle force against the lower first permanent molars and giving the lower lip a flexible appliance to work against. Or the wire framework may incorporate vertical loops, adjustable directly in the mouth (Fig. 4–34). Fränkel has emphasized the importance of breaking abnormal lip habits as early as possible.[11] The lip bumper, as well as the oral screen, is an excellent interceptive orthodontic appliance for this purpose. A removable appliance is shown in Figure 4–35. Muscle anchorage may also be used to exert a distalizing effect on the maxillary first molars, with and without fixed orthodontic appliances. The Denholtz appliance (Fig. 4–36) also uses a pliable plastic shield and coil spring elements to effect the maxillary molar retropositioning. Generally, however, the mandibular lip bumper is more effective, since the mentalis muscle is hyperactive, flowing into the excessive overjet, while the upper lip is hypotonic and likely to exert less force on the shield, without concerted muscle exercises.

References

1. Weinberger, B. W.: Orthodontics: An Historical Review of its Origin and Evolution. St. Louis, The C. V. Mosby Co., 1926.
2. Schwarz, A. M., and Gratzinger, M.: Removable Orthodontic Appliances. Philadelphia, W. B. Saunders Company, 1966.
3. Schwarz, A. M.: Gebissregelung mit Platten. Vienna, Verlag Urban und Schwarzenberg, 1938.
4. Nord, C. F. L.: Loose appliances in orthodontia. Trans. Europ. Orthod., Soc., 1929.
5. Taatz, H.: Kieferorthopädische Prophylaxe und Frühbehandlung. Leipzing, J. A. Barth, 1976.
6. Hotz, R.: Orthodontics in Daily Practice, Baltimore, Williams and Wilkins, 1974.
7. Kraus, F.: Prevence a naprava vyvojovych vad orofacialni soustavy. Prague, Statni Zdravotnicke nakladdatelstvi, 1956.
8. Kraus, F.: Vestibular and oral screen. Trans. Europ. Orthod. Soc., 1956, p. 217.
9. Fingeroth, A. L., and Fingeroth, M. M.: Early treatment: Theory and therapy. Orthod. Rec., *1*:87–99, 1958.
10. Garliner, D.: Some ancillary results of the correction of abnormal swallowing habits. N.Y. Dent., *39*:158–164, 1969.
11. Fränkel, R.: Funktionskieferorthopädie und der Mundvorhof als apparative Basis. Berlin. Veb Verlag Volk und Gesundheit, 1967.
12. Rokytova, K., and Trefna, B.: Use of a vestibular screen for rehabilitation of nasal breathing in children. Cesk. Otolaryngol., *9*:293, 1960.
13. Harvold, E. P.: The role of function in the etiology and treatment of malocclusion. Am. J. Orthod., *54*:883, 1968.
14. Linder-Aronson, S.: Adenoids: Their effect on mode of breathing and nasal airflow and their relationship to characteristics of the facial skeleton and the dentition. Acta Otolaryngol. (Suppl. 265), Uppsala, 1970.
15. Selmer-Olsen, R.: Personal communication, May 23, 1975.
16. Fränkel, R.: Technik und Handhabung der Funktionsregler. Berlin, Veb Verlag Volk und Gesundheit, 1973. 2nd ed., 1976.
17. Graber, T. M.: Orthodontics: Principles and Practice. Philadelphia, W. B. Saunders Company, 1972.

CHAPTER 5

The Guide Plane Plate and Propulsor in the Treatment of Class II, Division 1 Malocclusion*

This chapter is devoted to the discussion and illustration of the use of removable appliances as developed and modified by Professor Rudolph Hotz of Zurich, Switzerland, for the treatment of Class II, Division 1 malocclusion, primarily during the late transitional or early permanent dentition (late treatment, first phase, 10 to 14 years: Hotz).

THE GUIDE PLANE PLATE

This appliance has been referred to variously in the literature as the forward biting plate (Vorbissplatte) or the removable inclined plane plate. During the 10- to 14-year age range, Hotz often favors the guide plane plate over other appliances. Its mode of action is similar to that of the monobloc (activator) in that it allows for bite opening and forward mandibular displacement and development. It also utilizes an expansion screw and a labial bow. The chief difference between the guide plane plate and monobloc is that with the plate, the functional mandibular propulsion is not effective while the patient sleeps. But it is very effective for expansion of the upper arch, retraction of the maxillary incisors, and opening of the bite. In fact, bite opening may occur so quickly that it leaves the forward development of the mandible behind.

When this appliance is used correctly, with good growth timing, distoclusions can be corrected in a short time. Many Class II malocclusions with deep overbite, narrow maxillary arches, and protruding upper incisors respond well to the guide plane plate. It must accomplish the following four treatment objectives:
1. Opening of the bite
2. Mandibular propulsion

*Thanks is given to Professor Rudolph Hotz and Dr. Robert Shaye for their most generous and valuable advice and assistance in the preparation of this chapter, and to Verlag Hans Huber for permission to reprint text and illustrations.

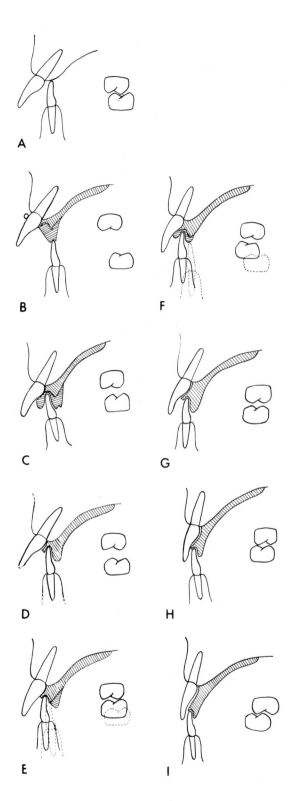

Figure 5–1. Construction and adjustment of the guide plane in the treatment of distoclusion with the guide plane plate. *A,* Distoclusion with deep bite and upper incisor protrusion. *B,* Plate with orientation ridge and self-curing acrylic. The edges of the lower incisors biting gently into the soft plastic indicate the crest of the plane. The mandible is in its maximum retrusive position. *C,* By biting forward slightly the bite groove is formed while the lingual surfaces of the incisors shape the forward slope of the plane. *D,* The guide plane after trimming excess acrylic. *E,* As the mandible becomes fixed in the forward position, the guide plane can be reduced from the palatal side. The posterior teeth erupt causing bite opening, and the incisors can be retruded by removing some plastic from their palatal surfaces. *F,* By applying fresh acrylic the bite groove can be moved forward and the plane itself reshaped. The former guide plane has been reduced to an orientation ridge *(B). G,* Form of the guide plane and amount of bite raising in the second and third steps of treatment. *H,* Guide plane and acrylic palatal to the upper incisors have been reduced according to the changes in occlusion and tooth position. *I,* Final form of the guide plane as a retention appliance. (From Hotz, R.: Orthodontics in Daily Practice. Baltimore, Williams and Wilkins, 1974.)

3. Transverse maxillary arch expansion

4. Retraction of the maxillary incisors and space closure

The guide plane is the most important part of the appliance. The form and construction are illustrated in Figures 5-1 to 5-6. It must be emphasized that the guide plane is not the same as a biteplane or biteplate or a simple inclined plane. Many treatment failures can be attributed to a lack of a full understanding of the philosophy of use and mode of construction of the appliance.

In the early years of use, the guide plane was fabricated in wax on the plaster cast first and then processed in vulcanite or a denture-base acrylic. The introduction of endothermic (self-curing) acrylic rendered this approach obsolete. The guide plane part of the appliance is now formed directly in the mouth. As treatment progresses and mandibular response can be demonstrated, the initial guide plane can be cut away and a new, more anteriorly placed guide plane can be constructed. This is usually necessary every 4 to 8 weeks.

The baseplate itself is fabricated without a guide plane, but with only a small ridge of plastic in its place (Fig. 5-1B). When the guide plane is added, the height, or vertical component, should be kept as low as possible to prevent

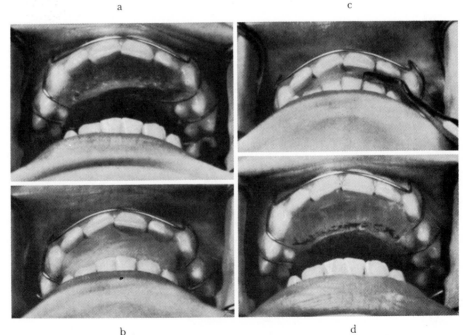

Figure 5-2. Forming the guide plane in the mouth. *A,* Plate with orientation ridge. As the jaws are closed the lower incisors must contact just anterior to the ridge. *B,* Self curing acrylic is applied to the plate. *C,* When the acrylic has achieved a firm consistency, the teeth close in the desired position. The labial part of the bite groove can be formed with a small spatula. *D,* Guide plane after acrylic has set. The black pencil line marks the height of the plane. The plastic behind this mark can be removed. The bite groove is widened slightly to give the lower incisors some freedom of movement. (From Hotz, R.: Orthodontics in Daily Practice. Baltimore, Williams and Wilkins, 1974.)

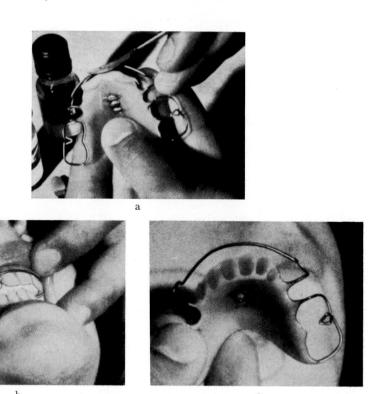

b   c

Figure 5-3. Moving the guide plane forward during treatment (reactivation). *A,* Applying soft acrylic to the former guide plane which has been roughened with a bur. *B,* Biting into the new position. *C,* The impression of the lingual surfaces of the lower anteriors in the soft acrylic. The interdental plastic is removed when set (the bite groove in this photograph is not deep enough). (From Hotz, R.: Orthodontics in Daily Practice. Baltimore, Williams and Wilkins, 1974.)

the bite from opening too quickly. This is difficult to accomplish initially in cases of very deep overbite since the groove anterior to the plane where the lower teeth contact the plate must have sufficient thickness, or the acrylic will be perforated. Later, as the guide plane is advanced, the bite opening can be more easily retarded in relation to the forward activation.

The mandibular response should become evident in 6 to 12 weeks. With the mandible in its most retruded position, the lower incisors no longer contact the edge of the guide plane, but anteriorly to it (Fig. 5-1E). As this occurs, the

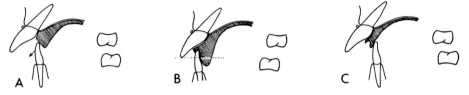

Figure 5-4. Common errors in guide plane construction. *A,* Lower incisors bite upon an inclined plane. Positive forward guidance is lacking, which can lead to dual bite and lower incisor tipping. *B,* Guide plane too large. Forward activation must be accomplished in small steps. The appliance becomes too uncomfortable for the patient to wear. *C,* Guide plane too small. The lower incisors bite behind the plane, tipping them lingually and increasing the distoclusion. (From Hotz, R.: Orthodontics in Daily Practice. Baltimore, Williams and Wilkins, 1974.)

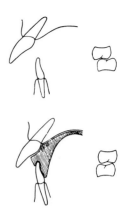

Figure 5-5. Guide plane plate in a case where no deep bite was present or bite opening occurred too rapidly. In such a case the guide plane would have to extend too far below the occlusal plane, making it impossible to wear the appliance during the day. It is assuming the form of a monobloc. (From Hotz, R.: Orthodontics in Daily Practice. Baltimore, Williams and Wilkins, 1974.)

plane is reduced from the palatal aspect with a vulcanite bur. As the mandible grows forward, the functional influence that is exerted by the guide plane (similar to the Oliver guide plane, monobloc, and propulsor) diminishes. The plane must be modified to re-establish optimum activation. As noted previously, the original acrylic plane is ground away and a new one is added with self-curing acrylic in a more anterior position (Fig. 5–1F and 5–3).

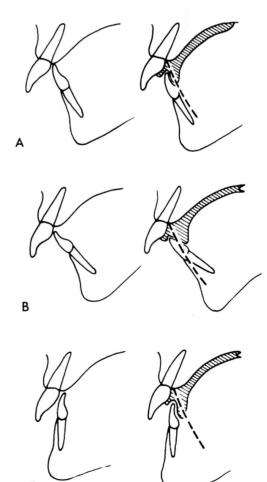

Figure 5-6. Effects of lower incisor axial inclinations on the form of the guide plane. *A*, Normal axial inclination results in good guide plane form. *B*, When the incisors are too procumbent, the guide plane becomes an inclined plane and should not be used. *C*, When the incisors are too recumbent, it becomes impossible to form a guide plane that can bring the mandible forward and still be tolerated by the patient. (From Hotz, R.: Orthodontics in Daily Practice. Baltimore, Williams and Wilkins, 1974.)

As treatment progresses, with the plane being moved forward in successive stages, care must be taken to coordinate vertical bite opening with anterior sagittal mandibular positioning. One must not let the vertical correction outdistance the horizontal change.

At the end of treatment, the same plate can be used also as a retaining appliance. Usually only a small guide plane is needed to hold the maxillomandibular sagittal relationship (Fig. 5–1*H*). The wearing time of the appliance is gradually reduced, being worn only at night, in much the same manner as conventional retention procedures with the Hawley retainer.

Treatment Response

As with any form of orthodontic treatment, treatment response is variable. Forward development of the mandible is dependent on growth increments and growth direction during appliance wear. If possible, treatment should be timed with the prepubertal growth spurt, to take best advantage of the postural guiding of the mandible. Despite the frequent individual unpredictability of growth potential, the pubertal growth spurt usually occurs between 11 and 13 years in girls, and between 12 and 14 years in boys. Simply stated, rapid Class II correction is probable evidence of a concurrent growth spurt and good treatment timing. This can be as short a time as 6 to 10 months. And yet other cases may well require several months before any improvement can be seen. In some instances, no response at all may be seen.

In slowly reacting cases, with minimal anteroposterior adjustment, where the growth spurt does not coincide with treatment or where the growth direction is more vertical, or down and back instead of down and forward, the danger exists that the guide plane plate may open the bite too quickly, disrupting the desired therapeutic coordination of anteroposterior and vertical changes. Bite opening that occurs through eruption of posterior teeth, increasing buccal segment height, is relatively independent of overall growth and age of the patient. It must be stressed again that the rate of vertical development must coincide with horizontal change and must be controlled by adjusting the height of the guide plane. Changing a Class II deep bite malocclusion into a Class II shallow bite malocclusion makes further treatment with functional appliances difficult, if not impossible (Fig. 5–5).

Morphologic and Functional Factors

In addition to horizontal mandibular growth components, remodeling of the gonial angle and ascending ramus may be considered as factors in Class II correction. These changes are difficult to assess cephalometrically as far as extent and effect are concerned. Hotz feels that deep bite cases with relatively flat mandibular and maxillary planes, with an acute angle between them, fare better than those cases where the angle of the mandibular plane and the angle between mandibular and maxillary plane are obtuse.

Another factor is the relationship of habitual occlusal position with postural rest position. Deep bite cases show a greater tendency to functional retrusion. This is particularly evident in Class II, Division 2 cases. Overclosure may result in habitual occlusion being posterior to centric relation and to centric occlusion. A functional analysis of the various mandibular positions is imperative. Only then can prognostic projections and assessments be made of the amount of correction to be obtained by growth as well as elimination of the functional retrusion. The mere correction of overclosure may eliminate posterior temporalis muscle activity and its retrusive effect on the mandible. Petrovic has shown the importance of external pterygoid influence in stimulating condylar growth. The reduction of the powerful posterior temporalis muscle action, which counteracts the effect of the external pterygoid muscle may allow full expression of all possible horizontal mandibular growth increments.

Auxiliary Elastic Traction

In addition to the roles of growth and elimination of functional retrusion in producing the anteroposterior correction, the guide plane can be coupled with the use of Class II intermaxillary elastics to exert a restraining effect on the growth direction of the maxillary complex. The effect is similar to that produced by the monobloc, propulsor, activator, and other functional appliances, which do not need to use intermaxillary elastics. Restriction of the forward growth of the maxillary complex by these appliances can be demon-

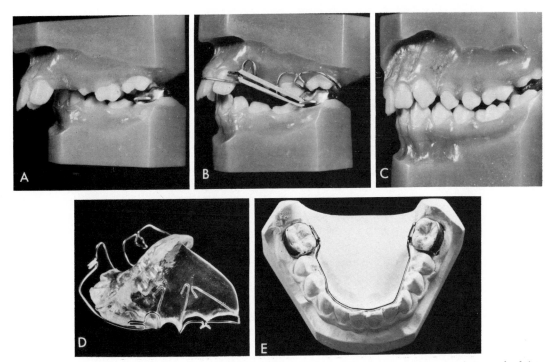

Figure 5-7. *A,* Class II, Division 1 malocclusion with deep bite and severe overjet toward the end of the second phase of the mixed dentition. *B,* Guide plane plate, lingual arch, and intermaxillary elastics in place. *C,* Same case at end of treatment. Overjet correction is attributable to growth and tipping of the upper incisors palatally. *D,* The guide plane plate with hooks for elastics bent into the vertical loops of the labial bow. *E,* Lingual arch for support of lower 6's. The arch wire must be well adapted to the anterior teeth. Mesiobuccal hooks have been welded to the bands to accept intermaxillary elastics. (From Hotz, R.: Orthodontics in Daily Practice. Baltimore, Williams and Wilkins, 1974.)

strated by serial cephalometric studies. How much of the change is actual withholding of forward growth and how much is redirection of growth is not known; perhaps it is a bit of both.

Where anteroposterior correction is proceeding too slowly, the effect of the guide plane plate may also be augmented by intermaxillary traction. This measure will remain effective during sleeping hours, when the functional effect of the guide plane plate is diminished. This becomes a valuable adjunct, particularly in severe cases of distocclusion. Elastic traction was described as early as 1890 by Case and Baker, and has been recommended in certain cases by Schwarz, in conjunction with removable appliances. As with all modifications of appliances, a careful differential diagnosis must be made. Elastic traction is a double-edged sword and can create undesirable movement unless used judiciously and observed carefully and frequently by both clinical and cephalometric assessment.

A well-adapted lingual arch, soldered to meticulously fitting lower first molar bands, is essential. The appliance must be passive. Buccal tubes are soldered on the molar bands to provide for elastic attachment. The maxillary end of the elastic attaches to the vertical loop of the labial bow (Fig. 5–7*B*). Light elastics are placed at bedtime and removed on rising.

Changes in the positions of the teeth within the jaws, as well as the basal skeletal changes, are necessary components of successful treatment. The teeth serve as anchorage units when intermaxillary mechanics are utilized as part of the correction. This is more obvious in fixed appliance mechanotherapy, but tooth positions are also amenable to change with functional appliances. Some functional appliances, such as the Fränkel Function Corrector (see Chapter 15) or the propulsor, are designed to direct their influence to individual teeth or groups of teeth where a change in position is desired. In the case where a guide plane plate is combined with the use of a mandibular lingual arch and intermaxillary elastics, as described above, the teeth become more important as anchorage units. The result may be tooth movement that is desirable or undesirable. Class II intermaxillary elastic traction exerts a distal force against the maxillary dentoalveolar complex but also produces a reciprocal mesial component on the analogous mandibular structures. Such movement can produce a much more rapid sagittal correction. How much of the change is basal, how much dental, and how much combined depends on the individual cases, the growth direction, the growth increments, the amount of functional retrusion, the amount and length of intermaxillary traction, the depth of the bite, the existence of mouth breathing, the presence or absence of tonsils and adenoids, the posture and function of the tongue, the original inclination of the mandibular incisor teeth, and other as yet unequated factors. A careful and complete diagnostic regimen is essential prior to treatment, to assign probable values to each potential conditioning factor. And diagnosis is a continuous decisional process during treatment, constantly modified by therapeutic feedback. Figure 5–8 illustrates a predominantly dental change for the correction.

While tooth movement due to intermaxillary change may be desirable in selected cases in the buccal segments, it can be quite hazardous in the mandibular anterior region. The maxillary incisors do not usually pose a problem and can usually be retracted quite successfully with most removable appliances, as long as torque is not needed (i.e., a simple tipping action instead of bodily movement). Labial tipping of the lower incisors, however, is to be avoided. This is the major danger in guide plane therapy. The correct shape and inclination of the guide plane is therefore of extreme importance.

Text continued on page 104

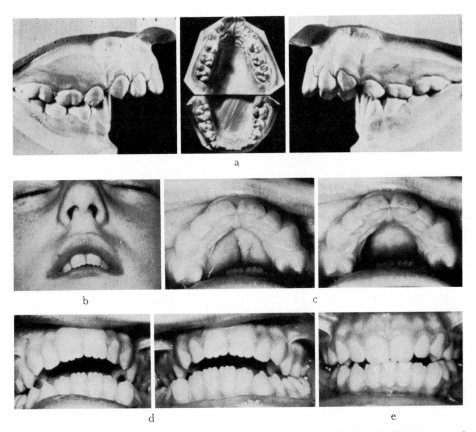

Figure 5–8. Extreme Class II, Division 1 in a 9-year-old girl. *A,* Class II, Division 1 malocclusion with an overjet of 18 mm. Successful treatment is dependent upon growth response. *B,* Poor labial position and tonus are present. *C,* The palatal vault is high, probably owing to abnormal tongue sucking and posture. *D,* As the mandible is protruded with the teeth in contact, an anterior open bite develops. As the mandible is carried farther forward, a crossbite develops on the right side, allowing the open bite to diminish slightly. An open bite can be anticipated upon upper expansion. *E,* Following one year of treatment with an upper expansion plate, lingual arch for lower anteroposterior expansion and intermaxillary elastics. Overjet is corrected. Open bite in the lateral incisor-canine area. *F,* Models corresponding to *E.* The arrowhead clasps have caused the upper 6's to move distally. The lower lingual arch with spring to expand the lower anteriors has been replaced by a retention arch.

Illustration continued on following page

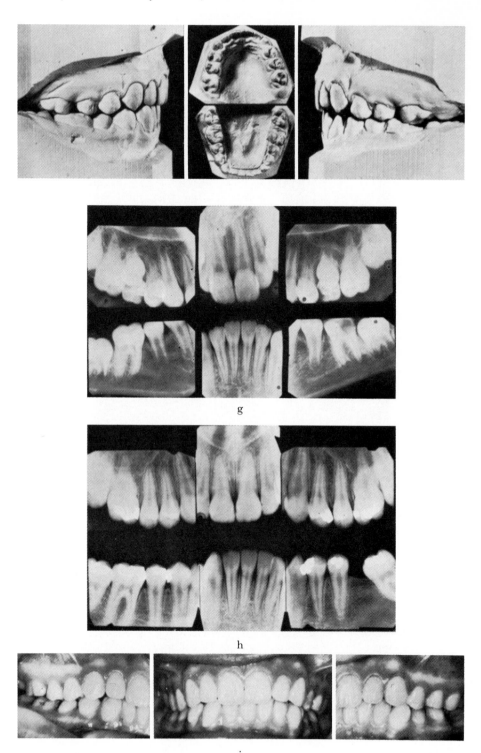

g

h

i

Figure 5-8 *Continued.* *G,* Radiographs corresponding to *A.* ⌐6 has deep caries with periapical involvement and will probably have to be extracted. *H,* Radiographs corresponding to *I.* Age 13, one year out of retention. 6 has been extracted. The patient declined prosthetic reconstruction. *I.* Age 13. Functionally and esthetically satisfactory result. The lower midline remains off to the left.

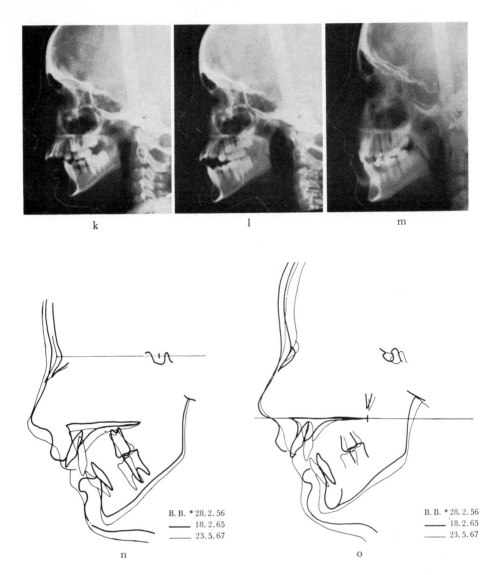

B. B. * 28. 2. 56
—— 18. 2. 65
—— 23. 5. 67

n

B. B. * 28. 2. 56
—— 18. 2. 65
—— 23. 5. 67

o

Figure 5–8 *Continued.* K, Pretreatment cephalogram. L, Cephalogram corresponding to D with resultant open bite. M, Cephalogram at age 12 after treatment, before extraction of |6, N, Tracings of pre- and post-treatment cephalograms superimposed on Se-N. It can be seen that the maxilla moved downward and backward. Anterior mandibular growth was limited. Tooth movement was largely responsible for the occlusal changes. The upper incisors were rotated around the apices, as were the 6's. More of a mesial bodily movement occurred in the lower. Intermaxillary elastics accounted for most

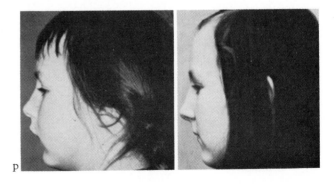

of the tooth movement. O, Tracings superimposed on the maxilla to show the extent of tooth movement. P, Profiles at the beginning and end of treatment show no dramatic changes except for lip posture. (From Hotz, R.: Orthodontics in Daily Practice. Baltimore, Williams and Wilkins, 1974.)

Structure and Treatment Details

The anterior slope of the guide plane derives its form from the lingual surfaces of the lower incisors as they bite into the soft acrylic mass. This allows for a definite forward positioning of the mandible. After a short period of time, this new position becomes an habitual accommodation, requiring a conscious forced effort to retrude the mandible and incisor teeth to a contact position that is posterior to the bite groove that has been established. It is important to note that the lower anterior teeth do not close on the slope of the plane itself, but into the bite groove that is anterior to the plane. This device is not an inclined plane upon which the teeth contact and glide; it is an appliance similar in form to the fixed and cemented metal occlusal guide plane as described by Oliver.

As the lower incisor teeth close into the incisal edge indentations of the bite groove immediately anterior to the guide plane, their labioincisal thirds are gripped by the acrylic, thus helping to prevent them from tipping labially. Figure 5–4 demonstrates the most common errors made in guide plane construction. Improper construction can cause the lower incisors to bite on the slope of the plane itself, thereby favoring labial tipping and possible dual bite. Occasionally, this may be beneficial and desired when lower incisors are lingually inclined and exacerbating the overjet. Improper construction can also produce too much forward mandibular positioning for patient tolerance by virtue of an excessively large inclined plane. The reverse occurs and the patient will be able to bite behind the plane, if it is too small, producing the opposite reaction—mandibular retrusion.

Use of the guide plane plate toward the end of the second phase of the mixed dentition, when canines, second premolars, and second molars are

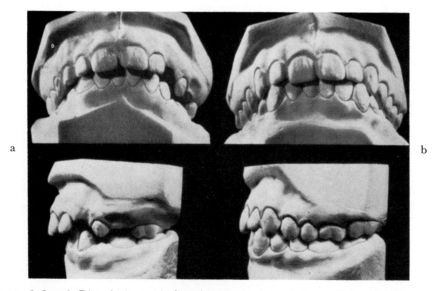

a   b

Figure 5–9. *A,* Distoclusion with deep bite in the second phase of the mixed dentition (eruption of canines and premolars). *B,* Same case four years later, three years after treatment with a guide plane plate. (From Hotz, R.: Orthodontics in Daily Practice. Baltimore, Williams and Wilkins, 1974.)

erupting (the transitional stage), can lead to a very rapid bite opening. The deep bite can be corrected within months, leaving the slower-correcting sagittal problem behind. The plate must be discontinued in these cases. This becomes clinically obvious because when the deep bite is no longer present, the guide plane, in order to contact the lingual surfaces of the lower incisors, must be extended vertically to the point where it cannot be tolerated by the patient (see Fig. 5–5).

Figure 5–9 illustrates a Class II case with a moderately deep overbite. It was treated with only a guide plane plate. In this case, the plate also acted as a space maintainer for the unerupted canines and premolars. Here, as in other examples, it should be clear that correction depends on the patient's own growth potential — the right amount of growth in the right direction at the right time. The clinician must search for all possible growth prediction clues before embarking on appliance guidance: familial pattern; timing of sexual development; changes in structural relationships as measured on the cephalogram, height and weight charts, wrist films; etc.

As has been pointed out already, the axial inclination of the lower incisors is critical to the construction of the guide plane itself. Extremes in inclination contraindicate its use. If the incisors are too procumbent, the guide plane assumes too flat an incline, which only enhances the existing procumbency (see Fig. 5–6B). Cases of severe incisor flaring are usually categorized as bimaxillary protrusions, as will be readily evident from a cephalometric analysis. In some cases, however, where lower incisor flaring is present, along with spacing, a lingual arch with a labial bow soldered to it may be used to upright the lower incisors first. This is done prior to guide plane plate use. In younger patients an alternative would be the monobloc (activator) with upper and lower labial bows to improve the incisor inclination. In older patients, where the premolars and canines have already erupted, treatment becomes more complex and the question of premolar extraction becomes a contingency. If such a decision is made after a thorough diagnostic study, other fixed or removable appliances are more effective in extraction cases than the guide plane plate.

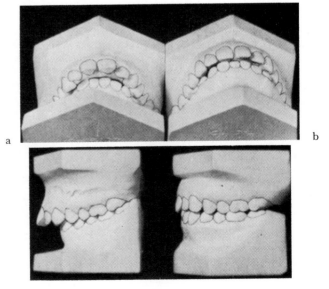

Figure 5–10. *A,* Distoclusion with deep bite and upper incisor protrusion at age 14. *B,* Same case after one year of treatment with a guide plane plate and intermaxillary elastics. (From Hotz, R.: Orthodontics in Daily Practice. Baltimore, Williams and Wilkins, 1974.)

Excessive lingual inclination of the lower incisors also can complicate guide plane plate construction. In such cases, it is advisable to upright the lower incisors first. One appliance of choice could be a fixed lingual arch with soldered loop springs. Or conventional banding, rotational control, etc., utilizing a light-wire labial arch, may be employed. The plate itself can be used as a simple bite-plate until the lower incisor correction has been achieved. Care must be taken that not too much bite opening occurs during this phase of treatment. Then, after lower incisor correction, the appliance is converted into a properly designed guide plane plate.

To take full advantage of muscle function, it is essential that the plate be worn at all times, especially while eating. Speech and eating difficulties are to be expected when the appliance is first inserted, but these problems disappear in a few days. Total patient compliance, together with favorable growth increments and growth direction, can actually correct some severe distoclusions in as little as 8 to 12 months (Figs. 5–10 to 5–12).

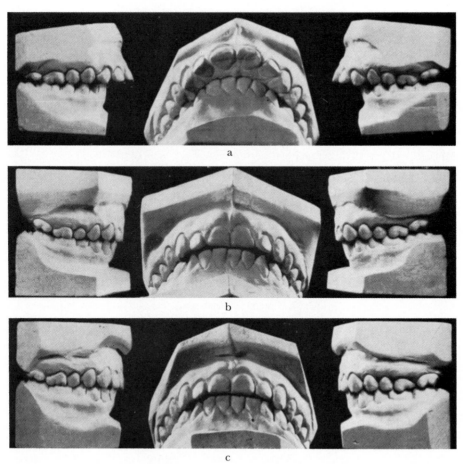

a

b

c

Figure 5–11. *A,* Distoclusion with deep bite and dentoalveolar protrusion of the upper anterior teeth. *B,* Same case following 16 months of treatment with a guide plane plate and intermaxillary elastics. *C,* Same case 15 months later, 10 months out of retention. (From Hotz, R.: Orthodontics in Daily Practice. Baltimore, Williams and Wilkins, 1974.)

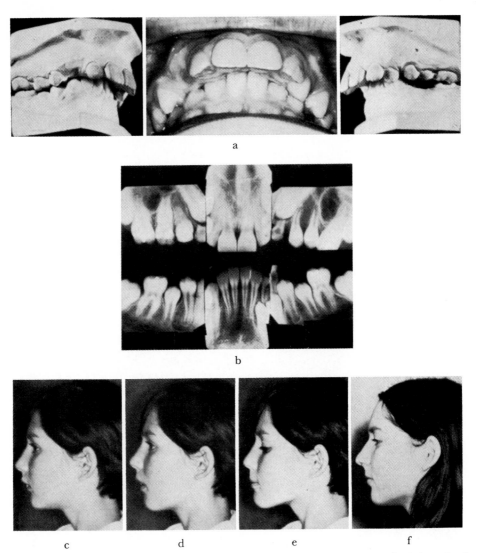

Figure 5-12.   Treatment of Class II, Division 1 malocclusion at the end of the mixed dentition period in an 11-year-old girl. *A,* Pretreatment records show the degree of overjet and overbite. The molar relationship is misleading because of mesial movement of the lowers. *B,* Radiographs taken several months before *A.* Adequate space seems to be present in the upper supporting zones along with a favorable path of eruption for the upper canines. There has been loss of arch length in the supporting zones. Sagittal expansion of the lower arch would lead to extreme labial tipping of the incisors. The arch length problem was solved by extraction of a lower incisor. A lower fixed appliance was used to close the space. Intermaxillary elastics were also used. *C,* Profile in occlusal position. *D,* Profile in rest position. *E,* Profile in maximum protrusive position. *F,* Profile one year out of retention. Extraction of the lower incisor is neither functionally nor esthetically disturbing. (From Hotz, R.: Orthodontics in Daily Practice. Baltimore, Williams and Wilkins, 1974.)

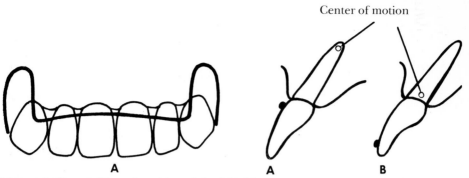

Figure 5–13. *A,* Normal position of the labial bow. It contacts the gingival third of the teeth ascending vertically at the mesial third of the canines. *B,* The labial bow is positioned incisally, causing a shift of the fulcrum coronally. (From Hotz, R.: Orthodontics in Daily Practice. Baltimore, Williams and Wilkins, 1974.)

Appliance Construction Modifications

As previously illustrated, the labial bow must be constructed properly. Resilient stainless steel wire is used and is formed around the maxillary incisor segment to approximate the cervical third of the incisor crowns (Fig. 5–13). The vertical loops on each end of the bow should be well rounded. Sharp bends are prone to breakage and tend to reduce the resiliency (Fig. 5–14). The curvature between the vertical loops should make a gentle and gradual curve and not compensate for individual irregularities and embrasure anatomy (Fig. 5–15). In cases where the maxillary first premolars are to be extracted, the labial bow must be constructed so that its insertions in the palatal acrylic will not

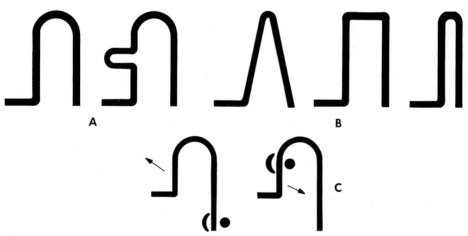

Figure 5–14. *A,* Correct form of the vertical loop, rounded and resilient. *B,* Sharp angles or very narrow loops reduce resiliency and lead to breakage. *C,* Making adjustments to the legs of the loop can effect changes in its position. (From Hotz, R.: Orthodontics in Daily Practice. Baltimore, Williams and Wilkins, 1974.)

Figure 5-15. *A,* Correct labial bow form. The bow is a regular continuous arc, contacting only the most anterior surfaces of the teeth. *B,* Incorrect form. The bow should not be adapted to the contours of the crowded anteriors. An exception would be the "Y-plate," in which the labial bow is used as a clasp. (From Hotz, R.: Orthodontics in Daily Practice. Baltimore, Williams and Wilkins, 1974.)

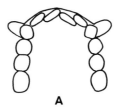
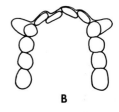

Figure 5-16. Position of the labial bow and arrowhead clasps where 4's have been extracted. 65⏌ are free to move mesially. This is not possible on the opposite side. (From Hotz, R.: Orthodontics in Daily Practice. Baltimore, Williams and Wilkins, 1974.)

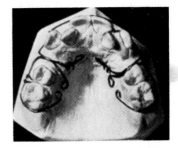

Figure 5-17. Trimming the plate for palatal movement of protruded incisors. *A,* By trimming the entire border away from the acrylic palatal to the incisors the fulcrum can be moved to the root apex. *B,* Incorrect trimming. The gingival border of the plate acts as the fulcrum. (From Hotz, R.: Orthodontics in Daily Practice. Baltimore, Williams and Wilkins, 1974.)

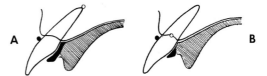

interfere with the distally moving canines (Fig. 5–16). Equally important is the judicious removal of acrylic from the anterior portion of the guide plane plate. To keep the center of incisor rotation (fulcrum) as apical as possible, the acrylic must be completely removed from the lingual surfaces of the upper incisors and from the palatal gingival margin (Fig. 5–17).

Retention of the guide plane plate becomes even more critical when using intermaxillary elastics. Arrowhead clasps are adequate retention elements unless the second deciduous molars are loose or the second premolars not fully erupted. If exfoliation of the maxillary second deciduous molars is imminent, it may be better to allow the second premolars to erupt first before applying intermaxillary traction.

The guide plane plate may also be used as a space maintainer when the maxillary second deciduous molars have been lost prematurely. One modifica-

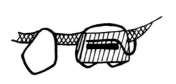

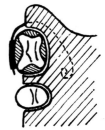

Figure 5-18. An alternative to the arrowhead clasp. The 6's can be banded with a short section of wire soldered to the buccal surfaces. These can be utilized as "artificial undercuts" for circumferential clasps. (From Hotz, R.: Orthodontics in Daily Practice. Baltimore, Williams and Wilkins, 1974.)

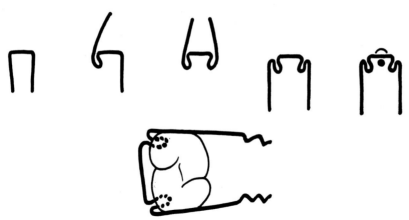

Figure 5-19.   The forming of an Adams clasp. Use of manufactured preformed clasps is recommended. (From Hotz, R.: Orthodontics in Daily Practice. Baltimore, Williams and Wilkins, 1974.)

tion may be to band the maxillary first permanent molars, with metal lugs soldered to their buccal surfaces. (0.045 inch round buccal tubes may also be used, if there is a possibility of using part-time extraoral force during treatment [see Chapter 16].) Circumferential clasps can then be used for the guide plane plate, snapping over the lugs or tubes for firm retention (Fig. 5-18). A further alternative is to use Adams clasps (Fig. 5-19).

In spite of good oral hygiene, a small percentage of children develop a palatal inflammation or an allergic response when wearing acrylic appliances constantly. In such cases, reducing the appliance wear to daytime only may be sufficient to overcome this reaction. Daytime wear makes maximum use of the functional influence. When elastics are used, a treatment compromise can usually be reached, where both optimum functional influence and nocturnal elastic traction achieve the therapeutic objective. Leaving the plate out for short periods of time after meals may be all that is needed.

Additional Appliance Wear

In many cases, it may be advantageous to complete treatment and retention with the monobloc (activator or propulsor). The choice of such an appliance depends on a number of clinical signs and progress of therapy attained with the guide plane plate alone. The basic monobloc, activator, or propulsor without wire clasps will often complete the anteroposterior correction and allow unhindered settling in. The guide plane plate clasps can at times interfere with settling in. It would seem, then, that the monobloc may be used both at the beginning and at the end of treatment, beginning in the early treatment phase of correction—7 to 8 years of age—and finishing at the end of the late treatment period—13 to 15 years of age. The guide plane plate serves in the interim period as a more active appliance.

As with all appliances, however, even this combination may not be successful in fully correcting all distoclusions. Functional jaw orthopedics can produce partial corrections, as can all orthodontic appliances. Sometimes, the answer may be to finish up with modifications as described above. Sometimes the use of extraoral force is indicated. Switching to full and complete fixed appliances may be the best choice, or a combination of fixed and removable appliances may provide the best answer in terms of both treatment result and treatment time. It is here that the diagnostic acumen and clinical experience of the orthodontist come into play. The orthodontist, like the orthopedic surgeon, needs a versatile armamentarium that is readily available to accomplish treatment objectives and conquer treatment problems as they arise. This point will be emphasized elsewhere again because of its importance. An orthodontist looking for the "easy way" of simple and uncomplicated answers to treatment questions will not find happiness in the world of removable appliances alone. No single panacea, fixed or removable, exists in this regard, despite the "Chamber of Commerce" propaganda seen in some of the literature, based on selected cases and partial practices.

Late Treatment of Class II, Division 1 Malocclusion (14 to 18 Years of Age)

Orthodontic treatment at this time is generally more difficult and demanding of the fullest measure of specialty diagnosis and therapeutic ministration. Morphologic, functional, psychological, and behavioral facets of the problem must be thoroughly studied before embarking on any form of mechanotherapy. As long as appreciable growth still remains, the chances of success may warrant the effort. Hotz feels that patients in this age range should be told that therapy is on a trial basis, if the guide plane plate is used. If, after a period of 3 to 4 months of intensive wear, a positive change is noted, then a lower fixed lingual arch can be placed and part-time elastic traction employed.

If no favorable reaction can be seen after the trial period, the treatment plan is changed. Basal adjustment no longer seems a valid treatment objective, and the changes that are effected are primarily within the tooth system to correct overbite and overjet as much as possible. One method of accomplishing this is illustrated in Figure 5–20, where the upper first premolars have been extracted. The maxillary canines are banded and a biteplate is used. The objectives are retraction of the maxillary anterior segment into the extraction spaces and reduction of the vertical discrepancy (overbite) with the help of the biteplate. Another treatment alternative is conventional multibanded therapy, probably with removal of four premolars. A final alternative is orthognathic surgery, with or without concurrent fixed orthodontic appliance treatment. The dramatic results of maxillary osteotomies, with removal of first premolars, often permit correction of both sagittal and vertical problems.

THE PROPULSOR

The propulsor, conceived by Mühlemann and refined by Hotz, is similar in its action to the monobloc or classic activator (Fig. 5–21). It can be described as a hybrid appliance, with features of both the monobloc and the simpler oral screen or mask (see Chapter 4). A definite advantage of the propulsor over other functional orthopedic, activator-like appliances is in its coverage of and ability to effect changes in the alveolar process, as well as the teeth of the maxillary anterior segment (Figs. 5–22 to 5–25). This makes the appliance particularly useful in cases of maxillary dentoalveolar protrusion.

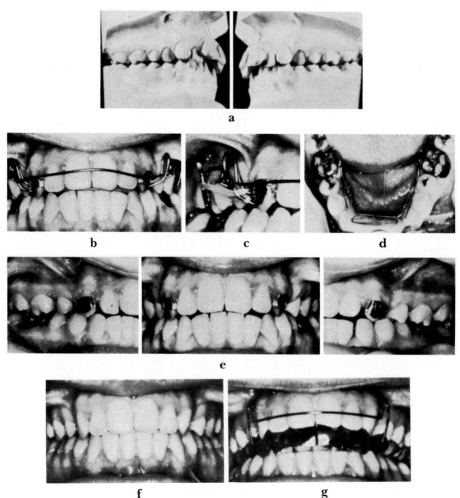

Figure 5-20. Treatment of Class II, Division 1 malocclusion in a nongrowing patient. *A,* Class II, Division 1 malocclusion with deep bite and crowded, protruded upper incisors. The patient is a 14½-year-old girl with no growth expected. Extraction of upper 4's will afford space for the canines and mesial movement of the 5's and 6's into a Class II inter-cuspation. The extracted teeth can be seen on the model. *B,* Distalization of the canines has begun. The incisors have been aligned with the labial bow. *C,* This close-up shows an elastic band used to move the canine. The elastic is passed to the outside of the labial bow arm to effect slight rotation. Distally, the elastic is attached to a special hook. The hook on the canine band itself should be attached toward the distal to avoid undesirable rotation. The labial bow guides the canine from the labial. *D,* The lower lingual arch serves to expand the lower arch, especially in the anteroposterior direction. Intermaxillary elastics may also be used from the upper labial bow to hooks on the lower molar bands. *E,* Photographs taken shortly before removal of the canine bands and lingual arch. The canines are in a Class I relationship. The 5's, 6's, and 7's must settle into a better Class II intercuspation. Bite open-ing is slightly overdone but will close as the occlusion settles in. *F,* Several months after the patient began wearing a retention monobloc, the bite has closed. *G,* The monobloc will be worn at least six months.

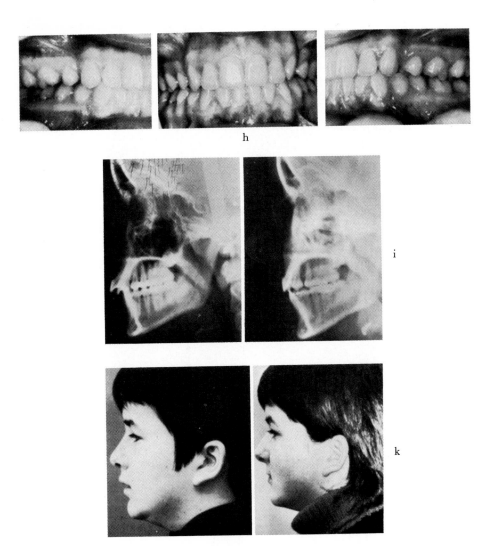

Figure 5–20 *Continued.* *H,* 10 months later. The right side occlusion is good; the left will continue to settle in and will be helped as the 8's erupt. *I,* Pre- and post-treatment cephalograms. *K,* Pre- and post-treatment profiles. (From Hotz, R.: Orthodontics in Daily Practice. Baltimore, Williams and Wilkins, 1974.)

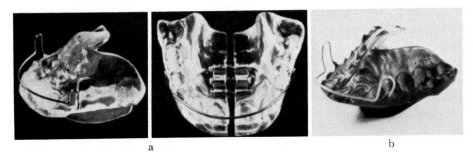

Figure 5–21. Plastic monobloc with expansion screw and labial bow. This is the most frequently used type of monobloc. (From Hotz, R.: Orthodontics in Daily Practice. Baltimore, Williams and Wilkins, 1974.)

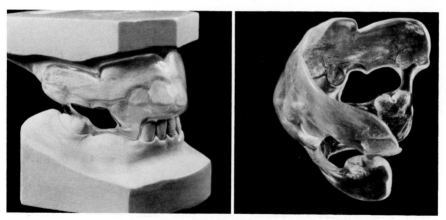

Figure 5-22. The propulsor. The plastic connecting the upper buccal to the lower lingual flanges also serves as occlusal support to stabilize the appliance in the beginning of treatment. As the muscles adapt to the appliance the interocclusal plastic is removed to allow for molar eruption. (From Hotz, R.: Orthodontics in Daily Practice. Baltimore, Williams and Wilkins, 1974.)

The construction bite is similar to that of the activator, but it is usually taken in a more forward position than that of the monobloc. As with the monobloc, the attempt of the mandible to return to centric relationship has a retruding effect on the maxillary arch. It also eliminates any functional retrusion tendencies, and offsets any functional dominance of posterior temporalis fibers, so often seen in classic Class II, Division 1 malocclusions. No wire configurations are used with the propulsor. As the intermaxillary relation improves, the appliance is reactivated or modified by adding acrylic to the area which contacts the upper anterior segment. Periodic modification is necessary because of the complete acrylic construction. This is simple to do, and patient compliance is usually good, because of the light weight and minimum bulk of the appliance.

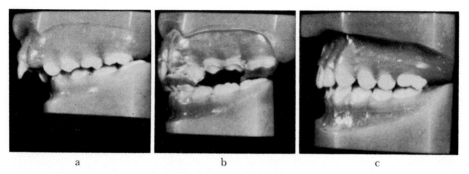

a   b   c

Figure 5-23. *A,* Class II, Division 1 malocclusion with a 15 mm. overjet at the end of the first phase of the mixed dentition. *B,* Propulsor in place. *C,* Same case after completion of propulsor therapy. For final occlusal correction a guide plane plate is indicated. (From Hotz, R.: Orthodontics in Daily Practice. Baltimore, Williams and Wilkins, 1974.)

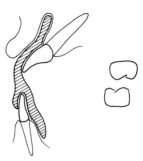

Figure 5-24. The broad surface support of the propulsor on the bucco-labial surfaces in the maxilla and the lingual surfaces in the mandible allow for pronounced forward activation in the construction bite. Note that the lower incisors are firmly grasped to prevent tipping. (From Hotz, R.: Orthodontics in Daily Practice. Baltimore, Williams and Wilkins, 1974.)

The acrylic between the occlusal surfaces of the first molars serves to stabilize the appliance when therapy is initiated. As treatment progresses, however, this acrylic is progressively removed to allow for unhindered eruption of the molars and resultant reduction of the deep overbite, if it exists. If selective eruption of mandibular teeth is desired, as recommended by Harvold and Woodside, to reduce the Class II buccal segment relationship by upward and forward eruption of the lower teeth while preventing forward eruption of the upper teeth, more acrylic can be removed opposing the lower molars, leaving them free.

The reader is referred to *Orthodontics in Daily Practice* by Rudolph Hotz, as translated and adapted by Robert Shaye, for more extensive discussions of both the guide plane plate and the propulsor. Both of the authors of this current text have seen first hand the successful results obtained by Professor Hotz and his colleagues. One of us (Graber) cannot forget an afternoon in 1964 when he saw 25 cases in succession of Class II, Division 1 malocclusion, all treated with the propulsor and all beautifully done. With a fixed appliance philosophy and training, a number of the cases would have been fully banded with extraction of premolars. All would have had some extraoral force guidance. A number of the cases seen were well out of any appliance guidance and were clearly stable. Obviously, essential ingredients of this success were case selection, good growth amounts and growth direction during treatment, and a high level of patient co-

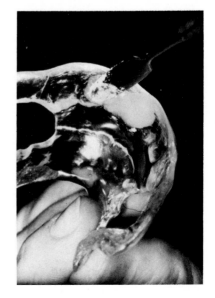

Figure 5-25. Reactivating the propulsor by adding acrylic to the area of the upper incisors. (From Hotz, R.: Orthodontics in Daily Practice. Baltimore, Williams and Wilkins, 1974.)

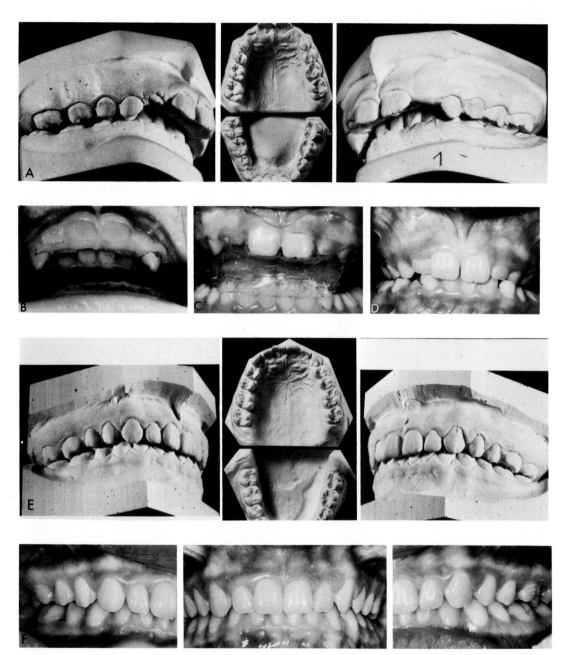

Figure 5-26. Severe Class II, Division 1 malocclusion with deep bite in a 7 1/2-year-old girl. *A,* Overjet measured 15 mm. Abnormal swallowing and sucking of the lower lip was present. *B,* This photograph shows the degree of overjet and overbite. *C,* Propulsor in place. The construction bite relationship was at its vertical and horizontal limits. *D,* Same case 10 months later. No dual bite present. The posterior teeth are almost in crossbite. The canines were reduced because they were causing premature contact. *E,* Same case at age 16. The propulsor had been worn only two years. *F,* Photographs corresponding to *E.*

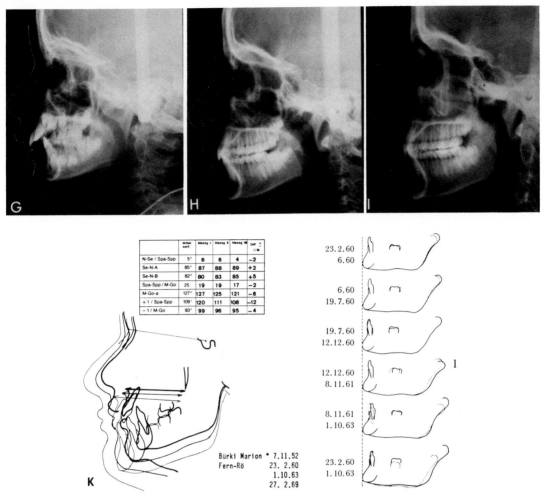

	Mittel- wert	Messg I	Messg II	Messg III	Diff + I/III
N-Se / Spa-Spp	5°	6	6	4	-2
Se-N-A	85°	87	88	89	+2
Se-N-B	82°	80	83	85	+5
Spa-Spp / M-Go	25	19	19	17	-2
M-Go-a	127°	127	125	121	-6
+ 1 / Spa-Spp	109°	120	111	108	-12
- 1 / M-Go	93°	99	96	95	-4

Bürki Marion * 7.11.52
Fern-Rö   23. 2.60
                   1.10.63
            27. 2.69

23.2.60
6.60

6.60
19.7.60

19.7.60
12.12.60

12.12.60
8.11.61

8.11.61
1.10.63

23.2.60
1.10.63

Figure 5-26 *Continued.* *G*, Cephalogram at beginning of treatment. *H*, Cephalogram at age 11, one year after discontinuing the propulsor. Second molars have not yet erupted. *I*, Cephalogram at age 16. *K*, Tracings at ages 7, 11, and 16. Forward mandibular development and retardation of maxillary growth during propulsor therapy are evident. It should be mentioned that such a good response to treatment cannot be expected in every case. *L*, Mandibular tracings, although limited in their ability to show growth changes, do give some indications as to treatment response. (From Hotz, R.: Orthodontics in Daily Practice. Baltimore, Williams and Wilkins, 1974.)

operation. It should also be emphasized that Professor Hotz was ready to change treatment plans in each case, if necessary, based on a continuing assessment of patient progress at each appointment. The Achilles' heel of removable appliances is that all too many dentists have learned to use only one or two types of removable mechanisms. The alternatives for change simply are not there, and the net result is a partial correction at best, with the dentist rationalizing that a little correction is better than none. This attitude is wrong and must not become prevalent in the United States, as it has in many parts of Europe, under socioeconomic stress. Hotz has been a strong force against this trend, as one of his treated cases shows (Fig. 5-26).

6

Functional Jaw Orthopedics: The Changes of a Concept

The activator and the appliances which appeared as changes of the original concept fill the greater part of this book. A systematic survey should be useful. The originally used designation, "functional jaw orthopedics," no longer has a clear meaning. It is retained here in memory. Some knowledge of the historical development of the appliances concerned and of their differences may help not only to understand better the present situation, but also to discern future trends. Also, there is the rather forlorn wish to stimulate students of our specialty to devote more attention to its history. For the future historian, the documentary evidence provided by publications will not be sufficient. Knowledge of the life and thoughts of the principal figures may be equally important, and with the passing of one generation after another, irreplaceable information will be lost.

THE PAST

Disregarding for the moment the living authors of currently used methods, we shall deal in this section with four men out of the past who came forward with a fundamentally new approach to orthodontic treatment. They were Norman W. Kingsley, who was the first in orthodontic therapy to use the forward positioning of the mandible;[1] Pierre Robin, who first designed a type of appliance that was later used to influence muscular activity by a change in the spatial relationship of the jaws;[2] Alfred P. Rogers, who recognized the importance of the whole orofacial system for the problems of orthodontic treatment; and Viggo Andresen, who took the decisive step of designing for the treatment of malocclusion an inert appliance that fitted loosely in the mouth and by its mobility transferred muscular stimuli to the jaws, teeth, and supporting structures.[5-8]

In 1879, Kingsley[1] described the bite plate he had designed. "It was adapted to the inside of the superior dental arch and the inclined surface marked 'A' projected below and caught the inferior incisors. The object was not to protrude the lower teeth, but to change or jump the bite in the case of an excessively retreating lower jaw." The original maxillary plate of Kingsley was modified and used by Ottolengui, combined with fixed appliances by Herbert A. Pullen, J. Lowe Young, and Oren A. Oliver.[9] Other constructions were designed for the same purpose. There was a sliding device of Edward H. Angle, generally fitted to the upper and lower first molars, named "the plane and spur retention."[10] A. M. Schwarz recommended crowns on upper and lower second deciduous molars—"Vorbisskronen."[12] A cone on the upper crown forced the Class II, Division 1 dentition into a Class I relationship. A massive pin and tube sliding device of Herbst was very popular in Europe.[12]

Early in this century, jumping the bite was a very popular method, but lack of success became apparent. "The treatment was to expand both the upper and lower arches and reduce the protrusion of the maxillary anterior teeth. . . . Then the mandible was moved forward by muscular action until they were in their proper mesiodistal relation. . . . However the trouble was that great difficulty was encountered in getting the mandible to stay forward after it had been moved. . . ."[9, 13] The introduction of intermaxillary elastics made the original appliance obsolete. It has survived, however, as the inclined plane of the maxillary Hawley retainer. A successor is the Hotz expansion plate with a guide plane.[14] This similarity, however, is deceptive. The Hotz appliance eases the mandible forward in stages and makes additional use of intermaxillary elastics worn during the night.

The term "jumping the bite" is widely used nowadays for the forward positioning of the mandible with functional appliances. It seems preferable, however, to apply the term as it was originally meant, that is, to let the mandible "jump" into the finally intended occlusion and to induce it to stay there. In contrast, the forward positioning by functional appliances is dislocating the mandible to stimulate alveolar or condylar changes, or both, to achieve the desired occlusion *by stages.*

In 1902, Pierre Robin published an article describing an appliance, the monobloc, to be used for bimaxillary expansion.[2] In 1923, according to Izard, Robin advocated its use for his "eumorphic method."[15] This was to correct "glossoptosis" and free the "vital functional confluent," meaning the throat, with its vital space, for the passage of air and food. He regarded glossoptosis as a very grave condition, threatening the very existence of the French people. In 1927 he wrote, "Any observer trying to diagnose glossoptosis will promptly detect that, whereas before the 15th year of age, three among four children will suffer from more or less grave glossoptosis, after 40 years not more than one of these has glossoptotic deficiency."[16]

Calculating these data, we deduce that three teenagers would have been free from glossoptosis for every nine suffering from it. Leaving only one survivor from these nine after 40 years, eight, or two thirds of the original 12, would have died prematurely. Izard pointed out that no statistics substantiated that death rate and that the French physicians seemed totally unaware of such a threat to the national health. An often-reproduced drawing of Robin shows where in the human body the sequelae of glossoptosis may be found. From headache to flat feet, no organ seems to be spared, with lung and heart diseases and appendicitis thrown in. The most curious fact is that the drawing was reproduced, apparently with approval, by Andresen in 1942 and Schwarz in 1956. Balters[17] founded his therapeutic concepts on an elaboration of Robin's views about glossoptosis. Robin's theories were not generally accepted in his own country. Izard's skeptical attitude has been mentioned already. Cauhépé and Coutand, analyzing Class II, Division 1 conditions, reached the conclusion that glossoptosis as described by Robin does not exist.[18] Nevertheless, his method was widely employed in France and Belgium.

The views of Robin and Balters, regarding malocclusion as part of a general pathologic condition of the human body, are too extreme to be acceptable. There are, however, prominent orthodontists who see, especially in Class II, Division 1 malocclusion, certain conditions connected with disturbances of posture and muscular behavior of the whole body.[19]

F. Watry used the monobloc with his physiotherapeutic treatment as a gymnastic appliance for "functional reeducation," according to his interpretation of Robin's teachings.[20] However, he was also influenced by Rogers' publications. Muscular exercises with the inserted monobloc, beginning with at least three daily half-hour sessions and then increasing in length, were meant to transform mandibular movements and transmit stimuli to the maxilla. When patients cooperated in this rather demanding treatment, satisfactory results were achieved. Watry thus came quite close to Andresen's activator. However, the muscle stimuli were provided by the patient's voluntary action, whereas Andresen made muscle action automatic with his loosely fitted appliance.

The bionator, according to Balters, is constructed to influence the position of the tongue.[17] Except for that and other miscellaneous ideological connections, it owes nothing to Robin's monobloc.

In 1918 Alfred P. Rogers recommended "exercises for the development of the muscles of the face, with a view to increase their functional activity." This was the title of an article in the *Dental Cosmos*.[3] He pleaded for "making facial muscles our allies in treatment and retention," again a title of an article in the *Dental Cosmos* in 1922.[4] There were exercises for the masseter-temporalis, pterygoid, mentalis muscles, tongue, orbicularis oris, and facial muscles. Orthodontists all over the world readily accepted the method. It was probably recommended in every textbook. An objective survey made 40 years ago, however, could not fail to observe that surprisingly few results were shown without the simultaneous use of appliances.[21] A few dissenting opinions could be found also. Dewey called attention to the fact that in Class II, Division 1 cases, habitually moving the mandible forward had a poor prognosis for treatment.[13] Although rare, there was frank condemnation, too, as in a book review in the *International Journal of Orthodontics* in 1931.[22] The author of the review claimed that these exercises were physiologically wrong and doing more harm than good.

Most of the exercises have become obsolete now. There apparently is not much need for them with the multiband techniques, which aim at fast alveolar adaptation, and no need with functional methods which have, in essence, incorporated them in the appliance. John Cleall recently has shown the very limited possibilities of changing form by voluntary muscular function alone.[23] Rogers, however, has proven to be right on two counts. The importance of lip exercises has been emphasized again and again by Hotz, Duyzings, Fränkel, and others. And Rogers was the first to recognize the fundamental importance of the muscles for the growth, development, and form of the whole stomatognathic system.

It has been said repeatedly that Viggo Andresen developed an appliance that was in some aspects identical with Robin's monobloc. Izard, however, stated correctly that although at first glance it seems to be a copy of Robin's construction, there are considerable differences.[15] Andresen himself declared that he had no knowledge of Robin's work when he made his first activator-like device in 1908.[5] The appliance was meant to serve as functional retention and to prevent mouth breathing. He made a maxillary plate[5] to which he added an extension behind the mandibular incisors. The lingual surfaces of these incisors were in contact with that portion of the appliance. He expressed his "special veneration for the biological ideas and work of John Nutting Farrar,"[24] when he wrote that "the apparatus fulfills the requirements laid down by Farrar in his day—but which seems to have been forgotten entirely—namely, that the apparatus is to be under the control of the patient just as much as that of the dentist, and that the apparatus is to work intermittently in accordance with Farrar's biological principle, 'labor and rest.'"[7] Also mentioned by Andresen in Farrar's recommendation to grind teeth interfering with the occlusion.*[6]

Andresen developed the activator from a plate devised by Norman Kingsley, to which he added lateral extensions to cover the lingual aspects of the mandibular teeth. The first appliance of this kind was constructed as a retainer, after the correction of distoclusion for his own daughter. The "biomechanical working retainer" was also designed to prevent mouth breathing.[5] Further use of the "retention activator," as Andresen later called the device, brought encouraging results. As was the custom of many orthodontists of that time, he removed fixed appliances from his Class II, Division 1 patients for summer vacations and inserted retainers. He found that the results of the previous treatment were not only preserved but, in many cases, actually improved during the vacation period.[25]

Andresen's activator was different from any other removable appliance in use up to that time. Entirely inert and lying freely movable in the oral cavity, it was set in motion by the tongue and oral musculature. Correction of the malocclusion was effected by the transmission of muscle stimuli to the teeth, the supporting tissue, and the jaws.

The novel device, based on strange new principles, was not likely to win adherents. Removable appliances were generally rejected at that time. In addition, against the current of the times, though not necessarily connected with activator treatment per se, Andresen advocated extractions. That subjected him

---

*John Nutting Farrar (1839–1913) wrote the first comprehensive and outstanding text devoted exclusively to orthodontics. The first volume of his *Treatise on Irregularities of the Teeth and their Correction* was published in 1888. Volume II was released nine years later, using the same title. Some 1400 hand-drawn sketches by the author illustrate the 1570 pages of the two volumes. Unfortunately, books by Angle have unduly overshadowed this tremendous work. Farrar's books still engender contemporary interest. Weinberger, the historian, elaborates on Farrar's contributions. "J. N. Farrar devoted all his life to perfecting appliances for the delivery of force to the movement of teeth as obtained from the screw. He was a mechanical genius and the correction of irregular teeth was to him an intricate mechanical problem, as may be seen by his complex mechanisms employed in the movement of teeth. Farrar developed the screw force for orthodontic treatment to such an extent as to give his appliances the most grotesque appearance. The 'law' which he formulated to guide orthodontic procedures is stated as follows: 'In regulating teeth, the dividing line between the production of physiological and pathological changes in the tissues of the jaw is found to lie within a movement of the teeth acted upon—allowing a variation which will cover all cases—not exceeding 1/240th or 1/160th of an inch every twelve hours.' Farrar was probably the first to recommend root movement of the teeth."

Angle took over and publicized many of Farrar's contrivances. In later years, Farrar's screw appliances for transverse expansion, combined with six miniature jackscrews, one for each anterior tooth, as illustrated in the Angle text, was better remembered than the biological principles developed by Farrar. Yet the tooth movement recommended above is 0.1 or 0.15 mm., which corresponds exactly to the research-validated guidelines of A. M. Schwarz, which limit the active force application to a distance smaller than the width of the periodontal membrane (0.2 mm).

Andresen's praise for Farrar's work, written fifty years after the first volume was released, is easier to understand if we remember that Andresen, who was born in 1870, was a dental student when Volume 1 of Farrar was published.

to the same ridicule that Tweed was to face later in the United States. Under the influence of Angle, extractions were totally rejected at that time. Furthermore, the Andresen concept of individual esthetic and functional optimum as the objective of treatment irreconcilably conflicted with the prevailing Angle idealistic dictum of perfect treatment results. Andresen also proposed "to replace the narrow-minded term 'orthodontia' which, so to say, has got an odious flavor among stomatologists, by the term 'eugnathics' or 'eugnathophysiognomics.'"[7] The activator was referred to occasionally as a miracle appliance. The greatest miracle seems to be that its value was recognized after all.

In 1925, Viggo Andresen, who had come from Denmark, became director of the orthodontic department of the Dental School in Oslo, and was appointed professor in 1927. It was here that he developed the system of functional jaw orthopedics. Another staff member of the same school, Austrian-born Karl Häupl, a pathologist and periodontist, was to become intimately involved. An eminent scientist, Häupl had not shown any interest in clinical orthodontics until this time. Thus he was not prejudiced against Andresen's unorthodox approach. He saw similarities in tissue changes induced by the activator and tooth migration, which he had studied.

Häupl then became director of the dental clinic of the German University of Prague. As one of the leaders of the profession in Central Europe, he was an enthusiastic advocate of the new method, and succeeded in convincing many orthodontists. He and Andresen regarded "functional jaw orthopedics," as they called it, as vastly superior to all previous methods, in bringing about growth changes in an entirely physiologic manner. Häupl justified his working hypothesis on the writings of Roux, who observed that "shaking the bone substance" will increase the activity of the osteoblasts, leading to increased formation of bone.[26] (See discussion in Chapter 1.) Andresen and Häupl claimed that the activator actually transmitted such stimuli to the bone.[8, 27]

These theories were argued forcefully and persuasively so as to convince the adherents of the new method that the activator was not only different from all other appliances but was also much superior from a biological point of view. It was fortunate that at the same time A. M. Schwarz introduced the new designs of the expansion plate.[11] Activator and plates complemented each other, making the treatment of most malocclusions possible. Certainly there was a great unsatisfied demand for simple and inexpensive orthodontic treatment. Thus, in spite of World War II and postwar conditions, use of the new methods spread rapidly, mainly in Central Europe, leading to a new development in removable appliances. It is worthwhile to know its history and to record it correctly.

As described earlier, the monobloc of Robin and the activator of Andresen are completely independent developments. Andresen had no knowledge of Robin's monobloc and did not modify it. It is grossly unfair to both men to write about a monobloc of Robin-Andresen. Technically the activator could be called a monobloc, but there is no reason to create an artificial confusion. The monobloc was Robin's and the activator Andresen's.

Though Andresen was the originator of the activator, the appliance was first discussed in an extensive and easily intelligible form in the textbook written by Andresen and Häupl. The designation "activator" apparently was first mentioned there. It does not seem right, therefore, to omit Häupl's name, as is done frequently. The activator, or whatever Andresen called his "apparatus," would have existed without Häupl. But we would hardly know about it. At a later time Häupl took an entirely wrong position on two important issues. His complete rejection of fixed devices led the profession astray for a time, as discussed in Chapter 1. He also refused to accept any further development of myofunctional devices. Yet one of the greatest achievements of the activator certainly is that it triggered a wealth of new constructions, as shown in the following pages.

THE PRESENT AND THE FUTURE

The introduction of Andresen's activator was a milestone in the history of orthodontics and epoch-making for the development of removable appliances. The results of treatment achieved by this simple device, only temporarily in contact with the teeth, were surprising. It soon became apparent, however, that the principle of the free mobility of the activator had its drawbacks. The patients too frequently lost the appliance during sleep.[28] That led to two further developments. By increasing the interocclusal distance with the construction bite, retention was improved. However, although the form of the appliance appeared to remain the same, the principles of the treatment according to Andresen were unwittingly abandoned. The other possibility was to increase the efficiency of the appliance. That was effected in two ways. The bulk of the device was radically reduced, making wearing around the clock possible, and the muscular impulses were reinforced by elastic elements incorporated in the construction.

The alternatives of the mode of action of the activator by muscular movement or muscular pressure, were, as shown in the following chapter, regarded as possible with use of the original activator of Andresen. During the last quarter of the century, however, treatment systems have evolved that rely almost exclusively on one or the other of these possibilities. To differentiate between them and to facilitate further discussion, it is proposed to name those relying on muscle mass and resting pressure "myotonic" and those using muscle activity or movement "myodynamic" appliances. The possible existence of a third group will be discussed in the section on Fränkel's function corrector.

It should be emphasized that the terms "myotonic" and "myodynamic" are suggested only as a temporary expedient and need not be regarded as a permanent addition to the orthodontic glossary. It must not be forgotten, either, that such a schematic division of the appliances will hardly take into account a number of variables, if an analysis of results achieved in individual cases is contemplated. These are the different reactions of the particular patient, structural differences of the skeletal parts involved which may result in different muscular reactions, the position of the head during sleep, the atmospheric pressure in the oral cavity, and others. More important is the fact that the mode of action ascribed to one group of appliances may, to some degree, be effective also with the other. Notwithstanding these limitations, an attempt to divide the multitude of activator derivates into defined groups should be plausible and useful. In fact, quite different systems of treatment have emerged. Furthermore, there are important differences in the mode of action of particular devices. These may produce a different reaction in the treated dentition also. Results of treatment reported are more easily accessible to scrutiny when examined in coherent groups according to the particular method.

Myotonic Appliances

A detailed description of the development of the activator is given in the following chapter. The initially small interocclusal distance with the construction bite was increased in each subsequent edition of the Andresen-Häupl text (see Chapter 7 by Slagsvold). However, Neumann, who was closely in touch with Häupl during the years after the first publication in 1936, does not have the impression that there was a hard and fast rule concerning the height of the construction bite. It was rather a recommendation that could be adjusted according to clinical judgment and the requirements of the particular case. The anterior dislocation of the mandible, certainly, was seen as more important and the interocclusal molar clearance may have varied according to the depth of the overbite and the position and inclination of the upper incisors. The vertical displacement of the mandible was increased first to prevent the loss of the appliance during sleep in some cases. The gradual increase during the years apparently was due to clinical experience. Thus, to use the terminology employed, the myodynamic activator of Andresen became the myotonic appliance of Andersen-Häupl-Petrik. The importance of that changeover escaped attention until it was pointed out by Slagsvold.[29]

This development points also to the fact that the original design of Andresen was not effective enough and that the increase in the interocclusal clearance was necessary. Simultaneously, as already pointed out, the theoretical superstructure built by Häupl lost any connection with actual treatment procedures.

The effect of muscular pressure is increased by immobilizing the activator. Herren achieved that by adding clasps on the lateral maxillary teeth and by the increased length of the lateral mandibular wings of the appliance[30] (see Chapter 8). The construction bite dislocates the mandible in a vertical and sagittal direction. Additional pressure is obtained by an increase of the dislocation in either direction. The activator of Herren makes use of maximal sagittal displacement. The designs of Harvold[31] and Woodside (see Chapter 12) increase the vertical dimension of the construction bite.

There are numerous reports about the working of the activator and the results achieved. Yet, as Ahlgren points out,[32] few systematic longitudinal studies of the treatment results with activators have been presented in the literature (Harvold and Vargervik, 1971;[31] Ahlgren, 1972;[32] Demisch, 1972[30]). Study of these reports is most productive, especially a detailed comparison of the peculiarities of the results achieved. Quantitative measurements, their frequency and distribution, should be scrutinized. With more such studies forthcoming, it should be possible to connect particular details of the appliance used with particular features of the results obtained. That will be even more productive later, when studies with myotonic and myodynamic appliances will be compared.

Myodynamic Appliances

The development of the myodynamic appliances is due to the ingenuity of H. P. Bimler. He was involved in the treatment of jaw injuries during World War II. One of his patients had lost the left gonial angle of the mandible, together with the adjacent soft tissues. The right side of the mandible had been provisionally fixed by wires to the maxilla, but the pull of the developing scar tissue had drawn the remaining part of the mandible to the left to such an extent that the lower right canine was touching the left upper canine. Bimler constructed an activator-like device, consisting of a thin maxillary plate with a splint, into which the patient inserted the remaining part of the mandible. In two weeks normal occlusion was re-established, but subsequently the muscular pressure led to a minor widening in the maxillary dental arch. From this observation Bimler deduced the possibility of expanding the maxillary arch by the crosswise transmission of transverse mandibular movements[33, 34] (see Chapter 13).

Attempts to apply these principles in the design of an appliance led Bimler to the construction of a number of prototypes, which he subsequently rejected.[35] Some of these may have influenced the making of other devices. In 1949, a description of his method was published in its final form. The appliance, then named "elastischer Gebissformer," had important new features. Its reduced size made possible its wearing during the entire day, thus preventing the "daily relapse" of the improvements obtained during the night. Its elasticity was meant to translate muscular movements in a more effective manner to the dentition and supporting structures. Furthermore, as the maxillary and mandibular parts of the device were connected by a wire, a gradual forward positioning of the mandible became possible. The feasibility of combining active and passive forces was shown.

Bimler and his appliances were furiously attacked by the functional jaw orthopedics establishment. Yet every functional appliance developed subsequently has made use of one or another of his innovations. These were not simply "skeletonized" activators but actual design changes. For example, the original activator was adapted by A. M. Schwarz as a bow activator to make a change in the relationship of the maxillary and mandibular parts possible. In a different form, other modifications were introduced by Karwetzky as a U-bow activator. Both are described in Chapter 8. It is noteworthy too that during the quarter of a century since the first description of it was published, the Bimler appliance has become more sophisticated and more varied, thereby permitting it to perform different tasks, but the principles have remained essentially the same.

The various methods described in this book bear witness to the variability of the principles underlying the myodynamic appliances. Stockfisch, originally a disciple of Bimler, has modified the "elastic bite former" and produced the Kinetor, which has the advantage of prefabrication of some of the critical parts, ease of assembly, modification, and repair, and the use of short rubber tubes between maxillary and mandibular appliance elements to stimulate the needed exercise (see Chapter 14). The Kinetor comes closer to being an active appliance. The elastic open activator of Klammt, combining features of different devices, is a more passive appliance (see Chapter 11). The bionator will be mentioned in another connection (see Chapter 9).

As stated above, there have been only a few satisfactory systematic studies of treatment results with the myotonic appliances. Apparently there are none dealing with the myodynamic devices. The most important reason for this may be that each of these appliances is used in a number of different designs to suit the purpose of the particular treatment. This makes the examination of closed groups treated in the same manner rather difficult.

The Function Corrector of Fränkel

Fränkel's appliance does not fit into either of the two groups of functional appliances described. The FR III, for the treatment of Class III conditions, is in part a myotonic device with an interesting different use of muscular pressure. That, however, is not the case with the FR I; moreover, muscular movements are not transmitted by this device. Consequently, his appliance requires a category of its own and must be studied separately (see Chapter 15)

A few decades ago, hardly anyone would have believed the possibility of the near-miraculous changes that the activator has been able to effect. An appliance that corrects malocclusions with practically no contact with the dentition still seems incredible. That, however, is exactly what the method of Rolf Fränkel does.

Fränkel's approach differs from other methods because he makes the oral vestibule the "operational basis" for his treatment. Oral screens or vestibular plates have been used for a long time. The propulsor, for example, designed by Mühlemann (see Chapter 5), combines them with an activator-like device. But these appliances, although very useful in some instances, have only limited possibilities.

There is only one precursor of Fränkel's ideas. Frantisek Kraus of Prague[36, 37] used the oral screens in a different way. His theories are not without interest in connection with the history of the Fränkel method. According to Kraus, the physiological development of the motor stereotype in muscular action in the orofacial system is interrupted by the results of a substitute, thumb, or tongue sucking, leading to a functional disturbance in the formation of the skeletal components.

Kraus believed that the discontinuation of the habit would in some cases bring about spontaneous rehabilitation of everything caused by the unnatural function. In others, "an inhibition of the initial cause" would be necessary. For that purpose, he used vestibular screens that were not allowed to touch the teeth anywhere and were extended to the transitional fold of the mucous membrane of both jaws (see Chapter 4). By inhibiting the unnatural causes, the development of the orofacial system is freed from both the functional and formative disturbances and it reverts to its normal physiologic trend.

Fränkel is in agreement with Kraus that malocclusion, especially that caused by crowding of the teeth, may result from a disturbance of the tonus as well as of the function of the perioral muscles, and this is the key problem for successful treatment. He does not, however, limit his appliances to inhibition and exclusion of the faulty muscular function only. Rather, he attempts to influence function in a more positive way, similar to that of orthopedic therapy, by utilizing some kind of exercises aiming at the re-education of the muscles concerned. By reducing the size of the vestibular screens, Fränkel has tried to overcome the narrow limits of an inhibitory therapy only, and to construct a device that may be worn during the day and thus make "jaw-orthopedic" exercises possible. Further study and experience and the analysis of the remarkable results of treatment have considerably broadened that original concept. Fränkel had already gained considerable experience through his original construction and use of buccal shields. Initially, his function corrector was nothing more than two buccal shields, connected by wires but without any clasps to fasten them to the teeth. Practical experience led to further reduction of the size of the shields and improved the shape of the connecting wires. Addition of other wire elements and acrylic parts served to augment the particular purpose of that kind of treatment. So gradually the function corrector acquired its present form.

Fränkel has clarified many details of the mode of action of the function corrector. It may, perhaps, be worthwhile to explore further by a deductive and speculative approach. In Chapter 15 the widening of the dental arches achieved by the function corrector is shown. The equilibrium of buccolingual muscle forces is controversial. Research indicates that it is not a simple one-to-one relationship. Yet, when the Fränkel appliance relieves the pressure exerted on the teeth and supporting tissues by the buccinator mechanism, the resultant widening of the dental arches and even the apical base could be regarded as proof that some sort of equilibrium existed before the insertion of the appliance and that it has been changed.

Expansion, for many years regarded as an essential part of treatment, has been shown to be made futile by a relapse in most cases. The stability of the results achieved by the function corrector may, therefore, be interpreted as connected with a change in the original muscular balance and the establishment of a new balance. If that can happen in the transverse dimension, the possibility of a similar occurrence in the sagittal and vertical dimensions has to be considered. It is, in fact, the professed aim of the FR I to achieve a new balance between the protractor and retractor ·muscles of the mandible. All myofunctional methods, which bring the mandible forward with the construction bite, keep it fixed in this protruded position by the appliance. The now more or less obsolete FR Ia, however, induces the patient to retain it in this position first by voluntary action, then subconsciously, helped only by wire loops barely touching the mucosa in the lower canine region. The therapeutic dislocation of the mandible has, however, a downward component also and, therefore, the sagittal and vertical dimensions must be considered in conjunction.

In 1952, Hotz and Mühlemann,[28] writing about the treatment of deep overbite, differentiated between two conditions, one with a small, the other with a large, interocclusal clearance between the posterior teeth in the rest position. They stated that the vertical development of the alveolar parts, under the influence of an appliance making use of an existing large freeway space, will remain constant. The same development, with a small freeway space, will leave no interocclusal clearance and relapse will follow. The same can be expressed in different terms. The oral functioning space is the space of the oral cavity with the teeth in occlusion increased by the additional space provided by the interocclusal clearance in the rest position. The functional space is thus determined by the postural position of the mandible and consequently cannot be altered. A. M. Schwarz[12] shrewdly remarked that that would be possible only by a change in the temporomandibular joint alone, which would be difficult to obtain.

It appears that the size of the functioning space is not likely to change subsequent to alterations brought about by treatment. The situation could be different if the desired change in the functioning space is effected first. That can be done, for example, by the insertion of a bionator, bringing the incisors into an edge-to-edge bite (see Chapter 9). Children tolerate the appliance very well when worn throughout the day. That may not be due solely to the reduced size of the appliance. The children seem to feel quite comfortable with the incisors in an edge-to-edge relationship. After all, this is the natural position for the incising and shearing of food and gives support to the opposing teeth. The organism is thus confronted with an enlarged functioning space which it does not need or want and must come to terms with it. Consequently, compensatory changes should follow.

Some observations appear to support such a supposition. S. F. Fish[38] examined the paired cephalometric radiographs of 55 edentulous patients, one pair with the dentures in place and the other with the dentures removed. In 71 per cent of the patients, a forward movement of the pharyngeal part of the tongue was observed after the removal of the dentures. The tongue moved forward to fill the enlarged space. Movements of other soft tissues as well as a closing movement of the mandible seem to serve the same purpose. The hypothesis is proposed by Fish that the "rest position" of the mandible is determined by the demands of the tongue in performing its respiratory function of completing the anterior wall of the pharyngeal part of the respiratory tract.

The surgical repositioning of the mandible for the correction of mandibular protrusion will decrease the functioning space. Some reports indicate that the simultaneous repositioning of the tongue is followed by adaptive changes. Grimm and Beitlich[39] found that after the operation, the hyoid-pogonion and hyoid-sella distances were increased, but after a time the pre-operative measurements were re-established. Sergl and Sitzmann[40] studied head plates to determine the effect of the operation on tongue position and pharyngeal air space. The results indicate that the pharyngeal space decreased through a repositioning of the tongue. Over a longer period the original spatial relationship was re-established by adaptive changes. It is not surprising, therefore, that Fromm and Lundberg,[41] two years after the surgical correction, found the position of the hyoid bone in relation to the cervical vertebrae and the reference point outside the mandible unchanged. They observed, however, a postoperative alteration of the head position. Solow and Tallgren[42, 43] found that even a slight change of the head position is reflected in the vertebral column. It is apparent that all of the muscular balance systems of the region are interconnected or perhaps part of one balance system. Some of the variations found by the investigations may be explained by the smaller or greater distance of the hyoid bone in relation to the mandibular plane. Cuozzo and Bowman[44] point out that the displacement of the base of the tongue with the hyoid bone could be limited by the stylohyoid ligament in instances of greater distance. The studies mentioned have been carried out with the teeth in occlusion. It would be interesting to ascertain whether findings would be different with the mandible in rest position.

Apparently there is some evidence that adaptive changes will follow alterations in the muscular balance system. It is suggested that such changes may be provoked by an appliance interfering effectively with the existing muscular balance. In addition to myotonic and myodynamic appliances there could be a third group. Until a more apt designation is found, they could be called appliances attempting postural guidance.

Growth and development are to a great extent determined by function. The part played by muscular balance is not well documented. Yet Bosma[45] stated, "Although there are mechanisms of autonomous development in these peripheral areas such as the growth and eruption of the teeth, the general form and arrangement of the mouth and pharynx *directly reflect their performances, particularly, I believe, the postural performance*" (italics added). It is not unreasonable to believe that an artificial change in the postural position could be exploited therapeutically.

Mandibular Growth

Controversy surrounds the question of whether additional mandibular growth can be induced by a myofunctional appliance. The affirmative answer of many leading European orthodontists is based on undeniable clinical experience. However, abundant reports of cephalometric studies attempting to give objective proof have failed to convince at least an equal number of investigators holding the opposite view. There seems to be no evidence, however, as to whether condylar adaptation is important from a practical point of view. In other words, will an otherwise perfect result lose its value if obtained without some change in the condyles? Apparently no systematic study has been published relating the achievement of condylar adaptation or the lack of such to a change in the physiognomy of the patient.

The result of the study undertaken by Harvold and Vargervik did not show condylar changes. Woodside, in Chapter 12 of this book, comes to the same conclusion. Demisch reported on the treatment of 28 children with Class II, Division 1 malocclusion with the activator of Herren (see Chapter 8). In four cases, treatment was abandoned for different reasons. In the remaining 24 patients, normal relationship of the dental arches was achieved entirely by activator therapy. In 16 cases, a preliminary observation period had been recorded. In half of these, treatment clearly induced an increased growth rate of the mandible, whereas in the other half the normal growth rate was maintained. No correlation with age or forward positioning of the chin was found.[30]

Stöckli and Dietrich[46] reported on an experimental and clinical investigation. In the latter, 25 cases of Class II, Division 1 malocclusions were treated with activators over a period of 18 months. After the successful treatment, there was a highly significant change in the SNA, SNB, and ANB angles, when pre- and post-treatment recordings were compared. In order to take into account the influence of normal growth, the results were compared with results in a group of untreated children observed by van der Linden. There was a significant decrease of the SNA angle of the treated children, but no increase of the SNB angle beyond the limits of normal variation. The authors concluded the following:

1. Activator treatment lacks the potential to induce adaptive tissue responses in the condylar cartilage and in the glenoid region. This would be necessary to produce the changes in vector of osseous tissue growth with a resultant translation of mandible downward and forward.

2. Tissue response may take place in the temporomandibular joint structures during activator treatment, but the reaction is so scanty in intensity, extent, and duration that, from a clinical standpoint, no significant increment in the desired direction can be obtained.

3. Histologic studies in monkeys indicate that the temporomandibular joint structures can be influenced by mechanical stimuli, but clinically we are still lacking the means to exploit this.

The arguments against condylar adaptation seem overwhelming. Nevertheless, some points can be made. The Harvold as well as the Woodside activator uses a very high construction bite. Thus, a considerable vertical pressure of the stretched muscles is evoked with practically no horizontal component. The Herren activator, with a maximal forward position of the mandible, yields somewhat different results. In the investigations, only activator appliances were tested. The results, therefore, need not apply to the myodynamic appliances. Finally, results of recent research by Petrovic and McNamara can be interpreted as indicating that a more favorable condylar response to treatment may be possible if, through action of the appliance, a proper stimulus is provided.

The research of Petrovic and his coworkers[47] has shown the great importance of the lateral pterygoid muscle for the forward growth of the mandible, and the possibility of its stimulation by changed function. To achieve that, the animal is forced by an inclined plane to move the mandible forward. Pulling the mandible in the same direction by elastics does not elicit the response.

A mandible brought forward will stay there after the conclusion of the experiment. It can be argued that such a result should be more stable when an artificial situation is not created but an abnormal Class II, Division 1 condition is rectified. Post-treatment "bounce-back" should be less.

The complexity of the neuromuscular and skeletal adaptation to altered orofacial function shown by J. A. McNamara[48] will discourage premature practical conclusions. Yet the extent to which mandibular skeletal adaptation is diminished in the older age groups of the animals could indicate the advantage of appliances which can be inserted at a very early age. The limitation observed in the amount and duration of the structural adaptation within the head of the condyloid process, however, need not apply to the orthodontic patient. In the experimental animal the mandible can be brought forward only comparatively little in comparison with the possibility in the human being with an overjet of 8 to 9 mm. The stimuli provided by the forward movement of the mandible should thus be of greater duration and intensity there. More research on the adaptive potential of the temporomandibular fossa itself is indicated. The membranous bone structure should be more amenable in guiding forces, with possible alteration of the articular eminence as well as the fossa during a rapid growth period. In the final analysis, the changes that occur may well be a combination of condylar, temporomandibular fossa, mandibular, basal bone, and alveolodental changes. The exact role of each structural modification will depend on a multiplicity of factors in each individual — morphogenetic pattern, age, sex, functional pattern, appliance control, orofacial habits, and other as yet unequated factors.

THE FUNCTIONAL MATRIX CONCEPT

It should be apparent that thoughts expressed in this chapter are closely related to the functional matrix concept evolved by M. L. Moss.[49-52] His concept provided the basis for the study of the problems and the comparison of clinical experience and theoretical considerations. The appliances attempting postural guidance could in more general terms be regarded as clinical applications of the functional matrix hypothesis. This, however, was not meant to be used as a blueprint or justification for any particular construction.

According to the theory, the functioning oral space is the capsular matrix in which the mandible is embedded. The expansion in volume of this space will lower the mandible and induce compensatory growth of the condylar process to keep intact its articulation with the articular eminence. It would seem at first glance that the passive "translation" of the mandible thus described could be reproduced by the construction bite of functional appliances. However, the corresponding growth of the condylar process presumed by the activator theories has not been clearly substantiated. That should not be surprising, as the primary factor is the expansion in volume of the oral space. The size of the functioning space, however, corresponds to the demands of function. Yet an alteration of the space, for example, by surgical correction of mandibular protrusion, does not impede breathing. No such disturbance is reported. That begs the question as to why the instantaneous adaptations observed seem to be of a transient nature. There may be a logical answer. The first compensatory changes do not provide an economical muscular balance. That would come by a more complicated readjustment. These considerations, although of uncertain value and validity, may yet be pertinent to the question discussed and should be pursued further.

The attempt to obtain condylar adaptation with the treatment of Class II, Division 1 malocclusion is apparently based on two dubious assumptions: the Class II condition is connected with an underdevelopment of the mandible, and additional growth to make up for the deficiency could be stimulated. Apparently, a majority, judging by the clinical results obtained, believed them to be insignificant. As pointed out earlier, however, recent research may give some pointers. Hyperpropulsion was shown to be effective in the experiments of Petrovic and coworkers. Used in conjunction with a suitable manipulation of the functioning space and an early beginning of treatment, it might bring about a more favorable reaction at the condyle. Treatment using the function corrector or the bionator may provide the opportunity for observations that might help to clarify these problems.

A number of functional methods are described in this book. A clarification of the differences among them seemed justified. A speculative approach to some problems was assumed to be of some use also. The next chapter will show the difficulty of reaching conclusions by a more customary review of the development.

References

1. Kingsley, N. W.: Oral Deformities. New York, D. Appleton & Co., 1880.
2. Robin, P.: Demonstration pratique sur la construction et la mise en bouche d'un nouvel appareil de redressement. Rev. Stomatol., *9*:561–590, 1902.
3. Rogers, A. P.: Exercises for the development of the muscles of the face, with a view to increase their functional activity. Dent. Cosmos, *60*:857–876, 1918.
4. Rogers, A. P.: Making facial muscles our allies in treatment and retention. Dent. Cosmos, *64*:711–730, 1922.
5. Andresen, V.: Beitrag zur Retention. Z. Zahnaerztl. Orthop., *3*:121–125, 1910.
6. Andresen, V.: Gnathologische Rhinologie. Die "Glossoptose" und die Funktionskieferorthopädie. Dtsch. Zahnaerztl Wochenschr., *45*:665–669, 1942.
7. Andresen, V.: The Norwegian system of functional gnatho-orthopedics. Acta Gnathol., *1*:5–36, 1936.
8. Andresen, V., and Häupl, K.: Funktionskieferorthopädie. Leipzig, H. Meusser, 1936.
9. Anderson, G. M.: Practical Orthodontics, 9th ed. St. Louis, The C. V. Mosby Co., 1960.
10. Angle, E. H.: Malocclusion of the Teeth, 7th ed. Philadelphia, S. S. White Dental Manufacturing Co., 1907.
11. Schwarz, A. M.: Gebissregelung mit Platten. Vienna, Urban & Schwarzenberg, 1938.
12. Schwarz, A. M.: Lehrgang der Gebissregelung II, 2nd ed. Vienna, Urban & Schwarzenberg, 1956.
13. Dewey, M.: Practical Orthodontia, 4th ed. St. Louis, The C. V. Mosby Co., 1919.
14. Hotz, R.: Die Grundlagen kieferorthopädischer Behandlung. Studieweek, 125–155, 1960.
15. Izard, G.: Orthodontie, 3rd ed. Paris, Masson, 1950.
16. Robin, P.: Die Pathogenie der durch die Glossoptosis beim Säugling, beim Kind und beim Erwachsenen verursachten Störungen. La Semaine Dentaire, 1926.
17. Ascher, F.: Praktische Kieferorthopädie. München, Urban & Schwarzenberg, 1968.

18. Cauhépé, J., and Coutand, A.: Die Fernröngenaufnahme. Leipzig, J. A. Barth, 1956.
19. Duyzings, J. C. A.: Form und Funktion in Zusammenhang mit dento-maxillarer, facialer, cranialer and zervikaler Orthopädie. Studieweek, 48–82, 1960.
20. Watry, F.: Die physiotherapeutische Behandlung der Kiefer-deformitäten. Fortschr. Orthod., *3*:196–200, 318–330, 1933.
21. Neumann, B.: Amerikanische orthodontische Behandlungsmethoden. Fortschr. Orthod. *2*:193–214, 1932.
22. Review of "Allied Orthodontia" by McCoy. Int. J. Orthod., *17*:801–802, 1931.
23. Cleall, J.: Malocclusions, orthodontic corrections and orofacial muscle adaptation. Angle Orthod., *40*:170–201, 1970.
24. Farrar, J. N.: A Treatise on Irregularities of the Teeth and Their Correction. New York, International News Co., 1888.
25. Häupl, K.: Personal communication, 1937.
26. Roux, W.: Beitrage zur Morphologie der functionallen Anpassung. Arch. Physiol. Anat., *9*:120–158, 1885.
27. Häupl, K.: Gewebsumbau und Zahnverdrängung in der Funkskieferorthopädie. Leipzig, J. A. Barth, 1938.
28. Hotz, R., and Mühlemann, H.R.: Die Funktion in der Beurteilung und Therapie von Bissanomalien. Schweiz. Monatschr. Zahnheilkd., *62*:592–606, 1952.
29. Neumann, B.: Funktionskieferorthopädie–Rückblick und Ausblick. Fortschr. Kieferorthop., *36*:73–85, 1975.
30. Demisch, A.: Effects of activator therapy on craniofacial skeleton in Class II/1. Trans. Eur. Orthod. Soc., 1972, 295–310.
31. Harvold, E. P., and Vargervik, K.: Morphogenetic response to activator treatment. Am. J. Orthod., *60*:478, 1971.
32. Ahlgren, J.: A longitudinal clinical and cephalometric study of 50 malocclusion cases treated with activator appliances. Trans. Eur. Orthod. Soc., 1972, 285–293.
33. Bimler, H, P.: Die elastisches Gebissformer. Zahnaerztl. Welt, *4*:499–503, 1949.
34. Bimler, H. P.: Personal communication, 1976.
35. Bimler, H. P.: Unpublished material.
36. Kraus, F.: Vestibular and oral screen. Trans. Eur. Orthod. Soc., 1956, 217–224.
37. Kraus, F.: Prevence a naprava vyvoijovych vad otofacialni soustavy. Statni zdravotnicke nakladatelstvi, Prague, 1956.
38. Fish, S. F.: The respiratory associations of the rest position of the mandible. Br. Dent. J., *116*:149–159, 1964.
39. Grimm, G., and Beitlich, E.: Kritische Bewertung der Operationsergebnisse von 101 Progeniefällen unter besonderer Berücksichtigung des Verfahrens nach Obwegeser-Dal Pont. Dtsch. Zahn. Mund. Kieferheilkd., *61*:295–313, 1973.
40. Sergl, H. G., and Sitzmann, F.: Zunge und pharyngealer Raum bei operativer Rückverlagerung des Unterkiefers. Fortschr. Kieferorthop., *36*:401–408, 1975.
41. Fromm, B., and Lundberg, M.: Postural behaviour of the hyoid bone in normal occlusion and before and after surgical correction of mandibular protrusion. Sven. Tandlak. Tidskr., *63*:425–433, 1970.
42. Solow, B., and Tallgren, A.: Postural changes in craniocervical relationships. Tandlaegebladet, *75*:1247–1257, 1971.
43. Solow, B., and Tallgren, A.: Head posture and craniofacial morphology. Am. J. Phys. Anthropol., *44*:417–435, 1976.
44. Cuozzo, G. S., and Bowman, D. C.: Hyoid positioning during deglutition following forced positioning of the tongue. Am. J. Orthod., *68*:564–570, 1975.
45. Bosma, J. F.: Form and function in the mouth and pharynx of the human infant. *In* McNamara, J. F., Jr. (Ed.): Control Mechanisms in Craniofacial Growth. Monograph No. 3, Craniofacial growth series, Center for Human Growth and Development, University of Michigan, Ann Arbor, 1975.
46. Stöckli, P. W., and Dietrich, U. C.: Sensation and morphogenesis: Experimental and clinical findings following functional forward displacement of the mandible. Trans. Eur. Orthod. Soc. 3rd International Congress, 1973, pp. 435–442.
47. Petrovic, A., Oudet, C., and Gasson, N.: Effets des appareils de propulsion et de rétropulsion mandibulaire sur le nombre des sarcomeres en serie du muscle pterygoidien externe et sur la croissance du cartilage condylien du jeune rat. Orthod. Fr., *44*:191–212, 1973.
48. McNamara, J. A., Jr.: Neuromuscular and Skeletal Adaptations to Altered Orofacial Function. Monograph No. 1, Craniofacial growth series, Center for Human Growth and Development, University of Michigan, Ann Arbor, 1972.
49. Moss, M. L., and Salentijn, L.: The primary role of functional matrices in facial growth. Am. J. Orthod., *55*:566–577, 1969.
50. Moss, M. L., and Salentijn, L.: The capsular matrix. Am. J. Orthod., *56*:474–490, 1969.
51. Moss, M. L.: Functionelle Schädelanalyse und die funtionelle Matrix. Fortschr. Kieferorthop., *34*:48–63, 1973.
52. Moss, M. L.: The primacy of functional matrices in orofacial growth. Dent. Pract., *19*:65–73, 1968.

CHAPTER 7

Activator Development and Philosophy

OLAV SLAGSVOLD

HYPOTHESES ON THE ACTIVATOR'S MODE OF ACTION IN CLASS II MALOCCLUSION TREATMENT

The Original Activator

According to the theories of Roux[112] and Wolff,[137] changes in function bring with them changes in internal bone structure and external bone form. In accordance with these theories, Andresen[5] aimed at correcting malocclusions by changing the functional pattern of the chewing apparatus. Thus, he claimed that a Class II relationship can gradually be changed into a Class I relationship by an appliance that makes the patient bite with the lower jaw in a normal relationship to the upper. Such an appliance will elicit increased activity in the protractors and the elevators, and relaxation and stretching of the retractors. Dysfunctions will be eliminated, and an adjustment of the complete orofacial muscle complex to the new functional pattern will be induced. An adjustment will also take place in bony structures. The teeth will be moved by intermittent forces generated in the muscles and transmitted through the appliance. Gradually the whole chewing apparatus will adapt to the jaw relationship prescribed by the appliance.[6, 7] Moreover, the changes brought about in muscular functional and structural patterns ensure a permanent retention of the improvements achieved in occlusion and craniofacial pattern.[8]

The appliance should in itself be passive (Fig. 7–1). To meet the theoretic requirements, it should force the mandible to assume a new closing pattern, bringing it into the desired relationship to the upper jaw (Figs. 7–2 to 7–4). Furthermore, it should be loose in the mouth in order to provoke the orofacial muscles, particularly the protractors and the elevators of the mandible, to bite it into place.[5, 6, 7] In other words, it was designed to change the functional pattern and also to activate the function. It was therefore named the activator.[8] It was recommended that the activator be used at night.[6]

Andresen[6] originally called his system biomechanical orthodontics. Later the name was changed to functional jaw orthopedics and then to the Norwegian system.[8] Andresen's hypothesis has been opposed by several authors.

133

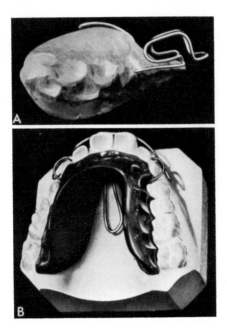

Figure 7-1. Activator designed for the treatment of a Class II, Division 1 malocclusion. (From: Andresen, V., and Häupl, K.: Funktionskieferorthopadie. Die Grundlagen des "norwegischen Systems," 2nd ed. Leipzig, H. Meusser, 1939.)

One of the first to reject it was Selmer-Olsen.[119] He stated that muscles cannot be stimulated to action at night, because Nature has designed them to rest during sleep. He believed that the mandible normally assumes a position of equilibrium between forces deriving from the oral and extraoral tissues: the opening and the closing muscles, the tongue, the cheeks, the fascial sheets, and the ligaments. An opening beyond this position requires active work from the opening muscles to overcome the resistance of the stretched fibers in the soft tissues. If a foreign body is inserted between the dental arches, the lower jaw is kept beyond the position of equilibrium, the closing muscles remain stretched, and a pressure is applied against the foreign body through the teeth. Hence, the tooth-moving forces in activator therapy are not brought into being by muscle function (kinetic energy), but by a stretching of the soft tissues (potential energy). Woodside calls this visco-elastic properties (see Chapter 12).

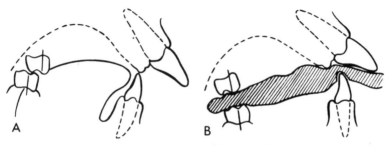

Figure 7-2. Construction bite (B) for Class II, Division 1 malocclusion treatment (A). (From Andresen, V., and Häupl, K.: Funktionskieferorthopädie. Die Grundlagen des "norwegischen Systems," 2nd ed. Leipzig, H. Meusser, 1939.)

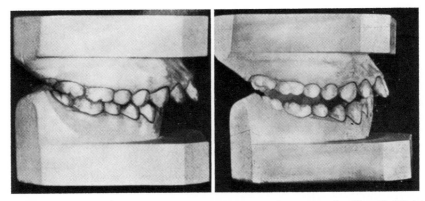

Figure 7-3. Mandibular displacement by activator treatment of a Class II, Division 1 malocclusion, as recommended by Andresen. (From Andresen, V., and Häupl, K.: Funktionskieferorthopädie. Die Grundlagen des "norwegischen Systems," 3rd ed. Leipzig, J. A. Barth, 1942.)

The disagreements between Andresen and Selmer-Olsen reflect current divergencies in the analysis of muscle response to the activator. In terms of present-day concepts, Andresen's interpretation presupposes freedom for the mandible to assume rest position. It does not appear from the literature that he considered the degree of mandibular displacement in relation to this position. Nevertheless, it would mean a violation of his principles to displace the mandible beyond it.

It may be added that Andresen taught a very moderate vertical displacement of the mandible with the appliance in place. Originally, he recommended an interocclusal molar clearance of only 2 mm., or the thickness of a match.[8, 9] Later he changed it to 2 to 3 mm.[10] and then to 2 to 4 mm.[11] Such a degree of displacement does not usually bring the lower jaw beyond rest position in a caudal direction, at least not in sleeping individuals, according to Andresen.

Selmer-Olsen's interpretation was based on the assumption that the mandible is displaced beyond rest position by the appliance. He had a well-defined view on this position. Furthermore, his interpretation of the dynamics of the various mandibular positions is in full agreement with findings made several years later.[2, 128, 135] He did not define and specify the freeway space, but it is im-

Figure 7-4. A Class II malocclusion profile with and without an activator inserted. (From Grude, R.: Myo-functional therapy. A review of various cases some years after their treatment by the Norwegian system had been completed. Nor. Tannlaegeforen. Tid., 62:1-28, 1952.)

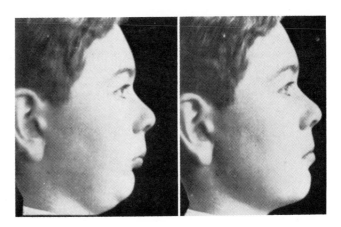

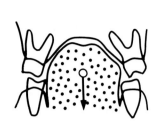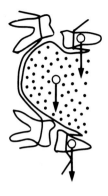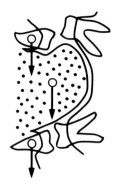

Figure 7–5. The mandibular rest position is influenced by gravity and varies with head postures.

plicit in his reasoning that it would be less than 2 mm. during sleep. On this assumption, the conclusion had to be that Andresen's hypothesis could not be true.

Thompson's studies[128] on the mandibular rest position also help delineate the degree of opening and had an influence on activator theories. Andresen's associate, Grude,[56] in his interpretation of the principles of activator therapy, concluded that the appliance works in the way postulated, provided that the mandible is not displaced beyond rest position. If it is deprived of the freedom of assuming this position its mode of action becomes fundamentally changed.[57]

Herren,[69] also analyzing the activator's mode of action on the basis of the spatial relationship between the mandible and postural rest position, came to the opposite conclusion: the activator does not work in the way postulated by Andresen, even if the caudal displacement of the mandible is less than 3 mm. Such an appliance does not increase the frequency of closing movements, and the tooth-moving forces are not brought into being by the activator in movement. An interpretation of his hypothesis follows.

The equilibrium between the forces acting upon the mandible in rest position is established and maintained by a continuous interaction between them. Gravity and air pressure are the dominant independent variables, muscle tension and muscle tonus the dominant dependent variables. When the equilibrium is disturbed by changes in the gravity vector and/or the intraoral pressure, the mandible is pulled to a location where these changes are compensated for by changes in muscle tension and muscle tonus (Fig. 7–5). Also, changes in muscle tonus are followed by a relocation of the mandible, whereby they are compensated for by changes in muscle tension.

The mandibular position prescribed by the activator is the desired postural rest position rather than the momentary rest position (Fig. 7–4). With an activator inserted, the mandible has a very limited mobility in all directions of space except caudally. It is more or less prevented from assuming any rest position lateral, anterior, or posterior to the position prescribed by the appliance. Hence, it is unable to assume most of the rest positions that occur during a night's wear. The forces which pull the mandible towards these rest positions are absorbed by the appliance and transmitted to the teeth and the alveolar processes (Fig. 7–6). These are the forces which move the teeth. Mandibular movements do occur, but the forces thereby created are of minor importance only, according to Herren.

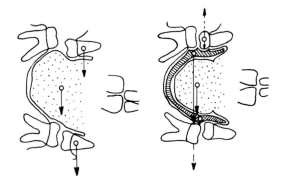

Figure 7-6. When the activator does not permit the mandible to assume rest position, forces are transmitted by the activator to the teeth and the alveolar processes. (From Herren, P.: Die Wirkungsweise des Aktivators. Schweiz. Monatsschr. Zahnheilkd., 63:829–879, 1953.)

The direction of the resultant force acting on the activator depends on the spatial relationship between the momentary rest position and the position in which the mandible is restricted by the appliance (Fig. 7–7). Accordingly, it varies from time to time. The location of the rest position depends on head and body postures (see Fig. 7–5), level of wakefulness, or sleep, state of mind, intraoral vacuum, etc. It cannot be controlled by the orthodontist. Only the position in which the mandible is kept by the activator is determined by him. It can be varied in all directions of space to meet the requirements of the treatment plan in question.

Although the operator does not have complete control of the direction of the forces which act on the activator and thereby on the teeth, the control is

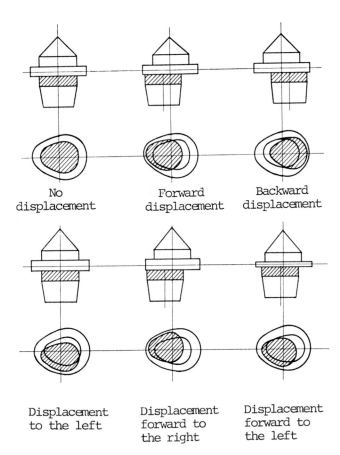

Figure 7-7. The direction of the force acting on the activator depends on the spatial relationship between the momentary rest position and the position prescribed by the activator. (From Herren, P.: Die Wirkungsweise des Aktivators. Sehweiz. Monatsschr. Zahnheilkd., 63: 829–879, 1953.)

No displacement Forward displacement Backward displacement

Displacement to the left Displacement forward to the right Displacement forward to the left

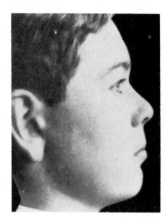

Figure 7-8. By an upright head position, muscle tension, muscle tonus, and air pressure balance the weights of the mandible, the soft tissues, and the activator. With an open mouth the weights are balanced by the muscles alone. (From Grude, R.: Myo-functional therapy. A review of various cases some years after their treatment by the Norwegian system had been completed. Nor. Tannlaegeforen. Tid., *62*:1–28, 1952.)

good enough to predict the direction of the tooth movements. In fact, the prevailing force direction is such that the dental arches adapt to the position in which the jaws are placed by the appliance.

The magnitude of the resultant forces acting on the activator depends on each and every one of the forces which act on the mandible, and on the interaction between them. The weights of the mandible, the tongue, and the appliance are constant. Herren[69] estimates the sum to be at least 250 grams. The forces deriving from muscle tension and muscle tonus vary in magnitude. Muscle tension, arising as a consequence of a stretching of the soft tissues, varies with the degree of the stretching, and accordingly with the degree of mandibular displacement and with head and body postures. Also, muscle tonus varies with the degree of muscle stretch. Furthermore, since it is controlled by the central nervous system, it varies with the state of mind, the level of wakefulness or sleep, etc., as previously pointed out. There is no doubt that muscle tension and muscle tonus constitute sources of considerable forces. Thus, by an upright head position and open mouth they balance the weights of the mandible and the tongue, and if necessary also the weight of the activator (Fig. 7–8).

In some head postures, the muscle tension, the muscle tonus, and the gravity vectors all act on the activator in the same direction. This is the case in a patient lying flat on his back with the mandible anteriorly displaced (Fig. 7–9). In other postures, the gravity vector and the muscle tension and the muscle tonus vectors act in different directions. They may even be diametrically opposed. This is the case in an upright head position (see Fig. 7–8). Accordingly, there is a considerable variation in the magnitude of the forces which act on the teeth.

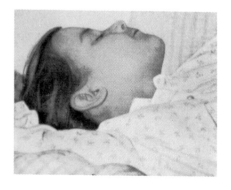

Figure 7-9. In a patient lying flat on his back, the muscle tension, the muscle tonus, and the gravity vectors all act on the activator in the same direction. (From Gerber, M.: Beobachtungen an schlafenden Aktivatorträgern. Fortschr. Kieferorthop., *18*:205–232, 1957.)

Although single teeth or tooth groups may be subjected to a continuous pressure for long periods of time, the forces are basically intermittent. The force application is interrupted every time the activator is removed from the mouth. The periodicity thereby introduced is called "the big intermittence." For the single teeth or tooth groups the forces may also be interrupted when the appliance is in the mouth. This shifting is called "the little intermittence."[70]

It appears that Herren has arrived at the same conclusion as Selmer-Olsen, although his reasoning is based on somewhat other premises.

In conclusion, there are two main theories concerning the original activator's mode of action. According to the first one, it is the activator in movement that moves the teeth. The forces are intermittent in nature, hitting the teeth as jolts. They are generated in the elevators of the mandible and other units in the orofacial muscle complex. The muscles are stimulated to action by an appliance that lies loose in the mouth, so that when it drops away from the upper jaw, it has to be replaced. It is a prerequisite for such a mode of action that the mandible is not displaced beyond postural rest position by the activator.[56]

The other hypothesis says that it is the activator at rest which moves the teeth. The appliance is squeezed between the jaws most of the time, and it is in this position that it exerts the tooth-moving forces. They vary in direction and magnitude. They may exert a continuous pressure against single teeth or tooth groups for long periods of time. However, the force application is also interrupted for periods of varying lengths.

Modified Activators

Some orthodontists have found the efficacy of the activator to be greater if the mandible is displaced farther caudally than indicated by Andresen (Fig. 7–10) (see Chapter 12).[2, 40, 138] Others believe that such a modification makes it easier for the patient to keep the appliance in the mouth.[77] While Andresen originally recommended an interocclusal molar clearance of a maximum of 4 mm., others have utilized clearances of 4 to 15 mm. or more.[2, 12, 14, 40, 54, 59-61, 74-77, 113, 114, 117, 127, 135, 138] Some authors state that they design their activators with a

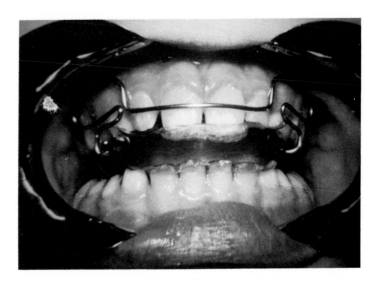

Figure 7–10. Activator with an interocclusal first molar clearance of 8 mm.

specified interocclusal molar clearance, exceeding the recommendations of Andresen by a varying number of millimeters.[12, 14, 40, 127, 135] Others claim that they displace the mandible a specified number of millimeters beyond rest position.[2, 3, 60, 61, 74, 75, 77, 138]

In accordance with the recommendations of Andresen,[6, 7] the activator is usually worn at night. Mandibular rest position during sleep will likely deviate from the rest position registered in the orthodontist's office during the day. As previously mentioned, it also varies with state of mind, level of wakefulness or sleep, and sleeping posture. Moreover, the height of the freeway space varies from individual to individual. Accordingly, it is not possible to define a circumscribed dimensional state between mandibular positions which are always and in all patients within freeway space, and mandibular positions which are always and in all patients beyond rest position. However, there can hardly be any doubt that many of the activators described in the literature displaced the mandible beyond rest position part of the time, most of the time, or all of the time they are in the mouth.

Despite this variance from Andresen's original theoretical appliance justification, such appliances are called activators. Many of the available reports on the activator's mode of action are based on studies of these modified appliances. Since they are commonly used, their mode of action is a matter of considerable interest.

Harvold[59] states that activators with a high construction bite spread the jaws apart. The effect is a stretching of the elevators and the retractors, as previously pointed out by Selmer-Olsen.[119] The forces thereby created are transmitted to the teeth. Woodside calls this visco-elastic force.

Similar thoughts have been presented by Herren and Ahlgren. Herren[69] based his hypothesis on studies of patients wearing activators that displaced the mandible 2 to 3 mm. below intercuspal position. As previously pointed out, he concluded that such activators are squeezed between the jaws most of the time they are inserted. That is true also for activators that displace the mandible beyond rest position, he says. Accordingly, the mode of action is in principle the same for all types of activators, regardless of the degree of vertical mandibular displacement. However, the forces are more constant in direction and more continuous in action on more pronounced displacements of the mandible. Furthermore, the force magnitude is greater, with one exception. With an open mouth the rest position is transferred farther down, and the pressure from the closing muscles on the appliance decreases.

Ahlgren[3] developed an hypothesis on the modified activator's mode of action, based on recent neurophysiologic research. In accordance with his findings in an electromyographic study of patients wearing activators which displaced the mandible beyond rest position, he presupposes that the elevators and the retractors are subjected to a stretch beyond their resting length as long as the appliance is in the mouth. Being elastically extensible, they respond by a passive tension. By increasing stretch, the tension increases exponentially, like a rubber band.

Stretching of muscles also gives rise to stretch reflex contractions, either of the tonic or the phasic type. A maintained stretch elicits a long-lasting tonic stretch reflex contraction, a momentary stretch gives rise to a transient phasic stretch reflex contraction. The stretch reflex elicited by the activator is of the tonic type.

The tonic activity varies with the level of wakefulness or sleep. In the waking state it is increased. In slow wave sleep it is depressed. In deep sleep it is completely abolished.

When worn during wakefulness, the activator elicits an increased frequency of swallowing movements, with an increased phasic muscle activity. Also, during deep sleep, phasic contractions of the tongue and the jaw muscles can be found.

In the waking state and during long periods of slow-wave sleep, the activator is squeezed between the teeth by the passive tension and the tonus in the stretched muscles. In this situation, it transfers a continuous force from the muscles to the teeth. During deep sleep, when the muscles are atonic, myoclonic twitches of the tongue and the mandible push the activator against the teeth, and thus intermittent forces are transmitted to them. Consequently, the activator works only sporadically in the intermittent fashion.

Schwarz[117] formed an hypothesis which seems to have been based mainly on studies of activators that have displaced the mandible farther caudally than recommended by Andresen. Activators create a stretching of various muscle groups, he says, and an active bite pressure, lasting for varying lengths of time, is elicited. It varies in magnitude with the blood pressure and with tetanic oscillations in the muscle contractions. The activator does not increase the frequency of mandibular movements.

Eschler,[39, 40] on the basis of electromyographic studies of the muscular response to activators with varying degrees of vertical mandibular displacements, developed an hypothesis that differs from those outlined above. He explains the response as a stretch reflex. Upon insertion of the appliance, the mandible is elevated by isotonic muscle contractions. These are succeeded by isometric, i.e., tonic, contractions, when the mandible assumes a static position in contact with the appliance. Because the mandible is prevented from reaching rest position, the elevators, and usually also the retractors, remain stretched. Fatigue sooner or later occurs, the contracted muscles relax, and the mandible drops down. When the muscles have recovered, the cycle starts over again.

Eschler[40] denies the activator's potential to activate the muscles, and particularly the protractors, directly. Its effect depends on the stretch reflex. Without a stretching of the muscles, there will be no effect of the appliance, and the effect is proportional to the degree of mandibular displacement. He recommends an interocclusal molar clearance of 4 to 6 mm. In agreement with Andresen, he believes in an increased frequency of mandibular movements when an activator is worn.

It thus appears that there are several hypotheses on the mode of action of activators which displace the mandible further caudally than recommended by Andresen. There is a good agreement between the hypotheses of Ahlgren,[3] Harvold,[59] Herren,[69] and Selmer-Olsen.[119] The disagreements between these authors and Schwarz[117] seem to be more attributable to differences in interpretation than in findings. In some respects there is also agreement with Eschler, but contrary to them, he claims that an increased frequency of mandibular movements is induced.

Most of these hypotheses have been based exclusively on observations and studies of activators that have displaced the mandible more than 4 mm. beyond intercuspal position. Still, they are claimed to be valid for all types of activators, regardless the degree of mandibular displacement.[100] As previously pointed out, it is implicit in Andresen's hypothesis that the mandible should not be displaced beyond postural rest position. It is a theoretic possibility that the original activator can act in the way postulated by Andresen, at least when the head is in an upright position. If the mandible is displaced beyond rest position, such a possibility does not exist. It is obvious that any hypothesis should be tested on its own premises. That also applies to Andresen's.

STUDIES ON THE ACTIVATOR'S MODE OF ACTION IN CLASS II MALOCCLUSION TREATMENT

The Original Activator

The activator's mode of action has been the subject of several studies.[1, 2, 14, 38-41, 47, 52, 69, 113, 114, 116, 117, 127, 133-135] Only few of them have been concerned with activators of the original design, with maximum interocclusal clearance of 4 mm.

Gerber[47] and Herren[69, 70] observed no increase in the frequency of mandibular movements in sleeping individuals wearing activators of the latter type. The muscles seemed relaxed. Aas[1] and Ahlgren[2] studied muscle activity in waking activator patients electromyographically. With the mandible at rest, Aas found a moderately increased activity in the posterior fibers of the temporal muscle, but the activity seems to have had the character of tonic stretch reflex contractions rather than phasic stretch reflex contractions (Fig. 7–11). Ahlgren found no evidence of an increased activity in the muscles studied. It should be noted that the lateral pterygoids were not included in any of these studies.

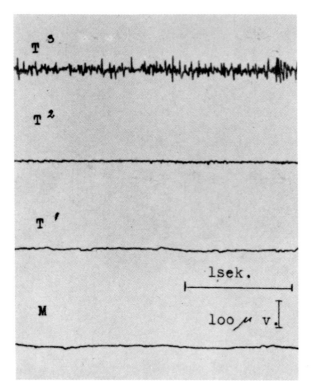

Figure 7–11. Activity in the masseter (M) and in the anterior (T^1), the intermediate (T^2), and the posterior (T^3) fibers of the temporal muscle in an awake patient, with the activator at rest. The mandible was displaced 3 mm. caudally and the width of a bicuspid anteriorly. (From Aas, B.: En elektromyografisk undersøkelse av m. temporalis og m. masseter ved forskjellige ortodontiske behandlingsmetoder. Nor. Tannlaegeforen. Tid., 70:85–103, 1960.)

The findings reported do not support the hypotheses of Andresen and Eschler, but they are compatible with those of Selmer-Olsen, Herren, and Ahlgren.

Modified Activators

Most of the studies on the activator's mode of action have been concerned with appliances that have displaced the mandible farther caudally than recommended by Andresen. Schwarz,[116, 117] watching patients during sleep, found no increased frequency in mandibular movements when such appliances were worn.

Eschler,[38, 40] on the basis of electromyographic studies, concluded that such activators, when worn during sleep, elicit a periodic shifting between isotonic contractions, isometric contractions, and relaxation in the retractors and the elevators.

Ahlgren,[2] in an electromyographic study, found no reflex biting on the activator or increased tonus during sleep. During waking hours, an increased tonus was observed in some of the muscles, especially when they were extensively stretched. Thilander and Filipsson,[127] also studying muscle activity electromyographically in waking patients, found only insignificant muscular activity when the activator was at rest (Fig. 7–12). During mandibular movements, an increased activity was observed, especially in the retractors (Fig. 7–13). Such

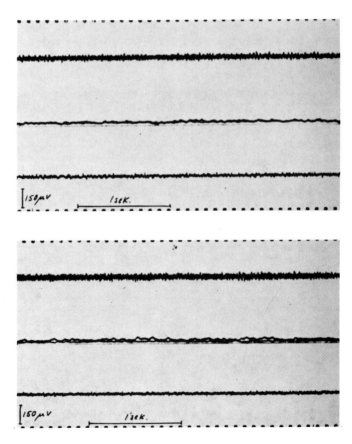

Figure 7–12. Activity in the suprahyoid (m.s.), the temporal (m.t.), and the masseter (m.m.) muscles in an awake patient with the activator at rest. The mandible was displaced more than 4 mm. caudally and the width of a cusp anteriorly. (From Thilander, B., and Filipsson, R.: Muscle activity related to activator and intermaxillary traction in Angle Class II, Division 1 malocclusions. An electromyographic study of the temporal, masseter and suprahyoid muscles. Acta Odontol. Scand., *24*: 241–257, 1966.)

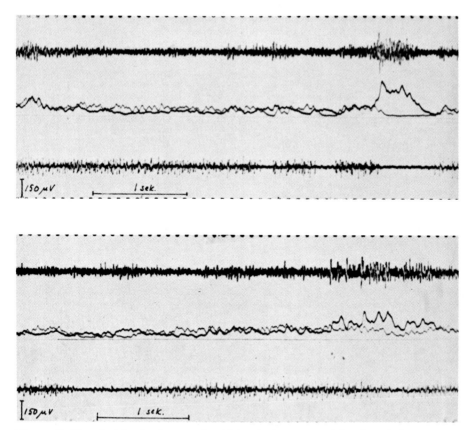

Figure 7–13. Activity in the suprahyoid (m.s.), the temporal (m.t.), and the masseter (m.m.) muscles in an awake patient with the activator "in function." Swallowing movements were performed spontaneously. The mandible was displaced more than 4 mm. caudally and the width of a cusp anteriorly. (From Thilander, B., and Filipsson, R.: Muscle activity related to activator and intermaxillary traction in Angle Class II, Division 1 malocclusions. An electromyographic study of the temporal, masseter and suprahyoid muscles. Acta Odontol. Scand., *24*:241–257, 1966.)

movements seemed to be provoked by the activator, presumably through an increased salivary production which required an increase in swallowing frequency.

Schmuth,[113, 115] Witt,[133] and Witt and Komposch,[135] evolving force curves by means of arrangements for pressure registrations (Figs. 7–14 and 7–15), found long periods of continuous pressure from the mandibular teeth against the activator when the mandible was displaced 4 to 6 mm. below intercuspal

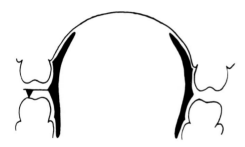

Figure 7–14. Transducer for the registration of vertical forces in activator therapy. (From Witt, E., and Komposch, G.: Intermaxilläre Kraftwirkung bimaxillärer Geräte. Fortschr. Kieferorthop., *32*:345–352, 1971.)

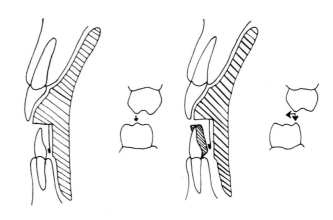

Figure 7-15. Transducer for the registration of the posterior forces against the activator, and the anterior forces against the lower incisors in activator therapy. The anterior mandibular displacement was increased by a splint on the lower incisors (right). (From Witt, E., and Komposch, G. Intermaxilläre Kraftwirkung bimaxillärer Geräte. Fortschr. Kieferorthop., *32*:345–352, 1971.)

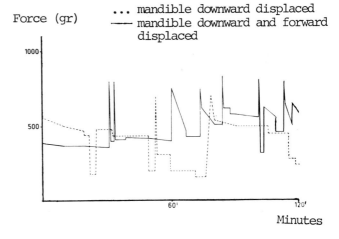

Figure 7-16. Variation in posterior forces against the activator during a two-hour period. (From Witt, E., and Komposch, G.: Intermaxilläre Kraftwirkung bimaxillärer Geräte. Fortschr. Kieferorthop., *32*:345–352, 1971.)

Figure 7-17. Variation in vertical forces against the activator during a two-hour period. (From Witt, E., and Komposch, G.: Intermaxilläre Kraftwirkung bimaxillärer Geräte. Fortschr. Kieferorthop., *32*:345–352, 1971.)

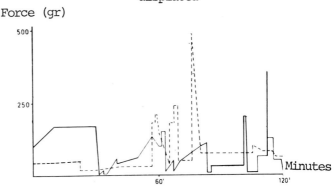

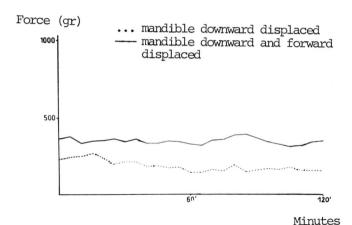

Force (gr)

... mandible downward displaced
—— mandible downward and forward
    displaced

Figure 7–18. Force curves based on the means for individual registrations every fifth minute during a two-hour period in 30 adult activator patients. (From Witt, E., and Komposch, G.: Intermaxilläre Kraftwirkung bimaxillärer Geräte. Fortschr. Kieferorthop., *32*:345–352, 1971.)

Minutes

position. The curves demonstrated varying frequencies of peaks, superimposed on the main level of the curves (Figs. 7–16 and 7–17). Witt[133] and Witt and Komposch[135] state that the forces consist of three components:

1. A basic component, varying with the degree of mandibular displacement, head posture, and level of sleep.

2. Oscillations, synchronized with breathing rhythm.

3. Oscillations, synchronized with blood pulse.

With a downward mandibular displacement of 4 to 6 mm. and a forward displacement of half the width of a premolar, Witt and Komposch[135] found

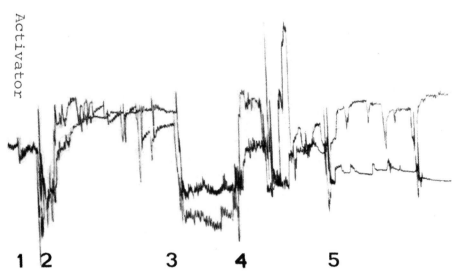

Figure 7–19. Variation in force application during a 15-minute period of restless sleep with changes in body postures. (Adapted from Witt, E., and Komposch, G.: Intermaxilläre Kraftwirkung bimaxillärer Geräte. Fortschr. Kieferorthop., *32*:345–352, 1971.) *1,* Body and head resting on the right side. *2,* Body turned to rest on the back. Face turned upward. *3,* Head turned to rest on the right side. *4,* Head turned to rest on the left side. *5,* Body turned to rest on the left side, head resting on the same side.

mean sagittal forces ranging between 315 and 395 grams for a group of sleeping adults. The means were calculated from individual registrations every fifth minute during two-hour periods (Fig. 7–18). With the same degree of downward displacement, but with no forward displacement, the means were significantly smaller, ranging between 145 and 270 grams (Fig. 7–18). The mean vertical forces ranged between 70 and 175 grams. In most individuals, they were greater when the mandible was displaced downward and forward than when it was displaced downward only, but calculations failed to show statistically significant differences. Corresponding studies on the effect of variations in the degree of vertical mandibular displacement do not seem to have been reported. However, Ahlgren[2] and Eschler[39] found in their electromyographic studies that the stretch reflex activity of the temporal and masseter muscles varies with the degree of vertical mandibular displacement.

Witt and Komposch could also confirm that the forces exerted on the teeth vary with the sleeping posture and the level of sleep (Fig. 7–19). In individuals sleeping on their backs they found relatively small tooth depressing forces, while the sagittal forces were relatively strong. During onset of sleep, the forces were large, generally speaking, but rather varying. During progressively deeper stages of sleep, the force curve gradually became smoother. In the stage of deep sleep the forces reached a minimum for the registrations.

Graf[52] and Witt and Komposch,[135] in the individual registrations, observed peaks of sagittal forces of more than 500 grams against the teeth (Figs. 7–16 and 7–17). The latter also made zero registrations, but only occasionally, and they covered only short periods of time. Hence, the forces applied to the teeth by the type of activator used by them are predominantly continuous when the appliance is in the mouth. However, there is pronounced variation in the force magnitude.

It may be concluded that the mode of action of activators which displace the mandible 4 to 6 mm. below intercuspal position is well documented. With such appliances inserted, the teeth or groups of teeth are subjected to forces that act almost continuously. There is a considerable variation in the force magnitude. The therapeutic forces are generated mainly in the muscles. By a stretching of different muscle groups, an increased passive tension, possibly also an increased tonus, is elicited, and these forces may be applied to different teeth or alveolar structures according to the treatment objectives.

The findings support the hypotheses of Ahlgren,[3] Harvold,[59] Herren,[59] and Selmer-Olsen,[119] and the thoughts of Ballard.[16] To a certain extent they are also compatible with the hypothesis of Schwarz.[117]

Based on these findings, it seems justifiable to state that orthodontic therapy based on removable appliances which displace the mandible more than 4 mm. beyond intercuspal position is not functional jaw orthopedics in the traditional sense. It appears that there also is justification for doubts regarding the nature of original activator therapy. Eschler[40] suggested the name "the muscle reflex method." Recent research implies that "the muscle stretch method" would be a more appropriate name.

The semantic and conceptual justification for the term "activator" may also be questioned. Hotz[76] uses the name "monobloc," coined by Robin,[110] to designate a block encompassing both dental arches. Although this would be a more appropriate name, the term "activator" is used in this chapter, since it seems to be so well established in the English literature.

STUDIES ON THE EFFECTS OF ACTIVATOR THERAPY IN CLASS II MALOCCLUSION TREATMENT

There is a great variation in the reaction to activator therapy. In some cases, occlusion improvements are remarkable; in others they are poor or even absent. Successfully treated Class II, Division 1 and Class II, Division 2 cases have been demonstrated by many authors.

A considerable number of studies have been conducted to analyze the effects of activator therapy. Practically all of them have been concerned with Class II, Division 1 malocclusions.

In some of the reports, the activators are described in detail. In others, the description is insufficient or absent. It is therefore difficult to relate the findings to different types of activators. However, conflicting findings may partly be ascribable to differences in activator design.

The activator was developed at a time when a widening of the upper dental arch was regarded as a proper procedure in the treatment of most Class II, Division 1 malocclusion cases. The appliance, usually split, was therefore routinely supplied with a so-called Coffin spring, usually activated for lateral expansion (Fig. 7–20). The lateral expanding effect of such activators has been documented in plaster cast studies.[56]

Slagsvold and Kolstad,[121] analyzing a group of Class II, Division 1 malocclusion cases, found increased dental arch widths at the upper first molars in all the cases studied (Table 7–2). This effect may be ascribable to a special spring, located mesiolingually to the upper first molars. Arch dimensions at the lower first molars remained essentially the same (Table 7–3).

A reducing effect on deep vertical overbites is regularly observed, particularly in young patients (Fig. 7–21). Such an effect has also been documented metrically in plaster cast studies (see Table 7–5).[4, 121] Criteria of a posterior (clockwise) mandibular rotation have been registered roentgencephalometrically.[61, 80, 122] Implications are that accelerated molar eruption contributes to the reduction of the vertical overbite. Considering the findings of Thompson,[128] it

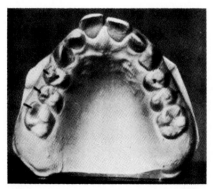 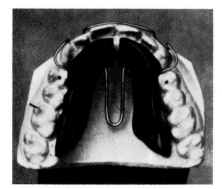

Figure 7–20. Activator designed for lateral expansion and retraction of the upper anteriors. (From Andresen, V., and Häupl, K.: Funktionskieferorthopädieae Die Grundlagen des "norwegischen Systems," 2nd ed. Leipzig, H. Meusser, 1939.)

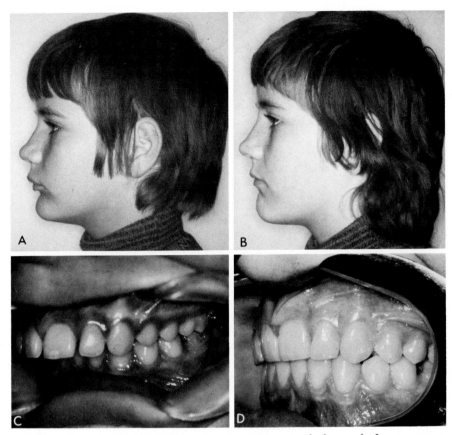

Figure 7–21. A Class II, Division 1 malocclusion case before and after treatment with activator and Kloehn headgear. Treatment lasted for 1.4 years.

seems reasonable to believe that depression of the incisors could also be expected if the appliances were worn more or less continuously. However, it is doubtful whether anterior tooth depression is a factor in regular activator therapy. It may be added that a reduction of the vertical overbite should hardly be expected in adult activator patients (see Fig. 7–39).

Anteroposterior tooth movements have been studied roentgencephalometrically by several authors. Bjork[25] and Parkhouse[102] found a forward displacement of the lower anterior segment, including the alveolar process, in relation to mandibular basal bone. Jacobsson[80] concluded that the lower incisors in his material were bodily displaced forward. Ascher,[15] Dietrich,[36] and Trayfoot and Richardson[129] found a labial tipping. Moss[97] reported a lingual tipping in nearly half his material. Demisch[33] registered an accelerated mesial drift of the lower molars, while Harvold and Vargervik[61] and Softley[122] concluded that the lower dental arch remained stable on its base. Hagerström[58] and Slagsvold and Kolstad[121] in plaster cast studies observed an increase in available space in the lower dental arch.

Considering the available information on the activator's mode of action,[135] it is advisable to expect a forward displacement of the mandibular teeth during therapy. If such a displacement cannot be tolerated, activator treatment should not be instituted, or steps should be taken to avoid or counteract anteriorly directed forces.

It has been shown in many case reports that the upper anterior teeth can be efficiently tipped lingually with activators. It has also been documented metrically in roentgencephalometric follow-up studies.[61, 80, 92, 107, 122, 129] Also, the axial inclination of lingually tipped upper anterior teeth can be corrected with activators (see Figs. 7–35 to 7–38).

Considering the activator's mode of action, it would be reasonable to expect the upper posterior teeth to migrate distally. Clinically, a space opening between them can frequently be seen, particularly in young patients (Figs. 7–22 and 7–23). They also assume a distal axial inclination (Figs. 7–22 and 7–24). Roentgencephalometric studies have produced controversial findings. Meach[92] concluded that the upper molars follow a normal path of eruption during activator treatment. Also, Harvold and Vargervik[61] were unable to confirm the hypothesis of a distal drift. Demisch,[33] on the other hand, found that the maxillary molars are either stopped in their mesial drift or moved distally.

A favorable change in the anteroposterior relationship between the apical bases of the two dental arches has been documented in several studies.[33, 36, 46, 66, 67, 92, 97, 122, 129] A restriction of the forward growth displacement or a backward tipping of the upper jaw may account for this, at least partly.[33, 36, 61, 66, 67, 80, 92, 97, 122, 129, 138] Many authors believe that accelerated mandibular growth is another contributing factor. This will be dealt with later in this chapter.

The reaction of the periodontal tissues to activator therapy has also been

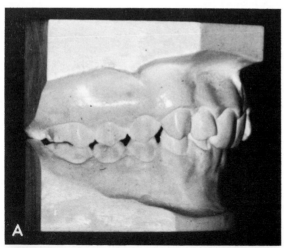

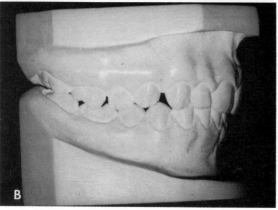

Figure 7–22. The upper posterior teeth seem to be tipped distally in Class II, Division 2 activator treatment. *A,* Before treatment; *B,* after treatment.

Figure 7-23. An activator (*B*) can be used for the distal-driving of upper bicuspids after loss of the first molars.

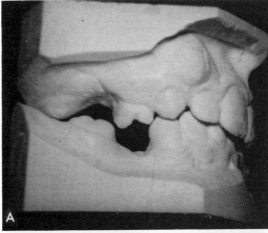

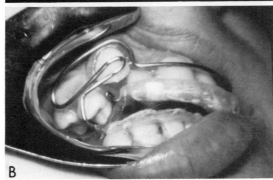

the subject of considerable interest. Häupl[63] maintained that the forces transmitted by the activator hit the teeth as jolts, causing vibrations which shake the periodontal tissues. Repeated jolts elicit tissue reactions which lead to tooth movements. These reactions are physiologic in nature, in contrast to the pathologic reactions found in fixed appliance therapy.

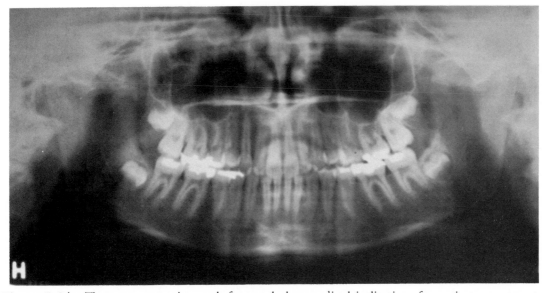

Figure 7-24. The upper posterior teeth frequently have a distal inclination after activator treatment.

The periodontal tissue reactions will not be dealt with further in this chapter. Suffice it to say that Reitan[108] was unable to confirm the conclusions of Häupl. Even though the intermittent character of the activator forces was reflected in a delay of certain reactions, the main pattern was essentially similar to that observed with fixed appliance therapy.

As pointed out previously, most of the analyses on the effects of activator therapy have been concerned with Class II, Division 1 malocclusions. It is reasonable to believe that most of the findings are applicable to Class II, Division 2 malocclusions as well.

HYPOTHESES ON CONDYLAR REACTION TO ACTIVATOR THERAPY

The Original Activator

The question of the long-term condylar response to activator treatment has been a subject of orthodontic research and writing for 40 years. As previously indicated, Andresen assumed that the adaptational processes to the functional pattern prescribed by his activator would also include the condyles and the muscles. Increases in phasic muscle activity in the protractors and relaxation and stretching of the retractors were supposed to be decisive factors in these processes. Fränkel has further elaborated these ideas and made them a principle in his therapy.[45] Recent research has interesting implications on potential adaptive response.

McNamara,[91] in experimental longitudinal electromyographic, roentgencephalometric, and histologic studies, tried to elucidate the relationship between muscle function and skeletal form by inserting a maxillary metal splint which displaced the mandible 2 mm. downward and 2 mm. forward. The appliance, being worn continuously, was found to change the behavior of the orofacial muscles, one of the manifestations being an increased activity in the superior head of the lateral pterygoids. A skeletal adaptation to the experimental conditions, followed by a progressive disappearance of the modified neuromuscular pattern, was observed.

McNamara maintained that the stimuli from the periodontal mechanoreceptors, and also from the articular and muscular receptors, may have prompted an anterior displacement of the mandible. The increased activity in the superior head of the lateral pterygoids may have been a manifestation of a reflex activity, first unconditioned and later conditioned, which assisted in the skeletal adaptation to the experimental changes in the environment. It should be added that the degree of mandibular displacement in McNamara's study corresponded closely to the recommendations of Andresen. However, the study was on small primates, not humans.

Studies by Petrovic et al.[105] also have bearing on Andresen's philosophy for functional jaw orthopedics. In accordance with previous findings of Baume[18, 19] and Koski,[85] Petrovic[103, 104] found that the phylogenetically and ontogenetically secondary cartilage of the mandibular condyles is morphologically and physiologically different from the primary cartilages in the epiphyses, the spheno-occipital synchondrosis, and the nasal septum. In contrast to them, it grows by division of undifferentiated cells, and the growth is to a higher extent regulated by local exogenous factors than by the growth hormones. Petrovic et al.,[105] on the basis of experimental studies, came to the conclusion that condylar growth is an expression of a locally structured homeostasis for the establishment and maintenance of a functionally coordinated chewing apparatus. The growth depends on continuous information from the teeth, the periodontal membranes, and the mandibular joint. The information is transmitted from receptors in these organs to the central nervous system, eliciting activity in the orofacial muscle complex. The activity in the lateral pterygoids stimulates the mitotic division of condylar prechondroblasts.

According to Petrovic et al.,[105] intermaxillary occlusal contact disturbances induce a functional displacement of the mandible. If optimal contacts can be re-established by a forward shifting of the mandible, activity in the lateral pterygoids is elicited. In young individuals such activity induces condylar growth. During the growth period, intermaxillary occlusal contact disturbances are repeatedly introduced by anterior growth displacements of the upper jaw. Similar disturbances can be created by orthopedic devices. Provided these devices have the ability of activating the lateral pterygoids, they can stimulate condylar growth. Appliances that hold the mandible in an anteriorly displaced position do not activate those muscles. Accordingly, they do not stimulate condylar growth.

Petrovic et al.[105] found a stimulating effect on condylar growth only in periods when the muscle tonus and the monosynaptic polysynaptic reflexes were maintained. In deep sleep, the appliance had no effect on the mitotic activity of the prechondroblasts.

The authors also demonstrated that intake of growth hormones increases the effect of the appliance. They concluded that the lateral pterygoids serve as a final common pathway to the condylar cartilage for hormonal and biomechanical stimuli.

The findings and conclusions of McNamara and Petrovic support Andresen's theory regarding the possibilities for inducing musculoskeletal adaptations by introducing a new closing pattern. Especially remarkable is the agreement regarding the pathway to condylar growth stimulation.

The conditions under which the experimental studies of McNamara and Petrovic were carried out deviated in several respects from the conditions under which activator therapy is applied clinically. A crucial question is whether activator treatment, as described by Andresen, meets the requirements of a therapy aimed at inducing skeletal adaptations. It seems particularly pertinent to ask whether the activator has the potential of activating the muscles, above all the lateral pterygoids.

The activator is traditionally worn at night. It is generally accepted that muscle activity is depressed during sleep. As previously pointed out, Herren[69] and Gerber[47] observed no increase in the frequency of mandibular movements in activator patients during sleep. Witt,[134] studying the response to another orthopedic appliance, the bionator, found that the mandible was moved reflexly forward when this appliance was used by day. It was also observed that the posteriorly directed pressure from the mandibular teeth against the appliance was much smaller in wakefulness than during sleep, implying that the protractors' level of activity was considerably higher. Petrovic and co-workers[105] in their experiments, found a high mitotic activity in the condylar prechondroblasts during wakefulness, but not during deep sleep. Accordingly, it may be questioned whether it is at all possible to stimulate muscle activity orthopedically during sleep.

No studies seem to have been reported on the response of the protractors to the activator during daytime wear. If the bionator has the potential to activate them, it is reasonable to believe that an activator of the original design has the same potential.

During the last 30 years, new types of removable appliances, based on functional jaw orthopedic principles, have been developed. The bionator of Balters[17] has already been mentioned. Others are the oral adaptor of Bimler,[22, 23] the functionator of Eschler,[42] the function corrector of Fränkel,[43, 44] the protractor of Gerlach,[48] the open activator of Klammt,[83] and the kinetor of Stockfisch.[123, 124] One of their characteristics being a light and open construction, they can more conveniently be worn by day than the original activator. If the hypotheses of McNamara and Petrovic are true, and if they have clinical application, these appliances may have advantages beyond the original activator in functional jaw orthopedics.

Modified Activators

Authors who deny the activator's potential to activate the protractors[40] and to induce functional mandibular movements[2, 69, 117] may still believe in its stimulating effect on condylar growth. It has been shown in a great number of experimental studies that condylar growth can be stimulated by a continuous wearing of devices which displace the condyles forward in the fossae.[20, 31, 32, 37, 65, 71, 91, 104, 125] There is evidence that a displacement of the condyles can also stimulate mandibular growth in man. Lund,[87] in a roentgencephalometric follow-up study of young individuals with unilateral condylar fracture, found extensive remodeling growth processes at the dislocated posterior fragment. Condylar growth was accelerated, and the condyle migrated back toward the glenoid fossa (Fig. 7–25). Hollender and Lindahl[72] observed apposition of bone also in the fossa in such cases (Fig. 7–26).

Petrovic et al. have given one explanation of the growth-stimulating effect of a therapeutic forward displacement of the mandibular condyles. It is also possible that the condyles "grow upwards and backwards so as to maintain the contact at the temporomandibular joints."[118]

If the latter hypothesis is true, activators with a more pronounced mandibular displacement may be expected to have a greater growth-promoting effect than activators which allow the mandible to assume only a postural rest position.

STUDIES ON THE EFFECTS OF ACTIVATOR THERAPY ON MANDIBULAR GROWTH

Great interest has been focused on the activator's effect on condylar growth. Several authors claim to have found criteria of a stimulating effect.[21, 34, 46, 53, 64–68, 84, 89, 90, 97, 101, 102] Others have been unable to draw such conclusions.[25, 36, 61, 80, 92, 107, 122, 138]

The matter is scientifically difficult to approach. As previously pointed out, the degree of success by activator treatment varies from patient to patient. In some individuals, no response at all can be observed. Therefore, if a group of successfully treated individuals is compared with a group of untreated indi-

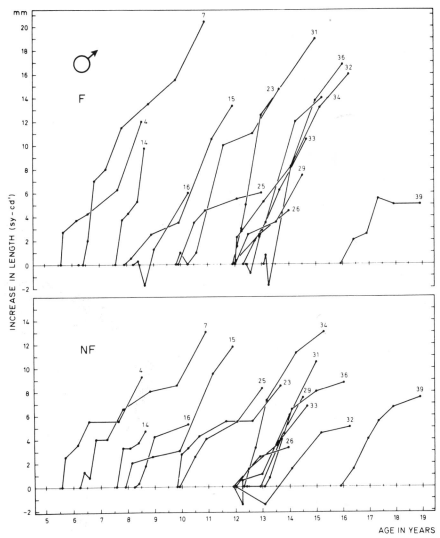

Figure 7–25. Cumulative growth curves for mandibular length on the fracture side (F) and the non-fracture side (NF) in 15 boys with unilateral condylar fractures. (From Lund, K.: Mandibular growth and remodelling processes after condylar fracture. A longitudinal roentgencephalometric study. Thesis. Acta Odontol. Scand., *32*:Suppl. 64, 1974.)

viduals, the study may be biased in that the former may constitute a selection of individuals with a specially favorable growth pattern. On the other hand, if the group of treated individuals also includes the unsuccessful cases, the mean changes may be too small to give significance in statistical tests.

Longitudinal studies have not solved the problem either, because accelerated growth in the treatment period, as compared to a pretreatment period, could be demonstrated in only some of the successfully treated patients.[33]

It seems justifiable to state that conclusive evidence of the activator's potential to accelerate condylar growth remains to be delivered. That applies to any type of an activator. However, the matter is not well enough elucidated to jus-

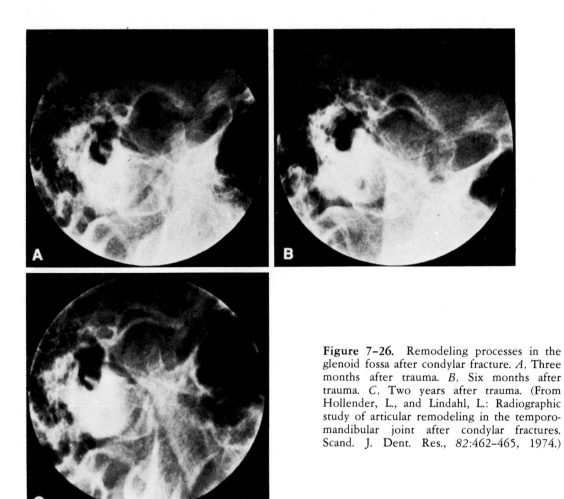

Figure 7-26. Remodeling processes in the glenoid fossa after condylar fracture. *A,* Three months after trauma. *B,* Six months after trauma. *C,* Two years after trauma. (From Hollender, L., and Lindahl, L.: Radiographic study of articular remodeling in the temporomandibular joint after condylar fractures. Scand. J. Dent. Res., *82:*462–465, 1974.)

tify the conclusion that such an effect does not appear in any type of a malocclusion, at any age, under any circumstances whatsoever.

HYPOTHESES ON THE MUSCULAR REACTION TO ACTIVATOR THERAPY

According to Andresen, in functional jaw orthopedics, changes in the occlusion and the craniofacial pattern should be induced by a re-education and a rebuilding of the orofacial musculature. It was postulated by him, and it has been claimed by his followers, that such a re-education and rebuilding can be accomplished through the introduction of a new mandibular closing pattern.

Even authors who reject Andresen's hypothesis believe in adaptational processes in the muscles.[2, 40, 69, 117] Ahlgren[2] assumes that the activator works like an interference which produces a new contraction pattern of the jaw muscles. Over a long period of time, the innervation pattern can be adjusted, and the mandible repositioned forward.

It is demonstrated in Class III surgical cases, it has been documented in groups of edentulous individuals,[126] and it has been shown in animals[120] that muscles adapt to a reduction in the distance between the points of insertion. It is reasonable to believe that they are also adaptive to increases in this distance, i.e., to a maintained stretch.

Andresen also believed that the exercise instituted by his activator will strengthen the muscles and thereby contribute to the development of a retention apparatus.[8] Harvold[60] states that isometric muscle contractions, elicited by the modified activator, change the muscle matrix in such a way that it becomes an effective retainer. Selmer-Olsen[119] agrees that muscles become strengthened by activity, but it remains to be shown that their form is permanently changed thereby. When the appliance is discarded, the muscular hypertrophy will vanish, he says.

STUDIES OF THE MUSCULAR REACTION TO ACTIVATOR THERAPY

With intensive activator wear, the mandibular intercuspal position sometimes seems to be transferred anteriorly after only a few months of treatment. Although the condyles rest anteriorly in the fossae or on the posterior slope of the articular eminences and there is a posterior open bite, it is not possible to force the mandible to bite further back. The situation may be seen as an expression of an adjustment of the functional matrix to the mandibular position prescribed by the appliance. It has been maintained that excellent conditions for condylar growth have thereby been created and that morphologic adjustments will follow.[136]

Ahlgren,[2] in electromyographic studies, found the postural muscle activity to remain essentially uninfluenced by activator therapy. The biting response, however, was found to change after one night's wear, although only temporarily. Upon removal of the appliance, the muscles, and particularly the temporal muscles, showed a sustained, erratic contraction pattern, much like the one found in individuals biting on severe occlusal interferences. Two hours later, the habitual contraction pattern had reappeared.

This pattern of reaction is characteristic also after six months of treatment. However, in a group of patients with Class II, Division 1 malocclusions, treated to correction with activators over a three-year period, Ahlgren[2] found the muscle patterns to be the same with and without the activators in the mouth. They closely resembled those observed at earlier stages of the treatment when activators were in the mouth.

Grossman et al.[55] made similar observations in a Class II, Division 1 malocclusion case. After two years of activator treatment, the patient showed a posterior temporal muscle activity, and a tendency to a protrusive biting. When the patient was instructed to perform an individual bite with increasing force, the posterior temporal muscle activity increased. The authors concluded that the bite of preference was the protrusive one.

Moss[98] found in individuals with Class II, Division 1 malocclusions a pattern of muscle activity which was significantly different from that of individuals with a normal occlusion. During and after activator treatment, the muscle activity approached that of adults with a normal occlusion.

Grossman et al.[55] and Moss[98, 99] also found changes in muscle activity of patients with Class II, Division 2 malocclusions subsequent to activator treatment. Before treatment many of them had a posterior path of closure from postural rest to intercuspal position. As a group, the patients of Moss had a muscle activity pattern which was significantly different from that of a group of individuals with normal occlusion. During treatment, it became essentially similar to it in most cases. Individuals retaining their original muscle activity pattern showed a tendency to acquire relapses in the occlusion when the appliance was discarded.

It should be added that Ahlgren and Moss, and probably also Grossman, used activators which displaced the mandible beyond rest position. Similar studies of patients treated with activators of the original type do not seem to have been reported.

Experimental studies of McNamara also have bearing on the muscular reaction to mandibular displacements. A maxillary splint, displacing the mandible 2 mm. downward and 2 mm. forward, was found to change the behavior of the orofacial muscles in young monkeys. A skeletal adaptation to the experimental conditions, followed by a progressive disappearance of the modified neuromuscular pattern, was observed.[91]

To this author, it seems an open question whether the findings reflect an adjustment of the muscles to the mandibular position prescribed by the activator, or just the elimination of disharmonies in the occlusion of the teeth.

It may be added that Moss[98] in his studies substantiated the assumption that muscle activity increases during activator treatment. Out of retention he observed a slight decrease, implying that the increase during treatment was not a result of maturing only, but also a product of the treatment.

ACTIVATOR DESIGN FOR CLASS II MALOCCLUSION TREATMENT

The activator is a one-piece removable appliance, encompassing both dental arches (see Figs. 7–1 and 7–27). Details in design have been varied greatly. The activator described in this chapter differs in various ways from the activator of Andresen. Readers who are interested in the latter are referred to one of the textbooks of Andresen and Häupl.[8-11]

The activator has a labial arch wire (0.032 or 0.036 inch) with hooks for

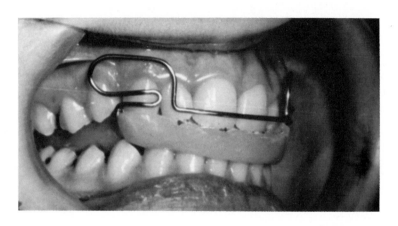

Figure 7–27. An activator for Class II, Division 2 malocclusion treatment in place.

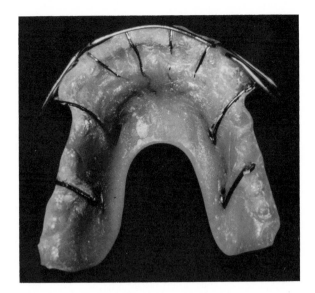

Figure 7-28. An activator for Class II, Division 2 malocclusion treatment before trimming.

the maxillary canines (Figs. 7-23 and 7-27). It has no spring for lateral expansion, unless there is a particular need for it (Fig. 7-20). Springs (0.028 or 0.032 inch), engaging the maxillary first premolars and first molars, are incorporated mesiolingually to the teeth in question (Figs. 7-23 and 7-28). The Class II, Division 2 activator has spurs (0.020 or 0.022 inch) behind the lingually inclined upper incisors (Figs. 7-28 and 7-29).

For the fabrication of the activator, a construction bite is needed. It may be produced on the plaster casts, but can be taken in the mouth more conveniently and with greater exactness. If a forward pull on the lower dental arch is indicated or can be tolerated, the construction bite is taken with the mandible anteriorly displaced to a normal sagittal relationship between the first molars. The displacement should not exceed the width of a premolar, and the lower central incisors should not bite anteriorly to the upper central incisors. If a forward pull on the lower dental arch is undesirable, the mandible is not brought forward.

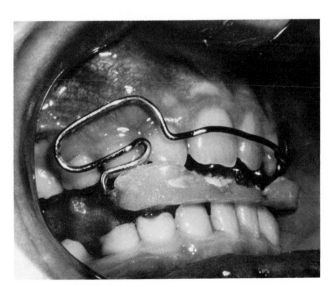

Figure 7-29. In Class II, Division 2 activator treatment, the upper central incisors are tipped labially by spurs lingual to them.

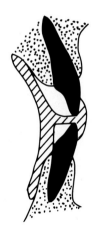 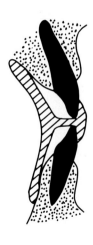

Figure 7–30. Trimming of the acrylic lingual to the incisors in a Class II, Division 1 malocclusion.

Vertically, it would be logical to relate the mandible to its postural rest position, and many orthodontists state that they do this. The author finds it difficult to determine mandibular rest position exactly and prefers to relate the mandible to the incisor overlapping. The vertical distance between the incisal edges of upper and lower centrals in the construction bite is about 1 mm.

Attention should be paid to the midline of the lower dental arch. A midline discrepancy caused by tooth migration cannot be corrected by means of an activator. However, in cases with a unilateral Class II relationship, the mandible is brought over to the side of the Class I relationship. It has been stated that such measures might create temporomandibular joint disorders.[131] The author has had no such untoward experiences.

The appliance is waxed on the plaster casts and processed on the cast of the lower jaw. The incisal part (3 mm.) of the labial surface of the lower incisors and canines is covered by acrylic (see Fig. 7–27). In Class II, Division I cases, the incisal part of the upper front teeth is also covered by acrylic.

In cases of deep vertical overbite, the activator is trimmed to allow eruption of premolars and molars in both jaws (see Fig. 7–23) The acrylic is also removed distally to the upper canines, premolars, and molars, and lingually to any upper tooth that should be moved lingually. Lingually to the lower incisors, the acrylic is trimmed to a one-point contact with each tooth, as close to the gingival border as possible, or to contact with the gingival surface of the alveolar process only (Fig. 7–30). Finally, any material that impinges on the gum tissue or conflicts with the opening and closing of the lower jaw is removed.

A certain increase in the height usually takes place during the processing. The interocclusal clearance in the first molar areas when the appliances are inserted varies with the degree of incisor overlapping. In cases of a deep overbite, it ranges between 4 and 8 mm.

POSSIBILITIES AND LIMITATIONS OF THE ACTIVATOR IN CLASS II MALOCCLUSION TREATMENT

In some cases of Class II malocclusions, a lateral expansion of the upper dental arch is one of the treatment objectives. Such an effect is probably inherent in all activator therapy. When the patient lies on his side at night, the rest position of the mandible is transferred to an excentric location, laterally to the median plane of the head (see Fig. 7–6). If an activator is inserted, the mandible is prevented from assuming this position. Diagonally directed, expanding forces, brought into being by gravity, are then applied to the dental arches (see Fig. 7–6).[69]

Additional lateral expanding forces may be induced by activation of incorporated springs. They are brought into action by a wedge effect within the upper dental arch when the appliance is bitten into place (see Fig. 7–20).

A reduction of the vertical overbite is one of the treatment objectives in many Class II, Division 1 cases and in practically all Class II, Division 2 cases.[13] Theoretically, such a reduction may be accomplished by an increased eruption of the posterior teeth, and/or an intrusion or an inhibition of eruption of the anterior teeth. If an increased eruption of the posterior teeth is intended, the activator is designed to relieve them from intruding forces. Normally, the teeth are in a state of vertical balance between inherent forces of eruption and intrusion, transmitted from the elevators through the occlusal contacts with the opposing teeth. With an activator inserted, the intruding forces are eliminated and the balance is broken. An accelerated premolar and molar eruption and a reduction of the vertical overbite may be expected.

As previously mentioned, a posterior rotation of the mandible has been registered during activator treatment of Class II, Division 1 malocclusions.[61, 80, 122] Similar studies of Class II, Division 2 malocclusions do not seem to have been reported.

With an activator inserted, forces deriving from the stretched elevators are concentrated on the anterior teeth (see Fig. 7–23). Even if they are incapable of intruding the teeth, such forces might be able to inhibit their eruption. Witt and Komposch[135] found the vertical forces to be smaller than the anteriorly directed forces which hit the lower teeth. It is conceivable that they vary with the degree of vertical mandibular displacement.[2, 39]

The efficacy of the activator in the treatment of deep vertical overbites has been documented in metric studies[4, 121] and in case reports. It should be pointed out that the effect varies from case to case.

The retraction of the upper anterior teeth in Class II, Division 1 malocclusions is accomplished by forces brought into being by a stretching of the retracting muscles of the mandible. The forces are transferred to the teeth by means of the labial arch wire, which is adjusted to lie tightly against their labial surfaces. If a retraction is attempted with an activator that does not displace the mandible anteriorly, the maxillary posterior teeth may be pulled mesially. Spaces can be closed. In any event, the axial inclination of lingually tipped upper incisors in Class II, Division 2 malocclusions can be corrected by a labial tipping of their crowns and a lingual torquing of their roots. In activator therapy, this is brought about by a combined effect of the lingual spurs and the labial arch wire. The spurs are activated to hit the teeth at their linguoincisal ridge (Fig. 7–31). The force is generated in the elevators, which press the appliance against the upper jaw and thereby press the spurs against the incisors (see Fig. 7–29). It has both a vertical and a labial component. By simultaneously pressing with the labial arch wire against the labial surface, as close to the gingival border as possible, a torquing of the teeth may be obtained (Fig. 7–31). If the labial arch wire is bent away from the teeth, a tipping movement will take place. The labial arch wire

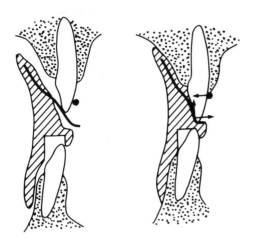

Figure 7–31. Trimming of the acrylic and activation of the spurs and the labial arch wire in a Class II, Division 2 malocclusion case. Torque is accomplished by the labial wire exerting lingual pressure at the gingival margin as the lingual spurs move the incisal edges labially.

may also be adjusted to tip protruding lateral incisors lingually. Space is a prerequisite.

The activator can be most efficient in tipping maxillary incisors one way or the other, but it gives no complete control of the root movements. Still, it is possible, as it also is in many Class II, Division 2 cases, to bring the upper incisors into a satisfactory position with this appliance (see Figs. 7–35 to 7–38).

The anteroposterior relationship between the dental arches may be normalized in Class II malocclusions by

1. A forward displacement of the lower dental arch, or of selected teeth or tooth groups in the lower jaw.
2. A distal driving of the upper molars, premolars, and canines.
3. An inhibition of the forward growth or a backward displacement of the upper jaw.
4. A stimulation of condylar growth.
5. A re-education or a rebuilding of the orofacial muscles.
6. An elimination of possible interferences which guide the mandible posteriorly during closure.

With an activator inserted, more or less continuously, anteriorly directed forces are applied toward the lower teeth, even if the mandible is not displaced anteriorly.[135] They can be directed against selected teeth or tooth groups, or against the alveolar process, by an appropriate trimming of the appliance. A certain command over the labiolingual inclination of the lower anterior teeth is obtained by a particular appliance design in relation to these teeth, as previously described.

Although conflicting findings have been reported, it should be anticipated that the lower teeth will come forward somewhat during activator treatment.

Action is equal to reaction. Posteriorly directed forces of the same magnitude and with the same variation are applied to the upper dental arch as the mandible is protracted. They can be guided against selected teeth or tooth groups by means of the incorporated springs.

With the Class II, Division 2 activator, distally directed forces can be applied to the posterior teeth also by a wedge effect within the upper dental arch. This effect arises when the appliance is pressed against the upper jaw, with the spurs lingual to the centrals, and/or the springs mesial to the first premolars and/or the first molars activated.

The posteriorly directed forces, brought into being by the stretching of the soft tissues, are transferred via the upper dental arch to the sutures. In young individuals, sutural growth seems to be inhibited by mechanical forces which act against the direction of growth.[104]

With the Class II activator inserted, the condyles are continuously held in a protracted position in relation to the fossae. The retractors and the elevators of the mandible are stretched. Whether it is possible by such a mechanotherapy to reposition the mandible forward permanently is still controversial.

Some authors have found an abnormal path of closure guidance to be a factor in many Class II relationships, especially in Class II, Division 2 malocclusions.[51, 55, 99, 128] Others have been unable to draw such a conclusion. An abnormal path of closure guidance is supposed to be attributable to overclosure of the anterior teeth or to cuspal interferences between the posterior teeth. Overclosure of the anterior teeth can be eliminated in activator treatment by a reduction of vertical overbite and a labial tipping and/or a torquing of the upper incisors. Cuspal interferences can be eliminated by a distal driving of the upper posterior teeth and/or a forward displacement of the lower jaw and/or the lower posterior teeth.

It is apparent that various types of tooth movements can be accomplished with activators. However, other types cannot be carried out. The activator is incapable of moving teeth bodily and of distally driving lower posterior teeth. It is most inefficient in the rotating of teeth, and in the closing of extraction spaces. It is less reliable in its action than are fixed appliances.

It has been speculated that if the activator is capable of moving teeth but incapable of repositioning the mandible, the dental arches may be adjusted to each other in a position outside the normal path of mandibular closure. A dual bite can be created, and serious temporomandibular joint disorders may arise. It is true that such discrepancies may be created, but it is equally true for fixed appliance therapy.[111] Generally speaking, no orthodontic treatment is completed until such discrepancies are eliminated. The activator is so constructed that it works until the mandibular position prescribed by the activator coincides with the rest position. A dual bite, therefore, is a transitional stage. It should be eliminated if the treatment is carried to its end.

Advantages

It is pertinent to ask whether the activator has advantages of any kind over fixed appliances. The activator allows a more efficient prophylaxis of caries and periodontal diseases during treatment. Generally speaking, it is less harmful to the investing tissues of the teeth. It is simpler to fabricate and manage, and activator therapy is less time-consuming for the orthodontist. For these reasons, some orthodontists feel that it has a definite place in orthodontics.

To others, the crucial question is whether it is possible with the activator to accomplish changes in the occlusion and the craniofacial pattern that cannot be made with other appliances. It appears that no definite answer can at present be given to this question.

As previously pointed out, it has been documented that it is possible to stimulate condylar growth by means of orthopedic devices in young animals. Furthermore, studies have been reported which show accelerated growth by condylar displacements in man as well.[87] These findings constitute a challenge to the orthodontic profession to find means and methods to take advantage of this potential. Although conclusive evidence on the potential of functional appliances to stimulate condylar growth is lacking, it may be stated that no other orthodontic appliance hitherto constructed offers a therapeutic approach more similar to the conditions under which condylar growth can be stimulated experimentally. It is a task for future research to penetrate and solve these problems.

APPLICATION OF ACTIVATOR THERAPY IN CLASS II MALOCCLUSION TREATMENT

The morphogenesis of the Class II malocclusions is not fully understood. However, there can be no doubt that many of them (Division 2 types) have suffered significant forward (counterclockwise) mandibular rotation with the center in the premolar area.

Bjørk,[29] in longitudinal roentgencephalometric studies with the aid of metallic implants, registered the following criteria for the forward rotation of the lower jaw (Figs. 7–32 and 7–33).

1. A forward inclination of the condylar head.
2. A greater curvature of the mandibular canal than of the contour of the mandibular border.
3. A downward convex mandibular border with a thick cortical layer in the anterior part.
4. A backward inclination of the symphyseal axis.
5. A large interincisal angle (more vertical).
6. Large interpremolar and intermolar angles.
7. A compression of the lower face with protruding lips and a deep mentolabial sulcus.

These are characteristics frequently found in Class II, Division 2 cases. There can be no doubt that a forward rotation of the mandible is an important feature in the morphogenesis of most malocclusions of that type.

Occasionally, some Class II, Division 1 cases exhibit signs of a forward mandibular rotation, although the interincisal angle in such cases usually is smaller than the average.

During a forward mandibular rotation, the chin is brought forward and upward. The mandible, therefore, looks well-developed anteroposteriorly, but the lower face appears vertically compressed. Accordingly, the profile presents a definite vertical problem. That also applies to the soft tissue (Fig. 7–33).

Therapy in cases with a deep vertical overbite and a forward mandibular rotational pattern (Class II, Division 2 problems) should aim at solving the vertical problem by an increased eruption of the posterior teeth. Such an eruption may transfer the center of the mandibular rotation forward, or even turn the forward rotation into a backward rotation. It has been shown in follow-up studies that such a change may be induced with activators.[61, 80, 122] Moreover, the vertical overbite seems to be rather stable in cases treated with activators.[4, 121]

It has been advocated that a biteplate be introduced early in childhood in cases of forward mandibular rotation, to intercept this developmental trend.[29] Such a trend may persist for a long period of time, from early childhood until late in adolescence. Biteplates, therefore, may be useful also in the later stages of growth. The activator meets the requirements of such a plate. If advantage

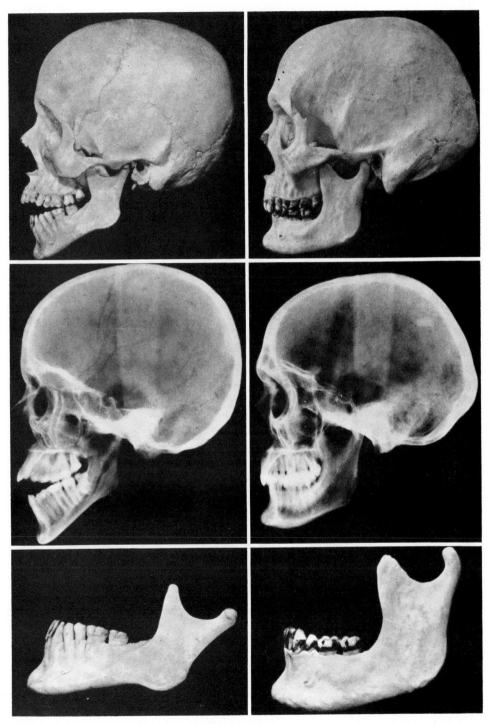

Figure 7–32. One case of backward mandibular rotation (left), and one case of forward mandibular rotation (right). (From Björk, A.: Käkarnas tillväxt och utveckling i relation till kraniet i dess helhet. Nord. Klin. Odontol., *1*:1–44, 1966.)

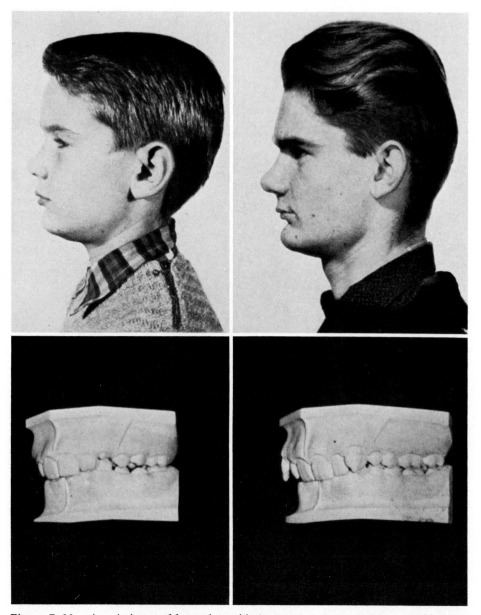

Figure 7-33. A typical case of forward mandibular rotation. (From: Björk, A., 1966: Käkarnas tillväxt och utveckling i relation till kraniet i dess helhet. Nord. Klin. Odontol., *1*:1–44, 1966.)

can be taken of other properties of this appliance, it might be preferable to a standard biteplate.

During a backward mandibular rotation, the chin is brought downward and backward. This is characteristic of most Class II, Division 1 malocclusions. The incisor overlapping in such individuals is usually small or nonexistent, the anterior face height is large, and the lips hardly meet (Figs. 7–32 and 7–34). Activators have no function in the treatment of such vertical problems. If an activator is indicated for other reasons, it should not be trimmed to allow eruption of the posterior teeth.

A deep overbite may be found also in individuals who have not had a forward mandibular rotation. In such cases, advantage may be taken of the bite-raising effect of the activator, unless signs of a backward mandibular rotational pattern are present.[29]

Most Class II malocclusions have an unfavorable relationship between the

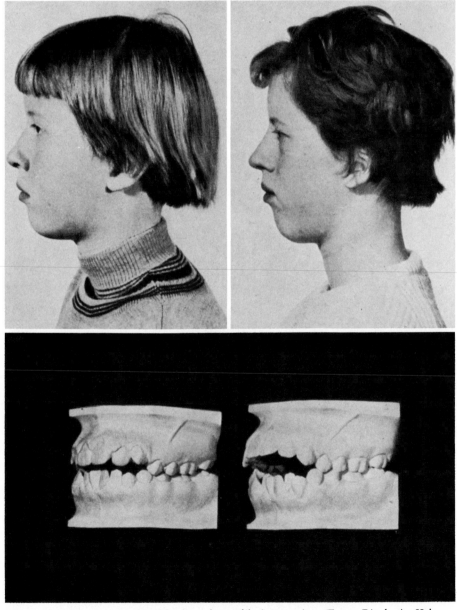

Figure 7-34. A typical case of backward mandibular rotation. (From: Bjørk, A.: Käkarnas tillväxt och utveckling i relation till kraniet i dess helhet. Nord. Klin. Odontol., *1*:1-44, 1966.)

apical bases of the anterior teeth in the two jaws, with a larger ANB angle than desirable. It has been shown that the activator has a favorable effect on such a relationship.[33, 36, 46, 66, 67, 97, 122, 129] Many individuals with a Class II malocclusion also have a receding chin. Again, this is primarily Division 1. Some orthodontists believe the activator has properties beyond those of fixed appliances in bringing the lower jaw forward. It should be remembered that an activator designed to change the relationship between the basal parts of the jaws may bring the lower dental arch forward on its base. Accordingly, it is hardly justified to institute activator treatment unless it is desirable, or at least permissible, to bring the lower dental arch forward on its base.

The positioning of the lower anterior teeth is a controversial question in clinical orthodontics. With a large ANB angle, the orthodontist frequently has to choose whether he will retract the upper anterior teeth extensively, protract the lower anterior teeth, or combine the two directions of movement. In some cases of Class II malocclusion, there is a surplus of space in the lower dental arch and the incisors are situated relatively far lingually. Occasionally they are located well behind the AP line. In such cases, it is permissible to tax the lower dental arch to correct the anteroposterior relationship between the two dental arches. In other cases, a protraction of the lower anterior teeth is undesirable out of regard for post-treatment stability.[81, 82, 86, 88, 93-96, 132] But slight lower incisor protraction may be necessary for a full correction of the axial inclination of the upper incisors, elimination of excessive overjet, and improvement of facial esthetics. Correspondingly, a retraction of the lower incisors may be desirable in consideration of post-treatment stability, but undesirable from an esthetic point of view. Under such circumstances, it may be justified to run a calculated risk of post-treatment crowding in the lower dental arch, to make it possible to give the upper incisors an acceptable axial inclination, and to improve facial esthetics.

The ideal Class II malocclusion case for activator treatment is a nonextraction, deep overbite case in which it is desirable or permissible to exert a forward pull on the lower dental arch. If there are no rotated teeth, such a malocclusion may be corrected without the use of supplementary appliances.

Many Class II, Division 2 cases belong to this group. It is the author's opinion that the activator is more efficient in the treatment of Class II, Division 2 malocclusions than in the treatment of any other type of malocclusion. The favorable prognosis is probably ascribable partly to the well-developed elevators of these patients and partly to the morphologic characteristics of the anomaly.

Since the tooth-moving efficacy of the activator increases with the degree of muscle stretch, the author finds it appropriate in cases of deep overbite to exceed the limit given by Andresen for the degree of vertical displacement. It is not necessary to exceed it extensively, i.e., by more than 8 mm., unless the freeway space is exceptionally large (see Chapter 12).

In cases of small vertical overbite, the vertical displacement of the mandible should be rather limited. Generally speaking, the activator is less efficient in the treatment of such cases.

Combination With Fixed Appliances

In the treatment of cases which cannot be brought to a satisfactory end result with activator treatment alone, a combination with other types of appliances frequently offers a good solution. As an aid in the correction of the Class

II relationship, extraoral forces against the upper first molars are often useful.[35, 62, 75, 106, 130] If cervical traction is chosen, the extraoral force will also have an elongating effect on the anchor teeth and thereby contribute to the opening of the bite.

By combining the headgear with a lip bumper or an E-arch in the lower jaw (bands on the first molars and a 0.032 inch labial arch wire), and Class III elastics, it is possible to upright and distally drive the lower molars. The effect on the vertical dimension is maximal if cervical traction is applied on the face bow, because the activator, the extraoral force, and the Class III elastics will then combine in reducing the vertical overbite.

If the Class II relationship is difficult to overcome, extraction of upper second molars may be resorted to, provided that third molars are present.[50] Such extractions, in combination with activator treatment, and possibly also extraoral and intermaxillary elastic forces, frequently give a good correction.

For the correction of rotated teeth, fixed appliances should be applied. Lateral crossbites can be efficiently treated with cross elastics. Appliances for such tooth movements may conveniently be combined with activators.

Since the activator cannot induce bodily movement of posterior teeth, it is not the appliance of choice for the closing of extraction spaces.

It should be mentioned that the activator can be used advantageously in the final stages of Class II treatment, after removal of the fixed appliances. The activator is not an efficient appliance in retaining rotations of teeth. However, it may be useful in the settling in of the posterior teeth and in the stabilizing of the vertical dimension.

In conclusion, the activator is not a universal appliance, by means of which it is possible to treat any malocclusion to a satisfactory end result. However, it may be a useful tool for the discriminant orthodontist in the treatment of many Class II malocclusions. The application of activator therapy should be based on a careful study of the case in question, and a detailed plan for the treatment objectives. Combination with fixed appliances may be the best approach in certain cases.

MANAGEMENT OF THE ACTIVATOR

For active treatment, the appliance should be worn at least 10 hours per day. There are no risks in using it more, and the more it is used, the better.

For the control of the appliance, it is not necessary to see the patient very often. However, the visits to the orthodontist stimulate and motivate the patient to wear the plate.

During the visits it should be emphasized that the molars and premolars are not to be prevented from erupting and that the soft tissues are not to be impinged upon. The activity of the springs and spurs should be checked. Careful scrutiny and periodic minor adjustments are frequently all that is necessary.

POST-TREATMENT STABILITY IN CLASS II MALOCCLUSION CASES TREATED WITH ACTIVATORS

Post-treatment stability is a neglected field in activator literature. A number of cases have been reported, but few systematic studies on represent-

TABLE 7-1. PATIENTS' AGE AT THE BEGINNING OF ACTIVATOR TREATMENT, AND LENGTH OF THE POST-TREATMENT OBSERVATION PERIOD (IN YEARS) IN A GROUP OF 13 CLASS II, DIVISION 1 MALOCCLUSION CASES

	Mean	Range
Age at the beginning of treatment	10.9	8.1 to 16.5
Duration of treatment	3.3	0.8 to 8.1
Length of post-treatment observation period	5.9	2.5 to 15.3

TABLE 7-2. CHANGES IN UPPER DENTAL ARCH WIDTH (in mm.) AT THE FIRST MOLARS DURING AND AFTER ACTIVATOR TREATMENT IN A GROUP OF 13 CLASS II, DIVISION 1 MALOCCLUSION CASES*

	Mean	Range
Treatment changes	+3.0	+0.5 to +6.0
Post-treatment changes	−1.7	0.0 to −4.0
Net changes	+1.3	−1.0 to +5.0

*+ designates increases; − designates decreases.

TABLE 7-3. CHANGES IN LOWER DENTAL ARCH WIDTH (in mm.) AT THE FIRST MOLARS DURING AND AFTER ACTIVATOR TREATMENT IN A GROUP OF 13 CLASS II, DIVISION 1 MALOCCLUSION CASES*

	Mean	Range
Treatment changes	+0.5	0.0 to +1.5
Post-treatment changes	−0.4	0.0 to −1.5
Net changes	+0.1	0.0 to +1.5

*+ designates increases; − designates decreases.

TABLE 7-4. VERTICAL OVERBITE (in mm.) AT THE BEGINNING OF ACTIVATOR TREATMENT, AT THE END OF TREATMENT, AND AT THE POST-TREATMENT CONTROL IN A GROUP OF 13 CLASS II, DIVISION 1 MALOCCLUSION CASES

	Mean	Range
At the beginning of treatment	5.5	3.5 to 7.5
At the end of treatment	2.9	1.0 to 4.0
At the post-treatment control	3.1	1.0 to 4.5

TABLE 7-5. CHANGES IN VERTICAL OVERBITE (in mm.) DURING AND AFTER ACTIVATOR TREATMENT IN A GROUP OF 13 CLASS II, DIVISION 1 MALOCCLUSION CASES*

	Mean	Range
Treatment changes	−2.6	−1.5 to −4.0
Post-treatment changes	+0.2	+1.0 to −0.5
Net changes	−2.4	−1.0 to −4.0

*+ designates increases; − designates decreases.

TABLE 7-6. HORIZONTAL OVERBITE (in mm.) AT THE BEGINNING OF ACTIVATOR TREATMENT, AT THE END OF TREATMENT, AND AT THE POST-TREATMENT CONTROL IN A GROUP OF 13 CLASS II, DIVISION 1 MALOCCLUSION CASES

	Mean	Range
At the beginning of treatment	8.0	5.5 to 13.0
At the end of treatment	2.9	2.0 to 3.5
At the post-treatment control	3.1	2.0 to 4.0

ative materials are available. To give the reader some information on the matter, the findings in a previously unreported study will be presented.[121]

The material consisted of series of plaster casts taken at the beginning of treatment, at the end of treatment, and at a post-treatment control. The cases were selected for exhibiting Class II, Division 1 malocclusions at the beginning of treatment and acceptable occlusions at the end of treatment, achieved by activators exclusively. Of 16 patients called back for post-treatment control, 13 responded. Information on the patient's age, the duration of treatment, and the length of the post-treatment observation period is presented in Table 7-1.

Treatment approach and appliance design were the same in all the cases. The construction bites were taken with the mandible displaced 4 to 6 mm. caudally and the width of one premolar anteriorly (8 to 10 mm.) The patients were instructed to wear the appliances at night, for a minimum of 10 hours in each 24. Retainers were not used.

An increased upper dental arch width at the first molars was registered at the end of treatment in all the cases. In the post-treatment period, a total relapse occurred in two cases, but in 11 cases there was a net gain between the beginning of treatment and the post-treatment control, ranging between 0.5 and 5.0 mm. (Table 7-2). Similar findings have been reported by Grude.[56]

Text continued on page 177

TABLE 7-7. CHANGES IN HORIZONTAL OVERBITE (in mm.) DURING AND AFTER ACTIVATOR TREATMENT IN A GROUP OF 13 CLASS II, DIVISION 1 MALOCCLUSION CASES*

	Mean	Range
Treatment changes	−5.1	−3.0 to −9.5
Post-treatment changes	+0.2	+1.0 to −1.0
Net changes	−4.9	−2.5 to −9.0

*+ designates increases; − designates decreases.

TABLE 7-8. CHANGES IN AVAILABLE SPACE (in mm.) IN THE ANTERIOR SEGMENT OF THE LOWER DENTAL ARCH DURING AND AFTER ACTIVATOR TREATMENT IN A GROUP OF 13 CLASS II, DIVISION 1 MALOCCLUSION CASES*

	Mean	Range
Treatment changes	+1.5	0.0 to +4.5
Post-treatment changes	−1.2	+1.5 to −4.5
Net changes	+0.3	−1.0 to +4.0

*+ designates increases; − designates decreases.

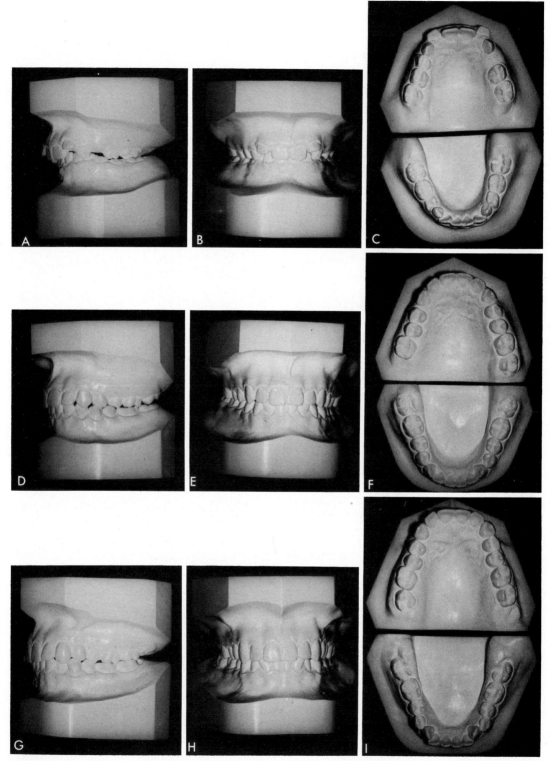

Figure 7-35. A Class II, Division 2 malocclusion treated with activator only. Treatment started at the age of 7.4 years (*A* to *C*) and completed at an age of 11.8 years (*D* to *F*). Post-treatment control at an age of 18.6 years (*G* to *I*).

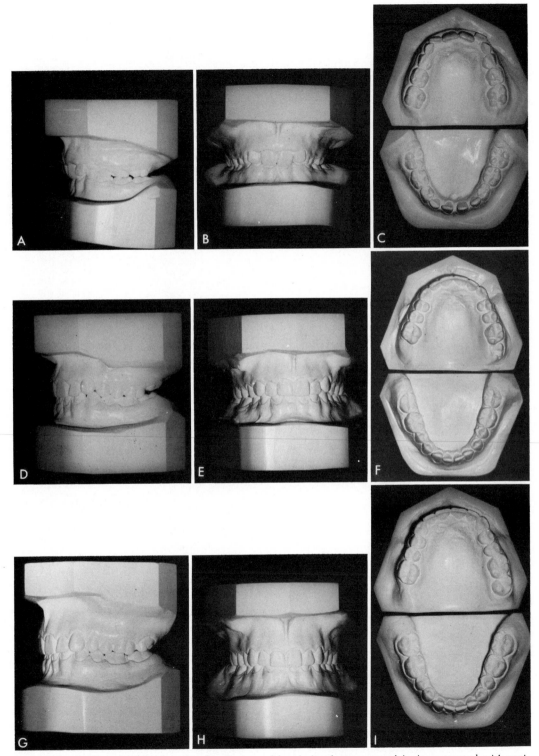

Figure 7–36. A Class II, Division 2 malocclusion with missing lower central incisors treated with activator only. Treatment started at an age of 8.0 years (*A* to *C*) and completed at an age of 13.7 years (*D* to *E*). Post-treatment control at an age of 18.5 years (*G* to *I*).

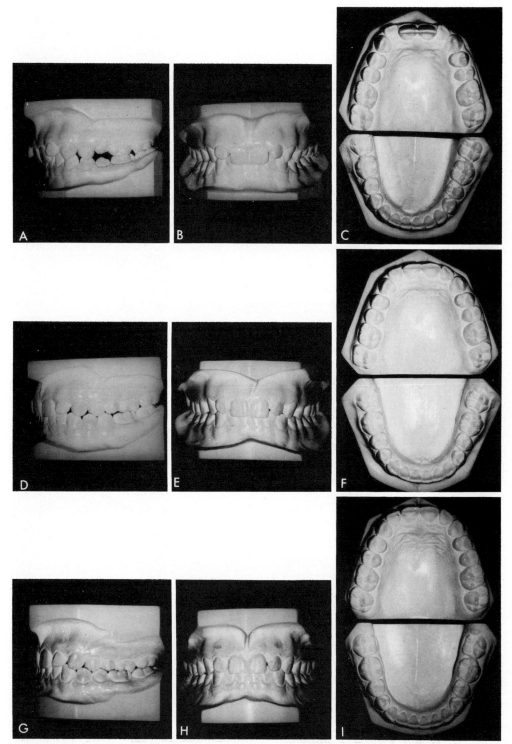

Figure 7–37. A Class II, Division 2 malocclusion treated with activator only. Treatment started at an age of 11.7 years (*A* to *C*) and completed at an age of 13.7 years (*D* to *E*). Post-treatment control at an age of 18.3 years (*G* to *I*).

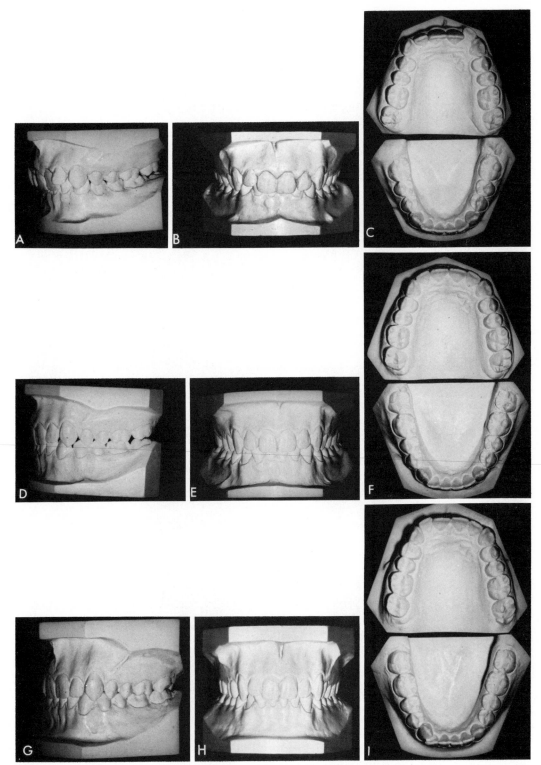

Figure 7–38. A Class II, Division 2 malocclusion treated with activator only. Treatment started at an age of 13.6 years (*A* to *C*) and completed at an age of 15.7 years (*D* to *F*). Post-treatment control at an age of 19.2 years (*G* to *I*).

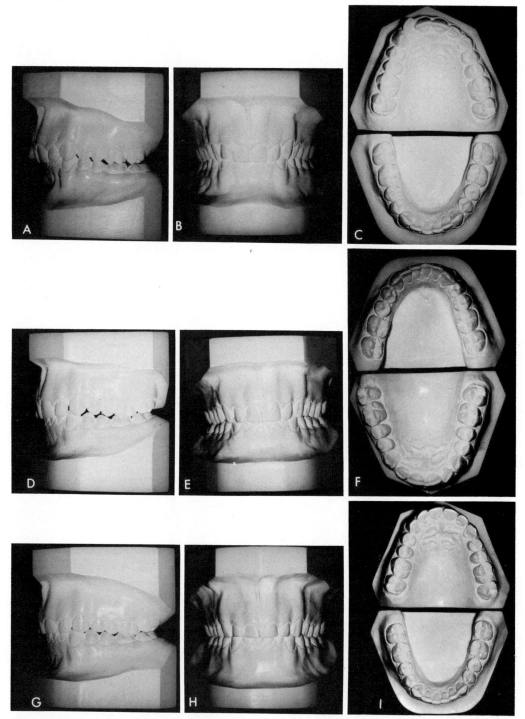

Figure 7–39. A Class II, Division 2 malocclusion treated with activator only. Treatment started at an age of 20.4 years (*A* to *C*) and completed at an age of 23.0 years (*D* to *F*). The occlusion was equilibrated one month later (*G* to *I*). Post-treatment control at an age of 36.7 years (*J* to *L*).

Illustration continued on opposite page

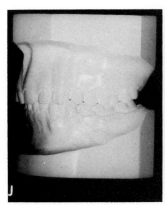
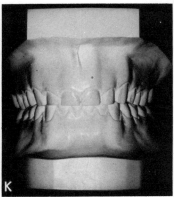
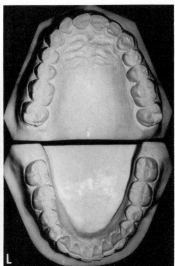

Figure 7–39 *Continued.*

The treatment changes in lower dental arch width at the first molars were small. So also were the post-treatment changes or relapse (Table 7–3).

The vertical overbite was reduced in all the cases during treatment. The post-treatment changes were small, and there was a net reduction from the beginning of treatment to the post-treatment observation period in all the cases (Tables 7–4 and 7–5). Similar findings have been reported by Ahlgren.[4]

The horizontal overbite was reduced in all the cases. The post-treatment changes were small, and in all the cases there was a net reduction between the beginning of the treatment and the post-treatment observation (Tables 7–6 and 7–7). Again, similar findings have been reported by Ahlgren.[4]

Available space in the anterior segment of the lower dental arch increased during treatment in 10 of the 13 cases, while it remained unchanged in three. In 12 cases it decreased during the post-treatment period, but it increased in one. In four cases, there was a net gain between the beginning of treatment and the post-treatment control visit. In five cases there was a net loss, and in four cases the available space was the same (Table 7–8).

No reports on studies of Class II, Division 2 malocclusion cases treated with activators seem to be available. A plaster cast series of five cases, treated with activators and chosen at random is offered as a source of information (Figs. 7–35 to 7–39). No supplementary appliances were used. It will be seen that the post-treatment change most frequently found was a crowding of the lower incisors.

It has been said that the orofacial muscle matrix is changed during activator treatment so that it becomes an efficient retainer. If this statement is meant to indicate that the occlusion of such patients is stable, the statement is not supported by the findings presented above. Post-treatment changes were common and usual findings in the group of patients studied. Similar observations have been made by Schmuth.[115] Systematic studies on the stability of results achieved by other types of activators do not seem to have been reported.

Bjørk[24, 26, 27] and Bjørk and Palling[30] found considerable changes in the occlusion and the craniofacial pattern also in random samples of orthodontically untreated individuals during adolescence. Hopkins and Murphy[73] and

Humerfelt and Slagsvold[121] made similar observations in individuals with good occlusions. It therefore appears unrealistic to expect orthodontically treated cases to remain stable during the same period when the normal occlusion also changes. Still, it must be an aim of the orthodontist to produce results of maximum stability. It has not been documented that the activator has advantages over other appliances in that respect. As pointed out by Graber,[49] the question of post-treatment stability deserves more attention than it has hitherto received, because information on this problem has a strong impact on orthodontic therapy.

References

1. Aas, B.: En elektromyografisk undersøkelse av m.temporalis og m.masseter ved forskjellige orthodontiske behandlingsmetoder. Nor. Tannlaegeforen. Tid., *70*:85–103, 1960.
2. Ahlgren, J.: An electromyographic analysis of the response to activator (Andresen-Häupl) therapy. Odontol. Revy, *11*:125–151, 1960.
3. Ahlgren, J.: The neurophysiologic principles of the Andresen method of functional jaw orthopedics. A critical analysis and new hypothesis. Sven. Tandlak. Tidskr., *63*:1–9, 1970.
4. Ahlgren, J.: A longitudinal clinical and cephalometric study of 50 malocclusion cases treated with activator appliances. Trans. Eur. Orthod. Soc., pp. 285–293, 1972.
5. Andresen, V.: Bio-mekanisk ortodonti. Et ortodontisk system for privatpraksis og skole-tannklinikker. Nor. Tannlaegeforen. Tid., *41*:71–93, 161–178, and 442–443, 1931.
6. Andresen, V.: Bio-mekanisk ortodonti. Et ortodontisk system for privatpraksis og skole-tannklinikker. Nor. Tannlaegeforen. Tid., *42*:131–138, 215–230, and 295–312, 1932.
7. Andresen, V.: Ueber das sogenannte "Norwegische System der Funktions-Kiefer-Orthopädie." Dtsch. Zahnaerztl. Wochenschr., *39*:235–238 and 283–286, 1936.
8. Andresen, V., and Häupl, K.: Funktionskieferorthopädie. Die Grundlagen des "norwegischen Systems." Leipzig, H. Meusser, 1936.
9. Andresen, V., and Häupl, K.: Funktionskieferorthopädie. Die Grundlagen des "norwegischen Systems." 2. Aufl. Leipzig, H. Meusser, 1939.
10. Andresen, V., and Häupl, K.: Funktionskieferorthopädie. Die Grundlagen des "norwegischen Systems." 3. Aufl. Leipzig, J. A. Barth, Verlag, 1942.
11. Andresen, V., and Häupl, K.: Funktionskieferorthopädie. Die Grundlagen des "norwegischen Systems." 4. Aufl. Leipzig, J. A. Barth, Verlag, 1945.
12. Andresen, V., Häupl, K., and Petrik, L.: Funktionskieferorthopädie. 6., umgearbeitete und erweiterte Auflage von K. Häupl and L. Petrik. München, J. A. Barth, 1957.
13. Angle, E. H.: Treatment of malocclusion of the teeth, 7th ed. Philadelphia, S. S. White Dental Manufacturing Co., 1907.
14. Arya, B. S., and Modi, A. B.: Changes in the electrical activity of the muscles due to insertion of the activator. J. Indian Orthod. Soc., *5*:35–40, 1973.
15. Ascher, F.: Kontrollierte Ergebnisse der Rückbissbehandlung mit funktionskieferorthopädischen Geräten. Fortschr. Kieferorthop., *32*:149–159, 1971.
16. Ballard, C. F.: A consideration of the physiological background of mandibular posture and movement. Dent. Pract. Dent. Rec., *6*:80–90, 1955.
17. Balters, W.: Eine Einführung in die Bionatorheilmethode. Ausgewählte Schriften und Vorträge. Heidelberg, C. Herrmann, 1973.
18. Baume, L. J.: The prenatal and postnatal development of the human temporomandibular joint. Trans. Eur. Orthod. Soc., pp. 63–73, 1962.
19. Baume, L. J.: Cephalo-facial growth patterns and the functional adaptation of the temporomandibular joint structures. Trans. Eur. Orthod. Soc., pp. 79–98, 1969.
20. Baume, L. J., and Derichsweiler, H.: Is the condylar growth center responsive to orthodontic therapy? An experimental study in macaca mulatta. Oral Surg., *14*:347–362, 1961.
21. Baume, L. J., Häupl, K., and Stellmach, R.: Growth and transformation of the temporomandibular joint in an orthopedically treated case of Pierre Robin's syndrome. Am. J. Orthod., *45*:901–916, 1959.
22. Bimler, H. P.: Die elastischen Gebissformer. Zahnärztl. Welt. *4*:499–503, 1949.
23. Bimler, H. P.: Prefabricated parts for oral adaptors. Trans. Eur. Orthod. Soc., pp. 355–358, 1960.
24. Bjørk, A.: A discussion on the significance of growth changes in facial pattern and their relationship to changes in occlusion. Dent. Rec., *71*:197–208, 1951.
25. Bjørk, A.: The principle of the Andresen method of orthodontic treatment, a discussion based on cephalometric x-ray analysis of treated cases. Am. J. Orthod., *37*:437–458, 1951.
26. Bjørk, A.: Variability and age changes in overjet and overbite. Report from a follow-up study of individuals from 12 to 20 years of age. Am. J. Orthod., *39*:779–801, 1953.

27. Bjørk, A.: Cranial base development. A follow-up x-ray study of the individual variation in growth occurring between the ages of 12 and 20 years and its relation to brain case and face development. Am. J. Orthod., *41*:198–225, 1955.
28. Bjørk, A.: Variations in the growth pattern of the human mandible: Longitudinal radiographic study by the implant method. J. Dent. Res., *42*:400–411, 1963.
29. Bjørk, A.: Prediction of mandibular growth rotation. Am. J. Orthod., *55*:585–599, 1969.
30. Bjørk, A., and Palling, M.: Adolescent age changes in sagittal jaw relation, alveolar prognathy, and incisal inclination. Acta Odontol. Scand., *12*:201–232, 1954–1955.
31. Breitner, C.: Experimentelle Veränderung der mesiodistalen Beziehungen der oberen und unteren Zahnreihen. Z. Stomatol., *28*:134–154 and 620–635, 1930.
32. Charlier, J.-P., Petrovic, A., and Herrmann-Stutzmann, J.: Effect of mandibular hyperpropulsion on the prechondroblastic zone of young rat condyle. Am. J. Orthod., *55*:71–74, 1969.
33. Demisch, A.: Effects of activator therapy on the craniofacial skeleton in Class II, Division 1 malocclusion. Trans. Eur. Orthod. Soc., pp. 295–310, 1972.
34. Demisch, A.: Auswirkungen der Distalbisstherapie mit dem Aktivator auf das Gesichtsskelett. Schweiz. Monatsschr. Zahnheilkd., *83*:1072–1092, 1973.
35. Dickson, G. C., Grossmann, W., Mills, J. R. E., Tulley, W. J., and Moyers, R. E.: Symposium on functional therapy. Dent. Pract. Dent. Rec., *15*:255–274, 1965.
36. Dietrich, U. C.: Aktivator-Mandibuläre Reaktion. Schweiz. Monatsschr. Zahnheilkd., *83*:1092–1104, 1973.
37. Elgoyhen, J. C., Moyers, R. E., McNamara, J. A., and Riolo, M. L.: Craniofacial adaptation to protrusive function in young rhesus monkeys. Am. J. Orthod., *62*:469–480, 1972.
38. Eschler, J.: Wesen und Möglichkeiten der Verwendung von kontinuierlicher und intermittierenden Kräften im Rahmen des Andresen-Häupl'schen Behandlungssystems. Oesterr. Z. Stomatol., *47*:53–76, 1950.
39. Eschler, J.: Die muskuläre Wirkungsweise des Andresen-Häuplschen Apparates. Oesterr. Z. Stomatol., *49*:79–105, 1952.
40. Eschler, J.: Die funktionelle Orthopädie des Kausystems. München, C. Hanser, 1952.
41. Eschler, J.: Elektrophysiologische und pathologische Untersuchungen des Kausystems, 4. Mitteilung. Elektromyographische Untersuchungen über die Wirksamkeit muskeltonussteigender Medikamente bei Anwendung des Andresen-Häupl Apparates. Dtsch. Zahnärztl. Z., *10*:1421–1428, 1955.
42. Eschler, J.: Die Kieferdehnung mit funktionskieferorthopädischen Apparaten: der Funktionator. Zahnärztl. Welt. *63*:203–207, 1962.
43. Fränkel, R.: The treatment of Class II, Division 1 malocclusion with functional correctors. Am. J. Orthod., *55*:265–275, 1969.
44. Fränkel, R.: Technik und Handhabung der Funktionsregler. Berlin, VEB Verlag Volk und Gesundheit, 1973.
45. Fränkel, R., and Reiss, W.: Problematik der Unterkiefernachentwicklung bei Distalfällen. Fortschr. Kieferorthop., *31*:345–355, 1970.
46. Freunthaller, P.: Cephalometric observations in Class II, Division 1 malocclusions treated with the activator. Angle Orthod., *37*:18–25, 1967.
47. Gerber, M.: Beobachtungen an schlafenden Aktivatorträgern. Fortschr. Kieferorthop., *18*:205–232, 1957.
48. Gerlach, H. G.: Muskeldynamik und Anomalien des Kauorganes. Fortschr. Kieferorthop., *23*: 184–192, 1962.
49. Graber, T. M.: Postmortems in posttreatment adjustment. Am. J. Orthod., *52*:331–352, 1966.
50. Graber, T. M.: Maxillary second molar extraction in Class II malocclusion. Am. J. Orthod., *56*:331–353, 1969.
51. Graber, T. M.: Orthodontics, Principles and Practice, 3rd ed. Philadelphia, W. B. Saunders Company, 1972.
52. Graf, E. Cited in Fränkel, R.: Technik und Handhabung der Funktionsregler. Berlin, VEB Verlag Volk und Gesundheit, 1961.
53. Gresham, H.: Mandibular changes in Andresen treatment of Angle Class II malocclusion. N. Z. Dent. J., *48*:10–36, 1952.
54. Grohs, R., and Petrik, L.: Die Funktionskieferorthopädie als Helferin der Prothetik. Z. Stomatol., *42*:160–178, 1944.
55. Grossman, W. J., Greenfield, B. E., and Timms, D. J.: Electromyography as an aid in diagnosis and treatment analysis. Am. J. Orthod., *47*:481–497, 1961.
56. Grude, R.: Myofunctional therapy. A review of various cases some years after their treatment by the Norwegian system had been completed. Nor. Tannlaegeforen. Tid., *62*:1–28, 1952.
57. Grude, R.: Ortodontisk terapi med avtagbar apparatur. Nord. Klin. Odont., 3/15/VI:1–31, 1966.
58. Hagerström, L.: Sex fall av distalbett med retruderade överkäksinsisiver behandlade med expansion. Sver. Tandlaekarfoerb. Tidn., *61*:826–833, 1969.
59. Harvold, E. P.: Distakokklusjon, Behandlingsmetodikk. Tandlaegebladet, *50*:146–155, 1946.
60. Harvold, E. P.: The activator in interceptive orthodontics. St. Louis, The C. V. Mosby Company, 1974.

61. Harvold, E. P., and Vargervik, K.: Morphogenetic response to activator treatment. Am. J. Orthod., *60*:478–490, 1971.
62. Hasund, A.: The use of activators in a system employing fixed appliances. Trans. Eur. Orthod. Soc., pp. 329–341, 1969.
63. Häupl, K.: Gewebsumbau und Zahnverdrängung in der Funktionskieferorthopädie. Eine funktionell-histologische Studie. Leipzig, J. A. Barth, 1938.
64. Häupl, K.: Transformation of the temporomandibular joint during orthodontic treatment. (Abstr.) Am. J. Orthod., *47*:151, 1961.
65. Häupl, K., and Psansky, R.: Experimentelle Untersuchungen über Gelenkstransformation bei Verwendung der Methoden der Funktionskieferorthopädie. Dtsch. Zahn. Mund. Kieferheilkd., *6*:439–448, 1939.
66. Hausser, E.: Wachstum und Entwicklung unter dem Einfluss funktionskieferorthopädischer Therapie. Fortschr. Kieferorthop., *24*:310–327, 1963.
67. Hausser, E.: Functional orthodontic treatment with the activator. Trans. Eur. Orthod. Soc., pp. 427–430, 1973.
68. Hausser, E.: Funktionskieferorthopädische Behandlung mit dem Aktivator. Fortschr. Kieferorthop., *36*:1–17, 1975.
69. Herren, P.: Die Wirkungsweise des Aktivators. Schweiz. Monatsschr. Zahnheilkd., *63*:829–879, 1953.
70. Herren, P.: The activator's mode of action. Am. J. Orthod., *45*:512–527, 1959.
71. Hoffer, O.: Les modifications de l'articulation temporomandibulaire par l'action des moyens orthopediques. Orthod. Fr., *29*:97–146, 1958.
72. Hollender, L., and Lindahl, L.: Radiographic study of articular remodeling in the temporomandibular joint after condylar fractures. Scand. J. Dent. Res., *82*:462–465, 1974.
73. Hopkins, J. B., and Murphy, J.: Variations in good occlusions. Angle Orthod., *41*:55–65, 1971.
74. Hotz, R.: Die funktionelle Beurteilung der Bisslage als Ausgangspunkt für die Prognose und die Begrenzung des Behandlungszieles. Fortschr. Kieferorthop., *16*:255–262, 1955.
75. Hotz, R. P.: Application and appliance manipulation of functional forces. Am. J. Orthod., *58*:459–478, 1970.
76. Hotz, R.: Orthodontics in daily practice. Possibilities and limitations in the area of children's dentistry. Bern, H. Huber, 1974.
77. Hotz, R., and Mühlemann, H.: Die Funktion in der Beurteilung und Therapie von Bissanomalien. Schweiz. Monatsschr. Zahnheilkd., *62*:592–606, 1952.
78. Humerfelt, A., and Slagsvold, O.: Changes in occlusion and craniofacial pattern between 11 and 25 years of age. A follow-up study of individuals with normal occlusion. Trans. Eur. Orthod. Soc., pp. 113–122, 1972.
79. Ingervall, B.: Relation between retruded contact, intercuspal and rest positions of mandible in children with Angle Class II, Division 2 malocclusions. Odontol. Revy, *19*:1–18, 1968.
80. Jacobsson, S. O.: Cephalometric evaluation of treatment effect on Class II, Division 1 malocclusions. Am. J. Orthod., *53*:446–457, 1967.
81. Johannesen, B.: Overjet and labio-lingual position of incisor teeth in treated Class II, Division 1 malocclusions. Thesis. University of Oslo, 1972.
82. Johannesen, B.: A critical evaluation of treatment planning Class II, Division 1 malocclusions. Studieweek, pp. 112–136, 1975.
83. Klammt, G.: Der offene Aktivator. Dtsch. Stomatol., *5*:322–327, 1955.
84. Korkhaus, G.: Ein kieferorthopädisch interessantes Zwillingpaar. Fortschr. Kieferorthop., *32*:257–263, 1971.
85. Koski, K.: Cranial growth centers: Facts or fallacies? Am. J. Orthod., *54*:566–583, 1968.
86. Litowitz, R.: A study of the movements of certain teeth during and following treatment. Angle Orthod., *18*:113–132, 1948.
87. Lund, K.: Mandibular growth and remodelling processes after condylar fracture. A longitudinal roentgencephalometric study. Thesis. Acta Odontol. Scand., *32*(Suppl. 64), 1974.
88. Martin, J. R.: The stability of the anterior teeth after treatment (Abstr.). Am. J. Orthod., *48*:788–789, 1962.
89. Marschner, J. F., and Harris, J. E.: Mandibular growth and Class II treatment. Angle Orthod., *36*:89–93, 1966.
90. May, J. F.: A laminagraphic and cephalometric evaluation of dental and skeletal changes occurring during activator treatment. M. S. thesis, University of Minnesota. Cited in Hirzel, H.-C., and Grewe, J. M. Activators: A practical approach. Am. J. Orthod., *66*:557–570, 1974.
91. McNamara, J. A.: Neuromuscular and skeletal adaptations to altered function in the orofacial region. Am. J. Orthod., *64*:578–606, 1973.
92. Meach, C. L.: A cephalometric comparison of bony profile changes in Class II, Division 1 patients treated with extraoral force and functional jaw orthopedics. Am. J. Orthod., *52*:353–370, 1966.
93. Mills, J. R. E.: The effect on the lower incisors of uncontrolled extraction of lower premolars. Trans. Eur. Orthod. Soc., pp. 357–370, 1964.
94. Mills J. R. E.: The long-term results of the proclination of lower incisors. Br. Dent. J., *120*:355–363, 1966.

95. Mills, J. R. E.: A long-term assessment of the mechanical retroclination of lower incisors. Angle Orthod., *37*:165–174, 1967.
96. Mills, J. R. E.: The stability of the lower labial segment. Dent. Pract. Dent. Rec., *18*:293–306, 1968.
97. Moss, J. P.: Cephalometric changes during functional appliance therapy. Trans. Eur. Orthod. Soc., pp. 327–341, 1962.
98. Moss, J. P.: Function—fact or fiction? Am. J. Orthod., *67*:625–646, 1975.
99. Moss, J. P.: An investigation of the muscle activity of patients with a Class II, Division 2 malocclusion and the changes during treatment. Trans. Eur. Orthod. Soc., in press.
100. Neumann, B.: Funktionskieferorthopädie. Rückblick und Ausblick. Fortschr. Kieferorthop., *36*:73–85, 1975.
101. Ozerovic, B.: Some changes in occlusion and craniofacial pattern obtained during treatment with removable orthodontic appliances. Trans. Eur. Orthod. Soc., pp. 329–337, 1972.
102. Parkhouse, R. C.: A cephalometric appraisal of cases of Angle's Class II, Division 1 malocclusion treated by the Andresen appliance. Dent. Pract. Dent. Rec., *19*:425–434, 1969.
103. Petrovic, A.: Recherches sur les mécanismes histophysiologiques de la croissance osseuse cranio-faciale. Ann. Biol., *9*:303–311, 1970.
104. Petrovic, A. G.: Mechanisms and regulation of mandibular condylar growth. Acta Morphol. Neerl. Scand., *10*:25–34, 1972.
105. Petrovic, A., Gasson, N., and Oudet, C.: Wirkung der übertriebenen posturalen Vorschubstellung des Unterkiefers auf das Kondylenwachstum der normalen und der mit Wachstumshormon behandelten Ratte. Fortschr. Kieferorthop., *36*:86–97, 1975.
106. Pfeiffer, J. P., and Groberty, D.: Simultaneous use of cervical appliance and activator: An orthopedic approach to fixed appliance therapy. Am. J. Orthod., *61*:353–373, 1972.
107. Qwarnström, K.-E., and Sarnäs, K.-V.: Röntgenkefalometriska studier av förändringar vid funktionskäkortopedisk behandling av distabett. 7 fall av Angle Klass II:1. Odontol. Revy, *5*:118–128, 1954.
108. Reitan, K.: The initial tissue reaction incident to orthodontic tooth movement as related to the influence of function. An experimental histological study on animal and human material. Thesis, University of Oslo, 1951.
109. Ricketts, R. M.: Analysis—the interim. Angle Orthod., *40*:129–137, 1970.
110. Robin, P. Cited in Hotz, R.: Orthodontics in daily practice. Possibilities and limitations in the area of children's dentistry. Bern, H. Huber, 1974.
111. Roth, R. H.: Temporomandibular pain-dysfunction and occlusal relationships. Angle Orthod., *43*:136–153, 1973.
112. Roux, W.: Gesammelte Abhandlungen über Entwicklungsmechanik der Organismen. Leipzig, W. Engelmann, 1895.
113. Schmuth, G.: Untersuchungen über die auf das FKO-Gerät einwirkende Kaumuskeltätigkeit während des Schlafes. Fortschr. Kieferorthop., *16*:327–331, 1955.
114. Schmuth, G.: Muskeltätigkeit und Muskelwirkung im Rahmen der Funktionskieferorthopädie. Dtsch. Zahn. Mund. Kieferheilkd., *32*:4–21 and 124–147, 1960.
115. Schmuth, G. P. F.: Behandlungzeit—Retentionszeit—Rezidive. Fortschr. Kieferorthop., *27*:22–31, 1966.
116. Schwarz, A. M.: Grundsätzliches über die heutigen kieferorthopädischen Behandlungsverfahren. Oesterr. Z. Stomatol., *47*:400–425 and 448–470, 1950.
117. Schwarz, A. M.: Die Wirkungsweise des Aktivators. Fortschr. Kieferorthop., *13*:117–138, 1952.
118. Scott, J. H.: The growth of the human face. Proc. R. Soc. Med., *47*:91–100, 1954.
119. Selmer-Olsen, R.: En kritisk betraktning over "Det norske system." Nor. Tannlaegefor. Tid., *47*:85–91, 134–142, and 176–193, 1937.
120. Sergl, H. G.: Changes in craniofacial pattern caused by functional adaptation—an experimental study in young rabbits. Trans. Eur. Orthod. Soc., pp. 197–209, 1972.
121. Slagsvold, O., and Kolstad, I.: Class II, Division 1 malocclusions treated with activators. A study of posttreatment stability. In manuscript, 1975.
122. Softley, J. W.: Cephalometric changes in seven "post normal" cases treated by the Andresen method. Dent. Rec., *73*:485–494, 1953.
123. Stockfisch, H.: Der Kinetor in der Kieferorthopädie. Die Praxis des polyvalenten bimaxillären Apparates und seine rationelle Technik mit Plastik—Fertigteilen. Heidelberg, A. Hüthig, 1966.
124. Stockfisch, H.: Possibilities and limitations of the kinetor. Trans. Eur. Orthod. Soc., pp. 457–460, 1973.
125. Stöckli, P. W., and Willert, H. G.: Tissue reactions in the temporomandibular joint resulting from anterior displacement of the mandible in the monkey. Am. J. Orthod., *60*:142–155, 1971.
126. Tallgren, A.: The reduction in face height of edentulous and partially edentulous subjects during long-term denture wear. A longitudinal roentgenographic cephalometric study. Acta Odontol. Scand., *24*:195–239, 1966.
127. Thilander, B., and Filipsson, R.: Muscle activity related to activator and intermaxillary trac-

tion in Angle Class II, Division 1 malocclusions. An electromyographic study of the temporal, masseter and suprahyoid muscles. Acta Odontol. Scand., *24*:241–257, 1966.

128. Thompson, J. R.: The rest position of the mandible and its significance to dental science. J. Am. Dent. Assoc., *33*:151–180, 1946.

129. Trayfoot, J., and Richardson, A.: Angle Class II, Division 1 malocclusions treated by the Andresen method. Br. Dent. J., *124*:516–519, 1968.

130. Tryti, T.: Angle Kl. II, 1 malokklusjoner korrigert med fasialbue og aktivator. Thesis, University of Oslo, 1974.

131. Tulley, W. J.: The scope and limitations of treatment with the activator. Am. J. Orthod., *61*:562–577, 1972.

132. Tweed, C. H.: A philosophy of orthodontic treatment. Am. J. Orthod. Oral Surg., *31*:74–103, 1945.

133. Witt, E.: Investigations into orthodontic forces of different appliances. Trans. Eur. Orthod. Soc., pp. 391–408, 1966.

134. Witt, E.: Muscular physiological investigations into the effect of bi-maxillary appliances. Trans. Eur. Orthod. Soc., pp. 448–450, 1973.

135. Witt, E., and Komposch, G.: Intermaxilläre Kraftwirkung bimaxillärer Geräte. Fortschr. Kieferorthop., *32*:345–352, 1971.

136. Witt, E., and Meyer, U.: Indications for and working action of bimaxillary appliances. Trans. Eur. Orthod. Soc., pp. 321–328, 1972.

137. Wolff, J.: Das Gesetz der Transformation der Knochen. Berlin, Hirschwald, 1892.

138. Woodside, D. G.: Some effects of activator treatment on the mandible and the midface. Trans. Eur. Orthod. Soc., pp. 443–447, 1973.

CHAPTER 8

The Activator: Use and Modifications*

The history of the activator has been described in the previous chapter. We shall never know the exact influence of Pierre Robin, who read a paper on his monobloc around the turn of the century, foreshadowing the shape, though not yet the function of the activator.[1] And, it has been said that Andresen was stimulated by Norman Kingsley and some of the ideas of John Nutting Farrar, who wrote one of the first books in orthodontics.[2, 3] Some observers feel that without the fortunate opportunity to join forces with Häupl, who was in Oslo at that time, Andresen's appliance might not have fared much better than Robin's.[4-7] The controversy over the actual effect of functional appliances stimulated Reitan to do his monumental research in the early 1950's, in which some of the early theoretical foundations of functional jaw orthopedics were refuted.[8] Yet, the simple but overwhelming fact is that a significant source of energy has been tapped by enlisting the orofacial musculature as a therapeutic adjunct. The Andresen-Häupl activator has held its own against the emerging multitude of similar apppliances and has not outlived its usefulness. Some of the modifications of the activator are described in this chapter, as well as those already discussed in Chapter 7. Special chapters are devoted to others.

The activator can be used for the correction of Class II, Division 1; Class II, Division II; Class III; and open bite malocclusions. It is best suited for achievement of gross changes in sagittal and vertical dimensions in the mixed and early permanent dentition period. Individual tooth movements are difficult to accomplish. The activator is, therefore, not generally recommended for the treatment of malocclusions with crowding and only rarely for those requiring extractions.

The mild to moderately severe Class II, Division 1 malocclusions with a deep bite and a horizontal growth direction respond best to the treatment with an activator. Figures 8–1 and 8–2 show activators and the cases treated with them. Since the most typical activator treatment is the treatment of the Class II, Division 1 malocclusion, the main emphasis of this chapter will be on the correction of this malocclusion.

---

*The authors are particularly grateful to Dr. Kaija Virolainen for her continuing advice and editorial assistance in the preparation of this chapter.

CORRECTION OF CLASS II, DIVISION 1 MALOCCLUSION

To correct the typical Class II, Division 1 malocclusion, or, in the language of functional jaw orthopedics, to change a "dysgnathia" into "eugnathia," all or most of the following transformations are necessary:

1. Expansion of the upper arch.

2. Retrusion of the upper incisors to form a normal arch.

3. Protrusion of the lower incisors in selected cases.

4. Reduction of a deep overbite:

    a. by intruding the incisors, or, at least preventing their normal eruption.

    b. by stimulating the eruption of posterior teeth, simultaneously guiding the maxillary posterior teeth distally and the lower posterior teeth mesially. There is, however, some divergence of views on this point (see Chapter 12). As for the lower arch, such movement may not be desirable in the case of present or foreseeable crowding of the lower incisors.

5. Forward positioning of the lower jaw from a full Class II position to one in a neutral (or Class I) relationship. In the language of functional jaw orthopedics, this is meant to stimulate additional development of the lower jaw in length by transforming the temporomandibular joint and elongating the ramus, possibly changing the angle of condyle to ramus. Such contentions, however, remain controversial.

The narrow V-shaped maxillary arch needs to be expanded to allow the forward movement of the mandibular arch. If much expansion is needed, it is advisable to expand the maxillary arch first with an active plate. Usually, expansion can be accomplished with the activator by incorporating an expansion screw in the palatal section. Some expansion can be achieved, even with a passive activator, by grinding off acrylic from the palatal roof so that the appliance can work as a wedge against the maxillary dental arches and alveoli.

Eruption of the posterior teeth (molars and premolars) is facilitated by grinding acrylic away from the occlusal aspects of the appliance contiguous to the teeth. The upper posterior teeth are guided distally and inferiorly by allowing contact with the appliance acrylic only at the mesiogingival aspects of these teeth. The lower posterior teeth are relieved to erupt occlusally and sometimes mesially and guided similarly by the appliance construction. In other words, with moderate expansion of the buccal segments, the maxillary buccal teeth are stimulated in a distal direction, while the mandibular buccal teeth have a slight mesial directional vector. Harvold has shown that normal eruption of the mandibular teeth is in an upward and forward direction. Hence, all efforts should be made to stimulate these physiologic and developmental phenomena[9] (see Chapter 12). Some authors, however, take special precautions to prevent any excessive mesial movement of lower buccal teeth, which might crowd the incisor segment.

The eruption of the lower incisors is prevented at the same time by letting the acrylic contact them incisally. If mesial tipping of lower incisors is not

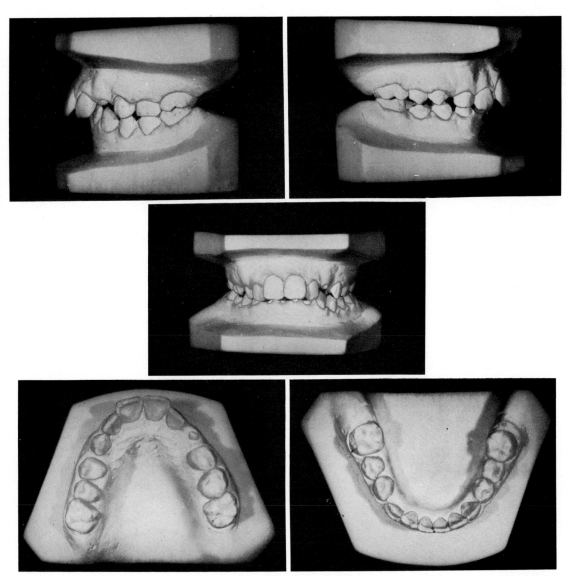

Figure 8-1. *A,* Female patient, 8 years, 8 months, with a Class II tendency, and the usual sequelae of excessive overbite and overjet, as well as abnormal perioral muscle function. If left unattended, the prospects are for the development of a full Class II malocclusion.

Illustration continued on following page

desired, the acrylic is extended over the incisal third of the labial surfaces. On the other hand, if forward tipping is indicated, acrylic is removed from the labial surfaces. The upper incisors are retracted by grinding acrylic away behind the incisors, including the alveolar portion, and by letting a stiff bow contact the teeth labially. Figures 8–1 and 8–2 illustrate response to activator therapy.

If the appliance is properly constructed, the muscles of mastication that are extended slightly past postural resting position are automatically stimulated to contract (stretch reflex) according to basic muscle physiologic principles. The same contractile tendency occurs when the sublingual muscles are extended by the forward positioning of the mandible, and they attempt to pull the lower jaw

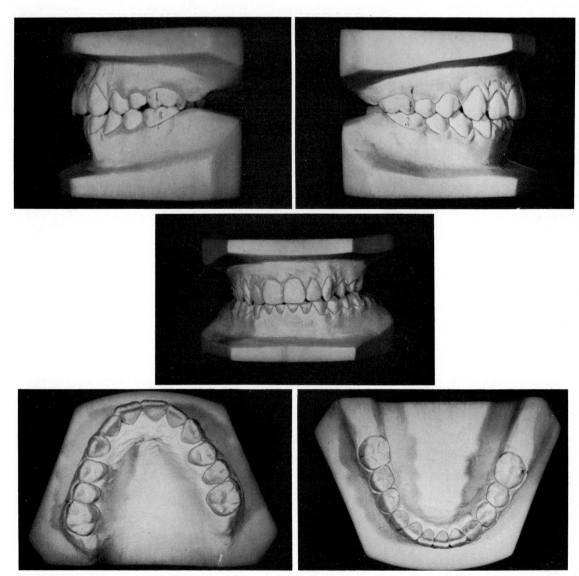

Figure 8-1 *Continued. B,* The same patient 10 months later, after the placement of an activator. Further correction of the overbite would require the continued wearing of an activator or a modified biteplate. But the intercuspation has been improved, overjet corrected, and the abnormal perioral muscle function eliminated.

Illustration continued on opposite page

back to the original position. The mandibular arch is, however, kept in a forward position by the appliance which, in turn, is buttressed against the maxillary teeth and alveoli. Thus, the lower incisor teeth, which are under pressure from the lingual, are able to move somewhat labially, and in so doing allow room for the lower posterior teeth to move upward and forward to a degree. At the very least, the physiologic mesial drift of the lower posterior teeth is brought to its fullest potential and increased during functional jaw orthopedic treatment. On the other hand, the maxillary arch is under pressure from the labial. This pressure stimulates retrusion of the anterior teeth and interferes

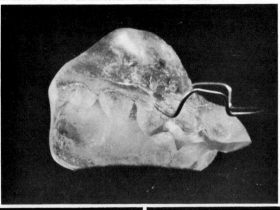

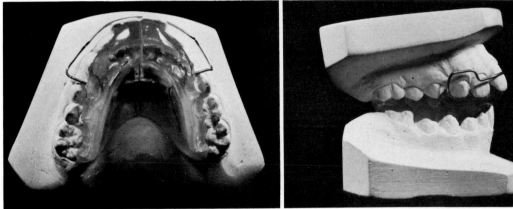

Figure 8–1 *Continued. C,* The activator used in treatment of this patient. *Lower left,* Appliance on mandibular plaster cast. *Lower right,* Upper and lower casts articulated with appliance in place. The labial wire on the maxillary portion assists in retention as well as in retracting maxillary incisors and closing spaces. (From Graber, T. M., and Swain, B. F. (Eds.): Current Orthodontic Concepts and Techniques, 2nd ed. Philadelphia, W. B. Saunders Company, 1975.)

with mesial drift of the maxillary buccal segments, possibly exerting an actual distal movement on these teeth as they erupt (Fig. 8–3). There is more frequent reflexive closing of the jaws during the sleeping hours. Some authors feel there is increased saliva flow during the wearing of the appliance. If this is true, it is evident that teeth are brought together more during appliance wear because of the greater demands of swallowing. If the mandible must be maintained in the forward position, then the muscles are subjected to more exercise. The resultant effect on the muscle-periosteum-bone interface, with resultant homeostatic adaptation, is favorable for correction of the malocclusion.

In the case illustrated in Figure 8–2, the movements listed above were simultaneously effected over a period of two and one-half years, using two activators which were worn during the night only. The second activator also was used as a retainer for one year following treatment. Although the changes that have been illustrated have been achieved with various orthodontic treatment philosophies, there is still controversy as to how they actually come about. As far as functional orthopedics is concerned, however, there is little doubt that most of the changes are instigated by the activator holding the mandible

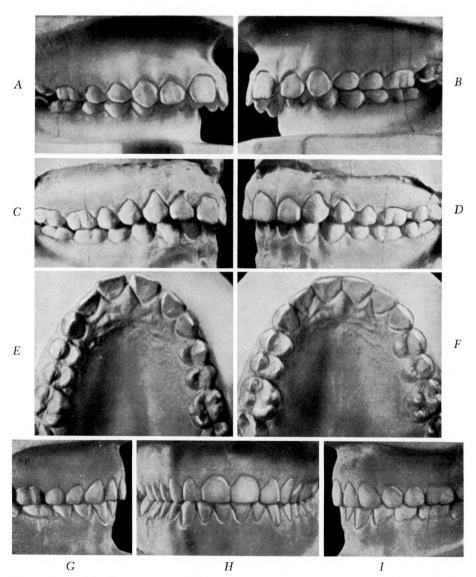

Figure 8–2. The first case treated by A. M. Schwarz. Activators were used exclusively as a test of functional jaw orthopedics. *A, B,* and *E,* Typical Class II, Division I malocclusion in a 12-year-old girl. *C* and *D,* Effect of the first activator, *J,* worn exclusively at night for 16 months. *F* to *I,* Effect of second activator, worn as retainer for an additional two and one half years. The model was made one year after removal of retention.

Illustration continued on opposite page

J

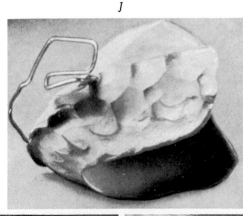

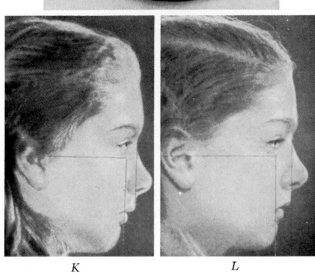

K   L

Figure 8-2 *Continued. J,* The first activator, made of vulcanite, with no expansion screw. (Canine loops, originally used by Andresen and Häupl, are rarely used now.) *K* and *L,* The patient before and after treatment. (From Schwarz, A. M., and Gratzinger, M.: Removable Orthodontic Appliances. Philadelphia, W. B. Saunders Company, 1966.)

Figure 8-3. The alveolar effect of the activator in the treatment of a Class II, Division 1 malocclusion. Arrow 1 demonstrates the retractive force of the sublingual muscles, which are extended while the lower jaw is kept in a forward position by the appliance. They tend to regain their original position. In this manner, they exert labial tipping force on the mandibular incisors. To offset this tendency, the acrylic encapsulates the lower incisor edges, so that, theoretically, only bodily forward movement is possible. The resistance of bodily movement is usually greater than the sublingual muscle retractive force. In most instances, the muscles accommodate to the forward position of the lower jaw. In some cases, however, minimal lower incisor bodily movement may occur (arrow 3). The weight of the lower jaw, which is partly absorbed by the appliance, and the retraction of the sublingual muscles (as long as it lasts) press the activator against the mesiolingual surfaces of the upper posterior teeth. This pressure induces a distal movement of the buccal segments in some cases (arrow 2), if it is not equalized by the resistance of the protruded upper anterior teeth. These should be simultaneously retruded by the labial bow of the activator. (From Schwarz, A. M., and Gratzinger, M.: Removable Orthodontic Appliances. Philadelphia, W. B. Saunders Company, 1966.)

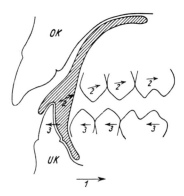

forward (hyperpropulsion) and the ensuing reaction of the stretched muscles transmitted to the periosteum, bone, and teeth. A restraining influence on maxillary growth and on the maxillary alveolodental complex, and a stimulating one on mandibular development with concomitant alveolar adaptation, are valid assumptions (Fig. 8–3). Various research endeavors tend to substantiate the claim that there is favorable change in the temporomandibular joint also. This possibility of induced change in the condyle is particularly likely in the prechondroblastic zone, as shown by Charlier, Petrovic, and Linck.[10] The improvement of a Class II, Division 1 malocclusion, without functional retrusion under activator therapy, is sometimes more rapid than is possible by alveolar adaptation alone. The frequently occurring transient appearance of a lateral open bite during activator treatment can also be interpreted as additional evidence of a skeletal change. It is believed by some that the functional matrix concept of Moss, the research of Moyers, McNamara, Stöckli, etc., support the interpretation that the artificial "translation" effected by the appliance could very well be responsible for the secondary adaptation in the temporomandibular joint.[11–14] An excellent discussion of this question is given in an article by Herren.[15]

Fabrication of the Activator

PRETREATMENT CONSIDERATIONS

Before the treatment with the activator is started, the forward movement of the mandible should be checked to see that it is not blocked by the occlusal interferences which make the correction of the distocclusion impossible. As previously mentioned, in Class II, Division 1 malocclusions, the width of the maxillary arch between the canines is often too narrow to allow the mandible to move forward. There are, however, instances when interference may be caused by a single tooth, and this may be overlooked easily. As a consequence, little or no progress may be achieved. For example, if the lower second molar is slightly overerupted distal to the first molar, it will impede the forward movement of the mandible. A similar condition may develop by the overeruption of the maxillary second deciduous molar into the space created by the premature loss of its antagonist. A quite common and easily overlooked cause for interference is the buccal crossbite of an upper premolar. The plan of treatment must take this into account. The buccal crossbite must be corrected first with an active plate. Other types of interferences, like narrow intercanine dimensions or lingually displaced upper lateral incisors, can often be corrected concomitantly with the activator treatment.

The Construction Bite

The purpose of the construction bite is to fabricate an appliance inducing the following effects: (1) to bring the lower jaw into a tolerable forward position with every occluding action of the mandible; and (2) to "block the bite," depressing the lower anterior teeth and stopping their eruption, while at the same time attempting to stimulate eruption of the posterior segments (raising of the bite).

Taking the construction bite, one should look at the bite in three different planes of space: sagittal, vertical, and frontal. It is, therefore, necessary first to clarify the following three points:

The Extent of Maximum Forward Movement of the Mandible. In the normal case, the maximum forward movement of the mandible averages about 10 mm. but may be as little as 7 or 8 mm. The optimal forward movement of the mandible for the construction bite usually is half the individual's maximum range. There are three reasons for this: (a) If the protrusive construction bite is more than half the maximum movement, it becomes more uncomfortable for the patient. He is less likely to keep the appliance in his mouth during the night, and he becomes less cooperative in general. As mentioned later, both Petrik and Herren do not subscribe to this limitation of forward positioning. (b) The distance of 5 mm. is approximately the same as that between the points of the buccal cusps of the first molars. This is the amount of distance necessary to change a Class II malocclusion into a Class I occlusion. (c) It is claimed that one of the best positions for obtaining the desired histologic transformation of the temporomandibular joint from a Class II to a Class I occlusion is approximately half the distance that the condyle can move forward along the anterior wall of the fossa to the articular tubercle. Movement greater than half the distance along the articular eminence might prevent any favorable anatomic rebuilding of the temporomandibular joint structures. The possibility of such happening is, however, controversial and denied by many.

The Extent of the Individual's Occlusal Clearance in Postural Resting Position. Clinical experience indicates that the opening of the construction bite by approximately 2 mm. in excess of the individual's postural resting position is optimal. Since in most individuals the interocclusal clearance (freeway space) amounts to 2 to 3 mm. in the molar area, and 4 to 5 mm. in the incisor area, an opening of 4 to 5 mm. in the molar area and 6 to 7 mm. in the incisor area frequently will be desired.

The Establishment of the True Midlines of the Upper and Lower Jaws. This determination is made in the original diagnostic study. When there is a lack of coincidence of the incisors and the true jaw midline, the latter is marked with a pointed pencil on the labial surface of the relevant incisor. The true midline of the jaws, marked carefully in this manner, must coincide when the construction bite is taken, except in instances of asymmetrical Class II malocclusions (see Fig. 3–8).

The rules outlined above have proved valid in clinical practice for many orthodontists. Ahlgren's exacting clinical and electromyographic studies have led him to recommend a construction bite that is 2 mm. below and 5 mm. in advance of postural rest position.[18] In the preceding chapter, the various types of activators discussed differed mainly in the way the construction bite was taken. It is apparent that this results in varied muscle reactions and the corresponding growth changes elicited.

There is some divergence of views on the extent of the forward movement of the mandible and the opening of the vertical dimension required for the construction bite. Many orthodontists bring the mandible forward as much as is needed to create a Class I molar relationship; and the bite is opened about 2 mm. beyond postural rest position to stimulate stretch reflex, as well as to hold the appliance in place at night when the patient is asleep. Clinical experience has shown, however, that good results are possible with smaller and larger displacements. The extent of the forward positioning of the mandible is related to the amount of bite opening. The greater the opening of the bite, the less should be the planned forward movement of the condyle for the construction bite.

As we know from the study of rest position, when the mandible is open beyond this position, the condyle moves downward and forward on the articular eminence. Thus, when the bite is open more than 5 mm. in the molar area, a forward movement of 4 mm. will suffice. Except in extreme cases, an opening larger than this is usually not tolerated well.*

Highly experienced clinicians such as Petrik or Herren entirely disregard the postural rest position. This might tend to facilitate the work of the operator, since rest position is variable and not easy to ascertain in young children. Petrik has also paid much more attention to the incisal relationship than to the posterior bite opening. The upper and lower incisal edges should meet as close to edge-to-edge as possible in a horizontal plane when viewed from the anterior aspect, according to Petrik. This maneuver will generally leave the incisors 1 to 4 mm. apart at most, with a posterior bite opening of 4 to 7 mm. This can vary from as little as 3 mm. to as much as 9 mm. posteriorly. With the establishment of an edge-to-edge construction bite, the minimal overbite of 2 to 3 mm. is generally compensated for by the condyle's moving downward and forward on the eminence. Some contact of the cusps of the posterior teeth can remain with small overbites of this magnitude. Beyond this, where there is a deeper original bite, the posterior teeth are separated varying amounts with the edge-to-edge incisal position. As Woodside has indicated, bite opening and forward position are related.

Contrary to many other clinicians, Petrik also has given preference to bringing the mandible forward the complete desired distance at once, and not in stages. Whatever advice the operator chooses to follow, he should be aware that there are no hard and fast rules. Rather, there are several clinical possibilities. The configuration of the original malocclusion and the movability of the mandible must be studied carefully before deciding which technique to follow. Taking the construction bite is a most important step in the treatment. It should be done directly in the patient's mouth. No articulator duplicates the exact condylar path of the patient.

The first step in taking the construction bite is the preparation of the plaster casts. Special care should be taken to extend the impression as deep as possible in the posterior lingual regions of the mandible, as these are important areas of anchorage for the appliance.

In our example, Figure 8–2, the maximum forward movement of the mandible was 10 mm. An overbite of 1 mm. in postural resting position was still present in this case. The incisor midlines and the true jaw midlines coincided in both jaws. Therefore, it was decided to move the mandible forward 5 mm. into a Class I relationship, and to establish a 1 to 2 mm. overbite between the upper and lower incisors. The upper and lower midlines should coincide also in the construction bite.

Before taking the construction bite, it is helpful to show the patient in the mirror where the mandible should be moved. In taking the construction bite, the patient can be instructed to move the mandible in the correct position with

---

*Activator Philosophy and Construction. University of Chicago, Center for Continuing Education, June 29–30, 1976.

the help of a mirror, but in most instances, it is speedier and more reliable if the operator guides the mandible forward with the assistance of the patient.

The following step-by-step procedure for taking the construction bite is suggested:

1. Reproduce the maximum forward movement of the mandible and the correct occlusal clearance of postural rest position. Observe whether functional lateral shift occurs and register true mandibular midline with a pencil on the labial surfaces of the upper and lower incisors on the casts and in the patient's mouth.

2. Determine the amount of mesial and vertical mandibular displacement necessary for the construction bite. It is helpful to mark the amount of mesial shift with a pencil on the buccal surfaces of the first molars.

3. Show the patient on the casts and in the mirror where the mandible should be moved. Practice the forward mandibular movement by gently guiding the mandible in the desired direction. Advise the patient to move the jaw slowly according to the verbal instructions and to stop movement immediately when asked to do so. Talk to the patient in a calm, reassuring manner.

4. Soften a sheet of beeswax and make a tight roll, approximately 1 cm. in diameter.

5. Shape the roll to conform to the lower arch, leaving the seam on the inside. Press the softened roll of wax on the lower arch so that only the buccal teeth are covered. In the front, the wax roll lies just lingual to the lower incisors. Make a groove on the wax to indicate the midline (Fig. 8–4). Remove any excess wax that extends onto the retromolar tissue. The distal half of the last molar tooth should not be covered with wax.

6. Transfer the wax to the patient's mouth, fitting it on the lower arch in the same manner that it was fitted on the plaster cast.

7. Move the mandible forward as it was previously practiced. If the registration fails, make a new wax roll and repeat.

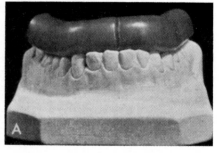

Figure 8–4. The wax roll for taking the construction bite. It is as thick as the little finger. *A,* The roll is formed and slightly impressed on the lower cast. Note that the edges of the incisors are not covered by wax. The lower midline is marked with a groove in the wax. *B,* Drawing of view of wax from above. The anterior section is positioned lingual to the lower incisors, hence the angular shape. The ends are shortened so that the distal halves of the last molars are not covered by wax. The wax roll, after the bite has been taken, must not touch the gingiva behind the last molars, because the soft tissue is compressed only in the mouth, not on the plaster casts. If compression of retromolar tissues occurred, the appliance would not fit exactly on the model. (From Schwarz, A. M., and Gratzinger, M.: Removable Orthodontic Appliances. Philadelphia, W. B. Saunders Company, 1966.)

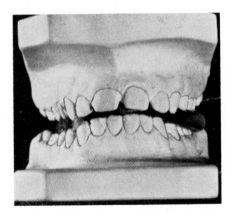

Figure 8–5. The chilled wax bite has been placed on the lower model and both casts are carefully occluded. The buccal excess is trimmed on the right side, so that the distance and relation between the molars can be seen. (From Schwarz, A. M., and Gratzinger, M.: Removable Orthodontic Appliances. Philadelphia, W. B. Saunders Company, 1966.)

8. Remove the wax bite from the mouth and chill it. With a sharp knife, trim the excess buccal wax until the occlusal surfaces of the molars are visible (Fig. 8–5). By carefully checking on the plaster casts, remove also all wax that is contacting the soft tissues, the interproximal papillae, and the palate. If this is not done, the wax bite cannot be seated properly on the casts.

9. Place the wax bite between the casts and check that the mandible is moved forward the desired amount in the three planes of space (Fig. 8–6). If the construction bite is incorrect, replace it on the lower cast, soften its superior surface, and add a layer of warm wax. Repeat the procedure from point 6 through point 10.

10. Replace the hard wax bite in the patient's mouth and have the patient close the jaw slightly more firmly to assure the correct fit.

CONSTRUCTION AND FITTING OF THE ACTIVATOR

The study casts and construction bite together with detailed instructions are then sent to the laboratory. (Laboratory procedures are explained on page

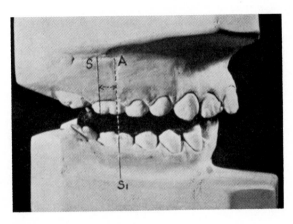

Figure 8–6. Measuring the distance that the mandible has been moved forward for the construction bite. The marks S and S₁ signify habitual occlusion and are extended gingivally on the models. After the wax bite has been cooled and the buccal excess removed, it is carefully placed between the upper and lower casts. The lower mark, S₁, is then extended to the upper cast (interrupted line A). The distance between S and A is then measured. In this case, it is 5 mm. The distance between upper and lower molars is also measured. Here the bite is opened 5 mm. in the molar region. Note that the end of the wax bite does not impinge on the retromolar soft tissue area. (From Schwarz, A. M., and Gratzinger, M.: Removable Orthodontic Appliances. Philadelphia, W. B. Saunders Company, 1966.)

201.) The technician should be informed as to whether an expansion screw is needed, what type of labial bow is needed, whether acrylic should extend over the labial surface of the lower incisors, etc. A regular labial bow of 0.8 mm. or 0.9 mm. with U-loops at the canine area is adequate. A bow with horizontal loop extensions against the mesial aspects of the canines is seldom used now (Fig. 8–2).

The activator can be fabricated of cold-cure acrylic directly on the models, or a wax matrix can be made first and then invested in the flask. The advantage with the latter method is that the wax matrix can be tried in the mouth for an accurate fit. This should be done regularly, at least by the beginner. The experienced clinician reserves the try-in for those cases in which no deep overbite exists. The wax-up must fit precisely. In case of a minor inaccuracy, the patient can be asked to bite into the wax to ensure proper adaptation. If this does not work out, or if the discrepancy is considerable, a new wax matrix has to be made. The wax model of the activator is then removed from the mouth, flushed, and chilled *without resetting on the model.*

After the activator has been processed in acrylic, the fit is again tested in the mouth. At this or the following appointment, the acrylic is ground off to achieve the desired tooth movement. It is advisable for the beginner to draw a

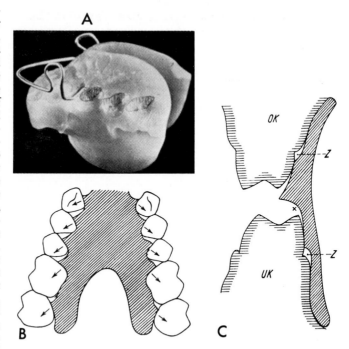

Figure 8–7. Freeing the way for stimulation of eruption of the posterior teeth, in cases of deep overbite. *A,* Mark directly on the activator with a soft pencil the mesiogingival areas of all the niches for all the teeth distal to the canines. These areas must not be touched by the vulcanite bur; all parts of the acrylic that may prevent the vertical movement of these teeth must be removed. *B,* The distal areas of the imprints of the upper teeth are removed to allow the teeth to drift distobuccally (arrows); expansion enhances these movements by pressing against the mesiolingual surfaces of the teeth, which can yield to the distal. It is important to remember that the whole tooth is moving, not only the crown. Therefore, free space must also be made for the gingiva by trimming these parts of the activator, if distal movement of the posterior teeth is intended. *C,* This drawing shows the trimmed buccal relief of the activator. OK, Upper jaw; UK, lower jaw; Z, free space for gingival margins; x, free interocclusal space for the lower teeth. The interocclusal projection shown in the drawing should be rounded off, not sharp, so as to prevent irritation. Where the appliance and teeth contact each other, shiny spots results from the sliding and indicate the correctly shaped relief; note the guiding surface for the upper teeth slanting buccally. This stimulates the upper teeth to expand more than the lower, so that both jaws will harmonize with width after the lower jaw has moved forward. (From Schwarz, A. M., and Gratzinger, M.: Removable Orthodontic Appliances. Philadelphia, W. B. Saunders Company, 1966.)

pencil line over those areas that should not be touched with a vulcanite bur. The guiding surfaces must be maintained exactly for the vertical movements of the posterior teeth as shown in Figure 8–7. These areas are the gingival halves of the dental embrasures. All other parts of the embrasure that could prevent the vertical movement of eruption of the teeth are to be removed, as shown in Figure 8–7. Even the sharply defined gingival margins should be rounded off (Fig. 8–7). The interdental crests of the posterior teeth also may be carefully reduced in areas where they touch the coronal portions of the teeth and possibly prevent continued eruption. Figure 8–7 demonstrates the dentoalveolar forces exerted by the activator, in addition to the anteroposterior change. If the operator wishes to retrude the maxillary buccal segments, the acrylic interdental projections must be reduced on the distal of each posterior tooth (Fig. 8–7). In this way, a distal tipping of the teeth is stimulated. This movement may be done in conjunction with expansion. In the lower arch, we usually relieve the buccal teeth for vertical movement only, to prevent the entire mandibular arch from moving forward on the base. Figure 8–8 illustrates some of the precautions required in handling the mandibular arch with the activator. When there is not a deep overbite, and when vertical stimulation is not desired, the activator is not relieved to allow eruption of the posterior teeth.

If one of the objectives is expansion, the acrylic projections in the interden-

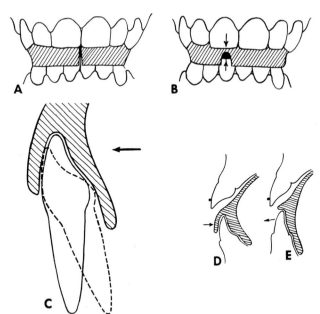

Figure 8–8. Periodic control of the activator's proper fit. *A,* When the activator is equipped with a screw for expansion, the incisal edges should be visible through the gap between the two halves of the activator. The distance between the edges of the upper and lower incisors (black area) is measured and recorded. *B,* When using an activator without an expansion screw, a narrow gap can be cut in the anterior overhang, in the region of the lower central incisors, making the edges visible. The distance can then be measured directly (arrows). The distance must remain the same during treatment, or it may be reduced while the labially inclined upper incisors are retracted and made more upright by the labial bow. *C,* If the distance recorded in *A* and *B* increases, it indicates that the lower incisors are no longer fitting exactly in the acrylic indentations of the labial construction. This means that the bodily restraint of the labial overhang is reduced, permitting labial tipping of the lower incisors (dotted line) by the lingual load of the appliance (arrow). In order to prevent this undesired tipping movement, the anterior overhang has to be relined again with self-curing acrylic directly in the patient's mouth. Then the distance between upper and lower incisors is recorded for future control. *D,* Correctly made covering for lower incisors, to provide maximum bodily resistance against labial movement. *E,* If labial tipping of lower incisors is desired (arrow), the labial surfaces of the lower incisors are not covered by acrylic. (From Schwarz, A. M., and Gratzinger, M.: Removable Orthodontic Appliances. Philadelphia, W. B. Saunders Company, 1966.)

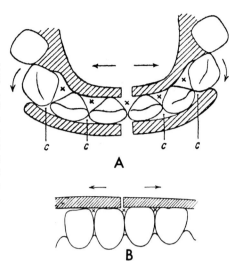

Figure 8-9. If the arch is to be expanded after the lower incisors are already correctly positioned, the interdental crests must be trimmed to prevent formation of spaces. *A,* Schematic section to show the labial and lingual crests (c and x), which must be removed. Thus the incisors remain in contact. The canines, under pressure linguodistally but retained mesiobuccally, are rotated from their more sagittal position into a more anterior position, compensating in this way the expansion of the arch (2 to 3 mm.) without spaces opening up between the incisors. *B,* The incisal crests, x, must also be removed. (From Schwarz, A. M., and Gratzinger, M.: Removable Orthodontic Appliances. Philadelphia, W. B. Saunders Company, 1966.)

tal spaces will move the incisors laterally with the turning of the screw. If the operator does not wish to move the incisors laterally, it is necessary to remove all interdental prominences by grinding them smooth (Fig. 8-9). To allow the maxillary incisors to retract, a space lingual to these teeth must be created (Fig. 8-10). The results of the grinding can be conveniently checked and rechecked by inverting the appliance on the upper and lower plaster casts. When the fit looks good on the models, it should still be checked in the mouth by placing the activator alternately on the maxillary and mandibular arches.

After the appliance is inserted, the patient is asked to open and close his mouth without loosening the appliance. It is important to note whether the labial bow slides automatically into its proper place on the maxillary anterior teeth with every closing movement of the mandible.

The labial bow, when used with the activator, has an effect similar to what is obtained with the active plate or Hawley appliance. The only difference lies in the kind of activation. The wire must barely touch the most prominent part of the teeth when the jaws are closed. The patient is admonished not to use the fingers to guide the appliance wire into place, since this may distort the wire. The biting function should properly seat the appliance without digital assistance.

The detailed steps in home care,[31] as outlined previously for other appliances, are explained to the patient. Masseter exercise is taught and prescribed to

Figure 8-10. Sagittal section through the anterior region of a Class II, Division 1 malocclusion, with the activator in place. The anterior space x allows the retrusion of the upper incisors; note that the free space reaches the apical third of the root, permitting the lingual movement of the alveolar process. A frequent error by the neophyte is to cut away acrylic only for the crowns of the teeth. The labial bow is positioned near the incisal edges to stimulate intrusion of the upper incisors if a deep overbite is to be corrected. S is the expansion screw, different from that in the active plate. It is placed between the upper and lower jaws to be equally effective for both jaws. The screw is placed as far anteriorly as possible, generally in line with the canine teeth. (From Schwarz, A. M., and Gratzinger, M.: Removable Orthodontic Appliances. Philadelphia, W. B. Saunders Company, 1966.)

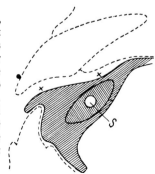

begin immediately. In fact, it is good procedure to have the patient go through the exercise to some degree before he leaves the office in order to detect potential sore spots. The patient is informed that the appliance may come out the first several nights until tongue control assists in holding it in place.

The patient who has trouble wearing the appliance through the night in the beginning is advised to wear it a few hours a day at first. Daytime wear of about three hours when doing homework or watching television is most important to speed up the progress of the treatment. Sometimes this makes the difference between success and failure.

In the routine case, the patient is asked to return in approximately a week. If he reports, as most patients do, that the activator is now kept in place all night, the first turn of the expansion screw may be made, and the patient is instructed to repeat this procedure once a week. The screw on the activator must be turned half the distance of the screw on the active plate, e.g., 45 degrees, or half a turn every week. Turning the screw must be coordinated with the expansion achieved. This must be checked clinically by the orthodontist at each office visit.

Sequential Treatment Procedures

The patient is usually checked every 4 to 8 weeks. At the return appointments, the fit of the appliance and the progress of the treatment are observed. The sagittal discrepancy should show some reduction as a result of retraction of the maxillary incisors and the forward positioning of the mandible. Actual growth increments are seldom of sufficient magnitude to produce a dramatic change. In an average case, the protrusion of the maxillary incisors should be reduced approximately 1 mm. every one and one-half to two months. The buccal segment interdigitation should be improved by 1 mm. every three to four months. It is, however, not infrequent that results do not show up for six months. According to Hotz, the best results of treatment with the activator are seen in about 20 per cent of the cases, where there is a large freeway space and a mandibular rest position that seems to be anterior to habitual occlusion (functional retrusion cases).[16] An additional factor mentioned by Hotz is the poor reaction of cases without deep bite, i.e., deep bite cases are likely to respond better, while shallow bite problems are likely to show a poorer sagittal change.

During the routine checkups, attention should be called to the following factors:

1. If there are any inaccuracies, the appliance should be ground down and stabilized by cold-curing acrylic, as indicated. This procedure may be done directly in the patient's mouth for greater accuracy. A major feature of the properly fitting appliance is the unaltered vertical relationship of the maxillary and mandibular arches as determined by the original construction bite. When the beginner experiences failure, it is often because he overlooks the increased vertical distance between the jaws, even though the patient may be attempting to close his mouth with the activator in place. The original vertical dimension should be maintained and not allowed to open. The best way to control this is to cut a narrow "window" in the labial acrylic over the lower incisors, as explained in Figure 8–8*B*. If an expansion screw is also used on the activator,

the vertical dimension becomes visible here after a few turns have created a gap (Fig. 8–8*A*).

The continual assurance of the activator's proper fit, as illustrated in Figure 8–8, is very important. The acrylic covering the lower incisors must fit exactly. If one of the treatment objectives is lateral expansion to make up for crowding in the lower anterior segment, the interdental acrylic projections between the incisors will literally move the incisors laterally as the expansion screw is turned — if the appliance fits properly. If, however, arch length is not needed in the lower anterior region as the buccal segments are expanded, it is necessary to remove the interdental acrylic projections by grinding and polishing the desired areas.

2. If careful observation indicates that the incisal margins of the mandibular anterior teeth do not fit properly into the niches created for them, it may be a disturbing indication of increased vertical dimension or excessive mandibular incisor procumbency. One reason for this may be that the expansion screw was turned too rapidly, before the alveolar process had a chance to respond completely and favorably. In this instance, the activator is too wide for the jaws, and the screw must be turned back until the appliance fits again. A possible cause for this retrogressive situation is that the appliance is not worn during the entire night, or that the mouth is kept open during the night, or that the masseter exercises are not being conscientiously followed.

3. A third point of concern during the routine checkup is the degree of expansion being accomplished by the appliance. The gap can be determined on a mark made near the expansion screw. Every 45 degree turn of the screw widens the gap 0.1 mm. when the Fischer screw is used. This means that if there is an interval of five weeks between observations, expansion of 0.5 mm. should have been obtained. If no measurable expansion is seen after some weeks of appliance wear, the turning of the expansion screw is slowed down or may even be abandoned for a while.

4. It is important to check the amount of space to the lingual of the maxillary incisors and to make sure that the acrylic in this area has been ground away, leaving an open space. If the progress in the correction of the incisor protrusion has been such that the space is reduced, more acrylic should be ground away leaving an open space (Fig. 8–10). Likewise, the labial bow should be adjusted at successive visits to ensure that it maintains contact in the desired position on the anterior teeth. If the correct position of the maxillary incisor segment has been achieved, cold-curing acrylic may be added on the lingual to stabilize the teeth in their proper relationship.

5. The appliance is adjusted not to interfere with eruption. As new permanent teeth erupt through the mucosa, the interfering acrylic should be ground away, and guide planes for the new teeth should be constructed by adding acrylic onto the appliance. Maxillary and mandibular second molars are usually not included in the appliance at the beginning of the treatment. Eruption of these teeth should be closely watched. If they start to overerupt, acrylic should be added occlusally to these teeth to allow the other teeth to catch up with the second molars.

6. A routine check is made of high spots and polished areas of "slides" caused by the contact between the appliance and the teeth. After the appliance

has been dried with compressed air, each polished area should be checked to determine whether it stimulates or retards the desired orthodontic movement. Those areas unfavorable to therapy should be removed. An absence of shiny areas may indicate improper or insufficient wearing of the appliance. If the appliance is too tight, this also may result in worn areas. Areas that tend to bind the appliance unduly should be eliminated.

7. The proper wearing of the appliance should be checked carefully. One method of checking whether the patient is wearing the appliance is to observe the character of the mucosa on the posterior periphery of the appliance. As with a full denture that is worn a great deal, there is an indentation that delineates the appliance margin. The presence of this tissue indentation is a fairly good sign that the appliance is being worn.

As the treatment progresses and the anteroposterior jaw relationship improves, the original activator occasionally seems to become ineffective. It is necessary, at that point, to change the construction bite by increasing the mandibular forward displacement. Most of the time, it is best to make a new activator. If, however, the activator still fits accurately in the mouth, the same appliance can be adjusted with a new construction bite. The following method for construction bite change is recommended by Kinast:

> Grind all interfering acrylic projections in the lower arch portion of the appliance so that the patient is able to move his mandible forward and keep the desired new construction bite position while the activator is firmly seated on the maxillary arch. The lower portion of the appliance may then be lined with soft wax. The appliance is replaced in the mouth, and a new construction bite is taken. After the wax has been chilled, it is cut off posterior to the premolar, and this area is thoroughly cleansed and roughened. When the jaws close, only the wax in the anterior portion is maintained in the new bite position. The uncovered areas are then filled with cold-curing acrylic, the lingual mucosa itself is covered with a thin layer of petrolatum, and the appliance is put in the mouth to allow the acrylic to harden. The appliance is removed when the material is nearly set and the surplus ground off and polished. The remaining wax in the anterior portion is removed, the area cleansed and roughened, and the procedure is repeated to complete the new construction bite.[17]

If the operator prefers to use an indirect method and readapt the appliance in the laboratory, impressions for new plaster casts and a new construction bite are first taken. The following laboratory procedure is recommended when an expansion screw is not used:

1. Place the plaster casts together with the construction bite in a fixator (articulator).

2. Cut the activator horizontally along the freeway space between the jaws.

3. Put the separated halves of the appliance on the casts.

4. Put a layer of cold-curing acrylic on the cut and roughened side of the appliance.

5. Put the casts with the halves of the appliances in place into the fixator and bring them together.

6. After the acrylic has set, remove the surplus and polish the appliance again.

Making an Activator in the Laboratory

The technician who has had experience in making a Hawley retainer or an active plate can easily construct an activator, since most of the steps are identical. The models, together with the construction bite, are placed in a fixator or in a simple articulator (Fig. 8–11). The height of the bite is marked exactly by fixing the distance from the lower to the upper half of the model (Figs. 8–11

A

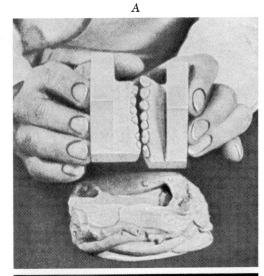

Figure 8–11. Fitting the models in the construction bite. *A,* The casts, assembled with the wax bite, to be set in soft plaster. *B,* The completed plaster fixator. *C,* The upper and lower models in a hinge-type articulator, with the incisors facing the hinge so as to facilitate lingual manipulation. One of the fixators used currently is shown in Figure 8–12. (From Schwarz, A. M., and Gratzinger, M.: Removable Orthodontic Appliances. Philadelphia, W. B. Saunders Company, 1966.)

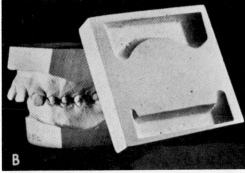

B

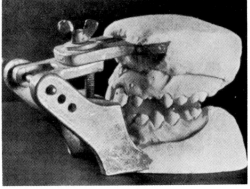

C

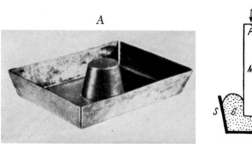

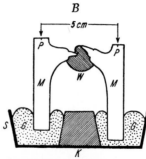

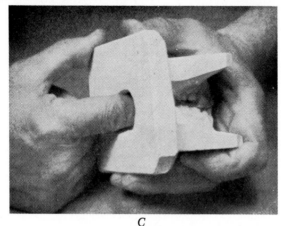

Figure 8-12. An expedient tray used for making a fixator, with a central opening to facilitate the molding of the appliance. *A,* Matrix made of metal; the side walls are not soldered at the angles, so they can be readily separated from the plaster after setting. *B,* Diagram of fixator fabrication: K, central cone of the metal material; S, sidewalls; G, plaster; M, upper and lower models; W, wax construction bite; P, marks made at the anterior surfaces of the bases to control the precise distance between the upper and lower models during manipulation. *C,* Shaping the wax in the lingual area of the activator, after the upper and lower halves of the appliance were separately molded and then set together. (From Schwarz, A. M., and Gratzinger, M.: Removable Orthodontic Appliances. Philadelphia, W. B. Saunders Company, 1966.)

and 8–12). According to the sketch prepared by the dentist, the wires are bent on the model, after which the model is painted with separating medium.

The first layer of wax is applied on each half of the model separately and carefully pressed into the interdental spaces. Half of the occlusal surfaces of the posterior teeth must be reproduced exactly.

The labial wire is placed in the same manner as for an active plate, except that the ends should be inserted into the acrylic halfway between the maxillary and mandibular teeth to avoid cutting off the wire as the teeth are relieved of acrylic. The working parts are free of wax and covered with modeling clay. The second layer of wax is then applied, forming a definitive outline of the margins.

The two halves of the activator formed in wax are now joined together by putting the model in the fixator (Fig. 8–12*A*) or by closing the articulator. Again, *carefully observe and check the distances between the upper and lower models.* Connect the two halves of the appliance with a small roll of soft wax and mold it into final shape, removing the modeling clay. The appliance is now ready for a try-in on the patient.

After the try-in and final minor adjustments to ensure wax adaptation, the appliance is invested in the flask, with the spaces left free by modeling clay covered with plaster. The appliance is placed obliquely in the flask, and as deeply as possible. An obliquely invested appliance can be more easily removed from the flask when it is finished.

The remaining steps are the same as those outlined for making an active plate. If an expansion screw is used, the procedure is also the same. The screw is placed in the waxed appliance before it is invested.

Treatment Considerations—Modifications of the Andresen-Häupl Activator

Most impressive results are achieved with the activator occasionally (Fig. 8–13). The array of functional devices filling several chapters of this book, however, tends to emphasize the preference given by many to appliances worn day and night. There is no doubt that favorable results of treatment are thus achieved with greater speed and certainty. Yet, more exact knowledge based on comparable investigations is needed for a definite judgment. Such has not been forthcoming, even after several decades of activator use. An immense number of publications have dealt with the technique and the results achieved. But, as Ahlgren points out, there is a lack of information about the proper selection of cases, duration of treatment, reasons for failure, etc.[18, 43]

In a clinical study undertaken by Ahlgren, 50 consecutive cases, 25 boys and 25 girls, were followed. The mean age of the group was 9 years, ranging from 7 to 14 years. Treatment time varied between 8 years and 1 year, with a mean of 3 years, 2 months. Results were negative in 12 cases.

The most obvious reason for unsuccessful treatment was poor cooperation—the appliances were not worn sufficiently. But, three additional factors were also decisive for the outcome of the treatment. Firstly, it was found that the habitual sleeping position of the patient was important to the result of the activator treatment. If the patient slept with his head bent backwards and his mouth open, the activator appliance became completely inactive most of the time. Secondly, some children had a very low threshold for oral and pharyngeal irritation and were unable to wear the appliance in the mouth during sleep. They lost the appliance involuntarily.

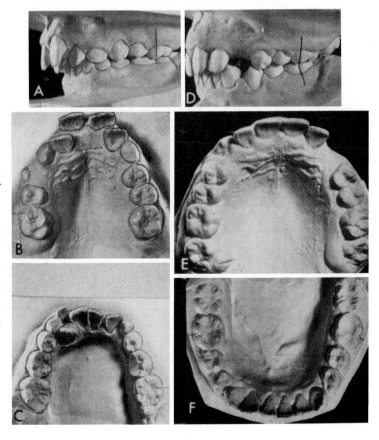

Figure 8–13. Significant expansion of dentoalveolar areas as a result of four activators. *A* to *C*, Class II, Division 1 malocclusion in a 10-year-old girl with a broad face. A bruxism habit was present during sleep. *D* to *F*, Result of treatment 3½ years later. The appliances were loose during the entire treatment, according to the strict rules of functional jaw orthopedics. Eruption of the buccally displaced upper canines is retarded. (From Schwarz, A. M., and Gratzinger, M.: Removable Orthodontic Appliances. Philadelphia, W. B. Saunders Company, 1966.)

The last factor mentioned by Ahlgren is an unfavorable growth period (amount) or unfavorable growth pattern (direction). If the treatment period could be correlated with favorable jaw growth, e.g., maximum pubertal growth, good treatment results could be expected.[44]

Within the limits specified above, activator treatment may give satisfactory results, especially for the correction of Class II, Division 1 malocclusion. Preference should be given to this appliance when wearing something else during the day is not feasible. Another special reason for its use is geographical distance making frequent activation of the appliance impossible. The slight adaptations

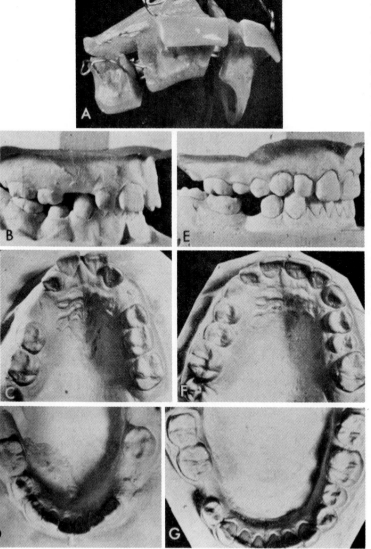

Figure 8–14. The distal screw on the activator. *A,* An activator used to expand both arches. At the same time a separate screw is inserted in the lower right activator flange to move the lower right molars distally. The screw retains the separated segment for the first molar; the occlusal surface of the tooth is freed of the acrylic to facilitate distal tipping. The arrow clasp must not be used to retain the appliance, particularly on the distal. The mesial arm and arrow should contact the tooth with every closing of the jaws, however. This intermittent stimulation follows the principles of functional jaw orthopedics. In addition, the screw opening jams the appliance into the space between the first premolar and first molar. In this regard, the force exerted emulates an active plate. *B* to *G,* The case treated with the modified activator in *A.* Views *B* to *D* are before treatment for a 13-year-old girl with a delayed dental eruption pattern (corresponding to 11 years). *E* to *G,* Twenty months later, with good cooperation, note the change. The space for the lower right second premolar has been opened. The premolar is lingually inclined, so it has not erupted yet. Distal tipping of the first molar occurred during eruption of the contiguous second molar. This is usually not a favorable factor. (From Schwarz, A. M., and Gratzinger, M.: Removable Orthodontic Appliances, Philadelphia, W. B. Saunders Company, 1966.)

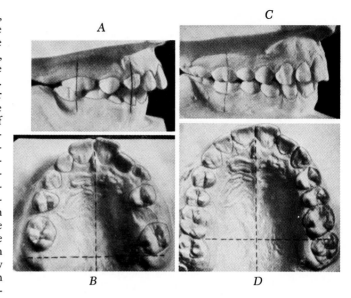

Figure 8–15. The effect of an activator, equipped with a distal driving screw in the upper right buccal segment. A and B, Before treatment in a 10½-year-old girl. A Class II, Division 1 malocclusion was present. The upper right first molar has shifted 4 mm. mesially. The distally drifting first premolar contributes to the space deficiency for the second premolar. C and D, One and a half years later, when a new activator was constructed to continue the expansion, the forward movement of the mandible and the remaining correction of the deep bite are evident. The first molar has moved distally despite the counteracting eruption of the maxillary second molar. The simultaneous eruption of the second premolar may have helped. The periodic turning of the screw creates an active pressure on the edentulous site, giving an active force to supplement the functional jaw orthopedic action of the activator. (From Schwarz, A. M., and Gratzinger, M.: Removable Orthodontic Appliances. Philadelphia, W. B. Saunders Company, 1966.)

needed for the treatment of simple cases will be possible, even if the interval between visits is three months or more. The sturdy construction will seldom require repairs.

The activator used for treatment of Class II, Division 1 malocclusion may be used for opening up space for the second mandibular premolar, or even a first premolar (Fig. 8–14). It is possible to insert jackscrews simultaneously on both sides. The screws should be turned alternately in that case, one week on one side, and the next week on the other, generally only half of the quarter turn of 90 degrees. To increase retention, the acrylic should be extended over the labial surfaces of the mandibular incisors. If more than half the space of the premolar is lost, correction is less likely, and another method of treatment should be used. It is not impossible to gain space for a maxillary premolar in the same way (Fig. 8–15). Active plates, however, especially in combination with a headgear, are preferable. The technique also is hardly suitable when the activator is used for the treatment of other types of malocclusion. In one way or the other, it will conflict with the construction of the appliance.

For the mesial or distal movement of incisors, canines, and occasionally the premolars, special springs have been designed by Petrik (Fig. 8–15B). The small U-bends serve to keep the spring in contact with the tooth being moved. They should not, however, be activated to exert pressure. For such a spring, the free end of the wire is bent into a closed loop to prevent irritation. For the closure of a diastema, the springs contacting the central incisors in Figure 8–15B may emerge from the opposite half of the activator. The turning of the screw will thus increase the contact and pressure on the incisor.

An activator used for treatment of any kind of malocclusion may simultaneously serve as a space maintainer. In the mixed dentition, the acrylic is extended into the space of the missing tooth or teeth. Care should be taken, however, to grind the acrylic away as the permanent teeth start to erupt. An alternative technique is to place a single or double wire anterior to the tooth or the teeth, the migration of which should be prevented. Devices worn day and night will, again, be safer and more effective. The use of the activator, reduced in size according to Schmuth, is recommended.[19] That is valid, too, for the retention of space gained by the extraction of the first premolar, to permit eruption of a labially erupting canine. Simultaneous improvement of a Class II, Division 1 condition can be achieved. Some loss of space, however, may occur.

CORRECTION OF CLASS II, DIVISION 2 MALOCCLUSION

The activator can be easily adapted for the treatment of Class II, Division 2 malocclusion when there is only slight crowding of the upper incisors. The upper central incisors are tipped labially by springs at the incisal. The labial bow exerts lingual pressure concomitantly at the labial gingival margin, to achieve lingual root movement (torque). Wires placed anteriorly to the upper first molar prevent the dislocation of the appliance in a posterior direction. The Herren activator described later is better suited to the task.[20-24] Another improved technique has been developed by Slagsvold and is described in Chapter 7.

CORRECTION OF OPEN BITE

The activator is not indicated for the treatment of skeletal open bite. It may be used for the treatment of open bites caused by tongue thrust and finger sucking. The activator is constructed so that eruption of the posterior teeth is prevented while elongation of the anterior teeth is encouraged. Therefore, the acrylic is not ground away from the occlusal surfaces of the posterior teeth, but the anterior teeth are allowed to erupt freely. Besides correcting the vertical development, the activator works as a habit appliance by intercepting the tongue-lip contact. The weakness of the appliance is that it is limited mainly to nocturnal use, which leaves the bulk of the 24 hours without appliance control. Other appliances worn continuously are, thus, more effective.

CORRECTION OF CROSSBITE

The activator has been recommended also for the early treatment of unilateral crossbites because both the maxillary and mandibular opposing dental arches and supporting structures can be used as bases for anchorage. The maxillary teeth in crossbite are moved laterally, the mandibular teeth lingually, with separate wire loops on each tooth, as shown schematically in Fig. 8–16. To

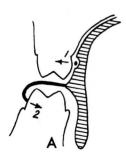

Figure 8–16. Activator modification necessary to correct a dentoalveolar crossbite in the molar area. A lingual bow spring (arrow 1) stimulates buccal movement of the maxillary molar. The bow (arrow 2) moves the opposing tooth lingually. (From Schwarz, A. M., and Gratzinger, M.: Removable Orthodontic Appliances. Philadelphia, W. B. Saunders Company, 1966.)

allow the mandibular teeth to move lingually, the acrylic on the lingual of these teeth is ground away. The acrylic must be sufficiently thick in the lower part of the activator to allow for this grinding. Correction of the abnormal jaw relationship in the construction bite is important. The procedure was described with the double plate used for this purpose (see Fig. 3–8). The construction bite must also establish at least 6 mm. clearance in the molar region for crossbite correction. Some other functional devices, however, are better suited for this treatment. Generally, active plates will be more effective, being worn all the time. (See the use of the active plate, Chapter 2).

CORRECTION OF CLASS III MALOCCLUSION

The true mandibular prognathism is undoubtedly one of the most difficult conditions to treat orthodontically. Nevertheless, the proponents of functional

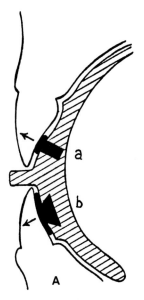

Figure 8–17. *A,* Labial movement of incisors with activator. Gutta percha or orangewood pegs are inserted into the labial surface of the activator immediately lingual to the teeth to be moved. In a, a hole the exact diameter of the orangewood stick is drilled and the peg inserted. The peg swells in width, binding it into the activator. It also increases in length when wet, pressing against the incisor. In b, the gutta percha is fixed into a cone shaped hole, but by an inverted cone bur. The warmed gutta percha is inserted and the excess cut away. Additional layers are added to induce labial movement of the contiguous tooth. *B,* The gutta-percha plugs are seen in the lingual indentations of the maxillary incisors. The mandibular labial bow exerts lingual pressure on the lower incisors. Wire spurs mesial to the maxillary first permanent molars are important, to prevent dislocation of the activator, *C.*

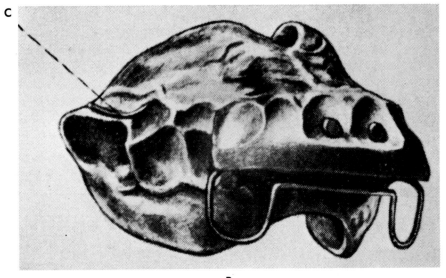

B

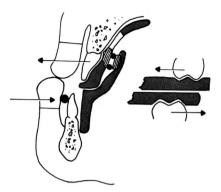

Figure 8–18. Wunderer modification of activator for Class III malocclusion. The appliance is split horizontally, with the upper and lower portions connected by a screw that is embedded in an acrylic extension of the mandibular portion behind the maxillary incisors. As the screw is opened, the maxillary portion moves anteriorly, with a reciprocal posterior thrust acting on the mandibular dentition (see arrows). Occlusal surfaces of the posterior teeth are covered with acrylic to enhance retention. (See Figures 8–19 and 8–20 for the jackscrew designed by Weise, which facilitates construction of the Wunderer activator.)

orthopedics claim that, if treated early, the development of a skeletal Class III malocclusion can be controlled with the activator. It is difficult to appraise results because most textbooks reproduce the initial and final models only in the forced occlusion and not in postural resting position. The results are naturally best in pseudo Class III problems. As in the treatment of the Class II malocclusion, the forces of the activator work reciprocally against both maxilla and mandible. The construction of the activator in the Class III treatment is, however, such that the restraining effect is directed toward the mandible instead of the maxilla. The construction bite for the Class III case is taken in the most retruded or hinge-axis position of the mandible, with the incisal edges 2 or 3 mm. apart. In addition to the maxillary labial bow, a mandibular labial bow is used to guide the mandible distally, as the teeth occlude. If lingual tipping of the mandibular incisors is desired, the acrylic is ground away on the lingual of the incisors. The maxillary labial bow is kept a slight distance away from the labial surfaces to relieve any lip pressure. The maxillary incisors are tipped labially with small screws, wooden pegs, or lingual springs, or by the application of gutta percha lingual to the incisors (Fig. 8–17). Regardless of the modification, distal dislocation of the activator should be prevented with the use of stabilizing wires just anterior to the maxillary first permanent molars.

Many will give preference to other appliances for the treatment of Class III conditions. The operator may, however, resort to the activator when an inclined plane or plate blocking open the bite has established only an edge-to-edge bite or a very slight overbite. The activator will then serve as retainer to improve this result. The incisor relationship may be improved, or at least maintained, until after the changing of the dentition treatment, when fixed appliances are feasible.

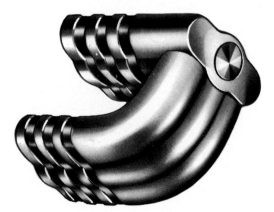

Figure 8–19. Jackscrew designed by Weise to effect horizontal and sagittal movements in activator or double plate construction. (Courtesy of Dentaurum Corporation.)

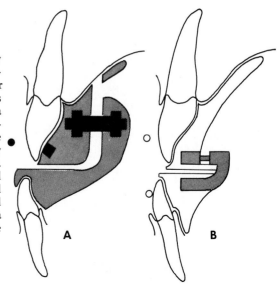

Figure 8.-20. *A,* Wunderer activator, modified by Weise screw. Labial wire stands away from maxillary incisors, while labial acrylic cap over lower incisors grasps the teeth tightly. As the screw is opened, the maxillary incisors move labially, with a reciprocal bodily lingual thrust to the lower incisors. To further expedite labial movement of the maxillary incisors, the use of orangewood pegs may be considered (black insert behind upper incisors). *B,* Weise screw placed in horizontally separated elements of an activator. As the screw is turned open, the maxillary incisors move forward toward the labial bow. The mandibular incisors receive a comparable posterior tipping force through the lower labial bow.

There may be a better case for the use of the activator designed by Wunderer[25] (Fig. 8–18), which is split horizontally. The upper and lower halves are connected with a screw, which is situated in an extension of the mandibular portion behind the maxillary incisors. By opening the screw, the maxillary portion is moved anteriorly, with a reciprocal backward thrust on the mandibular portion. To enhance appliance retention, the occlusal surfaces of the buccal teeth are covered with acrylic. The construction of such an appliance is facilitated by the screw designed by Weise (Figs. 8–19 and 8–20).[26] It connects the upper and lower portions of the activator, causing the reciprocal movement described. Mandibular prognathism frequently becomes progressive in the pubertal and postpubertal period of growth. By the action described, the activator may reverse or, at least, check this development. Opening the bite, however, must be avoided. This could make surgery, if ultimately needed, more difficult.

OTHER MODIFICATIONS OF THE ACTIVATOR

The Herren Activator

The principles of the Herren activator (Fig. 8–21) are based on the theoretical considerations, research, and practical experience of Paul Herren over a period of a quarter of a century.[20–24] Some of these aspects have been discussed in the preceding chapter. The method is in complete opposition to the kinetic concept of Andresen-Häupl, since observations on sleeping patients have revealed that there are relatively few movements of the masticatory apparatus, and therefore of the appliance itself. The movability of the appliance in the oral cavity is as little as possible, and active forces are applied wherever desirable. For the treatment of Class II, Division 1 and Division 2 malocclusions, the

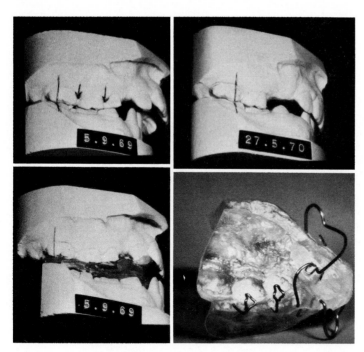

Figure 8–21. Herren modification of activator. *Upper left*, before, and *upper right*, after treatment. *Lower left*, construction bite with wax in place. *Lower right*, Herren appliance used. (Courtesy of Dr. A. Demisch, Berne, Switzerland.)

construction bite is taken in a strong mandibular propulsion, reaching sometimes almost the feasible maximum. Herren argues that the mandible, together with the activator worn during the night, will not retain the position it has with the patient sitting upright in the chair. Different postures assumed during sleep will change the relationship of the appliance to the surrounding structures in the oral cavity, with gravity playing an important role. A slight unconscious lowering of the mandible will detach the activator from the maxillary parts and lessen its effectiveness. The Herren activator, therefore, is fixed by clasps to the maxillary dentition. Screws and springs are employed as with active plates. The maximum forward positioning of the mandible by and for the construction bite is regarded as essential. Research undertaken by Graf[27] and Herren has shown that an advanced position of the mandible due to the inserted activator will, by the tendency of the stretched muscle to bring the mandible to the habitual position again, exert a pressure on the upper teeth in an occipital direction, and by means of reciprocal action, a mesial component on the lower teeth. This pressure is due to the increased tonus of the retractor muscles, although varied by different positions of the patient, with gravity playing some role too. With every millimeter increase of the forward position of the mandible, the sagittal forces on the jaws will increase too. For example, with a 5 mm. forward positioning, the pressure may be 500 grams. It will almost double when the mandible is brought forward 10 mm. Clinical experience is in accord with this evidence. Herren and Demisch observed six patients wearing activators, with the construction bite displacing the lower dentition in a forward direction by varying amounts of 4, 6, 8, and 10 mm. Taking into account clinically observable migration of teeth, the improvement in the distal relationship of the dental arches was correlated with the size of the anterior mandibular displacement. Two of those examined were identical twins. One, with 4 mm. anterior displacement of the mandible, had the Class II condition improved 1 mm. The other, with 10 mm. displacement, showed 5 mm. change, both after 10 months of treatment.

To test the effectiveness of treatment according to the principles described above, a nonselected group of 28 consecutive cases of Class II, Division 1 malocclusion (full Class II molar relationship on both sides) was followed by Demisch.[28, 29] In the course of treatment, four cases were lost (poor oral hygiene, unreliable wearing, unconscious removal of the appliance at night, and other reasons). In the remaining 24 cases, however, normal relationship of the dental arches, normal overjet, and normal overbite were achieved entirely by activator therapy. Average duration of active therapy was 14 months (range 5 to 28 months), exclusive of retention. Other details of the results have been described in Chapters 6 and 7.

The construction bite for the Herren activator is, as mentioned above, taken with an advanced position of the mandible and overcompensation of the postnormal occlusion (Fig. 8–21). Consequently, in a case of complete Class II relationship, the mandible is moved forward the width of a premolar plus an additional 3 mm. The edges of the incisors are kept apart a vertical distance of 2 to 4 mm. This opening will allow for sufficient thickness of acrylic covering the edges of the lower incisors and for the tipping back of the upper incisors, if necessary, with judicious removal of acrylic in the incisal region. For subdivision cases of Class II, Division 1 and Division 2 (unilateral Class II problems), the construction bite is taken with the mandible deviated to the normal side, overcompensating the original deviation.

As already mentioned, the Herren activator is fastened to the maxillary dentition by clasps. Triangular clasps are used for the case shown in Figure 8–21. Duyzings or Jackson clasps may be used as well. If deemed necessary, cemented bands with a piece of wire or a lug soldered to the buccal surface can be used to enhance the retention of the clasp. Mandibular mobility is restricted by extending the lateral parts of the activator lingually as far as possible toward the floor of the mouth. To regain freedom of movement for the mandible, an opening of about 25 mm. is necessary. Active parts deemed necessary, such as labial bows, screws, or springs, may be added as desired. These appurtenances will be more effective when the activator is fixed to the maxillary dentition.

To achieve the leveling of the bite, the impressions of the occlusal surfaces of the buccal teeth are removed from the acrylic (see Fig. 8–7). Also, the distal parts of the maxillary and the mesial parts of the mandibular occlusal indentations are ground off. The purpose is to facilitate tooth movement in a posterior direction in the upper and in an anterior direction in the lower jaw, as well as the expansion of both dental arches. The addition of clasps on the maxillary teeth should limit such tooth movements, except those induced by the action of the screw. Nevertheless, it is thought that, by activating the clasps distally, favorable migration of the teeth in conjunction with alveolar adaptation could be furthered with this type of appliance pressure.

For the Herren modification of the traditional activator, the lower incisors bite on a plane formed by the acrylic. Growth in an occlusal direction is thus impeded. This and the freeing of the occlusal aspects of the posterior teeth by grinding away the acrylic will assist eruption in the molar and premolar region, reducing the curve of Spee. A leveling of the occlusal plane is thus achieved. The edges of the incisors are covered by acrylic to prevent tipping. Acrylic is removed lingually, however, if lingual tipping of these teeth by a lower labial bow is desired.

Consistent and reliable wearing of the appliance for nine hours at night is regarded as sufficient by Herren. After an initial period of accommodation, patients are not required to insert the activator during the day. In spite of the extensive dislocation of the mandible by the construction bite, no sensitivity of the

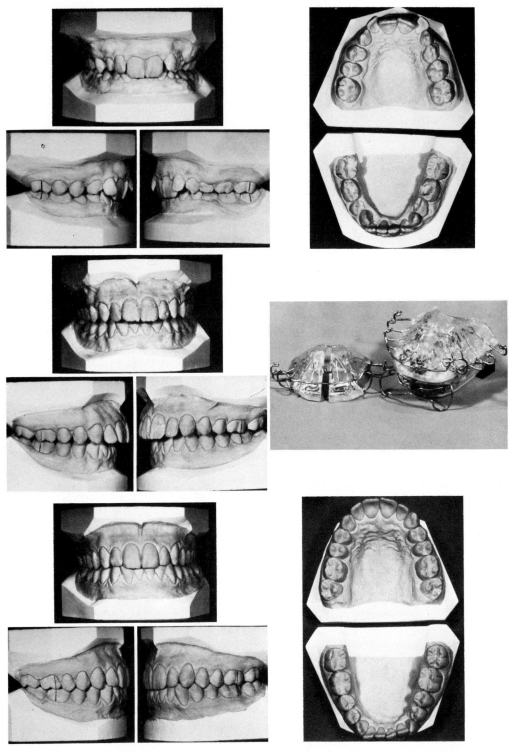

Figure 8–22.   Class II, Division 2, nonextraction case for 12-year-old boy. Both dentitions crowded. Original problem, *top*, treated with maxillary expansion plate. *Middle,* appliance at left used for 15 months, with incisors aligned by lingual springs and labial bow. Results of first phase of treatment shown in *middle* row. A Herren activator, *middle right,* was used for 46 months to achieve sagittal correction shown 5 months after appliance removal, *bottom*. Residual crowding of lower canines shows treatment limitations. A total of 24 sessions was needed. (Courtesy of Professor Paul Herren, Berne.)

temporomandibular joint is observed. Woodside makes the same observation in Chapter 12. Neither will it lead to a more frequent involuntary removal of the appliance by the patient during the night. Any lack of patient compliance would more likely be due to an aversion of the child to the appliance, and not to the magnitude of the mandibular dislocation created by the inserted appliance.

Class II, Division 2 malocclusion is equally amenable to correction by the Herren activator. A treated case is shown in Figure 8–22. The activator was inserted after an initial treatment of six months to relieve maxillary crowding and deep overbite, using an expansion plate. In simpler cases, the activator will suffice. The technique is similar to that recommended by Slagsvold in Chapter 7.

The Bow Activator of A. M. Schwarz

Schwarz was intrigued by the construction and elastic properties of Bimler's appliance, and he designed what he called the bow activator.[31, 32]

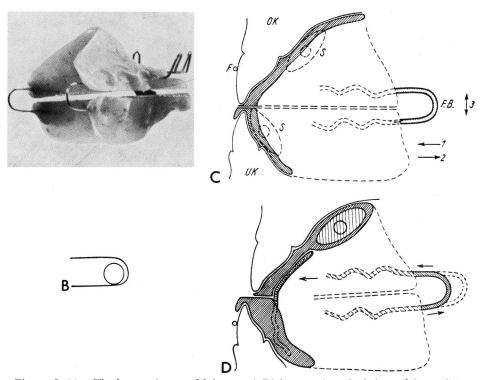

Figure 8–23. The bow activator of Schwarz. *A,* Right rear view; the halves of the appliance are connected with a simple bow or safety pin loop, *B,* made out of 0.9 to 1 mm. wire. In the anterior area between the halves, a layer of rubber is attached to act as a shock absorber and to open the bite in front (See Chapter 14 for similar use of rubber tubing.) *C* and *D,* Schematic drawings of sagittal sections. OK, Upper jaw; UK, lower jaw; S, expansion screws; F, labial bow; FB, elastic bow; arrows 1 and 3 show the different functions of the bow. *D,* Diagram of the bow activator designed to treat a Class III malocclusion. In addition, a lingual guiding bow for the upper jaw, as shown on the double plate for the lower, is also activated in the direction of the arrow (see Chapter 3). (From Schwarz, A. M., and Gratzinger, M.: *Removable Orthodontic Appliances.* Philadelphia, W. B. Saunders Company, 1966.)

Wunderer, as mentioned earlier, had already used a horizontally divided activator for the treatment of lower prognathism, joining the two parts by a screw.[25] The upper and lower halves of the bow activator are connected with an elastic bow (Fig. 8–23). It is thus possible to change the relationship of the two upper and lower halves of the appliance. With the treatment of Class II, Division 1 malocclusion, a beginning can be made with a small forward positioning, increasing this gradually by periodic adjustment. The transverse mobility was thought by Schwarz to provide an additional stimulus. There is the possibility, also, of activating only the bow on the side of a unilateral distoclusion. Finally, independent maxillary or mandibular expansion may be attempted by a screw incorporated in the particular half of the appliance. Experience by others, however, indicates that the results achieved may not come up to theoretical expectations. Such appliances are more easily distorted, and there may be some difficulty in adapting loops correctly. The additional hazard of breakage of the bow portion must be recognized.

Recently, it has been shown by Taatz[33] that the appliance is especially suited for the treatment of Class II, Division 1 malocclusion in the deciduous dentition. Small children will have the appliance in place for longer periods of

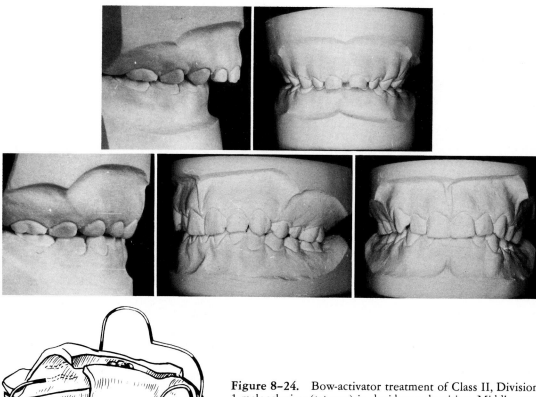

Figure 8-24. Bow-activator treatment of Class II, Division 1 malocclusion (*top row*) in deciduous dentition. Middle row, left shows correction, still in deciduous dentition. Middle and right show results in permanent dentition at 11½ years of age. Appliance configuration is shown below. (Courtesy Prof H. Taatz.)

time because they sleep more hours. They may also be induced to wear it during the day, accepting it as some kind of dummy or pacifier. Younger patients seem to adapt more easily to the gradual bringing forward of the mandible than to the sudden forward positioning. Necessary maxillary expansion will be achieved simultaneously by this maneuver (Fig. 8–24). The number of cases treated in the deciduous dentition is not high. Case selection must be done carefully. Treatment is discontinued if response or patient compliance is unsatisfactory.

The Reduced Activator of Schmuth

A simple but effective modification of the activator has been designed by Professor G. P. F. Schmuth, of Bonn (Fig. 8–25).[19] The acrylic part of the appliance is reduced in a similar manner, as with the Bionator. However, the customary labial wire of the activator is used, as well as most of the other simple appurtenances of this and other myofunctional appliances, including the Coffin spring, made of 1.1 or 1.2 mm. wire. As Schmuth points out, this is not a new appliance, nor a new method of treatment. It is an adaptation of the activator to use the principles of myofunctional treatment in the simplest manner. Saving of time and labor is only one of the advantages of this construction. The simple labial wire will not be damaged easily. The frequent breaking of the slender anterior acrylic part is avoided by splitting it in the midline. The judicious use of the Coffin spring, keeping the parts of the appliance in contact with the lateral teeth without pressure, will have a widening effect, especially when inserted during or soon after the eruption of the lower incisors. When not split, the appliance is stabilized and made more resistant by a lower labial bow wire.

Although the edge-to-edge bite of the Bionator may be used, Schmuth prefers the customary construction bite of the activator with an acrylic rim covering the lower incisors. Wearing during the entire day and night, except during meals, sports, or special demands at school, is requested. Most frequently, the appliance is used for part of the treatment. Simultaneously, with the changes brought about by the Andresen-Häupl activator, it may prevent the forward movement of permanent molars during the shedding of the deciduous molars or retract canines and retain posterior teeth after extractions. Also, it may be combined with fixed appliances of different kinds which can be worn simultaneously. The practical application of these versatile principles is shown in Figures 8–25 to 8–28).

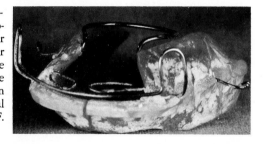

Figure 8–25. Schmuth modifications of activator (reduced activator or cybernator). Functional jaw orthopedic appliance with upper labial bow to hold out upper lip. Note protrusion loops for upper anterior teeth. Lower incisors are covered by acrylic to hold them in a stable position. A coffin spring is in the palatal portion and the lower acrylic structure is divided to permit expansion (transverse adaptation). Note spurs to prevent mesial drift of upper first molars. (Courtesy of Professor G. P. F. Schmuth.)

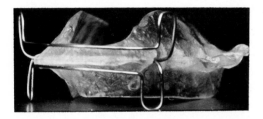

Figure 8-26. Schmuth type activator with two labial bows, without Coffin spring and without splitting of acrylic, since no expansion is planned. (Courtesy of Professor G. P. F. Schmuth.)

The Karwetzky Modification

The U-bow activator of Karwetzky is constructed quite similarly to the Schwarz bow-activator, but with an improved technique and an apparently increased efficiency. Since first published,[34] it has been perfected in a number of respects.[35, 36] It has stood up well, in comparison with other appliances,[37] and its use has been recommended in several recent textbooks.[38-40]

The Karwetzky appliance consists of maxillary and mandibular active plates, joined by a U-bow, in the region of the first permanent molars. In addition to acrylic covering of the lingual tissue aspects, gingivae, and teeth, the plates also extend over the occlusal aspects of all teeth (Fig. 8-29). The height of the construction bite, which seems to vary, depending on the modifier (Herren, Schwarz, Demisch, Woodside, Slagsvold, etc.), is that of the interocclusal space or clearance, with the mandible in postural resting position for the Karwetzky appliance. Thus, the space varies with the malocclusion treated and depth of the bite in the original malrelationship of upper and lower arches. In open bite problems, the construction bite slightly exceeds the postural resting position. For Class II, Division 1 malocclusions, the horizontal forward positioning is only part of the distance required to establish a normal interdigitation, usually not more than half of the anteroposterior correction required. A similar construction bite is made for Class II, Division 2 malocclusions. Further adjustments are made in stages (Figs. 8-30 and 8-31). In Class III, mandibular prognathism cases, the construction bite is taken in the most posterior position of the mandible possible in postural resting position. After mounting the casts on the articulator in the established initial construction bite, the interocclusal clearance created will become apparent (Fig. 8-32). It is then divided equally between the upper and lower plates.

The labial wires (0.9 mm.), wires for retention of spaces or those used to enhance the seating of the appliance (0.9 mm.), various closed springs (0.7

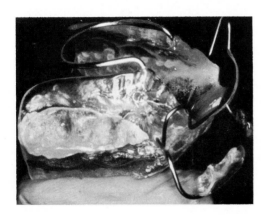

Figure 8-27. Schmuth type activator with one labial bow for upper jaw and with a Coffin spring. Note the combination with labial shields in the lower labial vestibule to hold out the lower lip, in a manner similar to the Fränkel function corrector. (Courtesy of Professor G. P. F. Schmuth.)

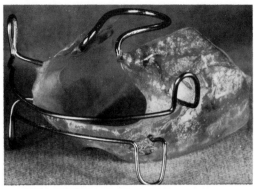

Figure 8–28. Schmuth activator with two labial bows and Coffin spring. It has not been necessary to cut through the acrylic of the lower part of the appliance for expansion adjustments. (Courtesy of Professor G. P. F. Schmuth.)

mm.), and any other appurtenances needed are fabricated and, together with any jackscrews that might be necessary, secured in place on the cast with sticky wax (Fig. 8–33). Cold-curing acrylic of putty-like consistency is then placed on the mandibular cast and the plate is formed with the appropriate thickness. While the acrylic covering the occlusal surfaces is still soft, it is pressed against a

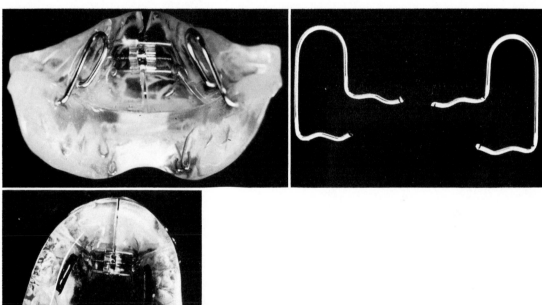

Figure 8–29. The U-bow activator of Karwetzky, type Ib. The longer leg of the U-bow measures 18 mm. from the top of the bow; the shorter leg is 11 mm. long.

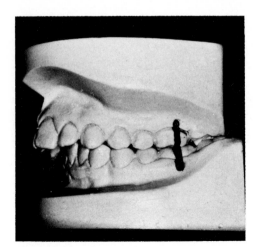

Figure 8-30. Plaster study models of a Class II, Division 1 case treated with the Karwetzky appliance.

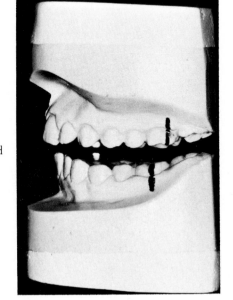

Figure 8-31. The same case as Figure 8-30, with casts related in the construction bite.

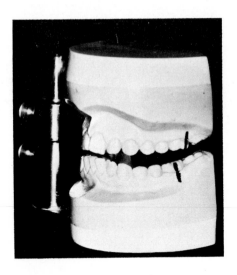

Figure 8-32. Casts in Figure 8-30, mounted on the articulator in the correct construction bite.

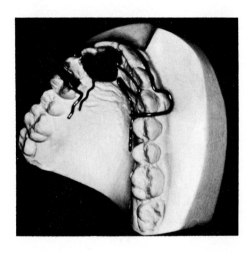

Figure 8-33. The upper cast with the wires in place.

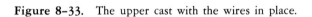

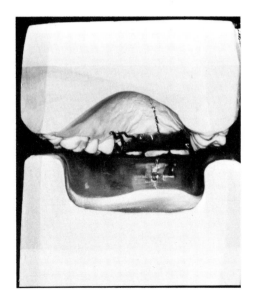

Figure 8–34. Lower plate finished and upper plate ready for addition of the acrylic portion.

small sheet of glass to give a smooth, flat surface. The relationship of this flat plane is checked with the casts properly related in the correct construction bite, and any adjustments are then made to insure the correct division of the interocclusal space between upper and lower appliances. After curing, the lower plate is polished in the usual manner and replaced on the lower cast (Fig. 8–34). The upper plate is made in similar manner, with its occlusal surface formed against the existing smooth and flat acrylic lower appliance occlusal covering. A thin layer of lubricant prevents the soft acrylic of the maxillary appliance from sticking to the lower surface while it is hardening.

Both finished plates are then joined by the U-bow, which is incorporated into the first permanent molar region by adding more cold-curing acrylic. Since the wire for the U-bow is 1.1 mm. in size, the acrylic must be of sufficient thickness to accommodate the horizontal parts of the wire to anchor the bow. To expedite this procedure, precise grooves are cut into the plates, deep enough to allow seating of the wires, and so no excess acrylic will be present after they are covered again with new acrylic. Though difficult, these areas must be carefully polished, as the rest of the surfaces have been. Small bends are made in the wires as they emerge from the plates so as to establish the appropriate distance from the acrylic surface and to permit adjustments that are described later. Replacement bows of the same size and configuration should be kept on hand, in the event that replacement is necessary later on, as the patient wears the activator.

Depending on where the ends of the U-bows are placed, three types of the Karwetzky activator may be created, each for a different treatment purpose. The U-bow has one longer and one shorter leg. The shorter leg is imbedded in the upper appliance, while the longer leg is attached to the lower plate. With the activator Type I, which is used for the treatment of Class II, Division 1 and Division 2 malocclusions, the longer lower leg is placed posteriorly. By constricting the bow, and thus narrowing the U-bend, the lower plate, which guides mandibular horizontal movements, is brought forward. This can be done unilaterally, by squeezing the U-bow on one side only (Fig. 8–35A). Type II of the Karwetzky activator is made by inserting the longer leg anteriorly in

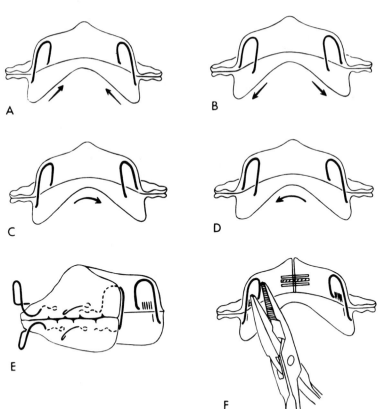

A

B

C

D

Figure 8-35. The mode of action of the U-bow activator: *A,* Class II, Division 1, type I. *B,* Class III activator, Type II. *C* and *D,* Designed for rotary movements of the mandible, type III. *E,* Marks made to control adjustments. *F,* Adjustment with flat, grooved pliers.

E

F

the lower appliance. It is used for treatment of Class III or mandibular prognathism cases, exerting a retrusive effect on the mandible as the U-bow is constricted by adjustments (Fig. 8–35*B*) Again, unilateral action is possible, or varied amounts of action transmitted to each side, depending on the degree of loop constriction. Type III is designed to influence the mandible in a transverse rather than sagittal direction, where there seems to be a displacement to one side or the other, i.e., a facial asymmetry or lateral crossbite. This is accomplished by placing the long lower U-bow leg anteriorly on one side and posteriorly on the other side. Consequently, the wire construction will tend to swing the mandible away from the side where the long leg is placed posteriorly (Fig. 8–35*C* and *D*). Scale markings may be inscribed between the legs of the U-bow, if desired, using a marking file, facilitating a more precise adjustment (Fig. 8–35*E*). Routine adjustments are made best with flat-nosed, grooved pliers (Fig. 8–35*F*). In the event that there are other treatment objectives, various appurtenances may be added (screws, springs, etc.) to accomplish the desired movement. As with all activators, however, care must be taken to keep the appliances as simple as possible, and to resist the temptation to do too many things at the same time.

Karwetzky feels that his design has inherent advantages over other activator-like appliances. The appliance exerts a delicate influence on the dentition and on the temporomandibular joint. The mobility of the parts allows various mandibular movements, which should make the activator more comfortable and should tend to reinforce the functional stimuli. The delicate forces, plus the gradual and sequential forward positioning of the lower jaw, will avoid the exertion of undue pressure. Experience gained over the last 12 to 15 years shows the possibility of treating the majority of malocclusions, including temporomandibular joint problems. The Karwetzky appliance may also be used to supplement treatment of certain types of jaw fractures.

The basic appliance action may be enhanced by combinations of different types of sagittal or transverse screws, labial wires, and springs. Such versatility permits use in 85 per cent of the cases treated, according to Karwetzky. The remaining 15 per cent will need treatment with an active plate first, or subsequently for retention. The U-bow activator may also be combined with the use of fixed appliances in these cases, particularly where there are severe rotations, or the need for selective extraction and uprighting of teeth contiguous to the extraction site. Another "plus" that provides an exciting potential for the appliance is the possibility of use with certain types of orthognathic surgery in adults. This is particularly true with corticotomies and subapical resections.[41]

With proper patient cooperation, correction may be achieved rather quickly, in as little as 5 to 8 months in favorable cases, and where growth direction and increments are optimal. Older patients naturally require a longer treatment time. The patients are required to wear the appliance for at least three hours during the day. This is absolutely essential. It allows the patient to get used to the appliance and not lose it during sleeping hours. The degree of patient compliance will influence the degree of success as well as the length of treatment in most cases. Karwetzky also feels it is important to use his appliance as the first one of choice. If attempts are made first with an active plate, which is smaller, the relatively greater bulk of the U-bow activator will seem uncomfortable to the wearer and increase the challenge of patient cooperation. Breakage may occur during treatment, but spare parts already fabricated and held in readiness are easily inserted in the appliance.

The following cases, using a modified vertical U-bow, have been treated by Dr. Karwetzky.[34–40] Treatment of the female patient, aged 26, whose casts are shown in Figures 8–36 and 8–37, was undertaken to relieve pains in the temporomandibular joint, to remove the disfigurement, and to facilitate prosthetic restoration. During the treatment, the pains in the temporomandibular joint initially increased but gradually reduced and disappeared. A U-bow activator Type I was used with the construction bite, creating an interocclusal clearance of 5 mm. between posterior teeth. Upper and lower labial bows were added, and a screw was incorporated to expand the maxillary plate. By repeated squeezing of the U-bow, the mandibular dentition was gradually brought forward. The result illustrated was achieved in one year. The re-examination of the patient five years later found the result satisfactorily maintained and apparently stable.

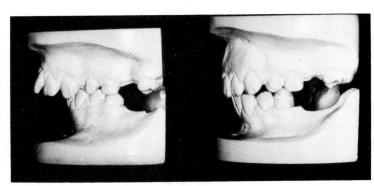

Figure 8–36. Casts of female patient with a Class II, Division 1 malocclusion aged 26 years, before and after one year of treatment with the Karwetzky U-bow activator.

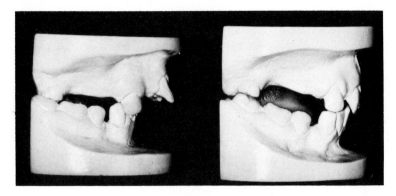

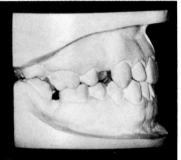

Figure 8-37. Right side of the patient in Figure 8-36.

Figure 8-38. Casts of female patient, age 17 years, with Class III malocclusion, before and after treatment.

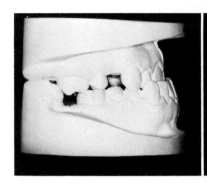

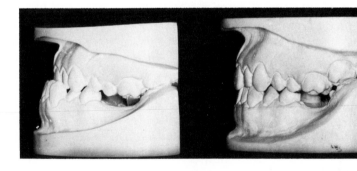

Figure 8-39. Same patient as Figure 8-38, before and after treatment with a Karwetzky-type activator.

Figure 8-40. Same patient as Figures 8-38 and 8-39, anterior views.

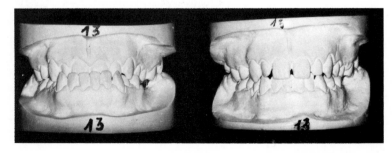

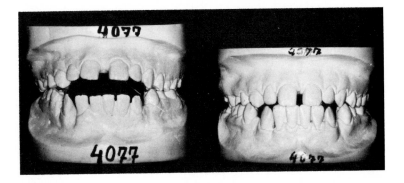

Figure 8–41. Casts of female patient, age 24 years, with open bite condition. Casts before and after treatment illustrate the change induced by the appliance, together with a corticotomy and excision of a portion of the tongue.

Treatment results with a case of Class III malocclusion are shown in Figures 8–38 to 8–40. When the patient, a girl aged 17, was first seen, attempts over a period of several years to achieve correction had failed. There was an apparent overdevelopment of the lower third of the face, in comparison with the middle third. Examination of the head plate showed a normal facial angle; the inclination angle, however, was 6 degrees smaller. The base plane angle was enlarged 10 degrees, the gonion angle 15 degrees. This also meant an enlargement of the SPP-A-B angle. The study of the casts revealed a slight maxillary underdevelopment in all three dimensions, and an excessive growth of the mandible only in a sagittal direction. There appeared to be an oversized tongue.

Treatment, therefore, was started with a V-shaped excision from the tongue to reduce its size. Then the U-bow activator Type II was inserted. An upper bow served to keep the upper lip away from the maxillary anterior teeth, which were moved labially by a continuous loop spring. A lower labial bow exerted pressure on the lower incisors to support the distal positioning of the mandible. After only a few weeks, a favorable change in the relationship of the

Figure 8–42. Cephalometric tracings made before treatment of patient in Figure 9–41. Note the procumbent interincisal angle.

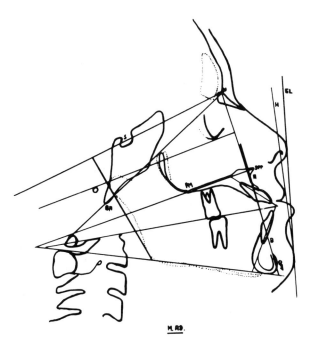

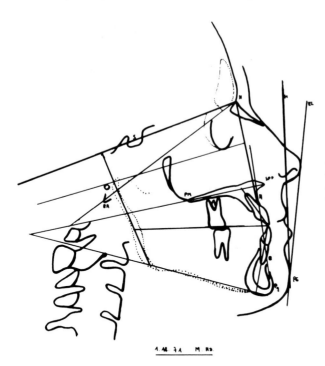

Figure 8-43. Same patient as Figures 8-41 and 8-42, with tracing showing the dramatic reduction of the interincisal angle following therapy.

incisors was observed, and after one year, the result shown was achieved. An examination four years later proved the stability of the correction.

When the treatment of a female, aged 24, was started, prolonged previous treatment had not improved the open bite of 11 mm. (Figs. 8-41 to 8-43). The vertical dimension of the lower part of the face was excessive. Lip closure was impeded, and mouth breathing enhanced frequent infections of the respiratory pathways. On the head plate, a minor enlargement of the base plane angle was seen, combined with a larger interincisal angle. There was an apparent bialveolar protrusion, attributable to an oversized tongue. No jaw orthopedic treatment had a chance of succeeding against the pressure of the tongue, which

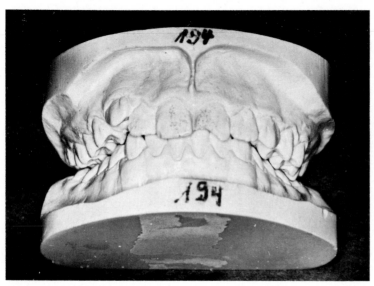

Figure 8-44. Casts of male patient, age 13 years, with "scissors bite." Double crossbite with maxillary buccal segments outside lower teeth. Upper right canine also has inadequate space.

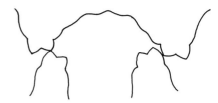

Figure 8–45. Cross-section (transverse) through casts before treatment of case shown in Figure 8–44.

would, inevitably, cause a relapse. In this case, therefore, the first step was a V-shaped excision from the tongue, followed by corticotomy in both anterior segments to lessen the resistance of the interdental septa.

The temporarily weakened support of the teeth facilitated their retrusion and the closing of the bite, without complications, using the U-bow activator Type I. Upper and lower labial bows, fitted in proximity to the gingival margins, effected this tooth movement in a little more than eight weeks. An observation examination three years later found the teeth in an entirely normal condition, with no sign of having suffered any damage. These cases demonstrate the potential of combined surgery and orthodontics in the treatment of older patients.

In a different manner, the U-bow activator was used in the treatment of a boy, aged 13, with bilateral nonocclusion (open bite) and the upper right canine crowded out of the dental arch. Even at this early age, there was sensitivity in the temporomandibular joint (Figs. 8–44 to 8–48). The design of the U-bow activator used after the extraction of the right upper first premolar is shown in the schematic drawing of Figure 8–46. It was fitted with both upper and lower labial bows. There was an expansion screw placed only in the mandibular plate. The acrylic was kept well away from the occlusal and palatal aspects of the posterior maxillary teeth, as well as from the lateral aspects of the palate. The displaced canine was aligned by the contact with the labial bow. The action of the screw, moving the mandibular teeth in a lateral direction, combined with the muscular pressure of the cheeks exerted on the maxillary dentition, achieved correction after a few months. The result was unchanged when the patient was seen three years later.

The modifications described in the last few pages show the potential versatility of the activator. The "individualizing" of the basic Andresen nighttime appliance has given a number of dentists the opportunity to express their own biomechanical ability and personal preferences for tooth-moving appurtenances. The problems created by such modifications, however, particularly in the hands of the neophyte, are not always so apparent. Yet this tendency to alter basic appliance design, without completely understanding the reasons for

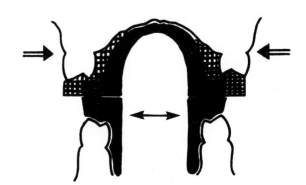

Figure 8–46. Schematic drawing of the U-bow activator used. Upper arch needs contraction while lower buccal segments require expansion.

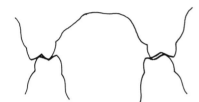

Figure 8-47. Transverse section through study casts after correction of scissors bite with U-bow activator.

appliance construction, has resulted too often in disillusionment of hundreds of dentists, and partial success, at best, for literally thousands of patients. It is almost a rule of thumb that the more complex the removable appliance, the greater the danger of patient discomfort, distortion of the appliance, and resultant noncompliance. For each force introduced in the appliance, there is an equal and opposite force. With several force vectors acting, the reaction may be partly successful, or actually harmful, introducing undesirable tooth movement or tissue damage.

It would be wise for any orthodontist, embarking on the use of removable appliances, to start with the simplest construction. It is better to construct two or three different appliances for a patient during treatment than to try to do everything with one. Experience will dictate subsequent modification and selective sophistication of functional appliances. It is better to turn to the developmental efforts of others who have had years of experience with such appliances. Thus, while this book has attempted to give the basic activator philosophy in Chapters 6 to 8 with modifications by Slagsvold, Harvold, Woodside, Hotz, Herren, Schwarz, Schmuth, Demisch, etc., other leaders in the field of functional appliances have started with the basic Andresen appliance and have produced their own unique combinations of structural and functional modifications. The remaining chapters of this book describe these efforts. Again, it is strongly urged that the orthodontist attempt to gain experience with these specific appliance constructions before attempting to make personal alterations and changes in form and action of the appliance, be it a Woodside

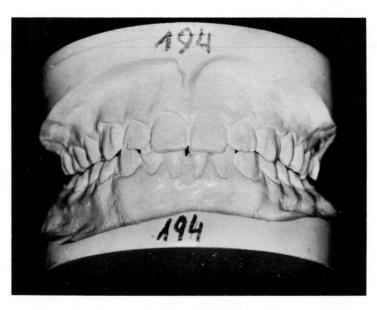

Figure 8-48. Plaster casts of patient in Figure 8-44, showing the results of successful treatment.

activator, a Bimler appliance, a Stockfisch Kinetor, a Klammt elastic open activator, or a Fränkel function corrector. A number of years ago, one of the authors of this book was taking a course with the developer of the Begg technique, P. Raymond Begg. In his inimitable style, Dr. Begg discouraged experimentation and change in the basic technique. He said, "Before disregarding my recommendations and making changes, first ask me why it failed when I tried it. After all, I have spent a lifetime trying and discarding alternate methods, selecting the best, the easiest, the most efficient way to do things."[42]

References

1. Robin, P.: Demonstration practique sur la construction et la mise en bouch d'un nouvel appareil de redressement. Rev. Stomatol., *9*:561–590, 1902.
2. Andresen, V.: The Norwegian system of functional gnatho-orthopedics. Acta Gnathol., *1*:5–36, 1936.
3. Farrar, J. N.: Irregularities of the teeth and their correction. New York, Farrar, 1888.
4. Andresen, V., and Häupl, K.: Funktionskieferorthopädie, lst ed. Leipzig, H. Meusser, 1936.
5. Häupl, K.: Gewebsumbau und Zahnverdrängung in der Funktionskieferorthopädie. Leipzig, J. A. Barth, 1938.
6. Andresen, V., Häupl, K., and Petrik, L.: Funktionskieferorthopädie, 6th ed. Munich, J. A. Barth, 1957.
7. Petrik, L.: Funktionelle Therapie-Spezieller Teil. *In* Häupl, K., Meyer, W., and Schuchardt, K.: Zahn-Mund und Kieferheilkunde, Vol. V. Munich, Urban & Schwarzenberg, 1955.
8. Reitan, K.: The initial tissue reaction incident to orthodontic tooth movement as related to the influence of function. Acta Odontol. Scand., Suppl. 1951.
9. Harvold, E.: The activator in interceptive orthodontics. St. Louis, The C. V. Mosby Co., 1974.
10. Charlier, J. P., Petrovic, A., and Linck, G.: La fronde mentonnière et son action sur la croissance mandibulaire. Orthod. Fr., *40*:100–113, 1969.
11. Moss, M. L.: The functional matrix. *In* Kraus, B. S., and Riedel, R. A. (Eds.): Vistas in Orthodontics. Philadelphia, Lea & Febiger, 1962.
12. Moyers, R. E., Elgoyhen, J. C., Riolo, M. L., McNamara, J. A., Jr., and Kuroda, T.: Experimental production of Class III in rhesus monkeys. Trans. Europ. Orthod. Soc., *46*:61–74, 1970.
13. McNamara, J. A., Jr.: Neuromuscular and skeletal adaptations to altered orofacial function. Ph. D. Dissertation, University of Michigan, 1972.
14. Stöckli, P., Hotz, R., Gisler, G., and Scheier, H.: Auswirkung der Skoliosebehandlung mit Extensions-korsetten auf den Kiefer-Gesichts Bereich. Schweiz. Monatschr. Zahnheilk., *77*:1029, 1967.
15. Herren, P.: Sagittaler Bissausgleich im Lichte einiger muskelfunktioneller Beobachtungen. Studieweek, 1965.
16. Hotz, R.: Die Beurteilung der Ruhelage bei der Behandlung der Klasse II. Fortschr. Kieferorthop., *26*:19–22, 1965.
17. Kinast, as quoted in reference 31.
18. Ahlgren, J.: A longitudinal clinical and cephalometric study of 50 malocclusion cases treated with activator appliances. Trans. Europ. Orthod. Soc., pp. 285–293, 1972.
19. Schmuth, G. P. F.: Kieferorthopädie. Stuttgart, Georg Thieme, 1973.
20. Herren, P.: Die passive Haltung und Bewegung des Unterkiefers. Schweiz. Monatschr. Zahnheilk., *63*:561, 1953.
21. Herren, P.: Die Wirkungsweise des Aktivators. Schweiz. Monatschr. Zahnheilk., *63*:829–879, 1953.
22. Herren, P.: The Activator's mode of action. Am. J. Orthod., *45*:512–527, 1959.
23. Herren, P.: Lecture notes (unpublished), 1974. Personal communication.
24. Herren, P., Weber, J., and Mueller, P.: The palpation phenomenon of the condyle at the external auditory meatus during treatment of Class II, Division 1 anomalies by means of activators. Trans. Europ. Orthod. Soc., pp. 295–310, 1972.
25. Wunderer, as quoted in reference 33.
26. Weise, W.: Die Behandlung. *In* Haunfelder, D., Hupfauf, H., Ketterl, W., and Schmuth, G. (Eds.): Kieferorthopädie, Praxis der Zahnheilkunde, Vol. IV. Munich, Urban & Schwarzenberg, 1969.
27. Graf, E. J.: Funktionelle Kräfte bei bimaxillaren Regulierungsapparaten. Doctoral Dissertation, University of Zurich, 1962.

28. Demisch, A.: Effects of activator therapy on the craniofacial skeleton in Class II, Division 1 malocclusion. Trans. Europ. Orthod. Soc., pp. 295–310, 1972.
29. Demisch, A.: Auswirkungen der Distalbiss Therapie mit dem Aktivator auf das Gesichtsskelett. Schweiz. Monatschr. Zahnheilk., *83*:1072–1092, 1973.
30. Taatz, H.: Kieferorthopädische Prophylaxe und Frühbehandlung. Leipzig, J. A. Barth, 1976.
31. Schwarz, A. M.: Lehrgang der Gebissregelung, 2nd ed. Vol. II. Vienna, Urban and Schwarzenberg, 1956.
32. Schwarz, A. M., and Gratzinger, M.: Removable Orthodontic Appliances. Philadelphia, W. B. Saunders Company, 1966.
33. Reichenbach, E., Brückl, H., and Taatz, H.: Kieferorthopädische Klinik und Therapie, 7th ed. Leipzig, J. A. Barth, 1971.
34. Karwetzky, R.: Ein neues funktionskieferorthopädisches Gerät nach Karwetzky. Dtsch. Zahnärztebl., *18*:419–423, 1964.
35. Karwetzky, R.: Der U-Bügelaktivator nach Karwetzky. Quintessenz, *21*:1–5, 1970.
36. Karwetzky, R.: Die Anwendung des U-Bügelaktivators in der zahnärztlichen Praxis. Dtsch. Zahnärztl. Z., *29*:891–93, 1974.
37. Dierks, P.: Das Wachstum des Gesichtsschädels unter dem Einfluss verschiedener Gerätetypen. Dissertation, University of Münster, 1974.
38. Schulz, H.: Der U-Bügelaktivator in Kieferorthopädie für Zahntechniker. Köln, Neuer Merkur, 1965.
39. Hennis, I.: Der U-Bügelaktivator nach Karwetzky. *In* Haunfelder, D., Hupfauf, L., Ketterl, W., and Schmuth, G. (Eds.): Kieferorthopädie, Praxis der Zahnheilkunde, Vol. IV, München, Urban & Schwarzenberg, 1969.
40. Rethmann, H.: Der U-Bügelaktivator. *In* Kieferorthopädisches Repetitorium. München, C. Hanser, 1970.
41. Köle, H.: Surgical operations on the alveolar ridge to correct occlusal abnormalities. Oral Surg, *12*:515–529, 1959.
42. Begg, P. R.: The Begg Differential Light Forces Technique. Technique Course, La Porte, Indiana, Oct. 6–10, 1962.
43. Ahlgren, J.: Late results of activator treatment: A cephalometric study. Br. J. Orthod., *3*:181–87, 1976.
44. Pancherz, H.: Long-term effects of activator (Andresen appliance) treatment. Odontol. Revy, Vol. 27, Suppl. 35, 1976.

CHAPTER 9

The Bionator

The Bionator, developed by Balters, has much in common with the Andresen-Häupl activator as well as other appliances that originated from it. These include those of Bimler, Klammt, and Van Thiel. All are functional jaw orthopedic appliances. Kantorowicz termed the Bionator "the skeleton of an activator from which there is nothing left but the naked embodiment of Robin's thoughts."

This assessment is essentially correct in two ways: (1) The Bionator is, in fact, considerably less bulky than the activator. It lacks the part covering the anterior section of the palate, which is contiguous to the tongue. Children are therefore immediately able to speak normally, although the appliance fits loosely in the mouth. This always surprises orthodontists who have had previous experience with the conventional activator or other removable appliances. Thus, it is possible to require that the Bionator be worn day and night except at meals. It is feasible for wear during school. An important feature of the Bionator is its freedom of movement in the oral cavity. It would be totally incorrect and detrimental to fix it by any device on either the maxillary or mandibular teeth. (2) The essential part of Robin's concept is function. To Balters, the essential factor is the tongue. To quote him, "The equilibrium between tongue and cheeks, especially between the tongue and the lips in the height, breadth and depth in an oral space of maximum size and optimal limits, providing functional space for the tongue, is essential for the natural health of the dental arches and their relation to each other. Every disturbance will deform the dentition and during growth that may be impeded too. The tongue is the essential factor for the development of the dentition. It is the center of the reflex activity in the oral cavity."

Eirew summarizes the Balters treatment objectives as follows:

1. In the labial area, the elimination of the lip trap and of the abnormal relationship between the lips and the incisor teeth.

2. The elimination of mucosal damage due to traumatic deep bite.

3. The correction of mandibular retrusion and associated malposition of the tongue.

4. The attainment of a correct occlusal plane, if necessary, by the screening of intrusive tongue and cheek musculature.

The Bionator is especially suitable to accomplish sagittal and vertical

The authors are indebted to Professor F. Ascher of Munich, who has supplied the material for this chapter, and to Urban & Schwarzenberg, the publishers of his book "Praktische Kieferorthopädie," who gave permission for use of the illustrations.

changes in the dentition. It is considered by many operators to be a most effective appliance for the treatment of the sequelae of a sucking habit. Here the spacing, protrusion of the upper incisors, Class II tendency, and narrow intercanine dimension are responsive to correction. In addition, with a deep overbite during mixed dentition and even at a later date, gratifying results may be achieved by the Bionator appliance as used in the treatment of bruxism, periodontal disease, and temporomandibular joint disorders. It should be stressed here again that, as with all appliances, success is not universal. Failures occur with any appliance, removable or fixed. Partial success is the more likely response. This can be due to lack of patient cooperation, wrong diagnosis, poor growth direction, inadequate growth increments, poor treatment timing, and the same multiplicity of factors that plague the correction of many morphofunctional malocclusions. Therapeutic modifiability is as important for removable as it is for fixed appliances. Treatment decisions and treatment mechanics are always subject to change and require constant vigilance on the part of the clinician, regardless of the appliance being used.

According to this view, the maximum power of the muscle activity is not so important as the orderly coordination of the manifold functions. Malocclusion thus must be regarded as a disturbance of that coordination. There may be a cause of the incoordinate activity. Of no minor importance may be the psychological component, producing parafunctional influences by which the action of the finger, tongue, lips, cheeks, etc., will produce deformation. For Balters, the Bionator will normalize function and lead to harmony of anatomic relations.

According to Balters, the essential points for treatment are: (1) to accomplish lip closure and bring the back of the tongue into contact with the soft palate; (2) to enlarge the oral space and to train its function; (3) to bring the incisors into an edge-to-edge incision or relationship. Like Begg, he feels that this is a natural bodily orientation; (4) By virtue of the above, to achieve an elongation of the mandible, which in turn will enlarge the oral space and make the improved tongue position possible; (5) An improved relationship of the jaws, tongue and dentition, as well as the surrounding soft tissues, will result.

All of the above will improve the muscular coordination and metabolism of the whole area in various ways. Balters feels that this frees the orofacial muscles of tension in the postural resting position and avoids the incoordinate muscle activity, which leads to deformation. According to Balters' philosophy, Class II malocclusions are a consequence of a backward position of the tongue, disturbing the cervical region. The respiratory function is impeded in the region of the larynx and there is thus a faulty deglutition. Concomitantly, there is mouth breathing. By the same analysis, Balters reasons that Class III conditions are due to a more forward position of the tongue and to cervical overdevelopment. He would explain Class I malocclusions as being due to lack of transverse development of the dentition, as a consequence of a weakness of the tongue in comparison with the strength of the buccinator mechanism. While much of this reasoning is teleologic and unsubstantiated by research endeavors, there is a certain degree of logic. The functional matrix concepts of Moss are strongly substantiated by Balters, and the neurotrophic elements of the functional matrix theory are consistent with much of the Balters philosophy.

If we are to accept these concepts, then the main objective of treatment for Class II, Division 1 malocclusions is to bring the tongue forward. This is achieved by stimulation of the distal part of the dorsum of the tongue. By developing the mandible in an anterior direction, to establish a Class I relationship, Balters feels that the cervical viscera may also be brought forward.

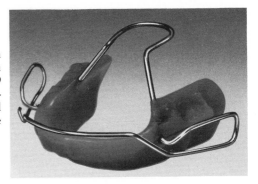

Figure 9-1. The standard Bionator appliance, used in the treatment of Class II, Division 1 malocclusions with excessive overjet and deep overbite. The labial wire (0.9 mm.) and the buccinator bends together form the vestibular wire. The palatal wire is heavier (1.2 mm.) and is curved in a distal direction. This type of Bionator may also be used in Class I cases with crowding of the anterior teeth.

Such change will enlarge the respiratory pathways and enhance the reflexes of deglutition, which will then become normal. Conversely, Balters wishes to get the tongue into a more backward and higher position for Class III malocclusions. Here, with the reduction of the anterior force vector, the mandible may return to a Class I relationship. Balters feels that the new posterior and superior tongue position will reduce cervical overdevelopment. For Class I malocclusions, transverse underdevelopment may be reduced by muscular training, which makes the tongue stronger. In such a matter, equilibrium between tongue and cheeks and tongue and lips may be established, with resultant dentitional equilibrium.

As might be expected, the Balters technique requires lip closure for the treatment of all kinds of malocclusion. Balters considers this a precondition for the free development of the growth potential, which has been impeded by abnormal function. This expression of uninhibited growth potential is made possible by the end-to-end incisal biting position.

There are three types of Bionator for carrying out the various malocclusion corrections: the standard, the Class III, and the open bite appliance. All have a vestibular wire and a palatal arch. In the original terminology, the palatal arch was termed "lingual" because its function is to stimulate the tongue. Since it is situated on the palate, the term palatal arch is preferred now to avoid

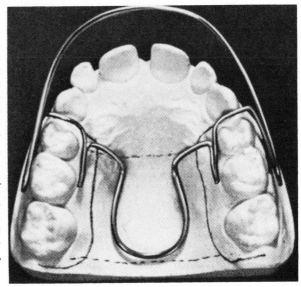

Figure 9-2. The maxillary cast, occlusal view, with the wires in place. The egg-shaped palatal arch (1.2 mm.) extends from a line connecting the distal surfaces of the first permanent molars anteriorly to about the middle of the first premolars. The vestibular wire (0.9 mm.) crosses slightly above the occlusal surfaces, then forms the buccinator bends in the deciduous molar area, passing anteriorly to form the labial wire. The buccinator bends are 2 to 3 mm. away from the teeth, on each side, similar to the Fränkel buccal shields. The labial wire, a continuation of the buccal bends, passes around the arch at a distance of 3 to 4 mm. from the mandibular teeth. Acrylic is added to this framework to finish the appliance. (From Ascher, F.: Praktische Kieferorthopädie. München, Urban & Schwarzenberg, 1968.)

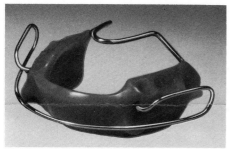

Figure 9–3. The Class III appliance. The labial wire (0.9 mm.) runs straight forward from the buccinator bends, so as to contact the lower lip. The buccinator bends are the same as for the standard appliance (see Fig. 9–1). The palatal wire (1.2 mm.) is curved anteriorly, however, with the opening to the distal. The acrylic construction is essentially the same as for the standard Bionator, except that it extends superiorly to the tips of the maxillary canines and 2 mm. beyond the incisal edges of the upper incisors. The construction bite is taken so as to provide a space of less than 2 mm. between the incisal edges of the upper and lower incisors. The acrylic may contact the upper incisors without pressure, but about 1 mm. of acrylic is removed from behind the lower incisors. The occlusal imprints of the buccal teeth are left in the acrylic, with only the sharp edges left by the fissures smoothed. If no opening of the bite is desired, the occlusal surfaces of the molars are also covered with acrylic. If the acrylic in the interocclusal space is thin, it may be reinforced by a thin wire or plastic mesh.

confusion. The arch must provide the essential stimulation in that particular region to strengthen the muscles of the tongue.

The standard appliance (Fig. 9–1) is used (a) for the treatment of Class II, Division 1 conditions to correct the backward position of the tongue and its consequences, and (b) for the treatment of narrow dental arches of a Class I malocclusion. Through continuous exercise, tongue function is stimulated and the volume or mass of the tongue is enlarged.

The Class III appliance is meant for the treatment of mandibular prognathism, to compensate for the forward position of the tongue (Fig. 9–3).

The open bite appliance is used to close the aperture formed in the anterior or lateral dentitional areas (Fig. 9–4).

STANDARD APPLIANCE

The standard appliance (see Fig. 9–1) consists of a relatively slender acrylic body fitted to the lingual aspects of the mandibular arch and part of the maxillary dental arch. As the illustration shows, it extends from somewhat distal to the first permanent molar on one side to a corresponding point on the other side. The maxillary part covers only the molars and premolars, however. The anterior maxillary part from canine to canine remains open. The relative position of the joined upper and lower acrylic portions is determined by the con-

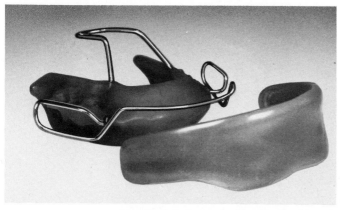

Figure 9–4. The open bite appliance. The vestibular and palatal wires are identical to the standard Bionator. The maxillary acrylic portion is modified, however, with acrylic extending up behind the maxillary incisors at the same level as it does for the posterior teeth. It does not contact the teeth or alveolus, however. Its purpose is to prevent the tongue from thrusting between the teeth. The construction bite leaves a rather thin layer of acrylic between all the posterior teeth. It may also be reinforced by meshwire. In a few cases, a vestibular screen may be added. It is attached to the distal bend of the buccinator wires by a wire hook or an acrylic extension. Its purpose is to prevent interference by the lips and cheeks.

TABLE 9-1. STABILIZATION OF THE BIONATOR

Teeth Present	Stabilization
1 2 III IV V 6	IV and V, upper and lower
1 2 III – V 6	V, upper and lower with space and time of eruption permitting; then the alveolar ridge may also be used for stabilization.
1 2 III – – 6	Upper and lower alveolar ridge
1 2 III 4 – 6	Upper 4 and alveolar ridge; mandibular alveolar ridge
1 2 3 4 5 6	Generally 4 and 5; different solutions may be necessary

In the late mixed dentition and in the permanent dentition with greatly elongated frontal teeth:

Elongated lower frontal teeth	Bite rim for lower incisors as used with the Andresen-Häupl activator
Elongated upper and lower frontal teeth	Bite rim for upper and lower incisors; all lateral occlusal surfaces remain free

The choice of teeth is given for stabilization with the standard appliance. For Class III and open bite Bionator other rules apply.

struction bite. This is generally taken in an edge-to-edge incisal relationship. The acrylic should extend about 2 mm. below the mandibular gingival margin and about the same distance above the maxillary gingival margin. It must remain rather thin so as not to interfere with the function of the tongue. The interocclusal space of some of the buccal teeth is filled with acrylic, extending over half of the occlusal surfaces of the teeth. The choice of these teeth is shown in Table 9-1. Depending on the size of the overjet, there are two alternatives for the anterior part covering the lower incisors:

1. The acrylic is extended to cover the lower incisors the same way as the activator does.

2. There is no acrylic covering necessary, because the incisors already will essentially meet in an edge-to-edge bite. This will be discussed in greater detail later, under the description of the construction bite.

The appliance is stabilized in the mixed dentition by having the upper and lower deciduous molars occlude on the acrylic. In the permanent dentition, this is accomplished by having the maxillary premolars occlude in the acrylic. The occlusal part of the acrylic bite block will, however, be ground flat, freeing the way for a transverse expansion of the dental arch. No acrylic covers the first molars. This permits further eruption and leveling of the bite in this region. The remaining permanent buccal teeth should subsequently follow suit. The acrylic covering these teeth, however, must be removed with caution, because after this, the appliance can be stabilized only by the contacting of the upper and lower incisors (Fig. 9-5). How stabilization is provided in the presence or absence of different teeth is shown in Table 9-1.

The other basic features of the Bionator are the palatal arch and the vestibular wire. The palatal arch is made from 1.2 mm. diameter hard stainless steel wire. It emerges from the upper margin of the acrylic, approximately opposite the middle of the first premolar. Then it follows the contour of the palate, at about 1.0 mm. distance from the mucosa. The arch forms a wide curve that reaches a line joining the distal surfaces of the first permanent molars, and it then follows an identical mirror image curve to insert on the opposite side. As Figure 9-2 shows, the configuration of the palatal arch is somewhat like the shape of an egg. As has been indicated, the theory of Balters is that the task of the palatal arch is to stimulate the distal aspect of the tongue. It is for this

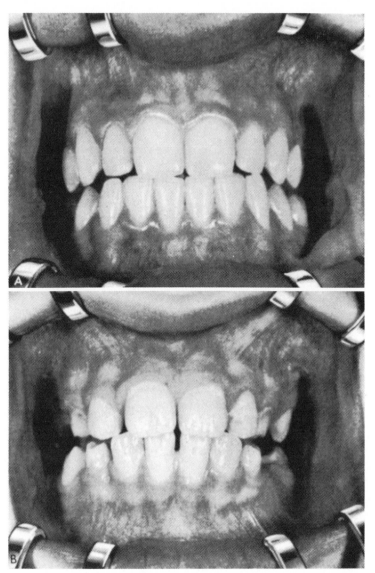

Figure 9–5. The construction bite is shown here in the standard position, in an edge-to-edge relationship of the central incisors. *B,* Where the maxillary central incisors are inclined too much labially, the construction bite is then taken with an edge-to-edge relationship on the lateral incisors. (From Ascher, F.: Praktische Kieferorthopädie. München, Urban und Schwarzenberg, 1968.)

reason that the curve of the arch is directed posteriorly. It should effect a *forward* orientation of the tongue, as well as the mandible, into a Class I relationship of the jaws. If the palatal vault is high, the tongue is prevented from touching the palate as it would usually do. It has been felt by disciples of Balters that there is subsequent flattening of the palate which, conceivably, would improve the breathing through the nose.

The vestibular wire is also shown in Figure 9–2 and is of 0.9 mm. diameter. It emerges from the acrylic below the contact point between the upper canine and the first premolar. The vestibular wire rises vertically and is then bent at a right angle to go distally along the middle of the crowns of the upper premolars. Just anterior to the mesial contact point of the first molar, the wire is fashioned in a round bend toward the lower dental arch. The wire, maintaining a constant level at the height of the papillae, parallels the upper portion anteriorly to the mandibular canines. At this point, the wire is bent to reach the upper canine, nearly touches the incisal third of the incisors, and from there, in a mirror image of the side already fabricated, proceeds posteriorly to the acrylic on the opposite side. The labial portion of the vestibular wire is kept away from the surface of the incisors by the thickness of a sheet of paper. The lateral portions of the wire are sufficiently away from the premolars to allow for expansion of the dental arch, but not enough to cause discomfort to the cheeks. Here again, the theory is that between the incisors and the mucosa of the lips a slight negative pressure is created. In the course of the treatment, this should help upright the incisors, provide space for them when the dental arch is widened laterally and sagittally, and probably favorably influence the development in the region of the apical base. The anterior portion of the vestibular wire is called the labial wire, while the lateral parts are called the buccinator bends. The buccinator bends have two treatment objectives:

1. To keep away the soft tissue of the cheeks, which is normally drawn into the interocclusal space. By keeping the cheeks away, the bite may be leveled and eruption will proceed in the buccal segments.

2. To actually move the surfaces of the orobuccal capsule (the cheeks) laterally, increasing the oral space by virtue of the forward positioning of the mandible, which relaxes the musculature while the vestibular wire holds it away from the alveolar mucosa. It is felt that the removal of this inhibitory influence will favor expansion or transverse development of the maxillary dentition. Fränkel has some very pertinent research which indicates that these objectives are attainable.

CLASS III APPLIANCE

The acrylic part of the Class III appliance (Fig. 9–3) is similar to that of the standard type. A mandibular plate and two lateral maxillary parts extending from the first premolar to the first premolar are joined together, opening the bite just enough to allow the upper incisors to move labially past the lower incisors. This opening of the bite should provide a space of less than 2 mm. between the edges of the maxillary and mandibular incisors. That space is covered, toward the tongue, by an extension of the mandibular portion of the plate from canine to canine. The edges of the upper incisors extend beyond the upper margin of acrylic about 2 mm. In this manner, the maxillary incisor teeth are positioned directly in front of an acrylic barrier which, however, does not exert any kind of pressure. About 1 mm. of the thickness of acrylic is removed from behind the mandibular incisors. This barrier blocks any forward movement of the tongue toward the vestibule. Its purpose is to teach the tongue by proprioceptive stimuli to remain in its retracted and proper functional space. It will now contact the uncovered anterior portion of the palate, stimulating the forward growth component in this area. This change in tongue function is strongly supported by the palatal arch, which is fabricated of 1.2 mm. wire as with the standard appliance. The round bend, however, is placed in an inverted position, extending forward to a line connecting the middle of the first premolars. From this point, the wire runs parallel on both sides to the upper margin of the acrylic, extending posteriorly to the distal surface of the first molar, where it enters the acrylic at a right angle bend. In the Class III type, the vestibular wire, also 0.9 mm. in diameter, is placed in front of the *lower* incisors. It emerges from the acrylic in the same manner as in the standard appliance, below the contact point of the upper canine and first premolar. The buccinator bend is fabricated the same as for the standard type. The wire goes in a distal direction until it reaches a point just behind the second premolar. From here, with the round bend, it runs forward again. As a labial wire, however, it is in proximity to the lower incisors, remaining the thickness of a sheet of paper away from the labial surfaces. The maxillary and mandibular premolar teeth occlude in the acrylic, as do first molars if their elongation is not desired.

OPEN BITE APPLIANCE

The purpose of this appliance (see Fig. 9–4) is to close the vertical space or open bite. It is recognized that in a great majority of cases the tongue is either causing or perpetuating the infraocclusion of the maxillary and mandibular incisor teeth, allowing overeruption of the buccal segments. In these cases, there is little or no interocclusal clearance because of the abnormal tongue function. It is necessary to prevent the tongue from inserting into the aperture. For this purpose, the maxillary parts of the acrylic are joined anteriorly, in contradistinction to the types just described where the acrylic is restricted to a contact with the buccal teeth only. As Figure 9–4 shows, however, the anterior part is not in contact with the teeth or alveolar bone, since it must not interfere with expected growth changes. As with the vestibular screen, which has already been described, it is hoped that the treatment response will not only improve the occlusion of the teeth but also transform the adjacent alveolar parts. The mandibular and maxillary acrylic portions are joined by slight bite blocks. With the open bite appliance, the small occlusal bite block used for stabilization has indentations of the teeth on the surface. The purpose of the lateral bite blocks is to prevent the posterior teeth from erupting while the anterior teeth are allowed to erupt freely. This should re-establish the interocclusal clearance and a postural vertical dimension that is in harmony with the occlusal vertical dimension.

The palatal and vestibular wires are the same as for the standard type of Bionator. However, in some cases the lips and cheeks, especially the lower lip, may be drawn into the open bite, which would interfere with the correction of the malocclusion. To prevent this from occurring, a lip shield may be added. The shield is placed in the vestibule and is loosely anchored to the appliance by an acrylic or wire extension over and slightly inside the buccinator bends. In this manner, an instant closure of the oral cavity is effected. Only seldom is this additional appurtenance needed.

THE BIONATOR CONSTRUCTION BITE

The importance of the construction bite has been sufficiently emphasized in the section dealing with activator. Detailed description has been given on just how to make it. With the standard type Bionator, it is also the objective to establish the dental arches in a Class I relationship. But most important is the position of the incisor teeth, as established by the construction bite. For this relationship there are several possibilities.

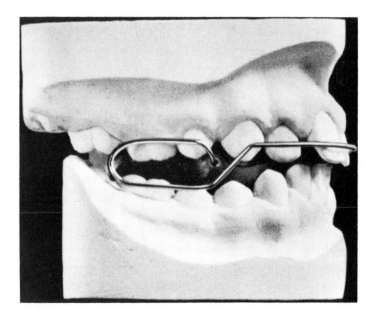

Figure 9–6. In cases of excessive overjet, the construction bite is taken with a correct sagittal relationship on the canines. The mandible is moved forward until the tip of the upper canine tooth is opposite the contact point between the lower canine and first premolar. The plaster casts illustrate such a relationship. Care must be taken to maintain the correct upper and lower incisor midlines during this maneuver, as shown in Figure 9–5. (From Ascher, F.: Praktische Kieferorthopädie. München, Urban & Schwarzenberg, 1968.)

1. Preference is given to an edge-to-edge relationship of all, or at least the lateral, incisors (Figs. 9–5 and 9–6). This will provide the maximum functional space for the tongue. The patient will also find the contact established between the incisors convenient.

2. In cases where the overjet is too large to allow an edge-to-edge incisal bite, these (the mandibular incisors) must be covered by a grooved rim similar to that of the activator (Figs. 9–7 and 9–8). In any event, an exaggerated forward movement of the mandible should be avoided. After the reduction of the overbite has been achieved, then a new appliance may be made with the incisors in an edge-to-edge bite, or step three below may be followed.

3. An additional maxillary incisal margin acrylic restraint may be used. This is fabricated by adding cold-curing acrylic on the mandibular incisor acrylic cover, right at the incisal margin (Fig. 9–8). The appliance is then placed

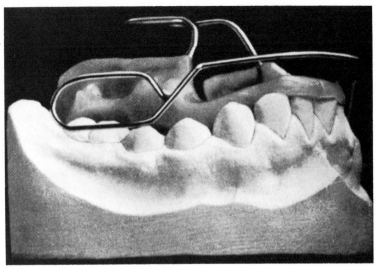

Figure 9–7. The appliance shown in Figure 9–6, seated on the mandibular cast. Instead of the usual edge-to-edge construction bite relationship, stabilization is provided in the anterior region by covering the lower incisors with an acrylic bite rim, similar to the Andresen-Häupl activator. When sagittal improvement has been achieved and overjet has been reduced, the incisors are then brought in an edge-to-edge relationship. For this a new appliance may be necessary. (From Ascher, F.: Praktische Kieferorthopädie. München, Urban und Schwarzenberg, 1968.)

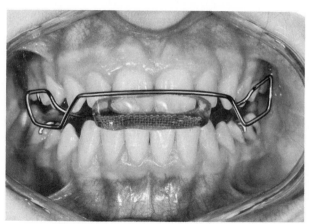

Figure 9-8. An alternative construction, adapted from Figures 9–6 and 9–7, is used in some cases. Acrylic is added to the lower incisor bite rim and the upper incisors bite into it when it is still soft. This kind of additional stabilization is preferred by some orthodontists at the beginning of treatment. This construction bite frees the occlusal surfaces of the buccal segments at an earlier stage of treatment, leading to more rapid leveling of the bite due to eruption of the posterior teeth. The wire hooks anterior to the first molars are for sagittal stabilization. The incorporation of mesh wire in the anterior acrylic construction prevents undue breakage.

in the mouth and the patient is instructed to close into the predetermined construction bite position, guiding the mandible carefully.

After the acrylic has hardened, it is cut down and polished, leaving just a groove with a thin 3 mm. wide cover for the maxillary incisors. The cover extends from the distal proximal surface of one lateral incisor to the corresponding surface of the other. This construction secures the position of the upper incisors. The intruding force exerted on them may be desirable also. Some operators prefer this modification of the Bionator for the construction bite right from the beginning. They are of the opinion that this frees the occlusal surfaces of the buccal teeth earlier, allowing a more rapid and reliable leveling of the bite. This modification also prevents any labial tipping of the mandibular incisors, as the mandible is led more positively into its new anterior position.

When incisors have been tipped labially from their original retroinclined position in the first stage of treatment, using an active plate, the groove with the cover for the maxillary incisors may be used to advantage for the stabilization and retention of these teeth. Figure 9–16 illustrates such a case. The groove for the upper incisors may also help in achieving better alignment of these teeth. For example, the lateral incisors sometimes interfere with the forward positioning of the maxillary centrals in Class II, Division 2 problems. In such instances, the acrylic lip on the labial is removed from the lateral incisal margin. Then a drop of cold-curing acrylic is placed on the lingual aspect of the groove, to contact the lingual lateral incisor surface. After the acrylic hardens, the appliance is replaced. A slight labial tipping pressure is then exerted on the lateral incisor.

Several factors have to be considered in the construction of the standard appliance for the treatment of Class II, Division 1 malocclusion. They are the size of the overjet, the distance the patient will be able to move the mandible forward comfortably, the presence or absence of deciduous molars and premolars, and the overbite.

In case of a slight overbite of the incisors, no lateral stabilization is provided. There is, in fact, no room for it. Further opening of the bite would be undesirable. It is worth mentioning that the Bionator is effective also in these cases, although for some reason such problems do not respond as well to treatment with the Andresen-Häupl activator.

Figure 9–9. *A,* When cold-cure (self-polymerizing) acrylic is used to fabricate the Bionator, the maxillary cast is covered with two or three sheets of base-plate wax. The wax is then cut out to permit selective application of acrylic. Half of the occlusal surfaces of the first permanent molar and the deciduous molars is uncovered, including also the distolingual third of the canines. Also, the wax is cut away from the gingival portion, to a distance of approximately 3 mm. beyond the gingival margin. The incisal edges are also uncovered, since they will contact the lower incisors when the construction bite is set up in the articulator. *B,* Wax is also applied to the mandibular cast, as in *A,* and cut away selectively for application of the cold-cure acrylic. The occlusal surfaces of all posterior teeth are exposed to the central fissures, as illustrated. Incisal edges are also free. As in the maxillary portion, the lower margin of the acrylic will be 3 mm. below the gingival margin. After both casts have been covered with wax, they are mounted in the articulator. The softened and slightly lubricated wax portions are pressed together to make sure that they are in the proper construction bite relationship. Then the casts are separated again and the wire elements are fixed in the maxillary wax covering. The wax portions of upper and lower parts are then joined and the acrylic is added in the parts where the wax has been cut away. During the setting process, the plaster casts are carefully withdrawn from the wax portion to make sure that there is no acrylic left in the undercuts. These would impede the insertion and removal of the appliance. (From Ascher, F.: Praktische Kieferorthopädie. München, Urban und Schwarzenberg, 1968.)

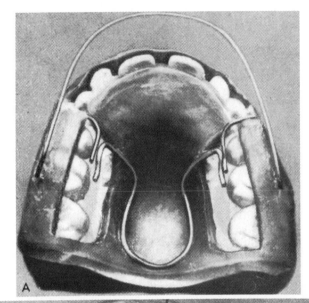

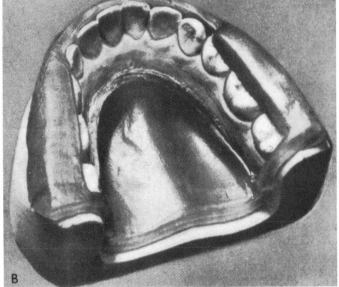

In presence of a deep overbite the lateral surfaces remain free also. If the elongation of the lower incisors is responsible for the overbite, stabilization is provided by the cover on these incisors, the same as used with the Andresen-Häupl activator (see Figs. 9–7 and 9–8). Deep overbite, associated with an elongation of the upper and lower permanent incisors, requires the Bionator with a bite rim for the upper as well as for the lower incisors. This latter construction (see Fig. 9–9) may be feasible sometimes only after reduction of the overjet has been achieved, with the Bionator covering the lower incisors only (see Fig. 9–7). It is possible occasionally to adapt this appliance for the upper incisors, too. Often a new appliance will be necessary.

If a Bionator with lateral stabilization has been used, the lateral surfaces are freed in the final phase of the treatment to facilitate the eruption of the lateral teeth.

When the appliance is fabricated without lateral stabilization, additional stabilization should be provided against sagittal displacement of the appliance. Wire hooks placed anteriorly to the first molars (proximally) may be used. These are illustrated in Figure 9–8. Care has to be taken lest they interfere with the further eruption of the molars. Short wire spurs, penetrating into the palatal side of the interproximal space, are also possible. Most often a projection of cold-curing acrylic, added to the appliance at the proper place, will serve the purpose.

With the very quick forward movement of the lower dentition, a lower buccal segment crossbite is sometimes produced. It may correct itself during the shedding of the deciduous molars. If persistent, it will need correction, but this is not difficult. The same rapid reaction may cause overcorrection of a Class II condition, producing a Class III malocclusion. This has to be watched.

For Class III malocclusions, which make up a very small percentage of cases treated, the construction bite is taken in the most posterior position that is possible for the mandible.

The technique for making the Bionator should not present any problems. The wires have been described both in the text and in the illustrations. The acrylic portions may be hot-cured in a flask, but they are made more easily with cold-curing acrylic. The most convenient way to do this is by covering the teeth and part of the wires with base plate wax, leaving little boxes for the acrylic. The upper and lower casts are then brought together in the fixator. The wax covering of both casts is then joined by melting the wax with a heated instrument, and cold-cure acrylic is applied. The appliance is then handled as any removable wire and acrylic combination and carefully polished so as not to distort the wire assemblage.

It has been emphasized previously that case selection is important. The Bionator appears to be especially useful for the treatment of Class II, Division 1 malocclusions or Class I with Class II, Division 1 symptoms, where the lower lip cushions to the lingual of the upper incisors constantly. The classic activator, which is only worn at night, would in this case be less successful. The Bionator intercepts the perverted perioral muscle activity during the day when it is most likely to deform the dentition. The Bionator may still be effective if worn only in the afternoon and during the night, and even when inserted only at night. Correction, however, will be slower, possibly incomplete, and sometimes not achieved at all. It is therefore in the best interests of the patient that he be persuaded to wear it day and night, except at meals and during sports. A few days of accommodation are, however, necessary before wearing it during school hours.

Children are advised to retain the appliance in the mouth when giving a short reply. If they have to read or speak longer and feel hampered, they should use the tongue to push the appliance out of the mouth into the left hand, which will hold it. They will learn to accomplish this maneuver quickly. The appliance is reinserted equally rapidly. This technique is preferable to using the fingers to remove the appliance, which necessitates grasping the labial wire. Even with care, the repeated manipulation will distort the wire.

After insertion of the appliance, a return appointment should be given in a week to check for sore spots. After this, appointments at 4- to 6-week intervals are quite adequate. In the average case, a year to a year and a half would be a reasonable estimate of the time needed to achieve correction.

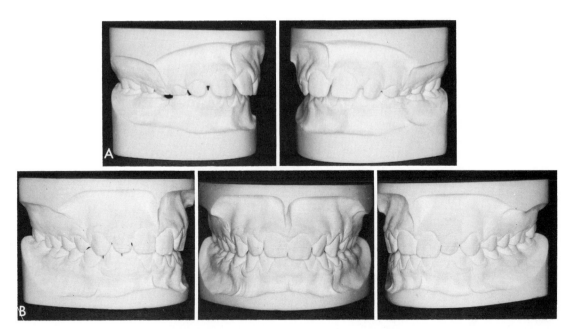

Figure 9–10. Male, age 9 years, 9½ months with a mild Class II, Division I malocclusion. The standard Bionator was used. Malocclusion characteristics were essentially eliminated after one year. Subsequent retention was followed by merely observing the changing dentition. The finished casts show the final result. (Courtesy of Professor F. Ascher.)

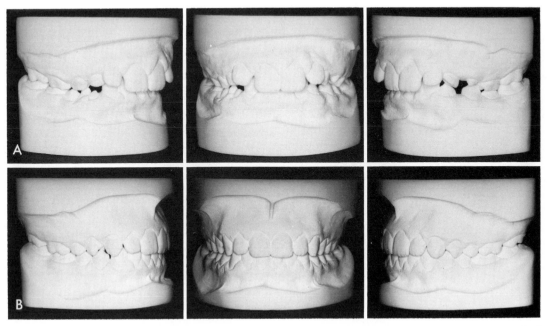

Figure 9–11. Interceptive treatment for a potential Class II, Division 2, malocclusion with a standard Bionator for a 9-year-old boy. Actual treatment was a year and a half. The finished casts are taken after eruption of the second molars.

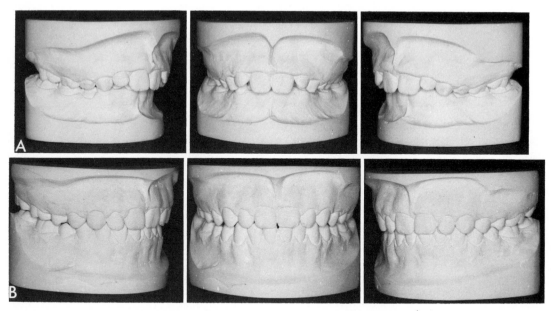

Figure 9-12. Class II, Division 2 malocclusion, treated with a standard Bionator. Beginning models are of a girl at 7 years, 4 months of age. Finished models are taken well after active treatment, with eruption of second molars. Note elimination of deep bite by the appliance.

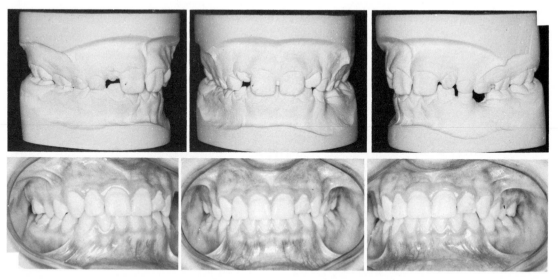

Figure 9-13. Patient, age 7½ years, with flush terminal plane, deeper than normal overbite, flaring of maxillary lateral incisors, and premature loss of a lower deciduous first molar. Post-treatment views demonstrate guiding effect of a standard Bionator, as malocclusion characteristics are eliminated.

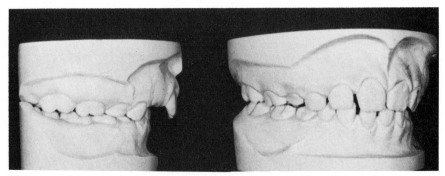

Figure 9–14. Before and after casts of seven-year-old boy, showing dramatic correction after one year of standard Bionator appliance control.

The same appliance is used for retention, worn only during the night. If correction was achieved very speedily, daytime wearing should not be abandoned at once. The orthodontist should always have in mind the problem of muscular adaptation involved in this kind of treatment. Therefore, the length of the retention period may vary from six months to one year, or even longer. The appliance is gradually worn less and less frequently at night. The patient must be instructed to wear the appliance more frequently again, if after an interval a slight muscular tension is felt when the appliance is inserted.

Relatively few problems should be encountered, even by the neophyte orthodontist. The Bionator is considered by many to be the best type of functional jaw orthopedic appliance to start with, because of its relatively simple nature. Daytime wear of the Bionator gives it an even better opportunity for correction and the prevention of subsequent relapse. Representative cases treated with the Bionator are shown in Figures 9–10 through 9–22.

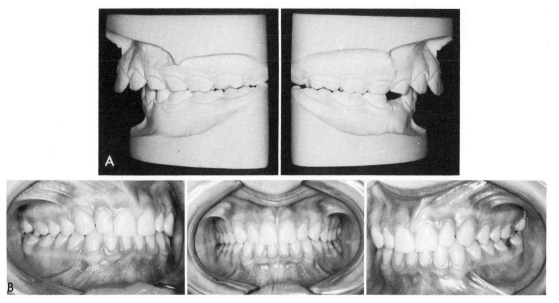

Figure 9–15. Class II, Division I malocclusion in an eight-year-old girl. Lower right deciduous canine has already been exfoliated. The intraoral views illustrate the final result of standard Bionator treatment.

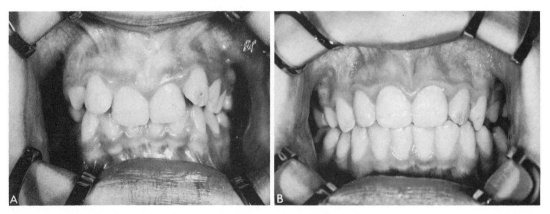

Figure 9–16. *A*, Before and (*B*) after intraoral views of a Class II, Division 2 malocclusion in an 11-year-old patient. The lingually inclined maxillary central incisors were first tipped labially with an active plate. Then a standard Bionator was worn for about a year and a half to produce the final result.

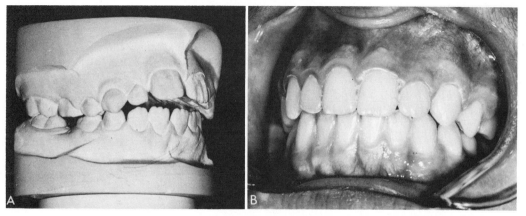

Figure 9–17. Open bite malocclusion in an eight-year-old girl. It was corrected with six months of treatment with an open bite Bionator (see Fig. 9–4). The intraoral view is taken after eruption of second molar teeth.

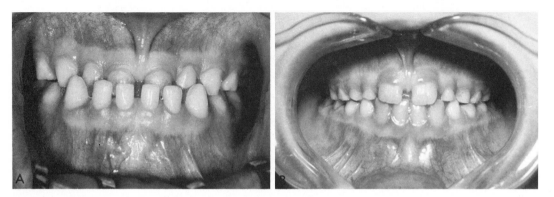

Figure 9–18. Class III malocclusion in a six-year-old girl, which was corrected by a Class III Bionator over a six-month period without any direct force application.

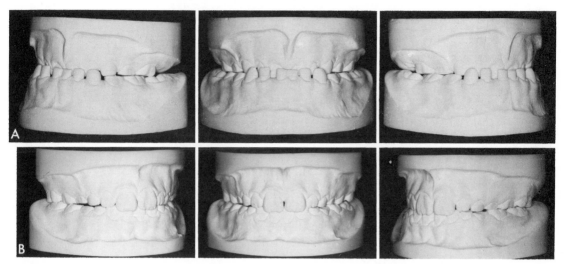

Figure 9–19. Class III malocclusion in a seven-year-old boy. The Class III Bionator was used during the shedding of the incisors. This patient, as well as the one illustrated in Figure 9–18, was not able to achieve an edge-to-edge bite prior to treatment, even with pressure against the chin, hence the likelihood of a true mandibular prognathism. Early treatment is thus highly desirable on a preventive basis. If an end-to-end bite is possible, success of therapy is almost certain. Even with the more severe problems, therapeutic success is still possible and depends on patient cooperation, the skill of the orthodontist in using the appliance, and his ability to influence both the patient and the parents.

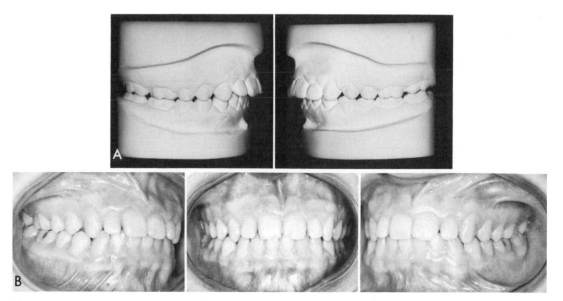

Figure 9–20. Class II type problem in the permanent dentition. Improvement of the occlusion and of esthetics was accomplished with good patient cooperation. Mixed dentition therapy is preferrable, however.

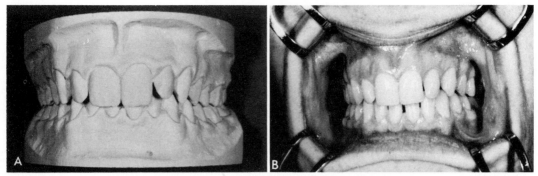

Figure 9-21. Deep bite in a 25-year-old woman, with occlusion improved and leveled by one year of treatment with a standard Bionator. The appliance was worn at night only as a retainer for an additional year. The intraoral view is four years out of active treatment. Patients often become so accustomed to wearing the appliance that they are reluctant to discontinue nocturnal wear. They complain they cannot sleep without the appliance.

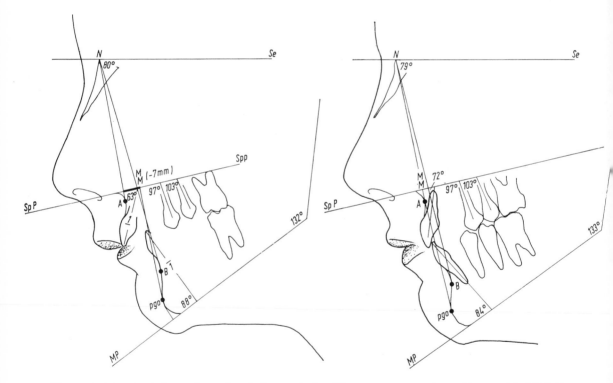

Figure 9-22. Cephalometric tracings before and after Bionator treatment in an 11-year-old girl. Evidence of condylar response and anterior mandibular development is presented. The elimination of the Class II, Division 1 malocclusion was of the magnitude of the width of a premolar. M-M, a perpendicular to the Spina-palate plane (Spp) from pogonion (pgo) is 7 mm. posterior to point A in the original tracing, but passes right through it in the final tracing. The forward positioning of point B is also indicated.

Reference

Ascher, F.: Praktische Kieferorthopädie. München, Urban & Schwarzenberg, 1968.

CHAPTER 10

Cutout or Palate-Free Activator

It is apparent that the original Andresen-Häupl activator has undergone a number of modifications by different clinicians. An additional modification has been made by Metzelder in an attempt to combine the advantages of the Bionator with some of those of the original Andresen-Häupl activator. The mandibular part is the same as the activator. In the maxillary portion, however, the acrylic covers only the palatal or lingual aspects of the buccal teeth and a small part of the adjoining gingiva. Thus, the palate remains free, making it easier for the patients to wear the appliance nearly continuously. The narrow anterior portion of the appliance is reinforced by a small screw. If expansion is not contemplated, then wires may be used for the same purpose. The labial wire is the same as that used with the activator and is made from 0.9 mm. diameter wire.

For the correction of a Class II, Division 1 malocclusion, the construction bite for the appliance is taken, if possible, in an edge-to-edge incisal relationship. Stabilization is provided by carrying the acrylic over the occlusal surfaces of some of the buccal teeth, or by a small rim of acrylic forming a little groove for the mandibular incisal margins. The technique is essentially the same as described for the Bionator and the choice between the different types of possibilities of treatment is made according to the principles established by Balters (Fig. 10–1). Some operators feel that the Bionator, with its thin mandibular portion, has a better chance of being worn continuously. They feel that the strong palatal arch will reinforce the Bionator and make it even less fragile than the palate-free modification. Metzelder's changes, however, do have some advantages. The appliance is easier to make and, what is more important, it may carry nearly all the appurtenances described for the activator. These include the jackscrew for expansion, the Petrik finger springs for moving of individual teeth (e.g., upper and lower canines after extractions), springs for the labial tipping of lower incisors, etc. It is quite appropriate to use the lateral jackscrew for opening space for one or two mandibular premolars, as described with the activator (Figs. 8–14 and 10–5). The acrylic portion above the screw must be reinforced by wires (Fig. 10–5). Even with the Andresen-Häupl activator, which is worn only at night, the lateral screw is often quite effective in reopening premolar space. This is particularly true if the loss does not exceed more than half the width of the tooth. Because of the greater amount of wearing time, success should be greater with the palate-free activator. It is important to note that the acrylic incisal coverage for mandibular incisors is necessary to prevent a procumbency developing in this area.

Figure 10–2 illustrates the appliance used for the treatment of Class II,

247

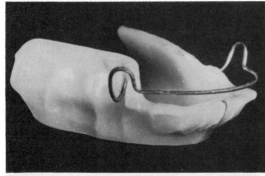

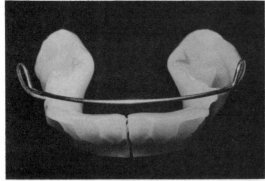

Figure 10–1. The palate-free activator for Class II, Division 1 treatment. (Courtesy of Dr. Klaus Metzelder.)

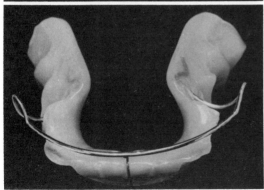

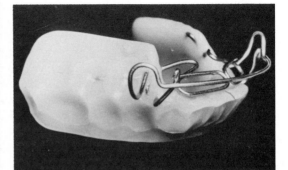

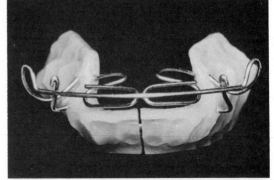

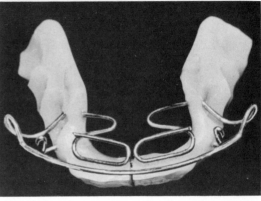

Figure 10–2. The palate-free activator for Class II, Division 2 treatment.

Figure 10-3. The palate-free activator for open bite treatment.

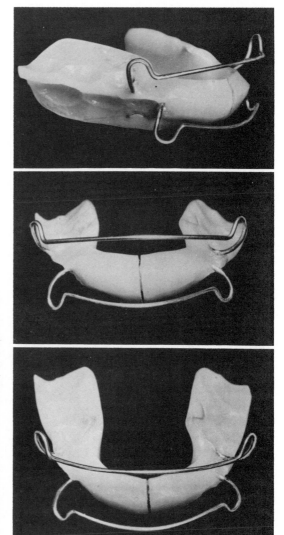

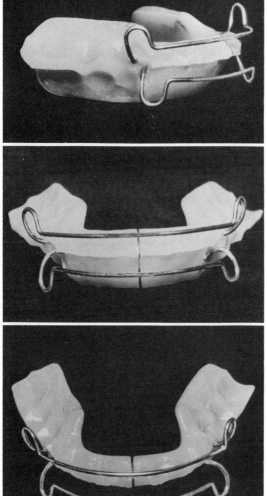

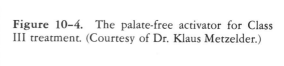

Figure 10-4. The palate-free activator for Class III treatment. (Courtesy of Dr. Klaus Metzelder.)

Division 2 malocclusions. Here, the occlusal surfaces of the buccal teeth are free of acrylic, to stimulate eruption and the leveling of the bite. Consequently, a bite rim with a groove for the incisal edge of the lower incisors may be used if desirable for stabilization. The labial tipping of the maxillary incisors may be achieved in a number of ways. The anterior portion of the acrylic may be added with a thin layer of cold-curing material, so that the teeth are contacted with appliance placement. This is then done from time to time as the teeth move labially. More effective is the use of springs. In Figure 10–2, springs designed by Bimler are shown. Smaller springs may be used for individual teeth as well and may prove more convenient. The labial wire has to be kept away from the labial surface of the incisors to permit the labial movement of these teeth. To reduce the chance of a posterior dislocation of the appliance as a result of the incisor spring adjustment, wires are placed mesial to the canines, as shown in Figure 10–2, or mesial to the first molars (Figs. 8–17*B* and 8–25).

In open bite treatment (Fig. 10–3), the acrylic again covers the occlusal surfaces of the buccal teeth. To provide the necessary space to add acrylic, the construction bite must open the interocclusal clearance 1 to 2 mm. The anterior part of the appliance is extended slightly upward, behind the maxillary

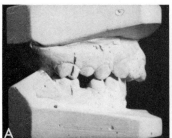
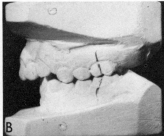
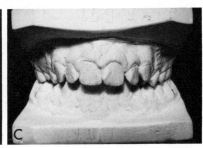

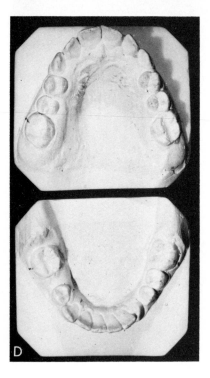

Figure 10–5.   Treatment of a Class II, Division 1 malocclusion for a 12-year-old girl, using the cutout activator as devised by Metzelder. *A, B, C,* and *D* are models of the occlusion at the time the appliance was placed.

Illustration continued on following page

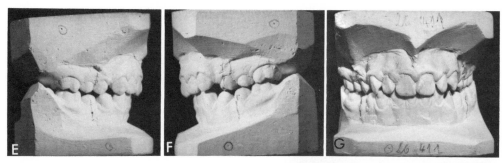

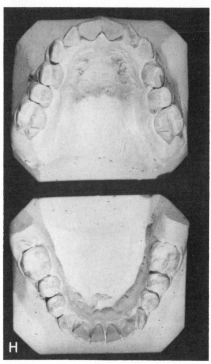

Figure 10–5 *Continued. E, F, G,* and *H* shows changes that have occurred after continuous day and night wear for a period of three and a half months. Widening of the dental arches between the maxillary first premolars is 3.4 mm.; between maxillary first molars, 4.7 mm.; between lower first premolars, 3.0 mm.; between lower first molars, 4.3 mm. The space for the lower right second premolars has been increased 3.9 mm., and the overjet was reduced 4.5 mm. *I* and *J.* The appliance that was worn during treatment. The construction bite is taken in a manner similar to that of the activator, with the mandible advanced approximately half a cusp in this case, with minimal vertical opening. The expansion screw is adjusted gradually. Note that the palatal portion has been cut out, with the maxillary flanges extending to basal bone, above the alveolar process limits.

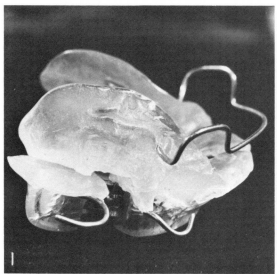

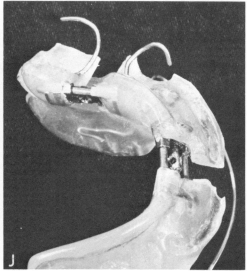

incisors. The acrylic is ground away behind the upper and lower incisor teeth to permit their elongation or eruption. An additional mandibular labial wire, as shown in Figure 10–3, may be used if desired.

The construction used for the treatment of Class III problems is illustrated in Figure 10–4. There is a broad acrylic anterior part which contacts the lingual incisal portion of the upper anteriors, which are to be moved forward by the frequent addition of cold-cure acrylic. Here again, as with Division 2 cases, a gentle "belly spring" may be used instead of adding the acrylic. Behind the lower incisors, the acrylic is ground away to permit retraction of these teeth. The maxillary labial arch must not contact the incisors, while the lower labial arch is in constant contact to enhance mandibular incisor retrusion. In the treatment of more difficult Class III malocclusions, an activator screw may be incorporated, according to Weise (Figs. 8–19 and 8–20). The increased bulk will militate against daytime wear for all but the most cooperative patients, however, and must be considered in the overall picture.

It has been mentioned frequently that patient cooperation is essential. The Metzelder modification may actually be used to enhance patient cooperation with the conventional Andresen-Häupl activator, which is worn only at night. When the appliance is frequently taken out, or pushed out with the tongue, cutting away the palate according to the Metzelder design may be efficacious in improving wear. Also, it then becomes possible to wear the appliance somewhat during the day to offset any lack of nocturnal wear. A good combination would be to wear the Metzelder modification during the day and a vestibular screen at night. This would then provide enough muscle power to effect the desired change.

The operator is encouraged to think of the broad functional implications of the appliances that have been described and to make use of a variety of appliances as the particular occasion demands. The chapter by Woodside on American modifications of the use of the activator will show additional means of enlisting muscle force for malocclusion correction.

Reference

Metzelder, K.: Ein modifizierter Aktivator und seine Anwendung. Fortschr. Kieferorthop., *29*: 273–278, 1968.

CHAPTER 11

The Elastic Open Activator

Another of the "daytime activators" is the elastic open activator designed by G. Klammt of Görlitz, GDR.* Klammt was first a disciple of Bimler, but he found Bimler's appliances too fragile for his use, and he tried to combine some of the elements with an activator which was cut out in front (Figs. 11–1 and 11–2). This modification has proved to be quite successful because of the reduced size, which has made it more agreeable for patients to wear. The modification has made it possible to insert the appliance for longer periods of time during the day. Further progress along these lines led to its present design. Although it was created quite independently, it became a parallel and similar development of the Bionator of Balters. Actually, it would appear that both constructions have mutually influenced each other, but with additional features being added to the elastic open activator as suggested by Werner.

The elastic open activator (Figs. 11–3 and 11–4) at first seems to resemble the Bionator, with no acrylic anteriorly and with more wires. There is, however, a substantial difference. The Bionator, although freely movable in the oral cavity, is carefully stabilized on posterior occlusal surfaces or the lower incisors, as the occasion demands. The Elastic Open Activator (EOA) almost completely

---

*This chapter is based on personal communication from Dr. G. Klammt, who also furnished all the illustrations except Figures 11–1 and 11–2. The authors are very grateful for his assistance.

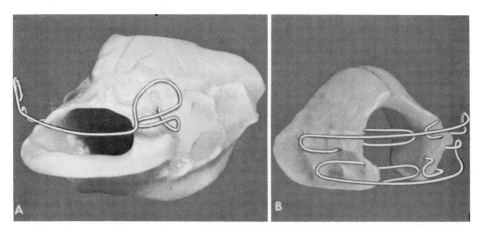

Figure 11-1. The open activator according to Klammt. *A,* Open in the upper anterior sector only; *B,* the entire front area open; labial bow and lingual loops to induce necessary movements of the anterior teeth in a given case; expansion screw in the palatal part. (From Schwarz, A. M., and Gratzinger, M.: Removable Orthodontic Appliances. Philadelphia, W. B. Saunders Company, 1966.)

253

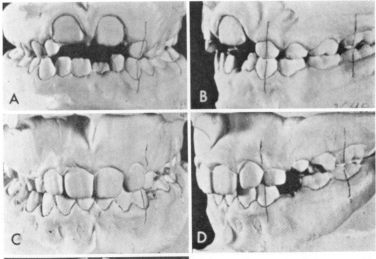

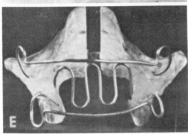

Figure 11-2. Alveolar open bite caused by sucking habit, combined with retroclusion, corrected with the activator. *A* and *B*, Cast of an 8-year-old girl before treatment; *C* and *D*, after treatment that lasted two years. *E*, The activator used, seen from the front. Note the open front part (according to Klammt; see Fig. 11–1) to permit the vertical growth of the incisors. The tongue is prevented from occupying the space between the incisal edges by a looped wire shield. From time to time the loops of the 0.8 mm. wire were opened a little to relieve the resistance against the expansion screw. (From Schwarz, A. M., and Gratzinger, M.: Removable Orthodontic Appliances. Philadelphia, W. B. Saunders Company, 1966.)

lacks such stabilization, and thus its vertical mobility in the mouth is unimpeded. There are two types of EOA. One type lacks any acrylic projections for the interproximal spaces, and it has a flat surface contacting the lingual surface of the buccal teeth (Fig. 11–3). The other type has acrylic projections contiguous to the entire lingual aspect of the teeth in the buccal segments (Fig. 11–4). In both types, the acrylic extends over a small part of the adjoining gingiva. The sagittal mobility is greater in the first type. If it is desirable during the course of treatment, the acrylic surface may easily be altered by grinding or by the addition of cold-cure acrylic.

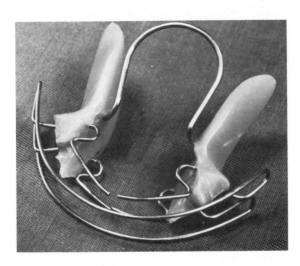

Figure 11-3. The standard type EOA (elastic open activator – Klammt) with flat acrylic parts. For further details see text.

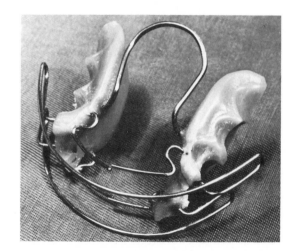

Figure 11-4. The standard type EOA (elastic open activator — Klammt) with contiguous acrylic parts (see text).

All activator devices are situated relatively loosely in the oral cavity, but none to such a degree as the EOA. After a short period of adjustment, the wearing of this appliance should not impede the speech, but its mobility seems to engage the tongue permanently. Because of the complete lack of appliance stabilization, the tongue has a close interaction with the appliance. Klammt notes that the appliance will react to most of the tongue movements, and so it must "come to terms" with the tongue. In other words, either the tongue or the appliance must adapt, with a good possibility that it is both.* In this manner, a great number of impulses are transmitted to the teeth, serving as the basis for transformative changes. Different designs of the appliance will make these impulses selective and capable of correcting a variety of malocclusions.

THE STANDARD EOA

The standard appliance consists of the bilateral acrylic parts, an upper and lower labial wire, a palatal arch, and guiding wires for the upper and lower incisors. These wires will have different designs, depending on the treatment objectives. The acrylic parts extend from the canine posteriorly to the point just behind the first or the second permanent molar, if it is present. The acrylic is quite thin in order to leave the largest possible space for the tongue. Stabilization of the acrylic portion is accomplished by means of contact with the lingual surfaces of the maxillary and mandibular canines.

The upper and lower labial wires emerge from the acrylic between the canine and first premolar. They must be constructed so as not to impede lateral expansion or vertical growth or eruption of any tooth. These wires proceed distally to the second premolar, then form a round bend and return to the anterior portion. The labial portion touches the incisors and proceeds to the other side, being adapted in an identical manner or mirror image. It is useful to put a small piece of plastic tubing over the wires where they emerge from

---

*The original concepts of Andresen and Häupl, stating that the activator is effective by virtue of the reflexly stimulated muscle contractions holding it, have not been accepted by many orthodontists. Reliable investigation of this point still must be done. It is possible that the mode of action of the EOA may be more in accordance with this postulated effect than the activator itself.

the acrylic. This makes subsequent adaptation easier and helps prevent breakage (as suggested by John Heath).

The palatal arch originates from the acrylic at the height of the upper first premolar. Rising steeply, it is soon bent at a right angle and formed into an oval shape, the most posterior part on a line that joins the distal surfaces of the first permanent molars. Klammt prefers that all parts of the arch be kept as close to the palatal surface as possible, leaving only sufficient distance to prevent it from impinging on the mucosa. If an adjustment is to be placed in the palatal arch to maintain expansion already achieved, this is done by flattening the posterior end of the loop with broad, flat pliers. If necessary, additional adjustments may be made at the bends opposite the premolars.

The guiding wires are placed in close approximation to the lingual aspects of the upper and lower incisors. The small bends visible in Figures 11–3 and 11–4 permit necessary adjustments. All wires are of 0.9 mm. diameter, with the palatal arch being 1.2 mm. in thickness. The construction bite is taken in the same manner as for the Bionator, with an edge-to-edge position of the incisors.

Figure 11–5 shows the wires held in place by sticky wax. The labial wires that cross the occlusion have small pieces of tubing. For the appliance modification with the acrylic in contact with the teeth, additional base plate wax may be used to limit the penetration of the acrylic so that it does not go beyond the

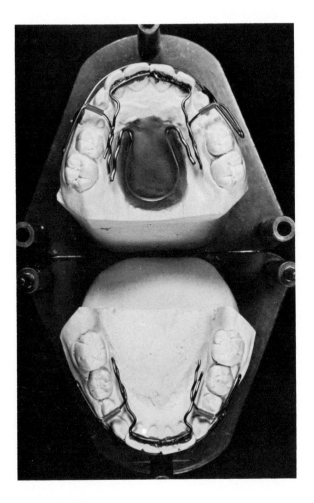

Figure 11–5. The standard type EOA in the articulator with wires kept in place by sticky wax before the application of the acrylic. Note the little pieces of tubing on the wires crossing the occlusion. For the appliance with contiguous acrylic, some more wax may be used to limit the penetration of the acrylic beyond the lingual cusps of the lateral teeth. For the flat acrylic surface, the interdental spaces and the interocclusal clearance are filled with wax. In both types, acrylic has access to the lingual aspects of upper and lower canines.

lingual cusps of the posterior teeth. For the appliance with the flat acrylic surface, the interdental spaces, as well as the interocclusal clearance area, are filled with wax. For both types, however, the acrylic has access to the lingual aspects of the upper and lower canines which are used to stabilize the appliance.

MODE OF ACTION OF THE EOA

Modifications and Treatment of Crowding Conditions

Figure 11–6 shows a drawing of the standard appliance with some of the modifications. If, for example, the second deciduous molar has been lost prematurely, its space is maintained by an extension of the contiguous acrylic (Fig. 11–6, *left*). With the flat acrylic surface, a double wire must be placed anterior to the maxillary first molar. Wires are added mesial to the first molar and distal to the first deciduous molar after the loss of the lower second deciduous molar (Fig. 11–6, *right*). The maxillary guiding wires are fabricated as indicated already. The rotation of the crowded incisors may be partly eliminated with the expansion of the dental arch. The mandibular guiding wires are so fabricated that they stimulate the lateral incisors to move with them when the dental arch is expanded (Fig. 11–6).

The standard appliance with the flat acrylic is used for expansion in Class I and for most Class II, Division 1 malocclusions. Treatment may also be undertaken during the shedding of the deciduous molars when active plates are not used. As with other functional jaw orthopedic appliances, completion of the

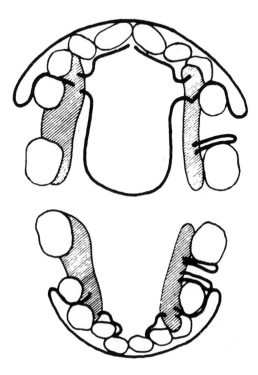

Figure 11–6. The standard appliance with some modifications. The mandibular guiding wires are fashioned so as to engage the lateral incisors when the arch is expanded. Different ways of space maintenance are shown. Contiguous acrylic is extended into the space (left). With flat acrylic flanges, a double wire prevents the upper first molar from drifting mesially after the loss of the second deciduous molars. An identical situation in the lower jaw requires a double wire behind the first deciduous molar too.

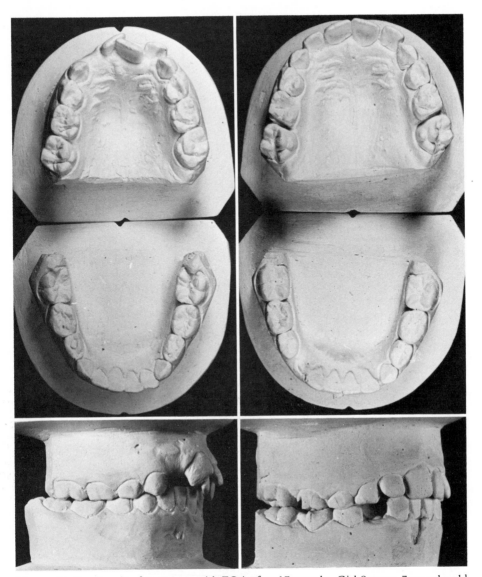

Figure 11-7. Result of treatment with EOA after 17 months. Girl 8 years, 7 months old at the beginning of treatment of a Class II, Division 1 malocclusion. Maxillary width increased 4 mm. and length 3 mm. It was necessary to grind grooves into the upper second deciduous molars for the placement of stabilizing wires (see Fig. 11–11*A*) to make the forward movement of the anterior teeth possible. To relieve the crowding of the upper central incisors, the upper labial wire, as shown in Figure 11–8, was used. For the treatment of crowding, vertical stabilization will generally be provided by the acrylic on the canines. Flat acrylic surfaces on the flanges are preferred, but contiguous acrylic is possible too.

treatment objectives with the use of active plates in the permanent dentition may also be necessary at times. This is not to be considered a limitation of the appliance but rather a therapeutic decision to best achieve the treatment objectives. The EOA may also be used in the presence of minimal overbite, in preference to an active plate that might create an open bite through conventional expansion procedures.

Figure 11–7 illustrates a case treated with the EOA. To achieve the increase in the maxillary arch length sagittally, stabilization was necessary. This

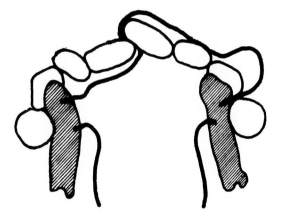

Figure 11-8. Maxillary labial and guiding wire as used for treatment of crowding. On one side the guiding wire is omitted, on the other the labial arch. Generally a double wire engages the crowded incisor.

was provided by wires lodged in grooves ground into the distal parts of the second deciduous molars (see Fig. 11–11*A*). To relieve the crowding of the maxillary central incisors, half of the maxillary labial wire was omitted, with the other half being used to engage the incisor. On this side, the guiding wire was used only for the opposite side (Fig. 11–8). With appropriate adjustments of the palatal arch and the labial wires, the appliance is thus adapted to follow the widening of the dental arches, but it should not be allowed to contact and press against the teeth. If the mobility of the appliance is reduced, it becomes ineffective and inconvenient to the patient.

Treatment of Class II, Division 1 Malocclusion

As with all functional jaw orthopedic appliances, it is the Class II, Division 1 malocclusion or the Class I with Class II symptoms that is most satisfactorily treated. Here, as with the Bionator, the appliance is especially successful when the condition has been aggravated by a sucking or a lip habit, which retrudes the

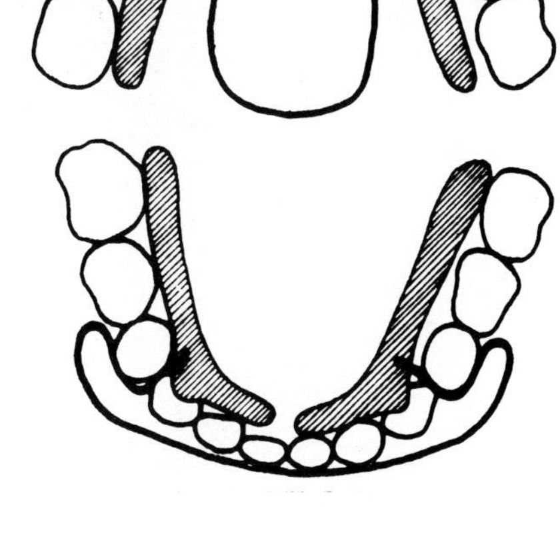

Figure 11-9. The EOA for the treatment of Class II, Division 1 cases. For detailed description see text.

lower incisors. The EOA with the flat acrylic surface is used. Maxillary guiding wires are not necessary and are thus omitted. They may be used temporarily when incisor crowding is present; in this instance, they engage the lateral incisors. As treatment progresses, they are removed or refashioned. If labial tipping of the mandibular incisors is not desirable, the mandibular portion of the acrylic is extended onto the anterior surface (Fig. 11–9). The acrylic should have minimal contact with the incisors, however, and then only near the gingival margin. As with the Fränkel appliance, which is discussed later, the patient may have difficulty accommodating all at once to the protruded position of the mandible, and then sore spots will appear on the gingival point of contact. If these spots cannot be eliminated quickly by grinding the acrylic, the protruded position has to be stabilized. Endothermic acrylic is added to the extension, securing its seat on the lower incisors and easing the mandible in its forward

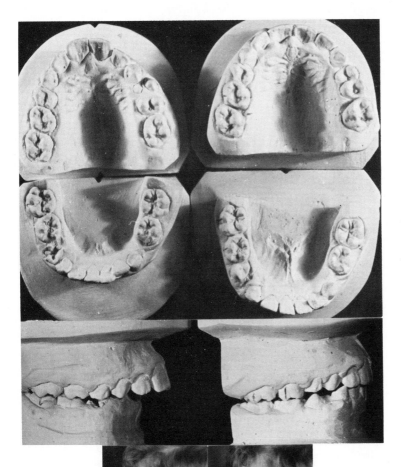

Figure 11–10. Boy aged 9 years at the beginning of treatment of Class II, Division 1 malocclusion with 11 mm. overjet. Progress after four months of treatment is shown, with maxillary arch widened 5 mm., canines in neutral occlusion, and overjet corrected. The distal inclination of 4 is retaining 6 in a distal relationship. Photographs show changes achieved by the four months' treatment.

position. Experience has shown that even with an overjet as large as 10 mm., it is usually possible to get the incisors into an edge-to-edge bite. Klammt indicates that he has never had any temporomandibular joint problems, even after such extensive forward positioning of the mandible. In the event that an edge-to-edge bite cannot be achieved, the mandible is brought into an intermediate position. During the progress of treatment, the appliance may then be modified to permit an edge-to-edge bite. It is preferable, however, to make a new appliance for this purpose.

As shown by the dotted line (Fig. 11-9), where the labial wire engages the upper central incisors, the wire may exert very slight pressure on the incisors. However, this should not be great enough to unseat the appliance. Figure 11-10 shows a case treated with EOA.

Treatment of Class II, Division 2 Malocclusion

The treatment of a Class II, Division 2 malocclusion, or *Deckbiss*, will generally require the labial tipping of the upper central incisors or possibly all incisors. Anchorage must be provided to prevent the appliance from being dislocated posteriorly. If the second deciduous molar is present, a groove is cut into the molar as seen on the cast shown in Figure 11-7. From the flat acrylic, a wire is placed in the groove (Fig. 11-11). In the presence of the permanent premolars, the acrylic will be contiguous, and a short piece of wire, placed just

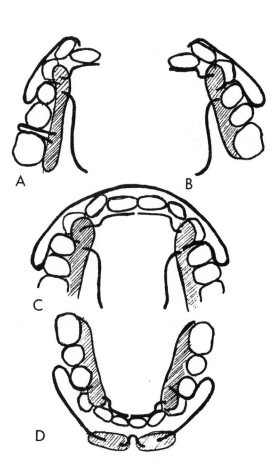

Figure 11-11. Drawings showing different arrangements for Class II, Division 2 treatment. *A,* For severe crowding in the presence of deciduous molars. Flat acrylic and stabilizing wire in a groove ground into the second deciduous molars. *B,* Severe crowding, premolars erupted; contiguous acrylic. *C,* Crowding not severe, standard type arrangement, contiguous acrylic. *D,* mandibular labial wire carrying lip pads. For further details see text.

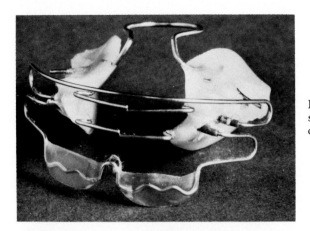

Figure 11-12. Class II, Division 2 appliance showing stabilizing wires omitted in the drawing of Figure 11–11*B*.

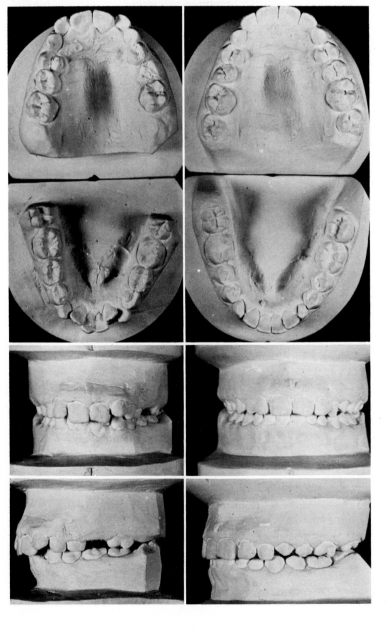

Figure 11-13. Girl 8 years, 8 months at the beginning of treatment. Second casts after seven months. Maxillary and mandibular arch widened 5 mm., crowding relieved, distal occlusion corrected.

mesial to the first molar, should be added to improve the stability of the appliance (Fig. 11–11). The maxillary labial wire is divided to engage the lateral incisors (Fig. 11–11*A* and *B*). If crowding is not severe, the usual labial wire construction will suffice (Fig. 11–11*C*). The mandibular labial wire carries lip pads, located as deep in the sulcus as possible. This is similar to the Fränkel function corrector (Function Regulator) construction. These lip pads are kept at a 1 mm. distance from the gingiva. Usually, no scraping of the model is necessary. But accurate impressions of this area are absolutely essential. The pads are used to counteract the pressure of the lower lip. Figure 11–12 shows the appliance with the stabilizing wire placed anterior to the first molars, which are not in the drawing of Figure 11–11. Figure 11–13 again shows a case that has been treated with the EOA appliance of Klammt.

Treatment of Class III Malocclusions and Anterior Crossbite

The design of the appliance here is with the acrylic contiguous to the buccal segment teeth.

The palatal arch is open to the distal, as shown with the Bionator, for Class III therapy. The maxillary labial wire carries lip pads similar to those of the Fränkel appliance. The mandibular lingual guidewires are kept a slight distance from the incisors and are formed without bends, since they are not to be activated. The maxillary guidewires may be covered with tubing as they emerge from the acrylic. They engage the maxillary incisors (Figs. 11–14 and 11–15). The construction bite is taken in an edge-to-edge bite of the incisors or in the most retruded mandibular position approaching it. It is advantageous to actually alter the construction bite by moving the maxillary casts approximately 1 mm. forward in the laboratory, when the models are mounted on the articulator. This stimulates the anteroposterior correction. Figure 11–16 illustrates a treated case.

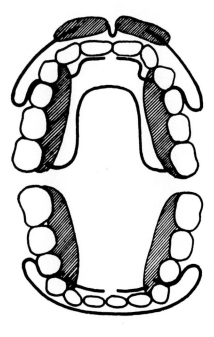

Figure 11–14. Schematic Class III appliance.

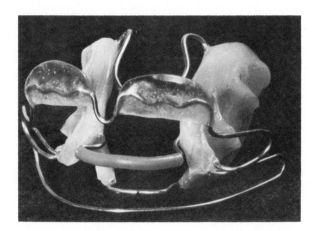

Figure 11–15. Class II appliance. For details see text.

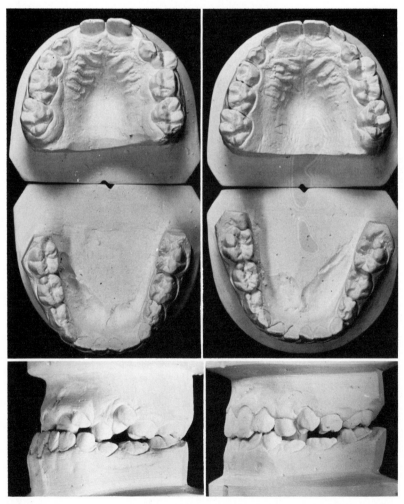

Figure 11–16. Treatment of Class III condition. Boy 8 years, 6 months; second casts after seven months. Slight widening and lengthening of maxillary arch. Inverted overbite corrected. Class III condition improved. ⌊4 nearly corrected.

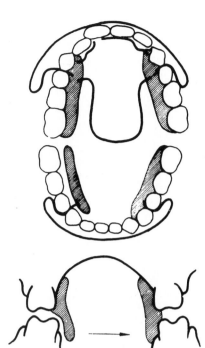

Figure 11-17. EOA for the treatment of crossbite. Construction bite is taken with a slight overcorrection of midline.

Treatment of Unilateral Crossbite

The appliance is constructed according to the diagram in Figure 11-17. The acrylic closely follows the teeth, except in the mandibular part that approximates the teeth in crossbite. It is advantageous to make the construction bite with a slight overcorrection of the midline. This maneuver helps to achieve the treatment result more quickly. Figure 11-18 illustrates a treated case.

Treatment of Open Bite

In the treatment of open bite malocclusions caused by abnormal perioral habits, the appliance is fabricated with acrylic contiguous to the teeth. The construction bite is taken with the buccal segments in contact. If there is a distoclusion, this may be simultaneously corrected by moving the mandible slightly forward. Guidewires are formed as illustrated in Figures 11-19 and 11-20. The vertical position of the wires is not discernible from the drawing. The wires originate from the maxillary part of the acrylic and are bilateral in order not to lessen the elasticity of the appliance. They keep the tongue away from the incisors and the open bite aperture. The wires should not contact the incisors, as this would be an obstacle to eruption and open bite closure. The condition of crowding, as well as the distoclusion already mentioned, may be corrected simultaneously with open bite treatment. A treated case is shown in Figure 11-21.

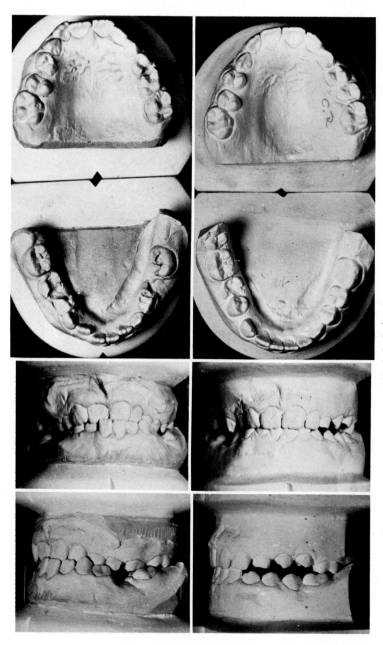

Figure 11-18. Treatment of crossbite. Girl 9 years, 1 month old. Second casts after 17 months of treatment. Maxillary arch widened 3 mm., lengthened 2.5 mm. Anterior and lateral crossbite corrected.

Treatment of Extraction Cases

The EOA is also useful in the treatment of extraction cases. The flat acrylic surface permits the closure of spaces created by the extraction, since there is no interference in the interproximal areas. This may be done in conjunction with the elimination of irregularities and Class II malocclusion characteristics. After the extraction of the first premolar, a wire spur may be necessary to retain the second premolar from moving mesially. This is to protect the canine space. In the event of an extraction of a mandibular first molar, for example, a wire spur may be added behind the second premolar to prevent it from tipping distally.

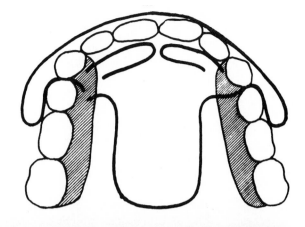

Figure 11-19. Drawing of EOA for treatment of open bite due to habits. The acrylic is contiguous. The vertical position of the guiding wires (see Fig. 11–20) is not discernible from the drawing. These wires emerge from the maxillary part of the acrylic and must not contact the incisors.

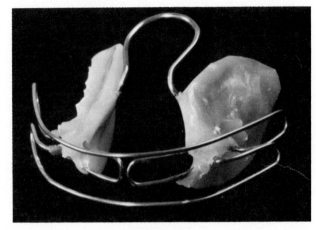

Figure 11-20. The EOA for the treatment of open bite due to habits. Vertical guide wires control tongue thrust.

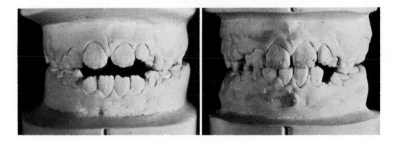

Figure 11-21. Treatment of open bite. Boy aged 8 years, 6 months. Second casts after eight months.

As with other removable appliances, common sense and ingenuity play a significant role.

Summary

The description of the elastic open activator has been kept to a minimum to avoid repetition. The principles are quite similar to those described for the Bionator. Indeed, it is wise for an operator to gain some experience first with the Bionator before turning to the EOA. However, the differences between the two appliances should again be emphasized. The Bionator is stabilized on selected occlusal surfaces. The EOA, even with the acrylic in contact with the lingual interproximal areas, has all the occlusal surfaces ground away so that there is no barrier to further eruption of the teeth in the buccal segments. The only occlusal stabilization is on the lingual surfaces of the upper and lower canines. In a case of a deep bite, even this area may be ground away to speed up the leveling of the bite, leaving it to the edge-to-edge construction bite for the incisors to sustain the tooth insertion and guidance with the appliance. As with other functional jaw orthopedic appliances, however, care must be taken to insure that stress on the incisors is vertical, not horizontal. As Björk has shown, when horizontal strain is created with the activator, there is a labial tipping or excessive procumbency of the mandibular incisors which may be undesirable. Routine cephalograms taken during therapy should be made to check progress and intercept any undesirable sequelae of this type. Such a record is imperative for all functional appliances, not only to intercept undesirable results but to check growth increments, direction, and tissue response.

Some operators have preferred to allow the lingual acrylic to contact the interproximal areas where Klammt has recommended a flat surface and only point contact. The claim is made that this permits better stabilization in some cases and allows for more precise adjustment for premolars. This is a personal preference, however. But close adaptation of the acrylic into the proximal areas is absolutely essential for Class III malocclusions, open bite cases, crossbite, and some Class II, Division 2 malocclusions.

It has been mentioned before, and is stressed again, that the operator should not be reluctant to make a new appliance when progress of treatment, growth, manipulation, etc., have made the current appliance fit poorly. It is better to fabricate a new appliance when modification cannot assure optimal fit. A poorly fitting appliance not only may interfere with correction but will often seriously deteriorate the level of patient cooperation. It is important to remember that the free mobility of the EOA is an important precondition for its effect. No adjustment of the appliance should exert positive pressure against the teeth. The appliance should be worn at all times except at meals, perhaps during contact sports, and for longer speeches at school.

After two weeks there should be no speech impediment; if there is, the operator may reasonably doubt that the patient has really followed the instructions and worn the appliance as prescribed. There is an adjustment period when the appliance is placed, however. It may be worn for three to four hours during the day and at night, gradually increasing the daytime wear over the next two to three weeks. Concerted motivational input is necessary for both the orthodontist and the parents. The free movement of the appliance makes it somewhat more difficult to become adjusted to it during the early stages of wear. Thus, if patient selection and psychological preparation are designed according to the precepts outlined above, gratifying results should be obtained in the great majority of cases.

CHAPTER 12

The Activator

DONALD G. WOODSIDE

As originally conceived by Andresen,[1] the activator was intended to correct malocclusion solely through the action of the muscles of mastication. Although its exact mode of action has not been clearly established, there is a sufficient body of clinical research and experience to present a rational approach to orthodontic treatment with the activator. This chapter will outline the possibilities and limitations of activator treatment, the clinical management of Class II and Class III malocclusions with the appliance, and the construction of the activator.

The activator or Andresen appliance (Fig. 12–1) and related appliances such as the Bimler (Fig. 12–2) and Fränkel appliances (Fig. 12–3) are removable functional orthodontic appliances, the first of which was the original monobloc designed by the French dentist, Robin, in 1902.[2-5] While each of these "functional appliances" employs the activation of neuromuscular reflexes to guide into more acceptable relationships the erupting teeth of children with malocclusion, each system emphasizes particular aspects of the neuromuscular physiology of the stomatognathic system which its originator considered impor-

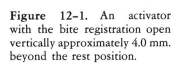

Figure 12–1. An activator with the bite registration open vertically approximately 4.0 mm. beyond the rest position.

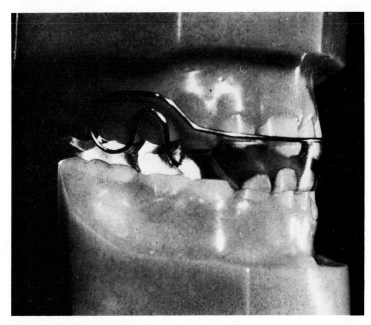

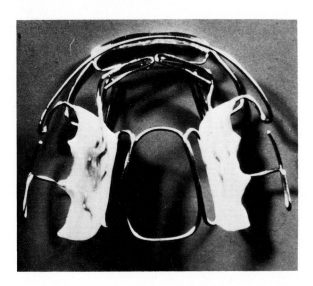

Figure 12-2. The Bimler appliance. This appliance may be described as a wire activator with accessory functions. One distinct advantage of this appliance is that it may be worn during the day as well as at night while sleeping.

tant. These time-tested and ingenious methods of orthodontic treatment provide useful adjuncts to the practitioner's orthodontic techniques. However, judged by the occlusal and facial esthetic standards currently demanded in North American orthodontics, the method used alone has serious limitations. The same statement, however, might be made about that other useful orthodontic adjunct, the headgear, which also cannot perform detailed tooth positioning by itself. The reader is therefore asked to forgo consideration of detailed tooth positioning and consider the gross occlusal and the facial changes which can be achieved by the "functional" appliances, which admittedly cannot

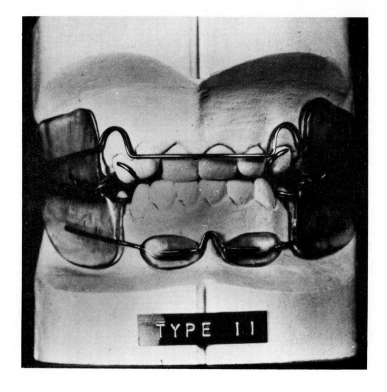

Figure 12-3. A typical Fränkel appliance for the correction of Class II, Division 2 malocclusion. The bite registration used in this appliance places the mandible downward and forward in relation to the maxilla. The mandibular labial portion of the appliance is used as a labial muscle appliance while the buccal acrylic portions act as an oral screen. This appliance may be worn during the day as well as at night while sleeping.

perform detailed tooth positioning. The reader might then consider how an ingenious system of European orthodontics might be adopted to assist in the attainment of occlusal and facial esthetic standards currently demanded in North America.

This chapter will discuss the activator only, and, after gaining a basic understanding of this appliance, the interested practitioner can proceed to study the variations in associated functional appliances (see Chapters 13 to 15).

The method is particularly useful in pre-orthodontic interception of malocclusion. It is also useful in the management of severely mutilated dentitions when the practitioner wishes to apply therapeutic procedures at the correct interval in the patient's growth cycle, but at a time when it may not be mechanically feasible to commence treatment by routine multibanded procedures, due to the premature loss of multiple teeth in the buccal segments. In these instances, the orthodontist routinely follows a period of activator treatment with a period of multibanded therapy to achieve a detailed alignment. It will be instructive to look at possibilities and limitations of activator treatment prior to proceeding to a detailed discussion of the treatment method.

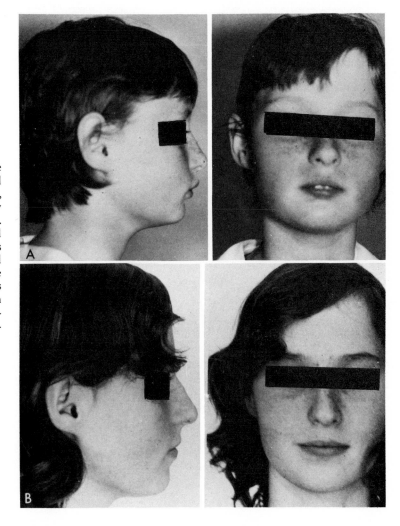

Figure 12-4. The soft tissue profile changes were obtained in the correction of a Class II, Division 1 malocclusion solely through the use of an activator. These pictures were selected to illustrate the potentialities and limitations of the method with respect to facial profile changes. While the patient is still moderately protrusive in the lip area following treatment, considerable improvement has been obtained.

POSSIBILITIES AND LIMITATIONS OF ACTIVATOR TREATMENT

Facial Changes

Figures 12–4 and 12–5 illustrate the soft tissue profile changes achieved through the use of the activator alone and the activator combined with premolar extractions followed by multibanded orthodontic therapy. As the figures illustrate, the method can assist in achieving marked facial changes through both nonextraction and extraction orthodontic therapy (see also Chapter 16).

Occlusal Changes

Figure 12–6 shows the occlusal changes achieved during a typical activator treatment and illustrates that the method can be used to achieve major mesiodistal and vertical changes. Although arch form can be restored, the ap-

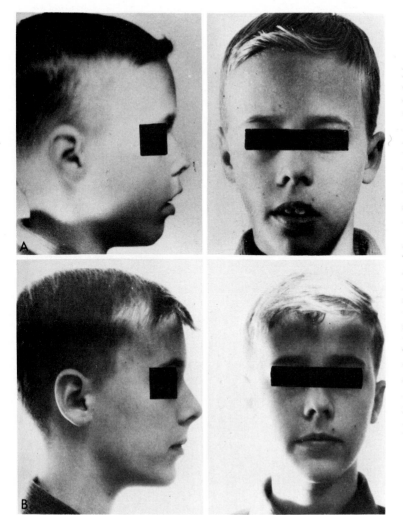

Figure 12–5. The profile changes obtained in a two-stage orthodontic treatment for a Class II, Division 1 malocclusion. The initial stage of treatment consisted of activator therapy in conjunction with serial extractions leading to the removal of four first bicuspid teeth. An initial reduction of apical base dysplasia and correction of the Class II, Division 1 malocclusion was obtained during this phase of treatment. The second phase of treatment consisted of a short period of multibanded edgewise mechanotherapy to achieve detailed alignment of the teeth and a second moderate reduction in apical base dysplasia. The activator is very useful when it is used in the mixed dentition to achieve an initial reduction in apical base dysplasia followed by a second reduction as the patient enters the prepubertal acceleration in facial growth.

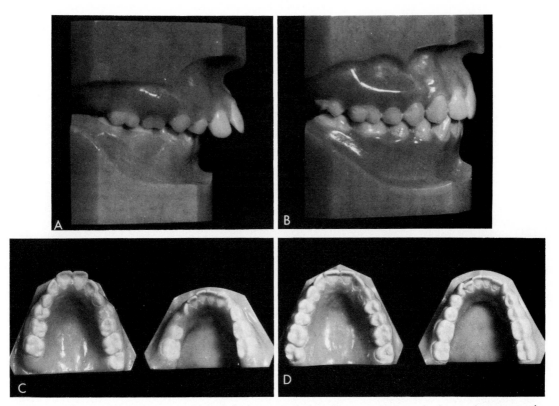

Figure 12-6. Occlusal changes achieved during a typical activator treatment. Activator therapy can be used to achieve major mesiodistal and vertical changes. Although arch form can be restored, the appliance cannot be used by itself to correct crowding.

pliance cannot correct crowding and does not perform detailed tooth positioning.

Skeletal Dysplasia Correction and Differential Control of Tooth Eruption

Cephalometric analysis of the results of treatment (Fig. 12-7) illustrates that the method can be used to achieve moderate reductions in skeletal dysplasia between the maxilla and the mandible but will not routinely reduce mandibular incisor protraction. Indeed, unless the clinician exercises considerable care, the mandibular incisors may move labially into an abnormal position relative to the lips and subsequently show a tendency to relapse. The tracings also show that it is possible to exert differential control over the eruption of teeth in the maxillary and mandibular buccal segments. By this means the maxillary buccal teeth may be permitted minimal eruption while the mandibular buccal teeth are allowed to erupt vertically in harmony with the vertical component of mandibular growth. The usefulness of this inhibition of maxillary buccal segment eruption will be discussed later under the heading "Functional Occlusal Plane."

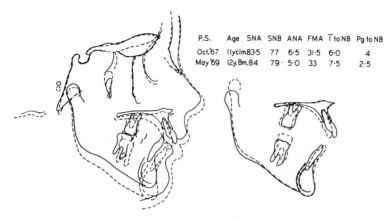

P.S.	Age	SNA	SNB	ANA	FMA	T̄ to NB	Pg to NB
Oct.'67	11yc1m	83·5	·77	6·5	31·5	6·0	4
May '69	12y.8m.	84	79·	5·0	33	7·5	2·5

Figure 12–7. The changes which took place during a typical Class II, Division 1 treatment. The tracings on the left have been superimposed on comparatively non-changing structures in the anterior cranial base. This tracing illustrates that the chin point descended in a much more vertical fashion than is usually seen with normal growth changes. In addition, the anterior nasal spine did not have a horizontal component of growth as is usual. This change at the anterior nasal spine would be considered desirable in the management of a Class II, Division 1 malocclusion while the change at the chin would be considered undesirable. The change at the chin is probably due to overeruption of the lower buccal segments which was accomplished with the activator. The tracings on the right illustrate the tooth movements accomplished in the maxilla and in the mandible separately. It can be seen that eruption of the maxillary buccal segment was inhibited while the maxillary teeth were tipped distally a small amount. The mandibular tracings show that the mandibular incisor teeth were displaced labially, and such loss of anchorage is considered undesirable. The mandibular tracings also illustrate the eruption in mandibular buccal segments which was permitted and is considered desirable provided this eruption is in harmony with the vertical component of mandibular growth.

Changing the Direction of Mandibular Growth

The activator can be used to alter mandibular growth directions to more vertical directions (Fig. 12–8). This measure assists in the conservative reduction of moderate mandibular prognathisms by a *vertical* manipulation of the jaws and dentition rather than by the conventional anteroposterior approach to the correction of Class III malocclusions in which the maxillary teeth are moved mesially and the mandibular teeth distally. This same vertical approach may be used to manage incisor crossbites with superimposed mesial functional displacement of the mandible.

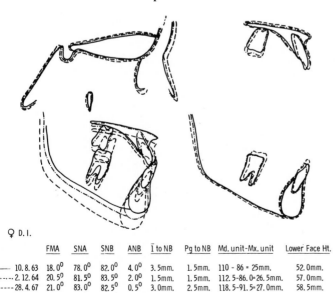

♀ D.I.

	FMA	SNA	SNB	ANB	Ī to NB	Pg to NB	Md. unit-Mx. unit	Lower Face Ht.
——	10.8.63	18.0°	78.0°	82.0°	4.0°	3.5mm.	1.5mm.	110 - 86 = 25mm.	52.0mm.
-----	2.12.64	20.5°	81.5°	83.5°	2.0°	1.5mm.	1.5mm.	112.5-86. 0=26.5mm.	57.0mm.
-----	28.4.67	21.0°	83.0°	82.5°	0.5°	3.0mm.	2.5mm.	118.5-91.5=27.0mm.	58.5mm.

Figure 12–8. The growth changes and tooth movements accomplished in the correction of a Class III malocclusion utilizing the activator. The tracings on the left illustrate that the activator may be used to alter mandibular growth directions to more vertical directions and thus assist in the conservative reduction of Class III malocclusions. This reduction is achieved by a vertical manipulation of the jaws and the dentition rather than by the conventional anteroposterior approach to the correction of Class III malocclusions in which the maxillary teeth are moved mesially and the mandibular teeth distally. The treatment consisted of two intervals of activator therapy. The tracings of the maxilla and the mandible on the right illustrate that the mandibular buccal segments were not permitted to erupt during the first period of activator therapy, while the maxillary buccal segments were allowed to erupt.

Intrusion of Teeth

While the activator is effective in the correction of overbite, it does not routinely achieve such correction through the intrusion of incisor teeth, but rather by permitting the eruption of teeth in the buccal segments. The activator thus stimulates active intrusion of incisor teeth by inhibiting their normal eruption. Because the teeth in the buccal segments are permitted to follow their normal eruption paths while the incisor teeth are not permitted to erupt, the effect of intrusion is achieved without actually intruding the incisor teeth.

Vertical Dimension

Figure 12–9 illustrates the soft tissue profile changes achieved during a 16-month treatment period in a patient who required no extractions and no space closures. The improvement in his facial contour was associated with marked increase in lower face height. This change illustrates a basic concept in activator therapy, namely, that the mesiodistal correction of Class II malocclusion is achieved through an apparent vertical manipulation of the dentition.[6,7] This vertical manipulation occurs most readily in those patients who have a vertical growth component accompanying the normal growth expressed at the chin. Indeed, the clinician may inadvertently increase the lower face height through careless manipulation of the activator (Fig. 12–7) by permitting the buccal teeth to erupt farther vertically than the vertical growth expressed in the mandible. Thus, excess lower face height at the beginning of treatment provides a definite contraindication to Class II activator treatment owing to the tendency for such treatment to inadvertently increase lower face height to levels that might result in a further deterioration in facial esthetics. Obviously, as Hotz has mentioned, individuals who have excess freeway space and reduced lower face

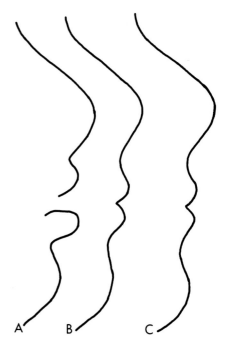

Figure 12–9. The soft tissue profile changes achieved during a 16-month activator treatment in a patient who required no extractions and no space closure. The improvement in the patient's facial contour was associated with an increase in lower face height. This change illustrates a basic concept in activator therapy, namely, that the mesiodistal correction of Class II malocclusions is achieved through an apparent vertical manipulation of the dentition. This vertical manipulation occurs most readily in those patients who have either overclosure or a vertical growth component accompanying the normal growth expressed at the chin.

A   B   C

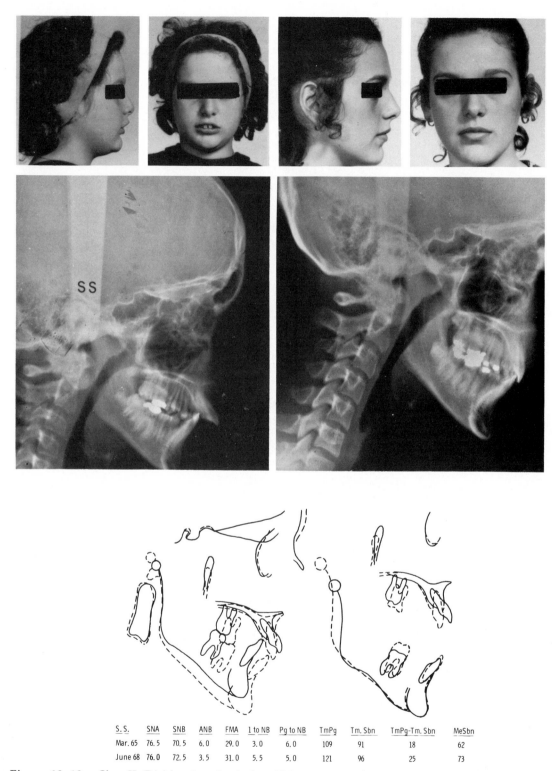

S.S.	SNA	SNB	ANB	FMA	1 to NB	Pg to NB	TmPg	Tm. Sbn	TmPg-Tm. Sbn	MeSbn
Mar. 65	76.5	70.5	6.0	29.0	3.0	6.0	109	91	18	62
June 68	76.0	72.5	3.5	31.0	5.5	5.0	121	96	25	73

Figure 12–10. Class II, Division 1 malocclusion. This case showed severe overclosure with an excess freeway space and moderately reduced lower face height at the beginning of treatment. Treatment was accomplished by lingual tipping of the maxillary incisors with removable Hawley appliance prior to activator therapy. Very favorable growth expressed at the chin relative to restricted development in the mid-facial area permitted satisfactory correction.

Illustration continued on opposite page

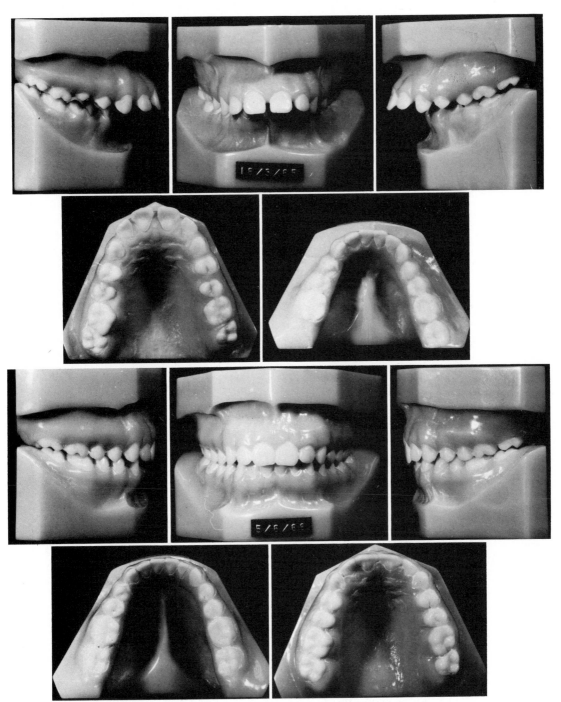

Figure 12–10 *Continued.* In overclosure cases such as this, eruption in both maxillary and mandibular buccal segments is permitted, and the vertical development is obtained wherever the clinician can obtain it. However, it is desirable to permit more eruption in the mandibular buccal segment than is permitted in the maxillary buccal segment, as was done in this case.

height due to mandibular overclosure make excellent cases to manage with the activator (Fig. 12–10).

Orthopedic Possibilities

Figure 12–11 shows that activator treatments accomplished with both small and wide vertical bite registrations may restrict midfacial development in the subnasal areas. Further investigations[8] have shown that while both small and wide vertical openings are equally effective in restricting midfacial development horizontally, bite registrations having wide vertical openings achieve this apparent restriction by a downward displacement of the midfacial area. Trayfoot and Richardson[9] and Harvold and Vargevik[7] have also shown restriction in the forward movement of the midfacial area in activator treatment cases.

Mandibular Growth

From the foregoing paragraphs it will be apparent that the activator controls alveolar growth and functions most effectively in those individuals who experience active phases of mandibular growth with a minimal forward component of growth in the midfacial area. Serial height recordings (Fig. 12–12) provide a useful method for determining how close the patient is to the prepubertal growth acceleration and hence how likely he is to experience a period of active mandibular growth during orthodontic treatment. The use of distance and velocity curves of mandibular length provides a further refinement

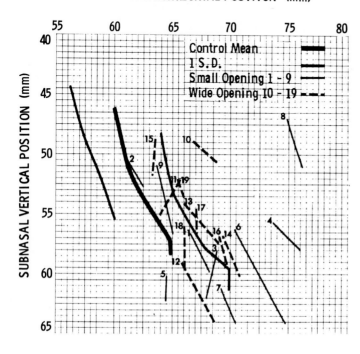

SUBNASAL HORIZONTAL POSITION (mm)

Figure 12–11. A comparison of the individual changes at subnasale of two activator-treated groups with the population standards for growth direction of the midface. Midface growth direction at subnasale has been superimposed on a millimeter grid system with SN as the horizontal axis of the grid. The fine solid lines and broken lines represent the growth direction followed by subnasale from the beginning to the end of a period of activator treatment. It can be seen that in cases 3, 5, 11, 15, 17, and 18 horizontal development of the midface was severely restricted in some cases and in these cases the midfacial area at subnasale was carried posteriorly.

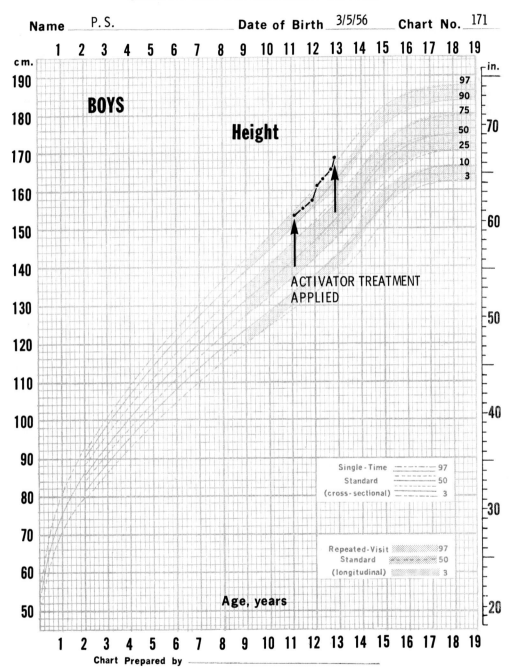

Figure 12–12. *A*, Tanner Growth and Development Record Chart for Boys. Serial height recordings on such growth and development records provide a useful method for determining whether the patient is likely to experience active facial growth during orthodontic treatment. Periods of accelerated physical growth are shown as areas of increased steepness in the growth channels.

Illustration continued on following page

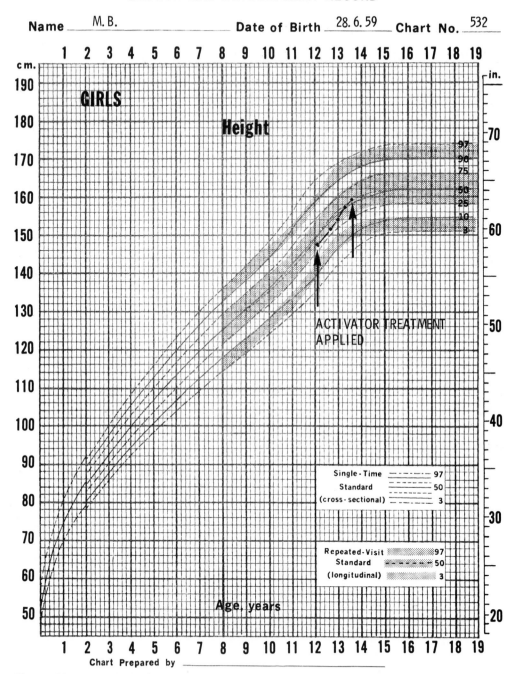

Figure 12–12 *Continued. B,* Tanner Growth and Development Record Chart for Girls.

of this technique (Fig. 12–13).[10] While there is considerable evidence to support the view that activators stimulate mandibular growth, the author feels that the best evidence does not support this view.[7] It is more likely that successful activator treatment coincides with normal periods of active mandibular growth.[8, 10]

	1 JAN.	2 FEB.	3 MAR.	4 APR.	5 MAY	6 JUNE	7 JULY	8 AUG.	9 SEPT.	10 OCT.	11 NOV.	12 DEC.
1	000	085	162	247	329	414	496	581	666	748	833	915
2	003	088	164	249	332	416	499	584	668	751	836	918
3	005	090	167	252	334	419	501	586	671	753	838	921
4	008	093	170	255	337	422	504	589	674	756	841	923
5	011	096	173	258	340	425	507	592	677	759	844	926
6	014	099	175	260	342	427	510	595	679	762	847	929
7	016	101	178	263	345	430	512	597	682	764	849	932
8	019	104	181	266	348	433	515	600	685	767	852	934
9	022	107	184	268	351	436	518	603	688	770	855	937
10	025	110	186	271	353	438	521	605	690	773	858	940
11	027	112	189	274	356	441	523	608	693	775	860	942
12	030	115	192	277	359	444	526	611	696	778	863	945
13	033	118	195	279	362	447	529	614	699	781	866	948
14	036	121	197	282	364	449	532	616	701	784	868	951
15	038	123	200	285	367	452	534	619	704	786	871	953
16	041	126	203	288	370	455	537	622	707	789	874	956
17	044	129	205	290	373	458	540	625	710	792	877	959
18	047	132	208	293	375	460	542	627	712	795	879	962
19	049	134	211	296	378	463	545	630	715	797	882	964
20	052	137	214	299	381	466	548	633	718	800	885	967
21	055	140	216	301	384	468	551	636	721	803	888	970
22	058	142	219	304	386	471	553	638	723	805	890	973
23	060	145	222	307	389	474	556	641	726	808	893	975
24	063	148	225	310	392	477	559	644	729	811	896	978
25	066	151	227	312	395	479	562	647	731	814	899	981
26	068	153	230	315	397	482	564	649	734	816	901	984
27	071	156	233	318	400	485	567	652	737	819	904	986
28	074	159	236	321	403	488	570	655	740	822	907	989
29	077		238	323	405	490	573	658	742	825	910	992
30	079		241	326	408	493	575	660	745	827	912	995
31	082		244		411		578	663		830		997
	JAN. 1	FEB. 2	MAR. 3	APR. 4	MAY 5	JUNE 6	JULY 7	AUG. 8	SEPT. 9	OCT. 10	NOV. 11	DEC. 12

Chart prepared by J. M. Tanner and R. H. Whitehouse University of London, Institute of Child Health, for The Hospital for Sick Children Great Ormond Street. London, W.C.1.

TABLE OF DECIMALS OF YEAR

DECIMAL AGE
The system of decimal age has been used in all charts. Thus the year is divided into 10, not 12. Each date in the calendar is marked (from the table below) in terms of thousandths of the year. Thus January 7th 1962 is 62.016. The child's birth date is similarly recorded, e.g. a child born on June 23rd 1959 has the birth day 59.474. Age at examination is then obtained by simple subtraction, e.g. 62.016—59.474 = 2.542, and the last figure is rounded off. This system greatly facilitates the computing of velocities, since the proportion of the year between two examinations is easily calculated.
Source of standards
The details of the source data and of the construction of these standards are set forth in J. M. Tanner, R. H. Whitehouse and M. Takaishi, *Archives of Diseases in Childhood* 1966 Volume 41. For the most part heights and weights for the age 0–5 are from the data of the University of London, Institutes of Education and Child Health, Child Study Centre, and the Oxford Child Health Survey, and for the ages 5½–15½ from the London County Council survey reported by Scott in 1959. Height attained and height velocity percentiles were calculated on the assumption of a Gaussian distribution at each age; weight attained and weight velocity percentiles were estimated directly from the frequency distributions. Smoothing was in general carried out graphically. The shape of the repeated visit standards are based on longitudinal data from the Harpenden Growth Study.

Figure 12-12 *Continued. C,* Tanner chart for expressing age as a decimal of a year.

In a study of the relationship between accelerations in mandibular velocity and periods of activator therapy, only one period of treatment out of thirty-two instances showed a coincidence between activator therapy and a concomitant increase in mandibular growth (Fig. 12-14).

In summary, activators can be used for the following purposes:

(a) To achieve major changes in facial esthetics.

(b) To achieve major occlusal changes in the mesiodistal, vertical, and transverse planes of space and to remodel arch form.

(c) To achieve moderate changes in apical base dysplasia.

(d) To increase the vertical dimension and hence to assist in the reduction of mandibular prognathism.

The appliance is limited in the following ways:

(a) It can slip the mandibular anchorage unless care is taken in appliance construction and manipulation.

(b) Active intrusion of teeth is difficult.

(c) It cannot be used by itself to correct crowding.

(d) It ideally should be used in growing individuals.

(e) It tends to produce moderate mandibular rotations and hence increase lower face height. This is desirable in overclosure problems and undesirable in patients with excess lower face height at the initiation of treatment.

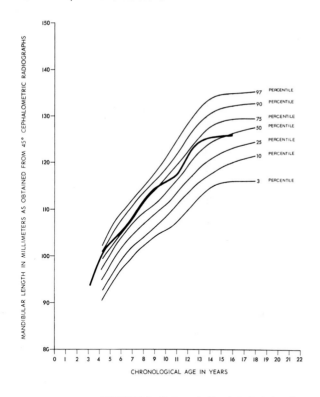

Figure 12–13. Case No. 416. This individual female mandibular distance curve is superimposed on the population distance standards. Periods of accelerated mandibular growth are shown in areas of increased steepness on the individual distance curve.

TYPES OF FACIAL MORPHOLOGY BEST MANAGED BY ACTIVATOR

Our knowledge regarding the nature of the Class II malocclusion has advanced surprisingly little since the early 1950's when surveys concerning the nature of the Class II malocclusion found conflicting results, asserting, for example, that the Class II malocclusion was characterized by a small mandible, or by a normal-sized mandible, or in others by a large mandible.[11] Such in-

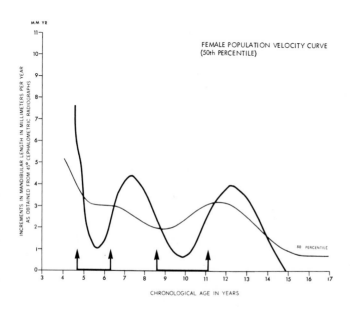

Figure 12–14. The graph illustrates a velocity curve of mandibular growth superimposed on a population standard for mandibular growth in females. There were two distinct accelerations in mandibular growth with peak velocity in mandibular growth occurring at 7.4 years of age for the first acceleration and at 12.3 years for the second acceleration. Two periods of activator growth were applied, with the first period initiated at 4.7 years of age and ending at 6.3 years. The second period of activator growth was applied at 8.6 years of age and ended at 11.1 years. It can be seen that the treatment had no effect on the mandibular growth rate during the treatment intervals. If treatment had been applied coincident with the two accelerations in mandibular growth there would be a great temptation to assume that the treatment was responsible for what, in effect, was a normal variation in mandibular growth rate.

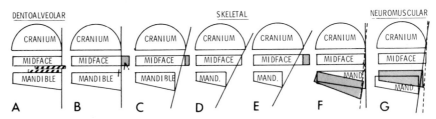

Figure 12–15. *A* represents a Class II, Division 1 malocclusion in which the parts of the face are harmoniously related while the teeth and alveolar bone have been distorted by environmental force. This represents a dentoalveolar malocclusion with excellent prognosis for a simple and successful therapy. *B* represents a Class II, Division 1 malocclusion due to the unfortunate combination of a very prognathic nasomaxillary complex superimposed on an orthognathic facial type to create a convex profile type too great to be compensated for by lingual adjustment of the maxillary incisors and labial adjustment of the mandibular incisors. Such skeletal malocclusions are very susceptible to the creation of overjet with the application of labially directed environmental forces to the maxillary incisors. *C* represents a Class II, Division 1 malocclusion due to the unfortunate random combination of a moderately retrognathic facial type with a moderately prognathic midfacial area to produce a total severe dysplasia. *D* represents a Class II, Division 1 malocclusion due to an extremely retrognathic facial type. The nasomaxillary complex may be back but the mandible is even more so. *E* represents a severe Class II, Division 1 malocclusion due to the superimposition of an extremely prognathic midfacial area on extreme mandibular retrognathism to create a very complex problem in facial structure. *F* represents a Class II, Division 1 malocclusion in which the midfacial area and the mandible were previously harmoniously related. With permanent alteration in the rest position of the mandible, as in chronic nasal obstruction, the mandible assumes an environmentally increased retrognathic position. This represents a neuromuscular malocclusion, since its origin involves the alteration of some very basic neuromuscular reflexes. *G* represents a Class II, Division 1 malocclusion with an excess freeway space which allows the mandible to overclose to an apparent orthognathic facial type. When such overclosure problems are examined at rest position, the mandibular retrognathism and the Class II malocclusion are revealed.

conclusive results will probably continue as long as samples for such studies are selected on the basis of occlusion, because Class II malocclusion is merely a common symptom of a large number of very different facial morphologies. The underlying cause of this symptom may be dentoalveolar, skeletal, or neuromuscular, but all produce the same Class II malocclusion even though the treatment and prognosis may differ markedly in the various facial morphologies. The orthodontic specialist uses static cephalometric radiography to assist him in distinguishing the different types of Class II malocclusions. Activators should not be used by clinicians who will not use cephalometric analyses to assist in establishing the nature of the facial morphology to be treated. Figure 12–15 illustrates seven types of facial morphology associated with similar Class II malocclusions. Some of these morphologic variations will respond better to activator treatment than others. For example,

1. The activator constitutes a form of Class II intermaxillary therapy and, if it is used correctly, can cause the mandibular dentition to slip labially. It follows, therefore, that it can easily be modified to slip the anchorage and thus correct dentoalveolar Class II malocclusions characterized by lingually positioned mandibular dentitions and labially positioned maxillary dentitions (Fig. 12–15*A*).

2. It is less appropriate in skeletal problems associated with extreme apical base dysplasias due to mandibular retrognathism. Unless the patient has favorable amounts and directions of growth in the midfacial and mandibular areas, the maxillary dentition must be retracted bodily to camouflage the skeletal dysplasia. The activator is not suited to perform active bodily retractions of incisor teeth (Fig. 12–15D).

3. The activator is more suited to the management of Class II malocclusions due to midfacial prognathism when amounts and directions of mandibular growth are favorable. In such children the clinician wishes to avoid retraction of the maxillary dentition in order to prevent over-emphasizing nose prominence. Because the activator does not perform active bodily retractions of teeth, it is suited for use in children who need minimal amounts of maxillary incisor movement while the mandible develops forward to camouflage the midface prognathism. However, children with midface prognathism frequently exhibit Class II, Division 2 malocclusions or environmental distortions of such malocclusions in which the maxillary incisor teeth have an upright axial inclination. Because the appliance does tend to incline the maxillary incisors lingually, it is not suited for use in children in whom the incisors are vertically upright or in a moderately lingual position at the beginning of treatment (Fig. 12–15) unless special modifications in design are used (Fig. 12–15C).

4. This appliance is well suited to the management of Class II malocclusions due to moderate skeletal dysplasias between the midfacial area and the mandible, where moderate amounts of mandibular growth and moderate amounts of maxillary incisor retraction may combine for successful treatment. It is not suitable for the management of skeletal dysplasias of any morphologic types that exhibit extreme dysplasia between the midfacial area and the mandible (Fig. 12–15B and E) unless it is to be used as the first stage of a two-stage orthodontic treatment.

5. It is ideal for the management of Class II malocclusions resulting from environmental influences such as thumb-sucking and chronic mouth breathing if some growth still remains and the oral habit can be eliminated. Many of our so-called skeletal Class II malocclusions are probably environmental simulations of skeletal problems (Fig. 12–15F). The exact prevalence of this type of Class II malocclusion is not known, but its presence should be suspected in any Class II malocclusion exhibiting excessive lower face height. The activator can be used to restore correct facial morphology in growing individuals where the environmental impact can be eliminated. However, if the excess lower face height is not due to environmental factors, the activator can produce further deterioration in facial esthetics as the Class II malocclusion is corrected.

6. Figures 12–15G and 12–16 show Class II malocclusions characterized by a normal path of closure, excess freeway space, and overclosure. In the overclosed position such malocclusions may appear to be Class I, but when examined in the rest position they are really Class II malocclusions with a total open bite superimposed. Such cases are obviously more retrognathic when examined in rest position and will be more difficult to correct if the excess freeway is reduced and eruption of teeth in the buccal segment is encouraged to restore a normal freeway space. Such overclosure thus complicates Class II treatment because the mandible must be treated closer to its rest position than to its overclosed position. The activator is an ideal appliance to effect the differential tooth eruption in the maxillary and mandibular buccal segments (Fig. 12–10). Such eruptive movements occur most readily in actively growing patients.

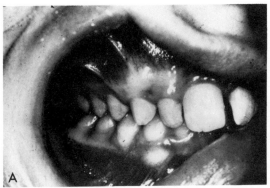
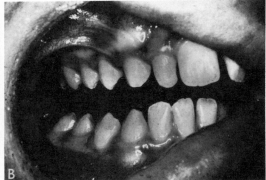
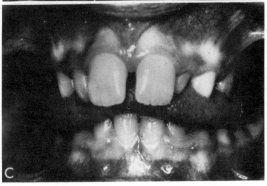
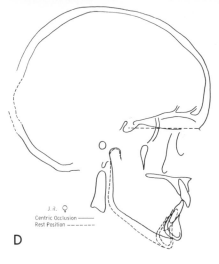

Figure 12-16. *A,* The photograph illustrates an apparent deep overbite when the occlusion is examined in centric occlusion. *B,* When the occlusion is examined in the rest position it can be seen that an excess freeway space exists. If the patient were permitted to close 2 to 3 mm. in the buccal segment area, an excess interocclusal clearance would exist and an edge-to-edge bite would still exist in the incisor area. Obviously, this is not a case of deep overbite but rather of apparent overbite. The case would more correctly be classified as a *complete open bite. C,* This photograph illustrates that the cause of the excess interocclusal clearance or the complete open bite is an abnormal posture of the tongue during rest in this individual. This condition is distinct from tongue thrust. Because the tongue rests between the occlusal surfaces of all teeth, the teeth are not permitted to erupt while the jaws continue their normal downward and forward growth. As growth continues, the inhibition of tooth eruption creates an increasing excess freeway space. When the patient closes, the tongue is withdrawn and the jaws overclose. *D,* The tracings illustrate the position of the mandible in this patient when the mandible is examined in centric occlusion and at rest position. Orthodontic treatment for this patient would more correctly be planned around the jaw relations indicated by the rest position tracing rather than the overclosed centric occlusion tracing, which gives a more prognathic position of the mandible than actually exists. Such vertical malocclusions are very suitable for treatment with an activator.

A differential assessment must be made for all Class II malocclusions with excessive interocclusal clearance and overclosure. Even as a skeletal mandibular retrusion can be masked when there is a normal upward and forward path of closure, so may a pseudo Class II be created by premature incisal contact, tooth guidance, and a resultant functional retrusion. Dominant temporalis muscle activity is often associated with this type of problem, exacerbating the mandibular retrusion. Thus a functional analysis is important in activator therapy. The rapid elimination of some sagittal malrelationships may be due partly to the correction of the functional retrusion and partly to growth. Prior knowledge of functional aberrations and compensations will permit more accurate therapeutic prognostications.

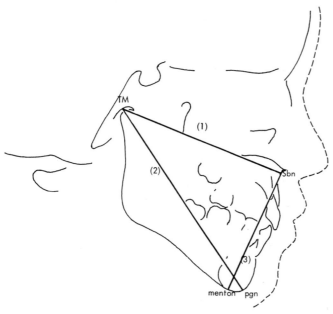

Figure 12–17. Harvold's[6,7] measurements for maxillary unit, mandibular unit, and lower face height.

1. Maxillary Unit Length
2. Mandibular Unit Length
3. Lower Face Height

TM = Temporo-mandibular point: A point in the articular fossa on the line from prognathion through the condyle which indicates the maximum length of the mandible.

Sbn = Subnasale: A point on the lower curvature of the spine where the vertical thickness is three millimeters

It should be repeated at this point that the clinician must have a thorough working knowledge of cephalometric radiography if he hopes to identify patients with severe skeletal dysplasia, excess lower face height, and overclosure characterized by reduced lower face height, and select suitable cases for activator treatment. Harvold[6,7,12] has provided data which are useful to assist in detecting the presence of problems in the vertical dimension (Fig. 12–17, Table 12–1). The use of these data will enable the clinician to avoid activator treatment in patients with excess lower face height and apply more suitable methods of orthodontic therapy for such problems. In addition, overclosure problems accompanied by short lower face height can be identified by clinical examination for excess freeway space and the use of Harvold's data. Activators may then be used in combination with mandibular labial muscle appliances and Class II elastics to elevate more actively the mandibular buccal segments to a new vertical level and assist in minimizing the overclosure and excess freeway space.

Harvold has provided additional data to assist in detecting the presence of severe skeletal dysplasia which may not be detected when routine cephalometric analysis is used. For example, patients may show ANB values usually associated with severe Class II malocclusion when in fact the maxilla and mandible match each other in size and no anomaly of the cranial base exists which would cause a skeletal dysplasia. This occurs in people who acquire severe clockwise rotations of the mandible through environmental impact (Fig. 12–15*F*). Measurements indicating excess lower face height assist in identifying the presence of such rotations while use of Harvold's skeletal unit matching data

TABLE 12-1. HARVOLD'S VALUES FOR LOWER FACE HEIGHT*

		Male						Female			
Age (years)	No.	Mini-mum (mm.)	Mean value (mm.)	Maxi-mum (mm.)	Standard deviation	Age (years)	No.	Mini-mum (mm.)	Mean value (mm.)	Maxi-mum (mm.)	Standard deviation
6	118	52	59	72	3.55	6	88	49	57	65	3.22
9	102	53	62	74	4.25	9	79	50	60	70	3.62
12	96	53	64	76	4.62	12	71	53	62	74	4.36
14	66	56	68	82	5.23	14	49	54	64	72	4.39
16	72	57	71	86	5.73	16	53	55	65	74	4.67

*Lower face height = anterior nasal spine − menton. Data by kind permission of Dr. Egil P. Harvold, Chairman, Section of Orofacial Anomalies, University of California, San Francisco, California.

(Fig. 12–17, Table 12–2) will show clearly that the parts of the face actually match each other well. Conversely, severe Class III malocclusions may be masked by such clockwise rotations of the mandible. Application of the data will show clearly that the parts of the face do not match each other and that dysplasia actually exists. The same principles are useful in the analysis of Class II and Class III problems complicated by overclosure because such overclosure masks the actual dysplasia when Class II malocclusions are analyzed from radiographs taken in centric occlusion, while the severity of Class III malocclusion is overemphasized when such malocclusions are analyzed from radiographs taken in the overclosed position.

FUNCTIONAL OCCLUSAL PLANE CHANGES IN CLASS II TREATMENT

Harvold[6, 7] has also emphasized the concept of the "functional occlusal plane" and the role played by its manipulation in the successful correction of Class II malocclusions. This plane represents the functional table of occlusion in the first permanent molar, second premolar, and first premolar areas. The level and inclination of the functional occlusal plane is the result of the

Figure 12–18. The diagram illustrates the different eruption direction of the maxillary and mandibular buccal segments relative to the functional occlusal plane. The functional occlusal plane is defined as the points of contact between the maxillary and mandibular first permanent molars, second bicuspid, and first bicuspid teeth. The type of occlusion which is established will be dependent upon the relative amounts of vertical eruption accomplished in the maxillary and mandibular buccal segments. For example, if there is minimum eruption of the maxillary buccal segments and over-eruption of the mandibular buccal segments, there will be a distinct tendency for the establishment of a Class III malocclusion as the functional occlusal plane stabilizes itself at a higher level. Conversely, if there is a minimal eruption of the mandibular buccal segments and over-eruption of the maxillary buccal segments, the functional occlusal plane will be established at a lower level and the mesial component of maxillary buccal segment eruption will be overemphasized. These changes may contribute to establishment of a Class II relationship.

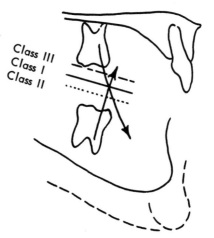

Class III
Class I
Class II

(Harvold, 68)

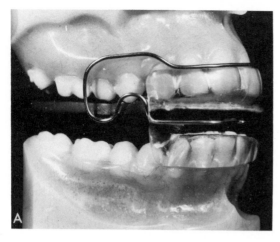

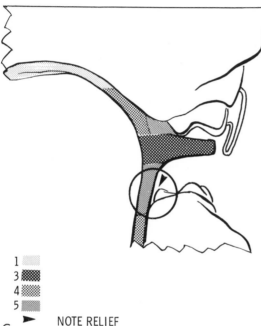

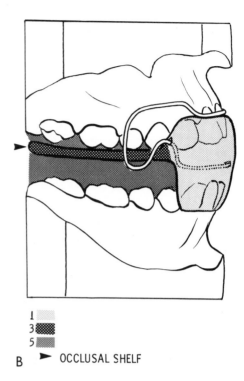

1 ▦
3 ▦
5 ▦
B ► OCCLUSAL SHELF

1 ▦
3 ▦
4 ▦
5 ▦
C ► NOTE RELIEF

Figure 12-19. *A,* A Class II activator. *B,* An activator trimmed to permit the desired vertical eruption of the mandibular buccal segments and to inhibit eruption of the maxillary buccal segments. 1 = Areas of hard acrylic contact with basal structures and also the labial surfaces of the incisor teeth. 3 = Acrylic which is left in contact with the occusal and also the mesial surfaces of the maxillary buccal teeth. 5 = Acrylic which is removed to permit eruption of mandibular teeth and distal movement of maxillary teeth. *C,* A view from the distal of a correctly trimmed activator. The lingual surface of the mandibular buccal segments should be clear of the acrylic the thickness of an explorer so that no friction stops will impede eruption of the mandibular buccal teeth. 1 = Areas of hard acrylic contact with basal structures and also the labial surfaces of the incisor teeth. 3 = Acrylic which is left in contact with the occlusal and also the mesial surfaces of the maxillary buccal teeth. 4 = Firm acrylic contact with the alveolar processes. 5 = Acrylic which is removed to permit eruption of mandibular teeth and distal movement of maxillary teeth.

neuromuscular, growth, and developmental forces acting on the dentition. The correct manipulation of the functional occlusal plane involves inhibition of eruption of the maxillary buccal segments, which normally follows a downward and forward curvilinear eruption path (Fig. 12–18). At the same time, the mandibular buccal segments are permitted to erupt vertically in harmony with the vertical growth of the lower face. Because the mandibular molars erupt roughly at right angles to the functional occlusal plane, a change from Class II to Class I malocclusion is facilitated.

This change may be achieved in nongrowing individuals if the mandible is rotated into a more vertical position and the occlusion allowed to adjust to the new mandibular position by differential control of tooth eruption. Because this

TABLE 12–2. HARVOLD'S VALUES FOR DIFFERENCES BETWEEN MANDIBULAR AND MAXILLARY UNITS*

	Male					Female			
Age (years)	*No.*	*Minimum (mm.)*	*Mean value (mm.)*	*Maximum (mm.)*	*Age (years)*	*No.*	*Minimum (mm.)*	*Mean value (mm.)*	*Maximum (mm.)*
6	118	10	17	27	6	88	10	17	24
9	102	13	20	28	9	79	13	20	28
12†	96	12	22	30	12†	71	16	23	36
14	66	14	25	38	14	49	18	26	39
16	72	17	27	39	16	53	19	26	39

*Data by kind permission of Dr. Egil P. Harvold, Chairman, Section of Orofacial Anomalies, University of California, San Francisco, California.

†At age twelve conservative Class II treatment will be difficult in growing children with difference values less than 16. Conservative Class III treatment will have a poor prognosis at difference values greater than 29. The values provide one indication of cases which might be considered for activator therapy.

change tends to increase lower face height and mandibular retrognathism, with unfavorable profile changes, it will not be the best procedure to follow in most nongrowing patients. Figure 12–19 illustrates an activator trimmed to permit the desired vertical eruption of the mandibular buccal segments and to inhibit eruption of the maxillary buccal segments. A vertical change of 3 to 5 mm. in the position of the buccal segments is usually considered adequate to effect the change from Class II to Class I occlusion. In the management of Class III malocclusions, buccal segment eruption is inhibited in the mandibular arch and encouraged in the maxillary arch. However, these changes cannot be used to achieve a total Class I relationship in Class II and Class III cases with severe skeletal dysplasias and steep occlusal planes (Table 12–2).

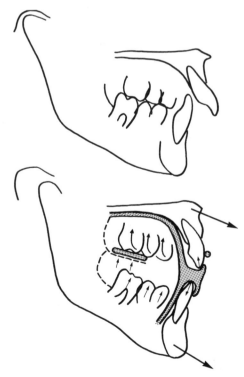

Figure 12–20. The working bite for a Class II activator. Bite registration places the mandible in such a position that any muscle and soft tissue action attempting to return the mandible to its normal position will apply intrusive forces to the maxillary and mandibular incisors. In addition, intrusive forces are delivered to the maxillary buccal teeth, which are in contact with an acrylic buccal shelf. The mandibular buccal teeth are free to erupt unimpeded. The intrusive forces generated by an activator do not usually cause active intrusion of teeth. Rather, these intrusive forces prevent eruption of teeth in growing individuals and hence obtain the effect of active intrusion.

THE WORKING BITE FOR CLASS II ACTIVATOR

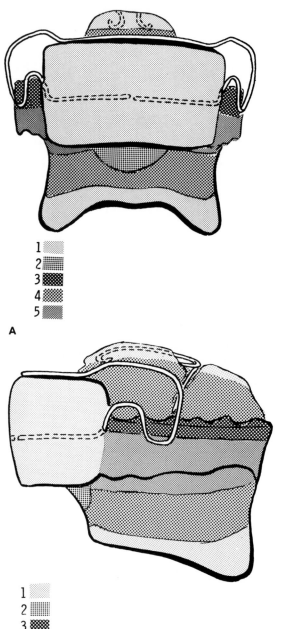

1 ▨
2 ▨
3 ▨
4 ▨
5 ▨

A

1 ▨
2 ▨
3 ▨
4 ▨
5 ▨

B

Figure 12–21. *A,* A frontal view of the activator. Note that the undercuts in the mandibular portion of the appliance are left in place to assist in retaining the appliance in position. The patient must insert the appliance sideways, and if he attempts to dislodge the appliance with his tongue these undercut flanges will rub on the lingual mucoperiosteum of the mandible. The patient quickly learns that he can avoid this discomfort by biting firmly on the appliance. 1 = Areas of hard acrylic contact with basal structures and also the labial surfaces of the incisor teeth. 2 = Areas of relief lingual to the maxillary and mandibular incisor teeth. 3 = Acrylic which is left in contact with the occlusal and also the mesial surfaces of the maxillary buccal teeth. 4 = Firm acrylic contact with the alveolar processes. 5 = Acrylic which is removed to permit eruption of mandibular teeth and distal movement of maxillary teeth. *B,* A lateral view of an untrimmed activator. Note that the acrylic is removed in the mandibular buccal segment in order to allow unimpeded eruption of the mandibular buccal teeth. The acrylic extends on the labial of the maxillary and mandibular incisor teeth to assist in anchorage control. The acrylic is extended deep into the mandibular retromolar area to assist in retaining the appliance in position. 1 = Areas of hard acrylic contact with basal structures and also the labial surfaces of the incisor teeth. 2 = Areas of relief lingual to the maxillary and mandibular incisor teeth. 3 = Acrylic which is left in contact with the occlusal and also the mesial surfaces of the maxillary buccal teeth. 4 = Firm acrylic contact with the alveolar processes. 5 = Acrylic which is removed to permit eruption of mandibular teeth and distal movement of maxillary teeth.

Illustration continued on opposite page

Because the direction of mandibular growth at the chin usually diverges from the inclination of the functional occlusal plane, any attempt to make the functional occlusal plane more closely parallel to the direction of growth at the chin will permit such direction to be expressed along the functional occlusal plane which is the plane of orthodontic correction and hence will enhance the effect mandibular growth has in correcting the malocclusion.

Figure 12–21 *Continued.* *C,* An inferior view of the trimmed activator. The acrylic that presses against the mandibular basal bone structure constitutes the sole anchorage because this acrylic presses firmly against basal bone structures. If this area is relieved, the appliance can move mesially and permit anchorage slippage. The area of alveolar relief lingual to the mandibular incisor teeth affords further protection against anchorage slippage in the mandibular incisor area. 1 = Areas of hard acrylic contact with basal structures and also the labial surfaces of the incisor teeth. 2 = Areas of relief lingual to the maxillary and mandibular incisor teeth. 3 = Acrylic which is left in contact with the occlusal and also the mesial surfaces of the maxillary buccal teeth. 4 = Firm acrylic contact with the alveolar processes. 5 = Acrylic which is removed to permit eruption of the mandibular teeth and distal movement of maxillary teeth. *D,* A superior view of the trimmed activator. This view illustrates the areas of hard contact (coding number 3) which are left in contact with the mesial of each maxillary buccal tooth. Coding number 5 indicates the areas of relief on the distal of each maxillary tooth. This trimming permits the maxillary buccal segments to be guided distally. Expansion may be achieved if the acrylic contacting the palatal vault is relieved moderately (coding number 1). The full thrust of the forces will then be dissipated laterally through the alveolar processes to those portions of acrylic (coding number 4) which are in contact with the buccal segment alveolar processes. The dislodging spring is activated approximately 0.5 mm. to provide continuous dislodging action and assist in activating the muscles of mastication.

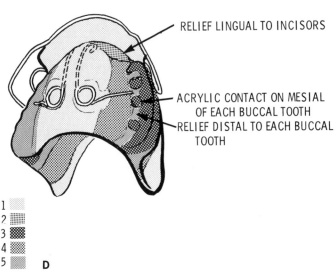

1
2
3
4
5

C ▶ NOTE THE ANCHORAGE WEDGE EFFECT AGAINST MANDIBULAR BASAL BONE FOR ANCHORAGE PURPOSES

RELIEF LINGUAL TO INCISORS

ACRYLIC CONTACT ON MESIAL OF EACH BUCCAL TOOTH
RELIEF DISTAL TO EACH BUCCAL TOOTH

1
2
3
4
5   D

BITE REGISTRATION AND THEORIES OF ACTION IN CLASS II MALOCCLUSION

The most important point in the construction of the activator is the registration of the wax bite which determines the relationship of the mandible to the maxilla when the appliance is in the mouth. The appliance consists of a maxillary and a mandibular plate joined together in the registered bite. Bite registration places the mandible in such a position that any muscle and soft tissue action that attempts to return the mandible to its normal position will apply an intrusive force to the maxillary and mandibular incisors which impedes further vertical alveolar development (Fig. 12–20). In addition, the appliance delivers intrusive forces to the maxillary buccal teeth, which are in contact with an acrylic buccal shelf. Because the activator shields the mandibular buccal segments from the forces delivered by the muscles of mastication at the moment of initial contact, these teeth are free to erupt unimpeded. Also, because the appliance contacts the mesial of all of the maxillary buccal teeth, any forces tending to retract the mandible and those forces delivered to the appliance from the labial tissues provide a distal thrust to the maxillary teeth and prevent their normal downward and forward eruption. Mesial thrusting forces directed at the mandibular dentition are intercepted by removing all acrylic contact with the teeth except at the mandibular incisal edges. Mesial forces directed against the mandible are delivered to the basilar structures to keep the mandibular anchorage from slipping (Fig. 12–21).

As originally designed by Andresen, the activator was intended to correct malocclusion solely through the action of the muscles of mastication. Although its exact mode of action still has not yet been clearly established, four basic neuromuscular concepts have evolved, which represent at least three different philosophies of bite registration.

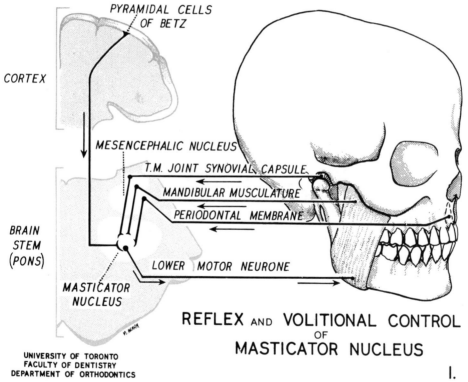

PYRAMIDAL CELLS OF BETZ

CORTEX

MESENCEPHALIC NUCLEUS

T.M. JOINT SYNOVIAL CAPSULE

MANDIBULAR MUSCULATURE

PERIODONTAL MEMBRANE

BRAIN STEM (PONS)

LOWER MOTOR NEURONE

MASTICATOR NUCLEUS

REFLEX AND VOLITIONAL CONTROL OF MASTICATOR NUCLEUS

I.

UNIVERSITY OF TORONTO
FACULTY OF DENTISTRY
DEPARTMENT OF ORTHODONTICS

Figure 12–22. The neural pathway for reflex and volitional control of the masticator nucleus (muscles of mastication). The proprioceptive fibers arising from the periodontal membrane, the muscles of mastication, and the temporomandibular joints ascend via the trigeminal nerve to the brain stem. Unlike the other sensory nerve tracts, the proprioceptive nerve tract has its cell body in the mesencephalic nucleus, which is located in the brain stem. The other sensory nerve tracts have their cell bodies in the trigeminal or gasserian ganglion (outside the brain stem). From the mesencephalic nucleus the tract descends to the masticator nucleus on the ipsilateral side, where it synapses with the lower motor neuron that carries the motor impulses to the muscles of mastication via the third division of the trigeminal nerve. The voluntary or volitional control of the masticator nucleus, and therefore the muscles of mastication, comes from the pyramidal cells of Betz, located in the cerebral cortex, and descends via the upper motor neuron. (By kind permission of Dr. M. Roberts.)

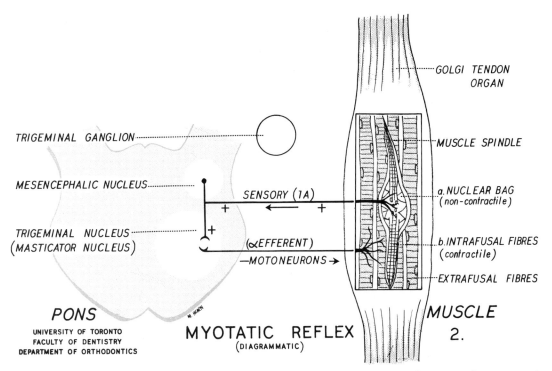

Figure 12-23. Reflex control of skeletal muscle contraction: Mechanism of the stretch or myotatic reflex. The stimulus for the stretch reflex is the stretch of the muscle. The stretch reflex, when elicited, causes contraction of the stretched muscle. *Muscle stretch receptors* are proprioceptive nerve endings called *muscle spindles.* The muscle spindle is located within the muscle itself and consists of a bundle of 2 to 15 thin intrafusal muscle fibers. The long slender ends of the intrafusal fibers are striated and contractile, whereas the central or *nuclear bag* region is noncontractile. The impulses arising from the muscle spindle (nuclear bag) are conducted by the Group 1A sensory nerve fibers. These sensory nerve fibers synapse with the motor neurons called *alpha efferents* that supply the extrafusal muscle fibers responsible for the contraction of the stretched muscle. The myotatic or stretch reflex is, therefore, a *monosynaptic reflex arc.* The *functional significance* of the stretch reflex is that it serves as a *mechanism for upright posture or standing.* Natural stretches are usually imposed on muscles by the action of gravity. During standing, the quadriceps muscles are subjected to stretch because the knee tends to bend in accordance with gravitational pull. The stretch of muscle acts as a stimulus to elicit the stretch reflex, causing a sustained contraction of the stretched muscle, so that the upright position is automatically maintained despite the action of gravity. The same stretch reflex acts in the mandibular musculature to maintain the postural rest position of the mandible in relation to the maxilla. (By kind permission of Dr. M. Roberts.)

1. A bite registration used commonly throughout the world registers the mandible in a position protruded approximately 3.0 mm. *distal* to the most protrusive position that patient can achieve, while vertically the bite is registered *within* the limits of the patient's freeway space (see Chapter 7). The proponents of this method believe that the presence of a loosely fitting activator increases the frequency of reflex contractions in the muscles of mastication against the appliance (Fig. 12–22). Intermittent movements of the appliance in swallowing and biting deliver distal and intrusive forces to the maxillary teeth engaged in the appliance.

Because the appliance is trimmed loosely, it will drop when the jaws relax. The patient must then be conditioned to bite into the appliance to keep it in position, and, if correctly motivated, soon develops a conditioned reflex and performs this act while sleeping. When the mandible moves mesially to engage the appliance, the elevator muscles of mastication are activated and deliver force to the teeth. Thus, when the teeth engage the appliance, the myotatic reflex (Fig 12–23) is activated so that, in addition to the muscle force delivered during swallowing and in biting, reflex stretch stimulation of the muscle spindles also elicits reflex muscle activity. The forces elicited result in tooth movement and bone remodeling and may either prevent further forward adaptation of the maxillary dentoalveolar process, move it slightly distally, or, more frequently, may direct its normal downward and forward mesial eruption distally. While these changes are proceeding, the mandible continues its normal rate and direction of growth. Obviously, if the change in direction of eruption is to be effective, the vertical component of mandibular growth must be adequate.

2. The bite registration, most commonly used in North America, registers the mandible protruded to a point approximately 3.0 mm. distal to the most protrusive position, while vertically the bite is registered approximately 4.0 mm. *beyond* the rest portion of the mandible (see Fig. 12–1). Clinicians using this bite registration maintain that the appliance induces activation of the myotatic reflex in the muscles of mastication and that the frequency of biting and swallowing increases only during the first few days of therapy. They thus maintain that the main force is provided through increased active tension in the stretched muscles of mastication (Fig. 12–23). In their view, this more extreme vertical separaton of the jaws is necessary because the appliance is worn mostly at night and the rest position of the mandible is altered during sleep,[13, 14] so that the freeway space may be approximately double what it is when the patient is awake. Thus, the more extreme vertical separation of the jaws ensures that the myotatic reflex will act when the musculature is more relaxed while sleeping.

Because the activator does not permit muscle shortening, the contractions produced are isometric rather than isotonic. During isometric contraction, muscle fibers develop higher tension, which is well sustained during the period of contraction. Studies conducted at the University of Toronto confirm that increased levels of masseter and digastric muscle activity are sustained to a high level during 10 to 12 hours of wear of the appliance.[15] It is for this reason that the activator is preferred by the author to the Bimler appliance. The compressibility of the Bimler appliance permits more isotonic muscle contraction and reduced force levels. However, the Bimler appliance has a distinct advantage in that the wearer is able to wear it more hours, which tends to initiate additional muscle activity. As a basic principle, activators should be constructed of a rigid material to obtain the force levels generated in isometric muscle contraction.

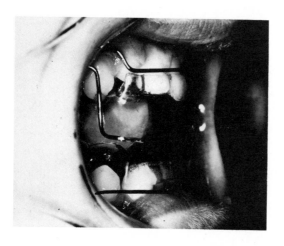

Figure 12–24. An activator with the bite registration opened vertically 21.0 mm. Such extreme bite registrations are utilized to take advantage of the forces generated when the labial musculature, skin, and other tissues are stretched. Greater force levels may be generated through the use of passive stretch rather than by the activation of the myotatic reflex in the various muscles of mastication.

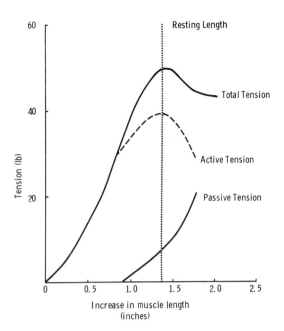

Figure 12-25. The total tension in muscle is the result of active tension from the myotatic reflex and passive tension from the viscoelastic properties of the tissues. Moderate bite registrations used in activator treatment attempt to use active tension to achieve correction of malocclusion. More extreme vertical openings in which the mandible is opened at least 8 to 10 mm. beyond the rest position use passive tension in the stretched tissues to achieve the correction. The diagram illustrates that the forces generated by a combination of active and passive tension may rise to higher levels than those generated by active tension alone.[17]

3. The third bite registration, which was originated by Harvold[7] and is gaining increasing acceptance, places the mandible approximately 3.0 mm. distal to the most protrusive position that the patient is able to achieve, while vertically, an extreme separation of the jaws is used so that the mandible may be opened 8 to 10 mm. beyond the freeway space. The author uses a vertical separation of approximately 12 to 15 mm. beyond the daytime rest position of the mandible (Fig. 12–24). The proponents of this concept contend that the use of the myotatic reflex and attempts to increase frequency of biting and swallowing should be largely ignored, letting passive tension (viscoelastic properties) (Fig. 12–25) in the stretched labial and oral musculature deliver the primary force to the appliance. Thus, the power to produce alveolar remodeling is obtained from the inherent elasticity of muscle, tendinous tissues, and skin without motor stimulation.[16, 17] Muscle spindles have not been clearly demonstrated in the labial muscles and therefore there seems to be no mechanism for turning off reflex muscle activity through a modification of myotatic reflex (Fig. 12–26). Thus, the more these muscles are stretched, the greater the force delivered to the activator. It is quite possible that the forces generated by this extreme bite registration represent a combination of forces generated by swallowing, biting, activation of myotatic reflex in the stretched muscles of mastication and the power delivered through the viscoelastic properties of stretched muscle, tendon tissue, skin, and musculature (Fig. 12–27).

The reason that the bite is registered for 3.0 to 4.0 mm. distal to the most protruded position which the patient is able to achieve in all three bite registrations is to avoid the possibility of initiating Golgi tendon organ activity (Fig. 12–26) and thus eliminate any undesirable myotatic reflex activity.

4. Schwarz[18, 19] believed that the patient could be conditioned to maintain a continuous sustained biting on the activator. He claimed to have recorded sustained tetanic contractions for up to four hours while the patient was sleeping. Figure 12–28 indicates that such hyperactivity is physiologically possible in properly motivated patients through the medium of signals from the higher

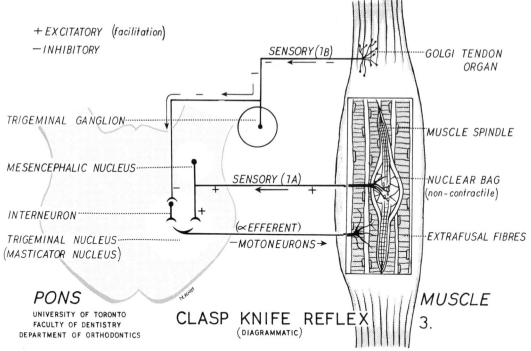

Figure 12-26. Mechanism of the clasp knife reflex or autogenic inhibition. If one attempts to flex forcibly the spastic limb of a patient, resistance is encountered as soon as the muscle is stretched throughout the initial part of the bending. This resistance is, of course, due to the hyperactive reflex contraction of the muscle in response to stretch (myotatic or stretch reflex). If flexion be forcibly carried further, a point is reached at which all resistance to additional flexion seems to melt, and the previously rigid limb collapses readily. Because the resistance of the limb resembles that of a spring-loaded folding knife blade, this phenomenon is called the *"clasp-knife"* reaction, i.e., *the muscle first resists, then relaxes.* The excessive or rapid stretch of the muscle brings into play some new influence which annuls the stretch reflex and allows the muscle to be lengthened with little or no tonic resistance. Thus, the stimulus necessary to elicit the clasp-knife reflex is excessive stretch and when elicited, it inhibits muscular contraction, thus causing the muscle to relax. The receptors for the clasp-knife reflex are the *Golgi tendon organs* located in the tendon of the muscle. The impulses are conducted by the Group 1B *sensory nerve fibers.* The impulses act on the motor neuron or *alpha efferent* supplying the stretched muscle. However, it is a disynaptic reflex arc because an interneuron is interposed between the sensory neuron and the motor neuron. It follows that during muscle stretch, the motor neurons supplying the stretched muscles are bombarbed by impulses delivered over two competing pathways, one facilitating and the other inhibiting muscle contraction. The output of the motor neuron pool depends upon the balance between the two antagonistic inputs. The *functional significance* of the clasp-knife reflex is to protect the overload by preventing damaging contraction against strong stretching forces. (by kind permission of Dr. M. Roberts.)

centers of the brain. Such activity would require conditioning of the patient and possibly autosuggestion.

In North America, bite registrations with the vertical dimension opened to the freeway space are not used extensively with activators. Most clinicians prefer[20] to use the alternate bite registrations to attempt to maintain better activity during the night when most activators are worn. The therapeutic importance of forces generated by the perioral musculature has also[21] been recognized. The true activator does not lend itself to long-continued daytime wear to provide biting and swallowing activity during the day as well as at night. The Bimler and Fränkel appliances are more suitable for daytime wear and for bite registrations opened vertically within the limits of freeway space (see Chapters 13 and 15).

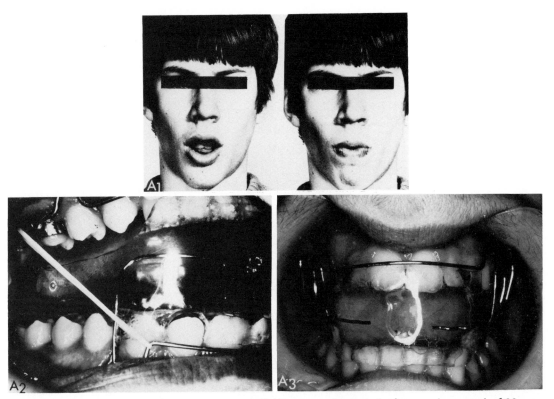

Figure 12–27. Two views of an activator opened 17 mm. at the incisal edges to give a total of 22 mm. opening are shown. Extreme bite registrations such as this were utilized to take advantage of the additional retractive forces to the maxilla generated by stretching of the lips, facial musculature, and the skin. The tension created in the orbicularis oris area is evident when the patient attempts to close his lips. This activator was used in combination with a mandibular labial muscle appliance to which Class II elastics were attached. This assisted in elevating the mandibular buccal segments, thus eliminating the excess freeway space in this overclosed patient. This also facilitated a vertical displacement of the functional occlusal plane. In addition, the mandibular labial muscle appliance created space in the mandibular arch for the alignment of moderate incisor crowding. Note that the second permanent molar teeth have been extracted to facilitate the elevation of the functional occlusal plane and the alignment of moderate incisor crowding. The tracings show that treatment was accomplished by a combination of restriction of forward development at ANS, excellent amount and direction of mandibular growth, and elevation of the mandibular buccal segments relative to the maxillary buccal segments. There was little tooth movement in the maxillary arch, and the mandibular buccal segments were directed distally by the mandibular labial muscle appliance. The soft tissue tracings are referred to the original nasion-pogonion line.

Illustration continued on following page

One point of caution should be noted in the use of the third bite registration. Activators tend to tip the maxillary incisor teeth distally. It follows, therefore, that they may tend to create an excessive lingual inclination of the maxillary incisor teeth. This tendency is emphasized with the third bite registration described previously because of the force levels applied with extreme vertical opening and because of the vertical tipping at the anterior end of the palatal plane which is created.[8] Therefore, the third bite registration should be used only where the maxillary incisor teeth are in pronounced labioversion. Where the maxillary incisor teeth are upright or have a very moderate lingual inclination, the practitioner should use the first or second bite registrations and attempt to treat the Class II malocclusion by utilizing available mandibular growth rather than by retracting the maxillary incisor area.

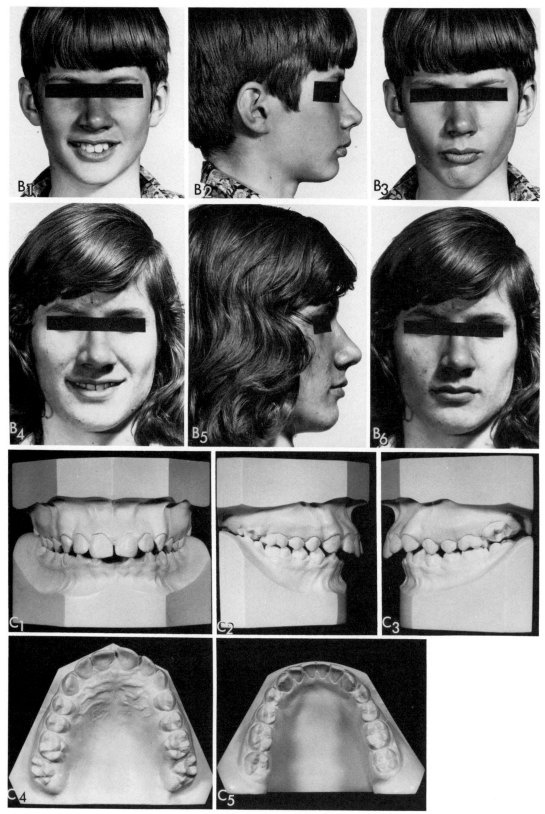

Figure 12–27 *Continued.*

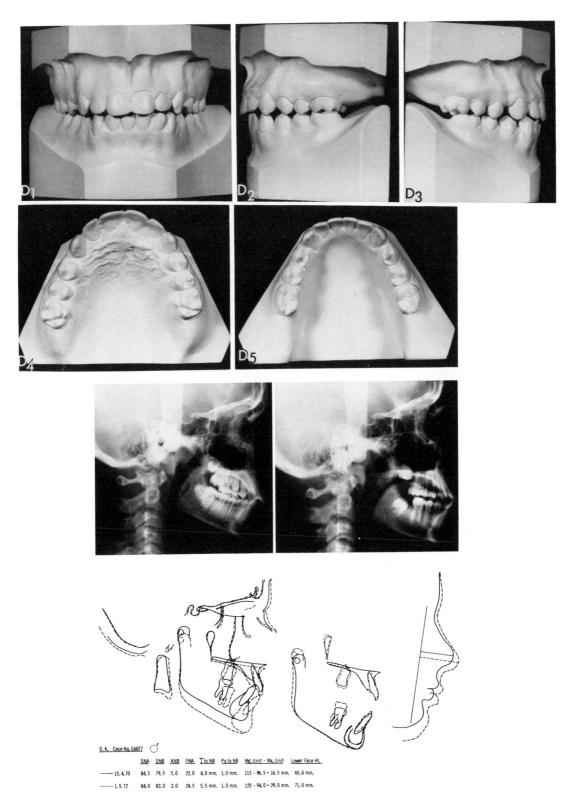

D. K.   Case No. G6077   ♂

	SNA	SNB	ANB	FMA	T̲ to NB	Pg to NB	Md. Unit - Mx. Unit	Lower Face Ht.
—— 15. 4. 70	84.5	79.5	5.0	22.0	4.0 mm.	1.0 mm.	113 - 96.5 = 16.5 mm.	65.0 mm.
------ 1. 5. 72	84.0	82.0	2.0	24.5	5.5 mm.	1.0 mm.	123 - 94.0 = 29.0 mm.	71.0 mm.

Figure 12–27   *Continued.*

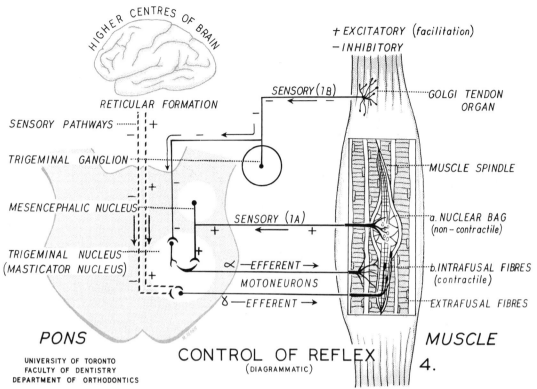

Figure 12–28. Regulation of the myotatic reflex from the higher centers of the brain via the reticular formation. In addition to the α (alpha) efferents or motor neurons supplying the extrafusal fibers of the muscles, smaller motor neurons or γ (gamma) efferents supply the intrafusal fibers of the muscle spindle (both contractile poles). Activation of the γ (gamma) efferents will cause polar contraction of the intrafusal fibers and therefore put the noncontractile nuclear bag region under tension. This will produce in the receptor endings a mechanical distortion indistinguishable from that occasioned by passive stretch of the whole muscle. In this way, the γ (gamma) efferents may initiate spindle discharge in the absence of external stretch, or, in the presence of stretch, so increase the sensitivity of the spindle that frequency of the sensory discharge is markedly increased. The γ (gamma) efferents thus serve as biasing mechanisms regulating the sensitivity of the muscle spindle receptors. It is through this γ (gamma) efferent system that the higher centers of the brain via the reticular formation influence the stretch or myotatic reflex. This is significant because it helps us explain how emotional or psychic disturbances affect the symptoms of temporomandibular dysfunction. The reticular formation influences the myotatic or stretch reflex mainly by facilitation or inhibition of the small γ (gamma) efferents, which cause contraction of the intrafusal fibers of the muscle spindles, thereby increasing the rate of the spindle firing, which in turn influences the amount of α (alpha) motor neuron firing. (By kind permission of Dr. M. Roberts.)

In summary, the various actions claimed by the proponents of the three bite registrations described here probably act cumulatively to a greater or lesser degree at various times; the greatest action probably results from the initiation of myotatic reflex activity and through the harnessing of the viscoelastic properties of muscle tissue. Because the muscles are not permitted to shorten, the muscle contractions generated are isometric rather than isotonic, with a greater resultant force.

Clinical Considerations in Bite Registration and Appliance Construction

In constructing the activator the mandibular impression should be extended deeply on the lingual side in the first and second permanent molar areas. The impression thus extends into an undercut area of the mandible to permit the construction of a deep lingual flange which assists in holding the appliance in position (Fig. 12–21*A*).

After deciding which of the three previously described bite registrations is to be used, the bite is registered using a thick roll of softened baseplate wax. A bundle of tongue depressors inserted into the wax in the incisor area will provide a guide for the patient's vertical closure (Fig. 12–29). The thickness of this bundle will be determined by the space between the maxillary and mandibular incisal edges when the patient's mandible is placed in the correct vertical and protrusive bite registration. After the bundle is inserted into the wax bite, the child is instructed to advance the mandible as far as he is able and then retract 3.0 mm. The patient then closes his mouth to the vertical dimension permitted by the tongue depressor bundle. Pencil marks can be made on the tongue depressor bundle at the points where the incisal edges contact it. Grooves may then be cut into the bundle at the pencil marks to provide definite anteroposterior and vertical guides to assist both patient and clinician to establish the correct bite relationship. After registering the bite, the assembly is removed from the patient's mouth and chilled. The tongue depressors are removed and the bite returned to the mouth to check that the midlines are correct. When the midlines do not match, they may be matched in the bite registration if: (a) the deviation is due to a lateral functional displacement of the mandible with the maxillary midline matching the midsagittal plane of the head when the mandible is at rest; (b) the discrepancy is not more than 2.0 mm. in midline deviations that are not

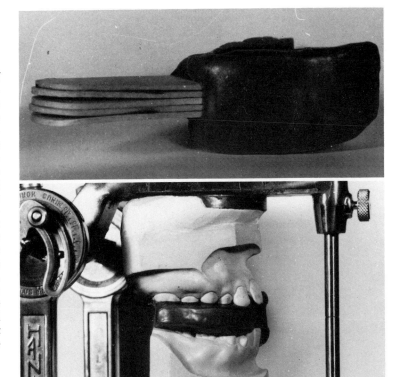

Figure 12–29. A bundle of tongue depressors inserted into a wax bite in the incisor area to provide a guide for the patient's vertical and anteroposterior closure during bite registration. The child is instructed to advance the mandible as far as he can, retract 3.0 mm., and close his mouth to the vertical dimension permitted by the tongue depressor bundle. Pencil marks are made on the tongue depressor bundle at the point where the incisal edges contact it. Grooves may then be cut into the bundle to provide definite anteroposterior and vertical guides to assist both patient and clinician to establish the correct bite relationship.

characterized by functional mandibular displacements. If the midlines are matched in the bite registration in patients with large midline discrepancies due to dental drift or skeletal asymmetry, as distinct from functional mandibular displacements, the treated result will show the midlines matching occlusally, but *both* the maxillary and the mandibular midlines may not match the midsagittal plane of the face.

The labial arch wire attached to the appliance is commonly of two designs, one as used in the construction of a Hawley retainer, and the other as used in the labial wire of an Andresen appliance. A modified Andresen design is used when there has been considerable narrowing of the maxillary arch in the canine area due to muscle contraction force. This design relieves the force of the cheeks from the maxillary canine area and permits normal arch form to be restored in this area (see Figs. 12–1 and 12–21*B*). The Fränkel appliance utilizes the same philosophy (see Chapter 15).

In the Class II activator, relief is placed lingual to the incisor teeth in both arches. In the maxillary arch a relief is carried lingually from the central incisors approximately 5 mm. on the same plane as the incisal edges, although a slight inclination from horizontal is sometimes used to control intrusion or extrusion of the incisors (see Fig. 12–21*D*). This relief permits remodeling of the alveolar process as the incisors are guided lingually. In the mandibular arch, the relief is in a level plane flush with the incisal edges of the central incisors and carried lingually for approximately 3 mm. (see Fig. 12–21*A* to *D*). It ensures that no force will be applied by the appliance to tip the mandibular incisors labially. It is essential that this mandibular relief not be carried any closer than 5 mm. to the deepest lingual edge of the appliance because the appliance must contact the tissue overlying basal bone in order to reinforce the mandibular anchorage.

TRIMMING PROCEDURE

An important step in the adjustment of a well-functioning activator is the correct trimming of the finished appliance. The following method must be carefully observed to direct the muscle and tissue forces to the maxillary teeth and to *avoid* applying these forces to the mandibular dentition in order to minimize anchorage slippage, a constant concern.

Mandibular Arch. In the Class II activator the basic aim in trimming is to remove all mesially directed forces from all mandibular teeth while permitting unimpeded eruption of the mandibular buccal teeth. To accomplish this, acrylic should rest only on the mandibular incisal edges, the most inferior portion of the mandibular alveolar processes, and as much as possible on the mandibular "basal" bone area to avoid delivering forces that might move the mandibular teeth labially. The lingual interproximal portions of acrylic in the buccal segments are trimmed so that the acrylic rests only on the soft tissue areas inferior to the teeth (see Fig. 12–19*C*). A 1.0-mm. clearance is left between the acrylic and the lingual surface of all mandibular buccal teeth to permit free eruption. Because the mandibular posterior teeth are allowed to erupt, the acrylic must be removed from the occlusal area.

Maxillary Arch. The basic trimming in this area is to prevent all eruption in the maxillary arch and, by the delivery of distal forces, to prevent further forward development of the maxillary dentoalveolar process. Because the forces must be directed against the maxillary incisors by the labial arch wire, against the molars by the dislodging spring, and against the mesiolingual sur-

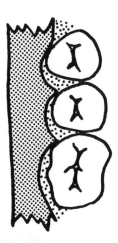

Figure 12-30. An occlusal view of the maxillary buccal segment with the acrylic of the activator contacting the mesial surface of each tooth and relieved on the distal surface. This trimming provides for posterior movement of the teeth in the maxillary buccal segment and wedges of acrylic are formed that can transmit a posterior force to the mesial of each buccal tooth in the maxillary arch.

faces of the other maxillary posterior teeth, the trimming of the maxillary portion of the activator must be precise.

To facilitate these changes the acrylic covering the maxillary incisors is left in contact with the labial surfaces of the incisors and covers the incisal edges to the level of the junction of the incisal and middle thirds of the central incisors.

A layer of acrylic is removed lingual to the maxillary incisor teeth and even with the incisal edges of the teeth, thus establishing a flat plane for the incisors to slide on as they are guided lingually and to provide room for remodeling of the lingual alveolar bone in the incisor area (see Fig. 12-43*B*).

An acrylic shelf is trimmed to inhibit eruption of the maxillary buccal teeth (see Fig. 12-19*A* and *B*). The interproximal portions of the acrylic in the maxillary buccal segments are also trimmed so that the acrylic will rest against the mesiolingual surfaces of the teeth. Thus, acrylic wedges are trimmed which can transmit a distal force to the mesial of each maxillary buccal tooth[21] (Figs. 12-21*D*, 12-30, and 12-45).

The Class III activator should arrest eruption of teeth in the buccal segments of the mandibular arch while permitting the buccal teeth to erupt in the maxillary arch. At the same time, it should provide for posterior movement of all mandibular teeth and anterior movement of all maxillary teeth. To facilitate these changes an acrylic shelf is trimmed to *inhibit* eruption of the mandibular buccal teeth (Fig. 12-31 *A* to *C*). Once again, acrylic wedges are trimmed which can transmit a distal force to each mandibular buccal tooth and a mesial force to each maxillary buccal tooth[21] (see Fig. 12-48*B*).

Much chair time can be eliminated if the trimming procedure is prefabricated into the construction of the appliance. The details of how this is accomplished are described in the Appendix under Details of Construction.

FURTHER POINTS IN APPLIANCE CONSTRUCTION AND MANIPULATION FOR CLASS II CORRECTION

A properly constructed activator maintains the predetermined bite registration vertically through contact between the acrylic of the appliance and basal bone structures in the maxilla and the mandible; hence, any vertical contact with the dentition is passive. The acrylic therefore should contact only the palate and those deepest points on the mandibular basal bone where there is no

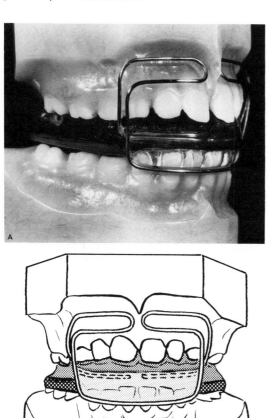

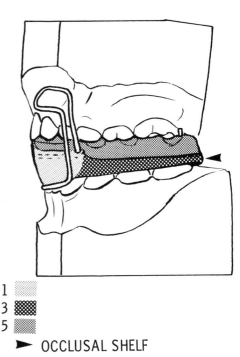

1 ░░
3 ▓▓
5 ▒▒

B ► OCCLUSAL SHELF

1 ░░
3 ▓▓
C 5 ▒▒

Figure 12–31. *A,* A Class III activotor. *B,* The lateral view of a Class III activator illustrates the acrylic shelf in the buccal segment which inhibits eruption of the mandibular teeth. The maxillary teeth are permitted unimpeded downward and forward eruption. In addition, the acrylic is trimmed so that the maxillary incisor teeth are totally free and contact is made only against the palate opposite the apical third of the maxillary incisor roots. The appliance is trimmed in the mandibular arch to permit only a distal eruption of the mandibular buccal teeth. 1 = Areas of hard acrylic contact with basal structures and also the labial surfaces of the incisor teeth. 3 = Acrylic which is left in contact with the occlusal and also the mesial surfaces of the mandibular buccal teeth. 5 = Acrylic which is removed to permit eruption and mesial movement of maxillary teeth. *C,* The figure illustrates that a total open bite is created by the bite registration, and the appliance is trimmed to permit downward and forward eruption in the entire maxillary arch to allow the therapeutically created open bite to close. 1 = Areas of hard acrylic contact with basal structures and also the labial surfaces of the incisor teeth. 3 = Acrylic which is left in contact with the occlusal and also the mesial surfaces of the mandibular buccal teeth. 5 = Acrylic which is removed to permit eruption and mesial movement of maxillary teeth.

frenum impingement (see Fig. 12–21*A* to *C*). Because the mandibular portion of the activator is wedge-shaped and fits accurately against mandibular basilar structures with no relief permitted, the mandibular anchorage is effectively controlled. Any forces which the appliance directs mesially against the mandible as the jaw attempts to retract to centric relation will be dissipated against basal bone rather than the teeth. Anchorage preservation is further reinforced through the relief afforded lingual to the mandibular incisor teeth (see Fig. 12–21*C*), and through the incisor protection obtained by covering as much as possible of the labial surfaces of the mandibular incisor teeth, the appliance can apply very little mesial force to the mandibular dentition even if the mandible drops out of it.

To further assist in retaining the appliance in position while sleeping, the mandibular lingual flange is extended (see Fig. 12–21 *A* and *B*) deeply lingual to the molars to condition the patient to retain the activator in his mouth. If he tries to remove it with his tongue, the deep flanges, which are undercut, will rub on the undercut surfaces of the mucoperiosteum and irritate the tissues. The patient quickly learns that he can avoid this discomfort by biting firmly into the appliance. The undercut lingual flanges are therefore another important conditioning device.

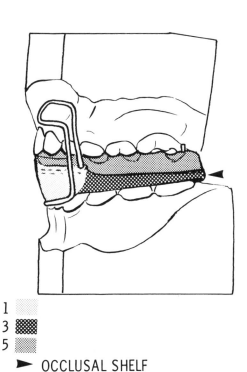

Figure 12–32. The configuration of the labial arch on the Class II activator may be altered to deliver a torquelike effect to the maxillary incisor teeth. Several degrees of torque may be obtained through the lingual activation of the torque extensions added to the arch wire, although it is difficult to obtain extensive torque with the activator.

LATERAL VIEW OF ACTIVATOR
FOR CLASS III CORRECTION

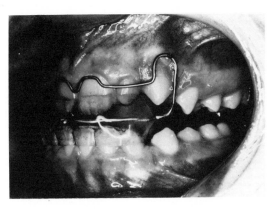

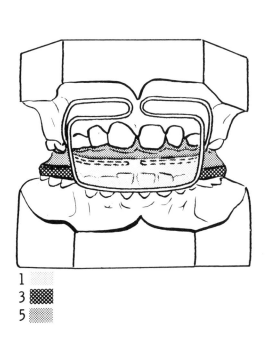

1
3
5

1
3
5

► OCCLUSAL SHELF

The maxillary labial arch extends from premolar to premolar and is in passive contact with the maxillary incisor teeth (see Fig. 12–19A). If the arch wire is kept as close as possible to the gingival margin of the teeth while the incisal edges are in firm contact with the acrylic on their labial surfaces, it will counteract the tendency for the incisor crowns to assume an overly upright position. Occasionally the configuration of this arch may be altered to deliver a torque-like effect to the maxillary incisor teeth (Fig. 12–32), and several degrees of torque may be obtained through the lingual activation of torque extensions added to the arch wire. It is, however, difficult to obtain extensive torque with the activator.

It is important to avoid relieving the palate in the maxillary arch because definite basal bone contact in the maxillary and mandibular arches is needed to assist in maintaining the stretch of muscles and associated tissues which provides the forces. If, however, one wishes to expand the maxillary arch, the palate may be temporarily removed so that the vertical thrust of the appliance is delivered against the lateral portions of the maxillary buccal segment alveolar process, which is then thrust laterally. Alternatively, the palatal acrylic can be shaved lightly with an acrylic bur to produce the expansion required to change an occlusion from Class II to Class I. The maxillary arch must expand approximately one-fourth inch to achieve this change. As an additional measure, the maxillary acrylic can be trimmed to an outward slope (Fig. 12–33) to allow the maxillary buccal teeth to erupt to a greater width. However, this is unnecessary because the width will change along the occlusal shelf (see Fig. 12–19) in activators that permit no eruption of the maxillary dentition. An elaborate wire configuration in the buccal area (Fig. 12–19) using heavy-gauge wire will hold the cheeks laterally and permit further expansion of the maxillary arch if this is desirable. This principle is similar to that employed by the Fränkel appliance. In addition, such a configuration will assist the cheeks to hold the appliance in position. Some practitioners routinely expand the palate with a removable expansion appliance before placing the activator in environ-

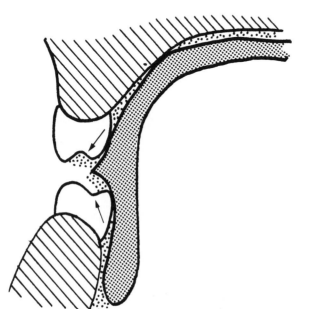

Figure 12-33. The maxillary arch may be expanded by cutting the buccal acrylic in the freeway space on an outward slope to allow the maxillary buccal teeth to erupt to a greater width. While many clinicians achieve expansion in this manner, this is unnecessary because the width will change along the maxillary shelf in activators that permit no eruption of the maxillary dentition.

mentally narrowed maxillary arches, but this is not necessary if the clinician pays attention to the details noted above.

Heavy-gauge dislodging springs are placed passively against the maxillary first permanent molars and adjusted distally 0.5 mm. These are not intended to move the molars distally but to create a dislodging action within the appliance. Such action conditions the patient to bite firmly into the appliance to keep it in position; for this reason, the dislodging springs act as additional activators of the muscles of mastication. They also provide friction against the mesial of the maxillary first permanent molar and, in activators where the acrylic has been trimmed occlusally in the maxillary buccal segments, tend to prevent its eruption. Thus, dislodging springs may assist in the correct manipulation of the functional occlusal plane (see Fig. 12–44).

In treated children with marked overclosure, wide interocclusal clearance, and resultant deep overbite, a vertical relationship of the teeth should be established in which the rest position lower face height approximates the occlusal position lower face height. To accomplish this treatment objective, considerable eruption must be obtained in the buccal segments to eliminate the excess freeway space maintained by these patients. In such cases, eruption is permitted in the maxillary buccal segments as well as the mandibular buccal segments, but the occlusal shelf should be removed in the maxillary buccal segment area only after considerable eruption has been obtained in the mandibular arch. Thus, the buccal teeth are permitted to erupt in both arches, but the mandibular buccal teeth are permitted to erupt 3 to 5 mm. more than the maxillary buccal teeth. This facilitates correct manipulation of the functional occlusal plane while at the same time enabling a practical closure of excessive interocclusal clearances. A lip bumper may be used in conjunction with light Class II elastics to assist in the required elevation of the mandibular buccal segments in such cases (see Fig. 12–27).

THE USE OF THE ACTIVATOR IN THE MANAGEMENT OF CLASS III MALOCCLUSIONS

The activator forms a useful method for intercepting moderate Class III malocclusions that exhibit normal or slightly less than normal lower face heights. The bite registration in such cases is obtained by rotating the mandible open the desired vertical amount, using one of the three vertical levels of bite registration described previously. No protrusive excursion of the mandible is desired or obtained in the Class III bite registration.

The appliance is trimmed to achieve a functional occlusal plane manipulation opposite to that encouraged in a Class II malocclusion. In other words, no eruption of the mandibular teeth is permitted while the maxillary buccal teeth are permitted an unimpeded downward and forward eruption. In addition, the acrylic is trimmed so that the maxillary incisor teeth are totally free and contact is made only against the palate opposite the apical third of the maxillary incisor roots. A total open bite is thus created by the bite registration, and the correctly trimmed appliance thus permits a downward and forward eruption of the entire maxillary arch to allow the artificially created open bite to close (see Fig. 12–31). The appliance is trimmed in the mandibular arch to permit only a distal migration of the mandibular buccal teeth. It is postulated that the vertical stretch created in all muscles affected by insertion of the appliance will cause a migration of either the origins or insertions of the muscles, at the bone-periosteum-muscle interface and will ultimately restore the resting length of the musculature. When such a change is accomplished in combination with vertical eruption of the maxillary incisor teeth, the direction of growth expressed at the chin may be altered from downward and forward to a more vertical direction, if the therapy is long-range and is carried through the prepubertal growth acceleration. Therefore, the appliance is used in an attempt to obtain a permanent alteration in mandibular posture and mandibular growth direction in the treatment of Class III malocclusions due to mandibular prognathism. Because such an alteration will increase the lower face height, it may enhance this dimension to undesirable levels in those patients who have excess lower face height at the beginning of treatment. Excess lower face height at the initiation of treatment is therefore a definite contraindication to Class III treatment with activators. Management of Class III cases with activators is much more effective in those patients who have Class III skeletal tendencies in combination with mesial functional displacement of the mandible and the overclosure which accompanies such conditions. In such children, the changes initiated by the activator will do much to resolve the total problem without causing further deterioration of the face in the vertical plane of space.

The labial wire configuration (see Fig. 12–31) is used in the maxillary arch as a maxillary lip bumper or labial muscle appliance. Fränkel utilizes the same philosophy in his appliance. At each appointment the maxillary labial portion is activated labially to hold the lips away from the maxillary teeth so that their downward and forward eruption may continue unimpeded. Thus, the labial musculature is utilized to provide additional thrust to the appliance. The appliance is relieved lingual to the mandibular incisors if the operator desires a moderate amount of lingual tipping of these teeth. The precautions relative to contact between maxillary and mandibular basal bone structures and the acrylic as outlined previously in discussing the Class II activator apply also to the Class III activator.

ADVANTAGES AND DISADVANTAGES OF ACTIVATOR THERAPY

The activator is a limited appliance for use in highly selected cases only. Careful case selection requires a clear understanding of the use of cephalometric radiography in assessing the facial morphology underlying the malocclusion and particularly an understanding of the assessment of excess lower face height, which constitutes a clear-cut contraindication to activator treatment in both Class II and Class III cases. While all orthodontic appliances require good cooperation, successful use of the activator requires superb patient cooperation. The practitioner should not spend undue time with uncooperative patients but, in his presentation to the parents, should make provision to change to headgear or multibanded therapy. However, the patient who does poorly with the activator will usually do poorly with other forms of orthodontic treatment unless the reason for lack of co-operation was allergy or nasal stenosis (inability to breathe with the appliance in place).

It was noted previously that the activator cannot produce a detailed precise finishing of the occlusion. In some instances, it is possible to refine the occlusion further through the use of a tooth positioner. If, before initial fabrication of the positioner, the positioner set-up is mounted on the articulator in vertically opened and protrusive bite registration, the positioner achieves an activator-like effect as well as a tooth-positioning effect. This effect can be used to correct a Class II malocclusion to the extent of one fourth to one third of a cusp. Such an articulator mounting must never be used where positioners are used to detail the occlusion in cases which were previously Class III. In such problems, the articulator pin is merely opened and the mandible is rotated vertically without the protrusive bite registration used in Class II bite registrations.

In most instances, the specialty-trained orthodontist uses the activator primarily for orthodontic interception and pre-orthodontic guidance in the management of major malocclusions. In such management, part of the original apical base dysplasia is corrected with the activator while the teeth erupt into improved positions, either in a nonextraction or an extraction treatment plan. The activator treatment is then followed by a short phase of multibanded therapy to detail the occlusion and obtain additional reduction in apical base dysplasia. The clinician should keep in mind that an occlusion finished to the standard customarily demanded in North America can be obtained only in highly selected activator cases and that accessory periods of multibanded therapy are frequently required to complete the result.

In spite of these limitations, the activator does have many advantages in the pre-orthodontic guidance of the occlusion. Its chief advantages are that it provides excellent control in the vertical dimension, particularly in overclosure cases (see Fig. 12–10), and, in the correction of malocclusion, uses the existing growth of the jaws to the maximum. During treatment, the patient experiences minimal oral hygiene problems and minimal tissue damage and tissue irritation. In addition, the intervals between adjustments may be longer than with multibanded orthodontic therapy, although it is advisable to see the patient briefly at six- to eight-week intervals to maintain an interested mental attitude and continued motivation in the patient. Such appointments are brief and usually consist of checking to make sure that none of the mandibular buccal teeth are impeded in their vertical eruption through contact with the acrylic on the lingual surfaces of these teeth, and recording the overjet so that its reduction may be checked from visit to visit. Because the initial appliance construction and the treatment appointments are brief, the method can provide more economical treatment in those cases that are suitable for activator correction. It is further useful in the correction of malocclusion with associated habits such as thumb-sucking and tongue-thrusting, and indeed the patient may obtain gratification from the activator instead of the thumb and obtain excellent action with the appliance.

SUMMARY OF INDICATIONS AND CONTRAINDICATIONS

The indications for the activator may be summarized as follows:

1. It is used primarily in actively growing individuals with favorable facial growth patterns (see Figs. 12–10, 12–27, 12–34 and 12–35).

Text continued on page 326

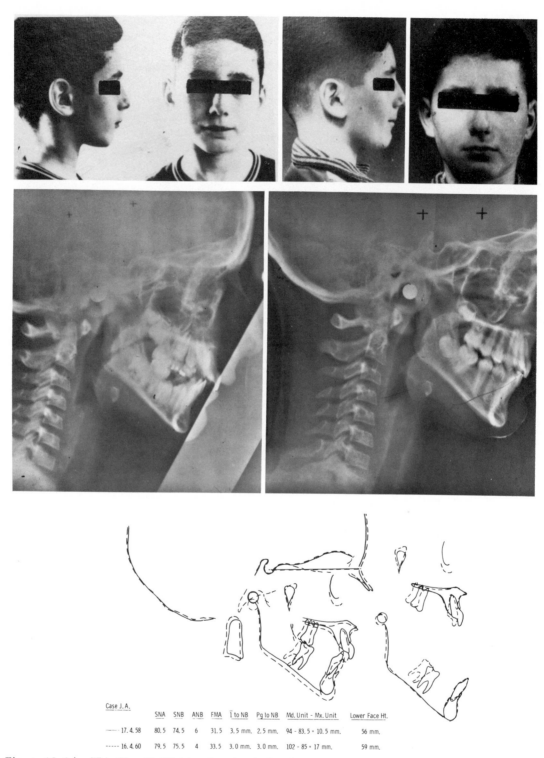

Case J.A.								
	SNA	SNB	ANB	FMA	Ī to NB	Pg to NB	Md. Unit - Mx. Unit	Lower Face Ht.
——— 17. 4. 58	80. 5	74. 5	6	31. 5	3. 5 mm.	2. 5 mm.	94 - 83. 5 = 10. 5 mm.	56 mm.
----- 16. 4. 60	79. 5	75. 5	4	33. 5	3. 0 mm.	3. 0 mm.	102 - 85 = 17 mm.	59 mm.

Figure 12–34. This Class II, Division 1, malocclusion illustrates the use of the activator in severely muti-
lated cases where it is not possible to use bands. The patient's family dentist removed $\frac{6E}{6ED} \bigg| \frac{E6}{ED6}$ immedi-
ately prior to the patient's presenting for treatment. An activator was used in the preorthodontic treat-
ment of this problem while waiting for $\frac{7}{7} \bigg| \frac{7}{7}$ to erupt. Correction was accomplished by a combination of

Illustration continued on opposite page

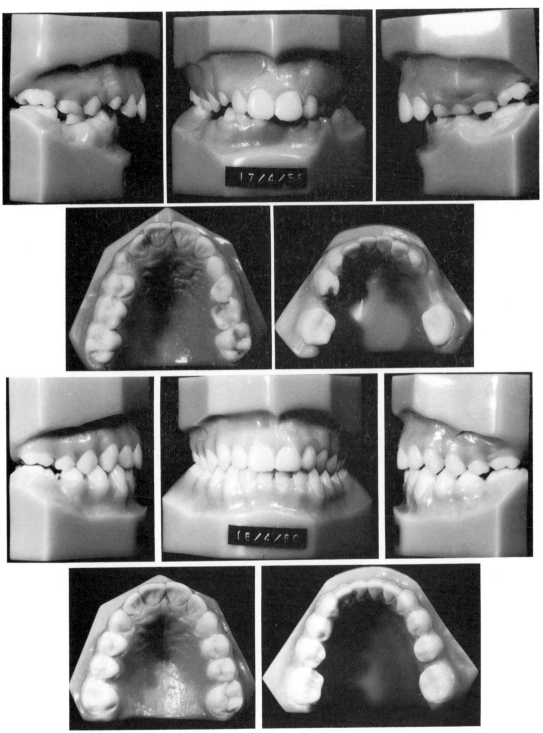

Figure 12-34 *Continued.*

favorable mandibular growth increment and direction relative to the midfacial growth. Correct manipulation of the functional occlusal plane and lingual tipping of the maxillary incisors assisted. The mandibular unit–maxillary unit difference of 10.5 mm. showed the presence of a severe mismatch in size between the maxilla and mandible. This did not show in the ANB difference of 6 degrees because the dentition was overclosed as indicated by the lower face height of 56 mm. prior to treatment. The patient's parents did not elect to have the second permanent molars uprighted following the activator treatment.

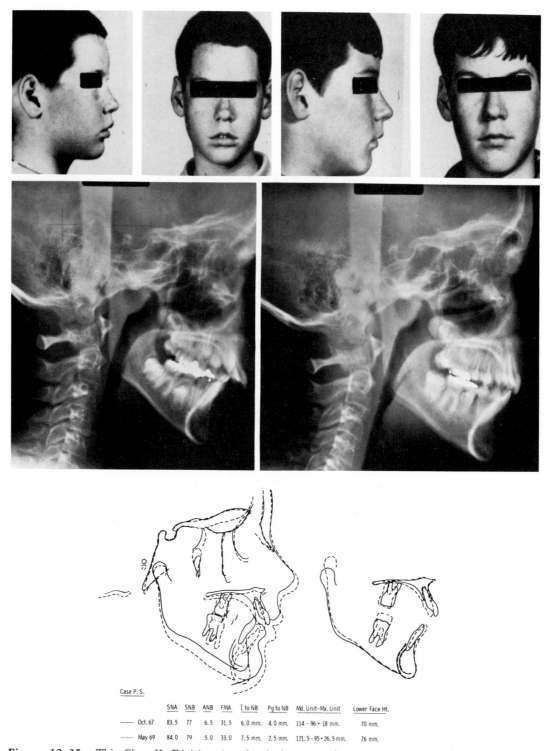

	SNA	SNB	ANB	FMA	Ī to NB	Pg to NB	Md. Unit-Mx. Unit	Lower Face Ht.
—— Oct. 67	83.5	77	6.5	31.5	6.0 mm.	4.0 mm.	114 - 96 • 18 mm.	70 mm.
----- May 69	84.0	79	5.0	33.0	7.5 mm.	2.5 mm.	121.5 - 95 • 26.5 mm.	76 mm.

Case P. S.

Figure 12–35. This Class II, Division 1 malocclusion treated with an activator illustrates the severe anchorage loss in the mandibular arch which may occur if the lingual flange of the appliance is not closely adapted to the lingual portion of the mandibular basal bone. The functional occlusal plane was treated correctly by restricting maxillary molar eruption and permitting the mandibular molars to erupt in harmony with the vertical component of mandibular growth. Retraction of the maxillary dentition assisted in the correction, although this amount of dental movement is not commonly seen by the author.

Illustration continued on opposite page

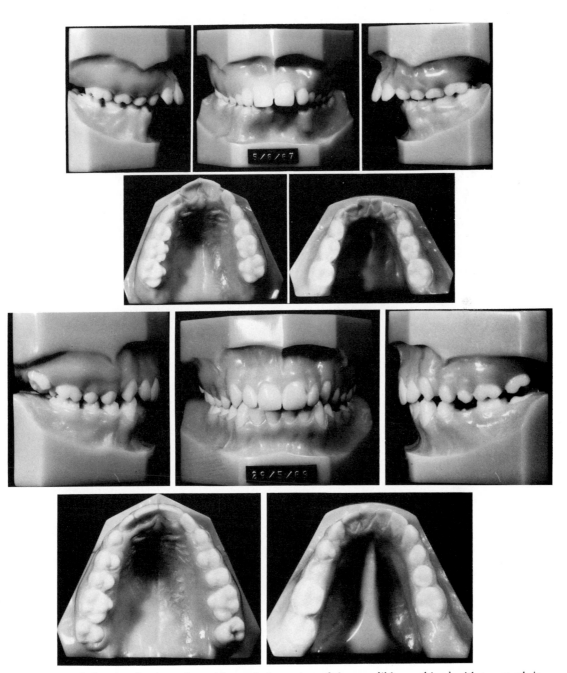

Figure 12-35 *Continued.* An unfavorable vertical rotation of the mandible combined with too much increase in lower face height occurred, and these are common sequelae to activator treatment. The author would probably not treat this case with an activator today owing to the large lower face height prior to treatment. The occlusal correction is unsatisfactory at this stage and requires other treatment procedures to complete it. The excessive lingual inclination of the maxillary incisors is another common unfavorable result of activator treatment.

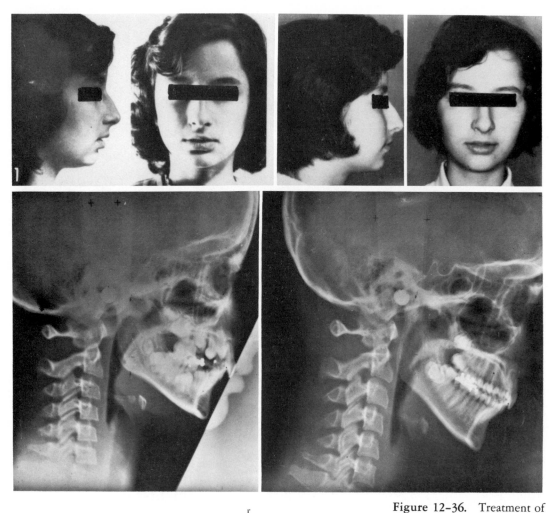

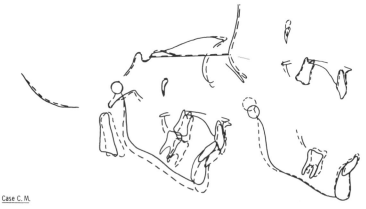

Case C. M.

	SNA	SNB	ANB	FMA	$\overline{1}$ to NB	Pg to NB	Md. Unit-Mx. Unit	Lower Face Ht.
—— 24. 1. 59	83.0	75	8.0	29	5.5 mm.	2 mm.	94.5 - 83.5 = 11 mm.	49.0 mm.
--- 4. 12. 62	83.5	77	6.5	26	6.5 mm.	2 mm.	102.5-85 = 17.5 mm.	52.5 mm.

Figure 12–36. Treatment of this Class II, Division 2 case took a long time to accomplish (3 years). This was because the skeletal dysplasia as indicated by the mandibular unit–maxillary unit difference (11.0 mm.) was extremely severe in this midface prognathism case. The dysplasia is more severe than is evident in the ANB difference of 8 degrees because the case was severely overclosed (lower face height 49.0 mm.), and this tended to mask the true extent of the dysplasia. Treatment was accomplished by holding the maxillary dentition in its original position while an orthognathically growing mandible advanced at a slow rate. The functional occlusal plane was handled correctly. Patient co-operation was average and the mandibular anchorage was slipped unfavorably. The case illustrates the difficulty in torquing maxillary incisor teeth with activators. Other methods of orthodontic management, including rhinoplasty, would have been more satisfactory for the management of this case of midface prognathism. The activator does have the advantage in such problems that the retraction of maxillary incisor teeth can be minimal and thus avoid further complicating the problem created by excess nose growth.

Illustration continued on opposite page

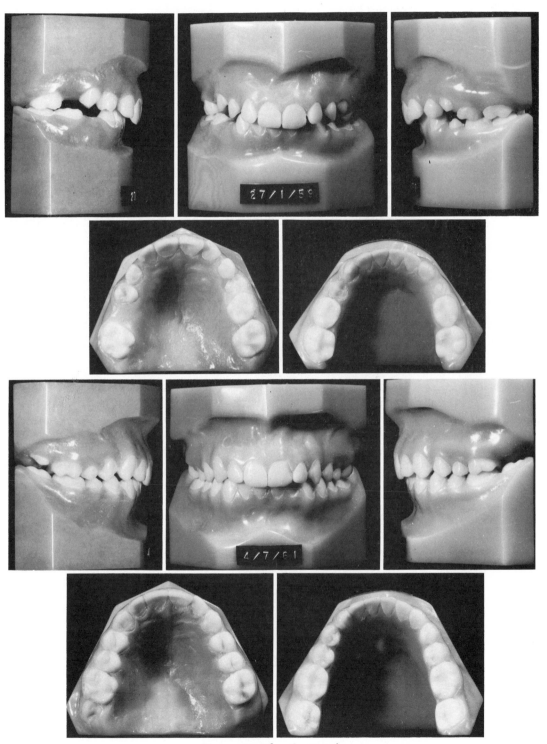

Figure 12–36   *Continued.*

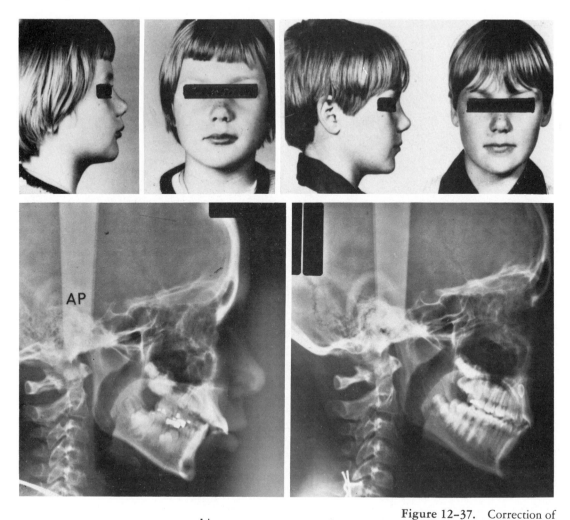

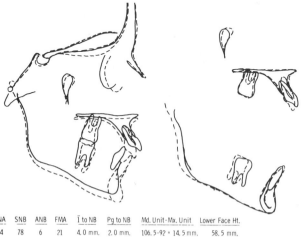

Case A.P.

	SNA	SNB	ANB	FMA	Ī to NB	Pg to NB	Md. Unit-Mx. Unit	Lower Face Ht.
——— May 66	84	78	6	21	4.0 mm.	2.0 mm.	106.5-92 = 14.5 mm.	58.5 mm.
------ Apr. 68	82	77	5	21	7.0 mm.	3.0 mm.	110-91.5 = 18.5 mm.	62.5 mm.

Figure 12–37. Correction of this Class II, Division 1 malocclusion was accomplished using an activator combined with a mandibular labial muscle appliance (lip bumper) and a mandibular leveling arch in the final two months of treatment. There was a good increment of growth expressed at the chin relative to minimal forward growth of the midface at ANS. The moderate amount of *vertical* growth expressed at the chin represents a problem which must be controlled by permitting minimal eruption of the teeth in the buccal segments to avoid creating a mandibular rotation. If measurements of the overjet made at the six-week check-up visits show the overjet to be stationary or increasing in spite of good appliance wear, the patient is either growing predominantly in a horizontal direction or is on a growth plateau. In such circumstances the eruption of teeth in both arches must be impeded by placing acrylic over the occlusal surfaces of the teeth in the buccal segments.

Illustration continued on opposite page

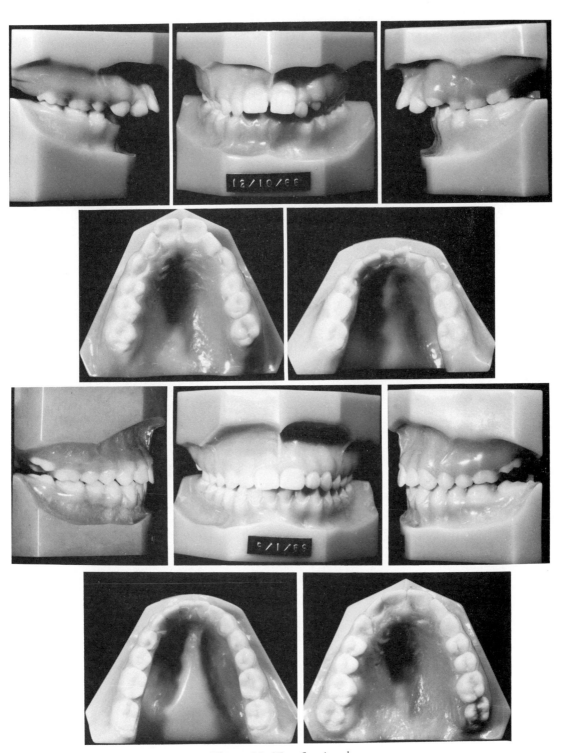

Figure 12–37 *Continued.*

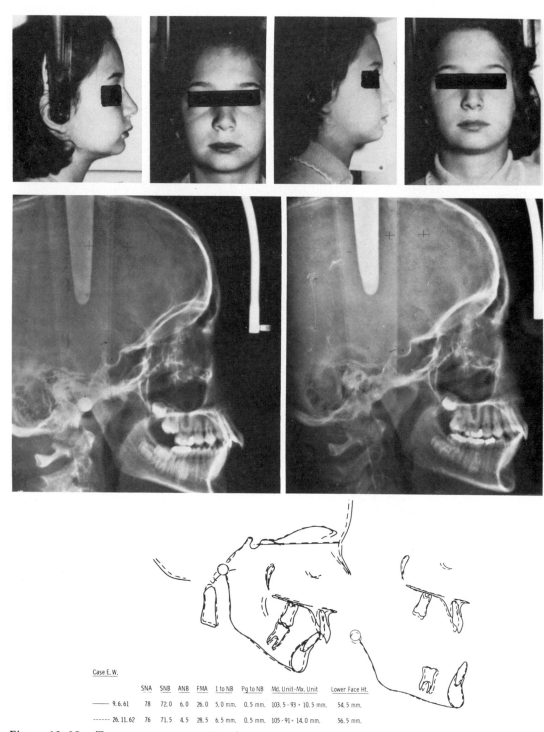

Case E. W.

	SNA	SNB	ANB	FMA	1 to NB	Pg to NB	Md. Unit-Mx. Unit	Lower Face Ht.
—— 9.6.61	78	72.0	6.0	26.0	5.0 mm.	0.5 mm.	103.5 - 93 = 10.5 mm.	54.5 mm.
------ 26.11.62	76	71.5	4.5	28.5	6.5 mm.	0.5 mm.	105 - 91 = 14.0 mm.	56.5 mm.

Figure 12–38. Treatment was accomplished primarily by lingual movement of the maxillary dentition in this nongrowing case. The mandibular anchorage was preserved. Moderate eruption of the maxillary molars occurred and probably contributed to the moderate mandibular rotation which occurred. Such successful results in nongrowing dysplasias with overclosure such as this are rare and the usual result is a reciprocal slippage of the alveolar processes in both jaws. (By kind permission of Dr. A. L. Posen.)

Illustration continued on opposite page

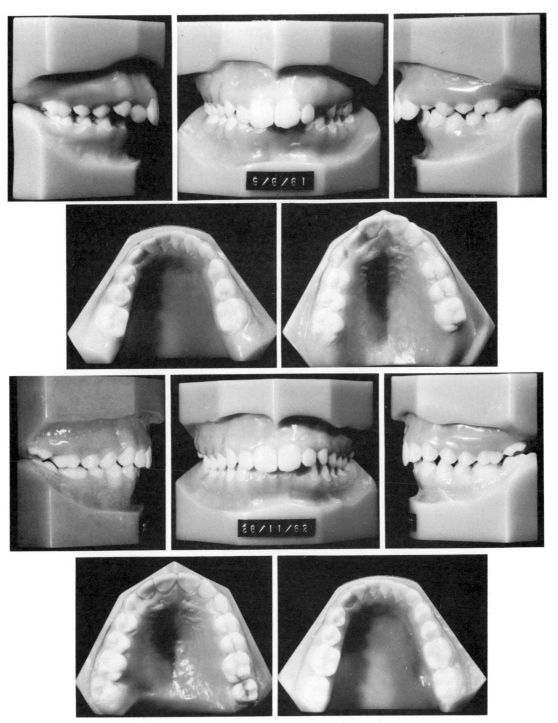

Figure 12–38 *Continued.*

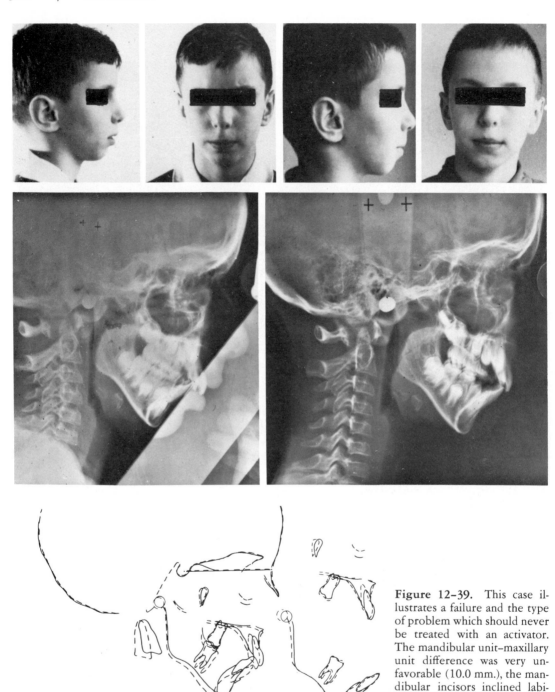

Case G. M.	SNA	SNB	ANB	FMA	Ī to NB	Pg to NB	Md. Unit - Mx. Unit	Lower Face Ht.
——— 22. 11. 58	78.0	70.5	7.5	37.5	7.5 mm.	- 1.5 mm.	90.5 - 80.5 = 10 mm.	59 mm.
----- 28. 5. 60	78.5	70.0	8.5	42.0	10.0 mm.	- 2.5 mm.	96.0 - 85.0 = 11 mm.	63.5 mm.

Figure 12-39. This case illustrates a failure and the type of problem which should never be treated with an activator. The mandibular unit–maxillary unit difference was very unfavorable (10.0 mm.), the mandibular incisors inclined labially off basal bone, and the patient was not growing rapidly. The functional occlusal plane was steep and where this occurs, very minor amounts of molar eruption in nongrowing patients create very large mandibular rotations at the chin, such as occurred here. The treatment failed aesthetically and occlusally owing to incorrect case selection.

Illustration continued on opposite page

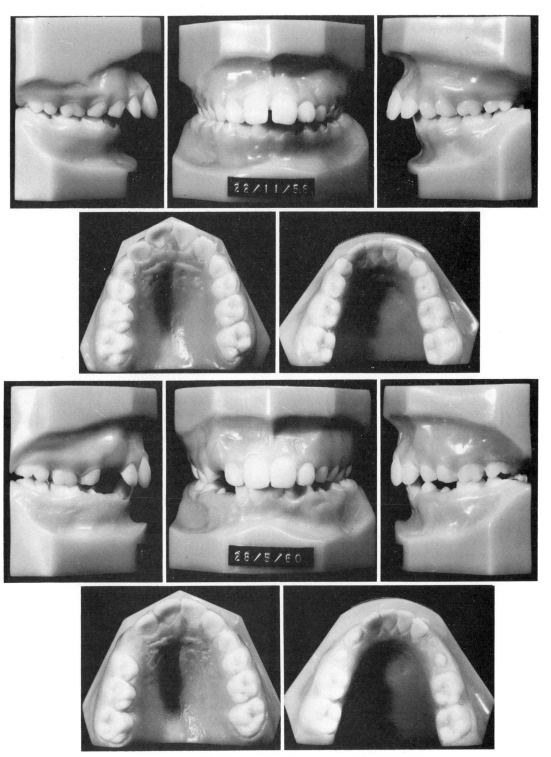

Figure 12–39 *Continued.*

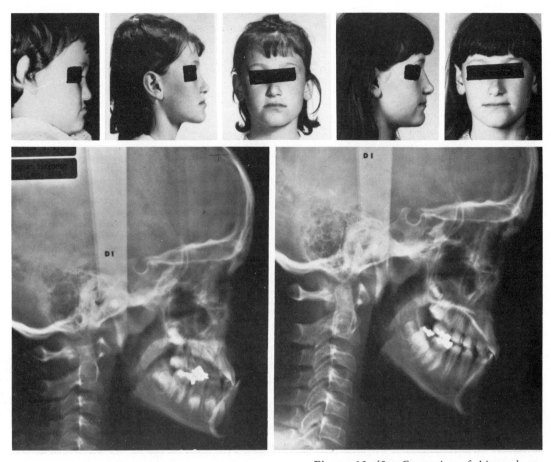

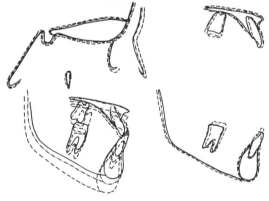

Case D. I.

	FMA	SNA	SNB	ANB	1 to NB	Pg to NB	Md. unit-Mx. unit	Lower Face Ht.
——— 10 8.63	18.0°	78.0°	82.0°	4.0°	3.5 mm.	1.5 mm.	110-86 = 25 mm.	52.0 mm.
------ 28.4.67	21.0°	83.0°	82.5°	0.5°	3.0 mm.	2.5 mm.	118.5-91.5=27mm.	58.5 mm.

Figure 12-40. Correction of this moderate Class III malocclusion was accomplished by two periods of interception with a Class III activator. Each period lasted approximately 18 months, and the tracings show a combination of treatment plus observations. The correction was accomplished by two purposeful vertical rotations of the mandible to create a retrognathic mandibular growth direction expressed at the chin. The maxillary buccal segments were allowed to develop vertically into the orthodontically created excess freeway space. During the final observation period the mandibular molars erupted, although this was not encouraged. This was not a case of mesial functional displacement of the mandible. Moderate labial tipping of the maxillary incisors was obtained by the periodic addition to acrylic to the activator in the area contacting the lingual apical areas of the maxillary incisors. At no time did the appliance touch the crowns of the maxillary incisors. Class III cases with excess lower face height prior to treatment are not suitable for this type of conservative Class III treatment.

Illustration continued on opposite page

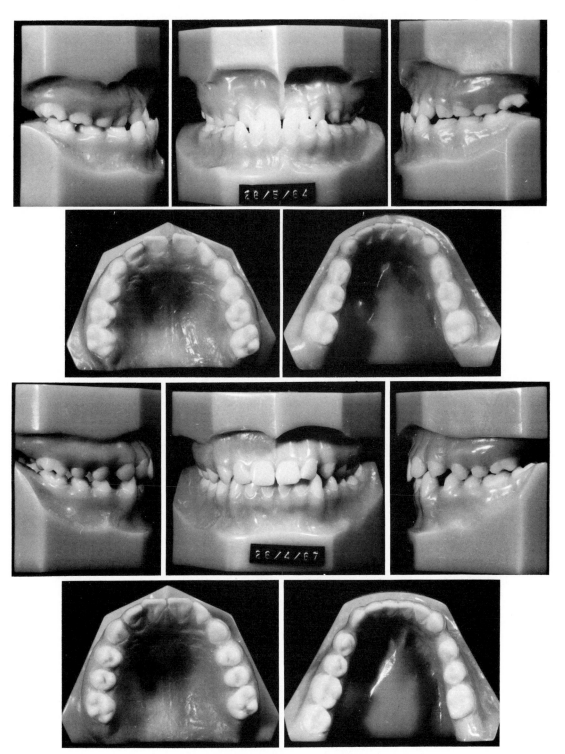

Figure 12–40   *Continued.*

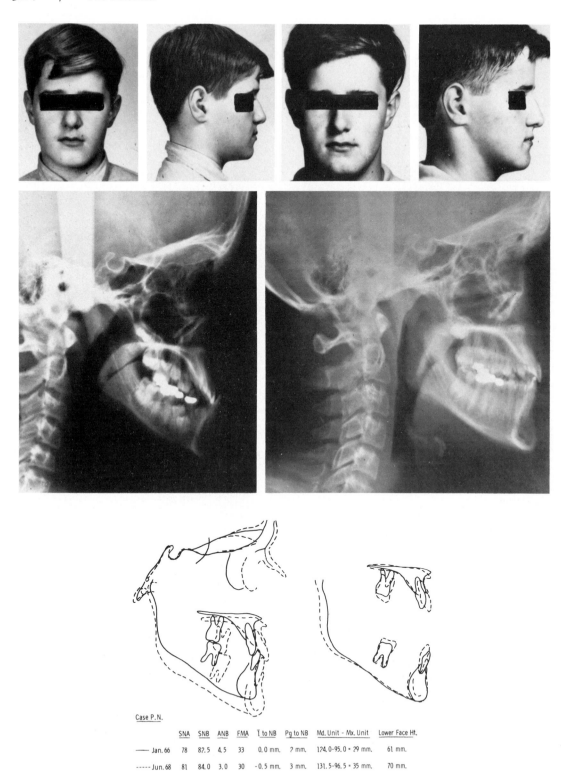

Case P.N.

	SNA	SNB	ANB	FMA	$\overline{1}$ to NB	Pg to NB	Md. Unit - Mx. Unit	Lower Face Ht.
—— Jan. 66	78	82.5	4.5	33	0.0 mm.	? mm.	124.0-95.0 = 29 mm.	61 mm.
----- Jun. 68	81	84.0	3.0	30	-0.5 mm.	3 mm.	131.5-96.5 = 35 mm.	70 mm.

Figure 12–41. This Class III malocclusion had a moderate mesial functional displacement of the mandible superimposed. While the prognathic mandible growth has been strong, favorable midface growth as shown at ANS aided in the treatment. An activator was worn on a reduced schedule at night as a retainer. Further detailing of the occlusion is required.

Illustration continued on opposite page

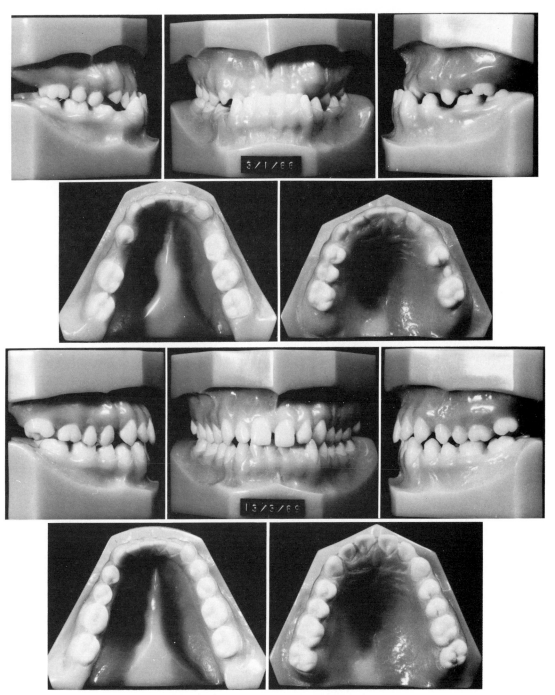

Figure 12–41 *Continued.*

2. The maxillary and mandibular teeth should be well aligned and the mandibular incisor teeth should be positioned upright over basal bone structures (see Figs. 12–10 and 12–34).

3. It provides a superb treatment in children with lack of vertical development in lower face height because differential vertical alveolar development can be readily obtained in either the maxillary or mandibular arch as desired (see Fig. 12–10).

4. It provides a useful preliminary treatment before major multibanded orthodontic mechanotherapy (Fig. 12–34).

5. It is useful for post-treatment retention in children with a deep overbite due to overclosure.

The appliance is contraindicated in the following situations:

1. The appliance is not useful in the correction of Class I problems of crowded teeth due to disharmony between tooth size and jaw size. It may, however, be used to assist in the correction of Class II malocclusions where disharmony between tooth size and jaw size has been superimposed and is being managed concurrently through serial extractions.

2. The appliance is contraindicated in children with excess lower face height and extreme vertical mandibular growth trends owing to the increase in lower face height which usually results if the use of the appliance is carried through and beyond the prepubertal growth acceleration. Because many problems of severe open bite are associated with excess lower face height, the appliance will not routinely be useful in the management of such problems (Fig. 12–35).

3. Because incorrect manipulation of the appliance tends to make mandibular incisor teeth more procumbent relative to basal bone, it should not be used in children who have even moderate amounts of such procumbency prior to the initiation of treatment (Figs. 12–35 and 12–36).

4. The appliance cannot be used effectively in children with nasal stenosis due either to structural problems within the nose or to chronic untreated allergy. Some clinicians routinely place breathing holes in the appliance to assist their patients during periods of temporary nasal stenosis associated with nasorespiratory infections.

5. The appliance has limited application in nongrowing individuals, although it may be used successfully in such individuals if the clinician has determined that the patient's facial morphology will tolerate an increase in lower face height. However, treatment changes tend to be slow in adults because the appliance makes use of vertical eruption of buccal teeth and such eruption may be very slow in nongrowing individuals (see Fig. 12–38).

A series of case reports (Figs. 12–10, 12–27, and 12–34 to 12–41) illustrates some of the uses of and contraindications to activator therapy. These cases have been selected for illustration purposes because they did not receive any multibanded orthodontic therapy. They will therefore illustrate not only the possibilities of activator treatment but also its limitations as a sole method of treatment. Several of the cases were selected to show situations in which activator treatment should not have been initiated (and represent distinct failures and misdiagnosis—Figs. 12–35 and 12–39).

Finally, it must be recognized that this method of orthodontic treatment is not a panacea; patients must be selected with care and attention paid to every detail in its manipulation. Indiscriminate application of the method will do much to discredit this useful addition to the clinician's orthodontic armamentarium.

APPENDIX

TECHNICAL DIRECTIONS TO TECHNICIANS REGARDING THE CONSTRUCTION OF THE ACTIVATOR

The activator is constructed of exothermic self-curing acrylic on stone models of the maxillary and mandibular arches. The mandibular impression should be extended deeply on the lingual side in the first and second permanent molar areas. The impression thus extends into an undercut area of the mandible to permit the extrusion of a deep lingual flange which assists holding the appliance in position (see Fig. 12–21A).

Decide whether to use bite registration 1, 2, or 3 as described previously and register the bite using a thick roll of softened baseplate wax. Wax bites should be kept in a jar of water at room temperature to minimize distortion until assembled on the casts for mounting on an articulator. In mounting the casts on an articulator the final coat of plaster on the upper articulator arm should never be more than one-fourth inch thick, because the setting plaster may distort the arm. All adjustments on the articulator should be locked in centric and the pin made even with the upper arm of the articulator. This is important because the pin may be removed during the construction of the wire work and then replaced accurately.

Design of the Labial Arch Wire

The labial arch wire and the dislodging spring wires are bent and fitted according to the needs of each case, using 0.036 inch stainless steel round wire, and put aside for future use. The labial arch wire is commonly of two designs, one as used in the construction of a Hawley retainer and the other as used in the labial wire of an Andresen appliance. A modified Andresen design is used when there has been considerable narrowing of the maxillary arch in the canine area due to muscle contraction force. This design relieves the force of the cheeks from the maxillary canine area and permits normal arch form to be restored in this area (see Figs. 12–1 and 12–21B). An adhesive tape relief will prevent impingement of the labial arch wire on the gingival tissues in the finished appliance. Therefore (a) place two layers of one-half inch wide adhesive tape on the soft tissue area of the model gingival to the canines, if the wire work is similar to a conventional Hawley appliance; (b) place four layers of one-half inch wide tape on any soft tissue area over which the Andresen design labial wire is to be shaped (Fig. 12–42B (c) if the wire work is to include the mandibular arch as in an activator for Class III treatment, the adhesive tape relief is placed accordingly (Fig. 12–42C).

Placement of Lingual Relief

In the Class II activator, relief is placed lingual to the incisor teeth in both arches. In the maxillary arch, this relief permits remodeling of the alveolar process as the incisors are guided lingually (Fig. 12–43A and B); in the mandibular arch, it ensures that no force will be applied by the appliance to tip the incisors labially (Fig. 12–43C).

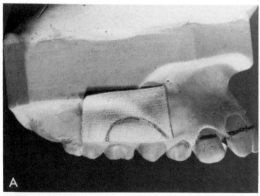
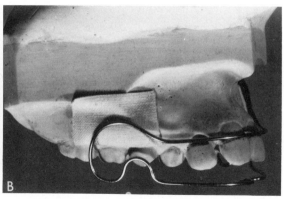
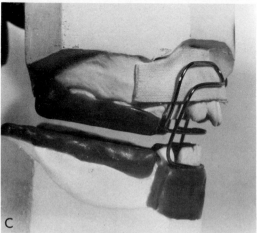

Figure 12-42. *A,* The form of the labial arch for a Class II activator is outlined on the relief tape and teeth. *B,* Four thicknesses of adhesive tape relief for the labial arch on a Class II activator. All bends made in the tag end for purposes of retention should be in the horizontal plane of space and are carried anteriorly in a symmetrical arc at the middle of the freeway space approximately 1 to 2 mm. labial to the maxillary incisors. *C,* Four thicknesses of adhesive tape relief for the labial arch on a Class III activator.

The relief in both arches is carried apically to a point approximating the junction of the apical and middle thirds of the roots of the incisors, tapering and blending in with the soft tissue at this point. It must not be carried any closer than 5 mm. to the lingual fold on the mandibular cast, because the appliance must contact the tissue overlying basal bone in order to reinforce the mandibular anchorage (see Fig. 12–21C). In a Class III activator, relief is placed on the lingual of the mandibular cast *only* and no relief is placed on the maxillary cast.

If exothermic self-curing acrylic is used, baseplate wax is adequate for the relief. If endothermic heat-cured acrylic is used, plaster of Paris should be used to afford a contrast with the stone cast.

Construction of Labial Arch

If the wire design is of the Hawley type, the tag ends are carried anteriorly in a symmetrical arc at the middle of the freeway space and kept approximately 1 to 2 mm. labial to the maxillary incisors. All bends made in the tag ends for the purpose of retention should be in the horizontal plane of space (see Fig. 12–42B).

If the labial wire is of the Andresen type, the form is outlined on the relief tape and teeth as illustrated (see Fig. 12–42A). The crest of the loop gingival to the canine areas should not be high enough to impinge on the mucobuccal fold.

A length of 0.032 to 0.036 inch wire is adapted to the labial surfaces of the incisors at the junction of the gingival and middle thirds of the crowns. This wire is kept straight in the horizontal plane from the junction of the middle and distal vertical thirds of one lateral incisor to the same location on the opposite side of the arch. The arch form should be kept symmetrical to avoid perpetuating minor irregularities in incisor alignment. Any loops lying over the canine area should have 1 to 1.5 mm. clearance to the labial to permit freedom for movement of the canine tooth. Such loops are occasionally used in the final stages of treatment to guide erupting canine teeth lingually when required.

The labial wire is checked for passiveness and sealed to the cast on the gingival side of the wire along the central incisors and at the loops over the premolar and canine areas. Wax should not be permitted to flow incisally to the wire.

Dislodging Springs

Dislodging springs (Fig. 12–44*A* and *B*) are made of 0.035 to 0.036 inch wire so that they can apply an undermining force to the molars and intermittently dislodge the appliance from close contact with the teeth. The diameter of the helix is established by shaping the spring around the round beak of a pair of 139 or 390T pliers at a point near the throat to produce a coil with an outside diameter of 8 to 9 mm. The straight

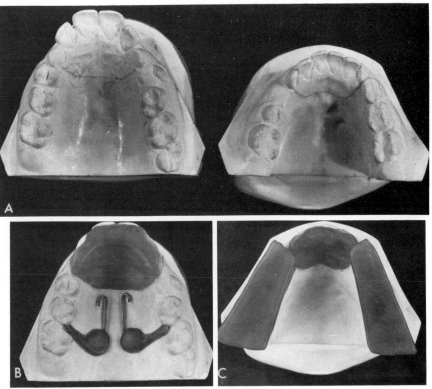

Figure 12–43. *A*, The pencil outline for relief areas lingual to the maxillary and mandibular incisors. *B*, The wax relief lingual to the maxillary incisors is illustrated. This relief is carried lingually from the central incisors approximately 5.0 mm. on the same plane as the incisal edges and usually in a horizontal plane. A slight inclination from horizontal is sometimes used to control intrusion or extrusion of the incisors. The relief is carried from cuspid to cuspid in an arc which provides about 2.0 mm. lingual relief when the distal of the cuspid is reached. The illustration also shows wax placed over the active arm of the molar springs. *C*, The wax relief lingual to the mandibular incisors is illustrated. This relief is in a level plane flush with the incisal edges of the central incisors and is carried lingually for approximately 3.0 mm. arcing from the distal of each cuspid with a lingual extension of approximately 2.0 mm. The illustration shows that the occlusal surfaces of the buccal teeth in the mandibular cast are prepared with a wax platform which is carried occlusally to an approximate height of 5 to 7 mm. and is as wide as the buccolingual width of the buccal teeth. This platform should be parallel to the wax on the maxillary cast.

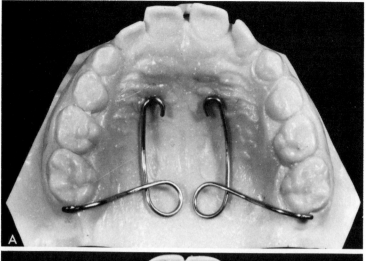

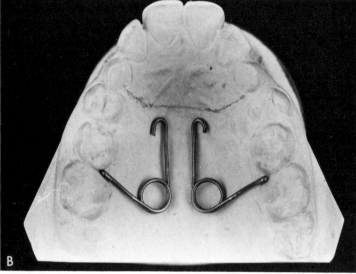

Figure 12–44. *A,* The dislodging spring design used in a Class II activator. *B,* The dislodging spring design used in a Class III activator.

part of the lever arm should be approximately 15 mm. long. The end of this arm, which fits into the embrasure, should be bent back vertically on itself for approximately 2 mm. to afford more contact against the proximal surface of the tooth and eliminate any sharp ends.

The spring for a Class II activator is placed over the palate, with the anterior arc of the coil opposite the mesioproximal surface of the first permanent molar. The only part of the spring that touches soft tissue is in the embrasure and at the helix, the rest having a 0.5 to 1.0 mm. palatal relief. The active arm of the spring always rests on the occlusal side of the helix so that the helix will unwind when activated. The spring for a Class III activator is the reverse of that for a Class II. It unwinds with the thrust in a mesial direction and, in its placement on the palate, the distal part of the helix lies in line with the distoproximal surface of the first permanent molar (Fig. 12–44B).

The tag end of the dislodging spring, which will be embedded in acrylic, extends approximately 15 mm. anteriorly where it terminates in a hook for retention. It is shaped to the contour of the palate with 0.5 to 1.0 mm. relief at all points. If exothermic acrylic is to be used, enough baseplate wax is placed (Fig. 12–43B) on the active arm and helix of the spring to secure it to the cast and to prevent acrylic from contacting these parts. Wax must be kept away from the tag end, which is to be embedded in the acrylic. If endothermic acrylic is to be used, the spring is held in place with temporary cement or plaster of Paris.

Prefabrication of Trimming

A considerable amount of chair time can be eliminated from the trimming procedure if areas are blocked out on the casts, using wax for exothermic acrylic appliances or plaster for endothermic acrylic appliances. The activator will then have the trimming processed into it. The method is described using wax to provide for inhibition of eruption of the maxillary buccal teeth and at the same time to provide for posterior movement of these teeth. The occlusal surfaces of the buccal teeth in the maxillary cast are covered with baseplate wax and this is built up occlusally until only the cusp tips are exposed. Wax, approximately 1 mm. thick, is flowed on the entire distolingual surface of each posterior tooth into the center of each embrasure. No wax is applied on the mesiolingual surface of these teeth. Thus, when the acrylic is applied, wedges are formed that can transmit a posterior force to the mesial of each buccal tooth in the maxillary arch (Fig. 12–45).

The occlusal surfaces of the buccal teeth in the mandibular cast are prepared in a similar manner with the wax carried occlusally to an approximate height of 5 to 7 mm.; this builds a flat platform which is as wide as the buccolingual width of the buccal teeth. This platform should be parallel with the wax on the maxillary cast (see Fig. 12–43C). If the above steps have been followed, there should be a space of 2 to 3 mm. between the two arches in the buccal segments (Fig. 12–46A and B). When the acrylic is applied, it forms a shelf in the space between the maxillary and mandibular casts in the area of the buccal segments. It is this shelf that inhibits the eruption of the maxillary buccal teeth (see Fig. 12–19A to C). The embrasures on the lingual surfaces of the mandibular buccal teeth are filled with wax so that no acrylic contacts the lingual surfaces of the mandibular buccal teeth. Figure 12–47 illustrates the placement of wax on the lateral portions of the labial arch to prevent this part from becoming embedded in acrylic.

The Class III activator should arrest eruption of teeth in the buccal segments of the mandibular arch while permitting the buccal teeth to erupt in the maxillary arch. At the same time, it should provide for posterior movement of all mandibular teeth and anterior movement of all maxillary teeth. To facilitate tooth movements and avoid tedious chairside trimming, the occlusal surfaces of the buccal teeth of the mandibular cast are covered with baseplate wax and built up occlusally. The remaining detailed waxing is described and illustrated in Figure 12–48A. The occlusal surfaces of the maxillary buccal teeth are waxed similarly, and this is described and illustrated in Figure 12–48B. If these steps have been followed, a space of 2 to 3 mm. remains between the two arches in the buccal segments and when the acrylic is applied, wedges are formed that can transmit a mesial force to each maxillary tooth (Fig. 12–48A to C).

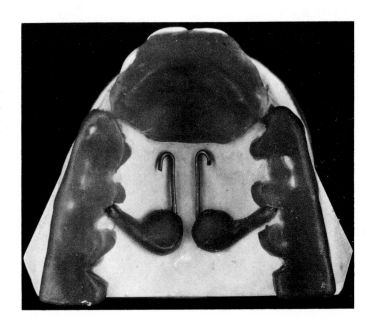

Figure 12-45. The figure shows wax, approximately 1.0 mm. thick, flowed onto the entire distolingual surface of each posterior tooth into the center of each embrasure. No wax is applied to the mesiolingual surface of the teeth. Thus, when the acrylic is applied, wedges are formed that can transmit a posterior force to the mesial of each buccal tooth in the maxillary arch.

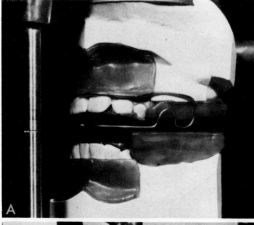
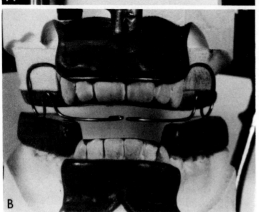

Figure 12-46. *A,* The maxillary and mandibular casts mounted on an articulator in the bite which was registered previously. Wax reliefs have been placed on the maxillary and mandibular casts lingual to the incisor teeth, occlusal to the mandibular buccal teeth, and distal to the maxillary buccal teeth. In addition, wax strips have been placed on the labial surfaces of the gingival portions of the incisor teeth to prevent acrylic from extending beyond these areas when the appliance is processed. Acrylic will extend into the space between the maxillary and mandibular occlusal wax platforms to form an occlusal shelf that will inhibit the eruption of the maxillary buccal teeth. In addition, acrylic will flow between the incisal surfaces and encompass the retentive portion of the labial arch wire which is centered in the interincisal freeway space. *B,* The frontal view illustrates the build-up of wax in the mandibular arch and the lack of occlusal wax build-up in the maxillary arch. This will permit eruption of the mandibular buccal teeth.

Extension of Acrylic for Incisor Protection in Class II Activator

The acrylic of the Class II activator is extended through the incisor freeway space from the distal of one canine to the distal of the other in both arches. Thus, acrylic is carried gingivally on the labial surfaces of the maxillary and mandibular teeth to a distance equal to two-thirds the height of the crowns of the central incisor teeth (see Fig. 12–19*A*). The vertical height of these labial acrylic extensions is obtained by softening a one-half inch wide strip of double-thickness baseplate wax and adapting it over the la-

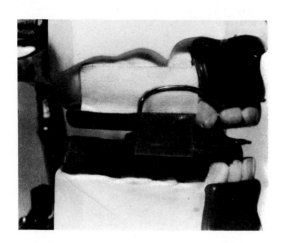

Figure 12-47. The illustration shows the placement of a piece of wax over the lateral portion of the labial arch in order to prevent this part of the arch wire from becoming embedded in the acrylic.

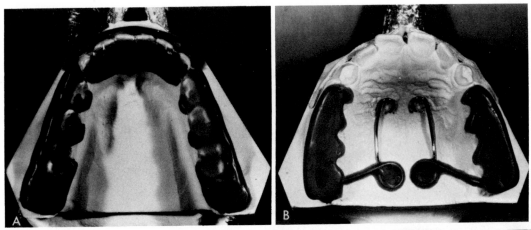

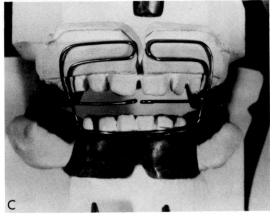

Figure 12–48. The occlusal wax-up of the mandibular arch for a Class III activator. The occlusal surfaces of the buccal teeth of the mandibular cast are covered with baseplate wax, and this is built up occlusally until only the cusp tips are exposed. Approximately 1.0 mm. thickness of wax is flowed on the entire distolingual surface of each posterior tooth to the center of each embrasure. No wax is applied on the mesiolingual surface of these teeth. Thus, when the acrylic is applied, wedges are formed which can transmit a posterior force to each mandibular tooth. *B,* The wax-up for the occlusal surfaces of the maxillary arch of a Class III activator is illustrated. The wax is carried to an approximate height of 3 to 5 mm. and a flat platform shaped to the buccolingual width of the posterior teeth. This platform should be parallel with the wax on the mandibular cast. Wax approximately 1.0 mm. thick is flowed on the entire mesiolingual surface of each maxillary buccal tooth to the center of each embrasure. No wax is applied to the distolingual surface of these teeth. Thus, when the acrylic is applied, wedges are formed which can transmit a mesial force to each maxillary tooth. *C,* If the wax-up in the maxillary and mandibular arches has been performed correctly, a space of 2 to 3 mm. remains between the two arches in the buccal segments. An acrylic shelf will flow into this space and will remain in occlusal contact with the mandibular arch while the maxillary buccal segments are permitted to erupt occlusally.

bial surfaces of the six maxillary anterior teeth and the labial wire. The incisal two-thirds of the crowns are left exposed, and the wax is sealed to the cast with a hot spatula. Similarly, a one-half inch strip of double-thickness baseplate wax is adapted over the labial surfaces of the six anterior mandibular teeth and the incisal and middle two thirds of the crowns are left exposed and the wax is sealed to the cast with a hot spatula (Fig. 12–46*A* and *B*).

The acrylic of the Class III activator is extended through the incisor freeway space from the distal of one canine to the distal of the other in the mandibular arch only. The acrylic is carried over the labial surfaces of the mandibular incisors for a distance of two-thirds the height of the crowns where it approximates the labial wire. Acrylic should not cover the labial surfaces of the maxillary incisors (see Fig. 12–31).

Design of Labial Arch Wire for Class III Activator

The 0.036 inch labial wire for the Class III activator (see Fig. 12–42*C*) is designed to recurve on itself in the maxillary incisor vestibule. The maxillary portion of the labial wire acts as a lip bumper to hold the lip away from the maxillary incisor teeth and facilitate their downward and forward eruption. The arms lie on each side of the frenum parallel with the occlusal plane approximately 2 to 3 mm. gingival to the incisors and recurving about 2 mm. short of the frenum. These arms recurve in a distal direction approximately 5 mm. gingival to and parallel with the lower arm. The upper portion of the arm is bent occlusally at the distal embrasure of the canine or further distally if muscle attachments permit; this portion continues to the middle of the freeway space where it is bent horizontally and carried to the midline. The retention tags provided on this arm should lie in the middle of the freeway space over the incisor teeth.

The vertical extension of the lower arm is bent occlusally about 1 mm. anterior to the vertical part of the upper arm. This arm must have room to move posteriorly without contacting the arm behind, and yet it must not be placed so far anteriorly that it impedes the anterior movement of the canine. This arm is carried from the maxillary to the mandibular arch, where it turns at right angles to the junction of the gingival and middle thirds of the mandibular incisors. At this point, it is shaped symmetrically over the labial surfaces of the mandibular incisors to the canine on the opposite side where it again returns vertically.

Application of Separating Medium

The casts and articulator are soaked in water at room temperature for five minutes and the excess water shaken off before applying the separating medium. Two thin coats of separating medium are brushed on the casts, allowing the first coat to dry before applying the second and seeing that the separator flows over the labial surfaces of the incisors and that any excess is drained off.

Add Wax Sheet on Labial to Mold Labial Extension

A wax shell to contain the acrylic is formed around the buccal and labial surfaces of both arches by shaping a strip of baseplate wax over the mounted casts from the posterior of one side to the posterior of the other (Fig. 12–49).

Sprinkle Acrylic on Casts

Liquid and powder are applied in the incisor protection section. The mixture should be fluid enough to flow around the labial surfaces of the incisors and thus not trap air. Powder and liquid are added to the exposed occlusal surfaces of the wax over the buccal teeth and around the lingual surface of the mandibular arch, finally filling in the palate. The articulator should be turned continuously during the application of powder and liquid to keep an even thickness of acrylic, and sprinkling should be continued until the acrylic reaches an even thickness equivalent to two sheets of baseplate wax (Fig. 12–50).

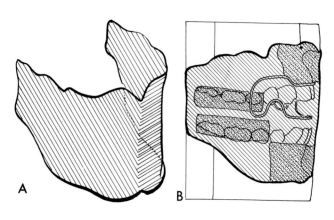

A   B

Figure 12–49. A wax shell to contain the acrylic is formed around the buccal and labial surfaces of the maxillary and mandibular arches by shaping a strip of baseplate wax over the mounted casts from the posterior of one side to the posterior of the other. The wax strip should be wide enough to cover the crowns of the teeth on both arches, and the wax on the labial surfaces should not touch the maxillary and mandibular incisors but rather bridge the gap between the jaws. The wax is sealed around the entire border with a hot spatula.

Figure 12-50. The photograph illustrates the completed sprinkling of acrylic monomer and powder over the various relief areas illustrated previously. An undercut area is sometimes present in the gingivolingual area of the mandibular molars and must not be relieved, because its presence provides one of the key methods by which the patient is conditioned to retain the appliance in position while asleep. When such an undercut is present the appliance must be inserted sideways. The lingual flange should be kept as deep as possible in this area in order to obtain maximum use of the undercut. Extra thickness should be left in this area for strength. The acrylic shelf extending into the freeway space is also illustrated. This shelf will impede eruption of the maxillary buccal segments but will allow eruption of the mandibular buccal segments.

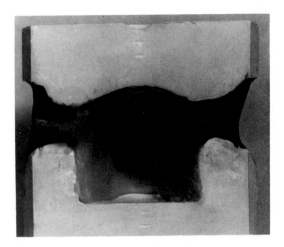

Curing the Acrylic

Separating medium should be applied to the surface of the acrylic with a brush as soon as the excess monomer has evaporated. The casts are then immersed in room temperature water in the pressure cooker, at a pressure of 30 lb. per square inch for 30 minutes. (The temperature of the water in the cooker must not exceed room temperature. Any greater temperature may soften the wax bites and distort the appliance.) The usual safety precautions should be observed when releasing the air after curing. This method of curing prevents excessive evaporation of monomer and produces increased density and decreased porosity.

Remove Appliance from Casts

The sheet of wax which was placed on the labial surfaces of the casts is removed, and the labial and buccal extensions of the acrylic are inspected for any large air bubbles. Such spaces are repaired with acrylic powder and liquid. It is not necessary to return the appliance to the pressure cooker to cure such a repair. The appliance is carefully pried from the casts with a plaster knife that is placed under the posterior border of the palate and under the lingual border of the mandibular portion. Where possible the acrylic is trimmed to a thickness of one sheet of baseplate wax to reduce bulk. The appliance is then polished.

References

1. Andresen, V., and Häupl, K.: Funktions-kieferorthopädie. Die Grundlagen des Norwegischen Systems. Leipzig, H. Meusser, 1936.
2. Robin, P.: Demonstration practique sur la construction et la mise en bouche d'un nouvel appareil de redressement. Rev. Stomatol., *9*:561–590, 1902.
3. Watry, F. M. A.: Dix ans de traitement physiotherapeutique. J. Dent. Belge, 1934.
4. Watry, F. M. A.: Die physiotherapeutische behandlung der Kieferdeformitäten. Fortschr. Orthod., 1933.
5. Watry, F. M. A.: A contribution to the history of the physiotherapeutics in maxillofacial orthopedics. Dent. Rec., *68*:192–196, 1948.
6. Harvold, E. P.: Some biologic aspects of orthodontic treatment in the transitional dentition. Am. J. Orthod., *49*:1–14, 1963.
7. Harvold, E. P., and Vargevik, K.: Morphogenic response to activator treatment. Am. J. Orthod., *60*:478–490, 1971.
8. Woodside, D. G., Reed, R. T., Doucet, J. D., and Thompson, G. W.: Some effects of activator

treatment on the growth rate of the mandible and position of the midface. Trans. Eur. Orthod. Soc., in press.

9. Trayfoot, J., and Richardson, A.: Angle's Class II, Division 1 malocclusions treated by the Andresen method. Br. Dent. J., *124*:516–519, 1968.

10. Woodside, D. G.: Distance, Velocity and Relative Growth Rate Standards for Mandibular Growth for Canadian Males and Females, Aged Three to Twenty Years. Thesis submitted in partial fulfillment of the requirements for certification by the American Board of Orthodontics, 1969.

11. Fisk, G. V., Culbert, M. R., Grainger, R. M., Hemrend, B., and Moyers, R.: The morphology and physiology of distoclusion. A summary of our present knowledge. Am. J. Orthod., *39*:3–12, 1953.

12. Harvold, E. P.: Personal communication, 1972.

13. Storey, A. T.: Physiology of a changing vertical dimension. J. Pros. Dent., *12*:912–921, 1962.

14. Tallgren, A.: Changes in mandibular rest position in adults. Trans. Eur. Orthod. Soc, 1958.

15. Boucher, G.: An Electromyographic Study of the Effect of Monobloc Therapy on the Activity of the Temporalis, Masseter and Digastric Muscles. Thesis submitted in partial fulfillment of the requirements for the Diploma in Orthodontics, Faculty of Dentistry, University of Toronto, 1965.

16. Ahlgren, J.: An electromyographic analysis of the response to activator (Andresen-Häupl) therapy. Odontol. Revy, *11*:125–151, 1960.

17. Ganong, W. F.: Review of Medical Physiology, 5th ed. Los Altos, California, Lange Medical Publishers, 1971.

18. Schwarz, A. M.: Grunsätzliches über die heutigen kieferorthopädischen Behandlungsverfahren. Z. Stomatol., *47*:400, 1950.

19. Schwarz, A. M.: Die Wirkungsweise des Aktivators. Fortschr. Kieferorthop., *13*:117–138, 1952.

20. Posen, A. L.: The monobloc. Angle Orthod., *38*:121–128, 1968.

21. Posen, A. L.: The influence of maximum perioral and tongue force on the incisor teeth. Angle Orthod., *42*:285–309, 1972.

22. Björk, A.: The principle of the Andresen method of orthodontic treatment, a discussion based on cephalometric x-ray analysis of treated cases. Am. J. Orthod., *37*:437–458, 1951.

CHAPTER 13

The Bimler Appliance

H. P. BIMLER, M.D., D.D.S.

In 1949, the first results of an orthodontic treatment of Class II, Division 1 cases with an unconventional appliance were published in Germany. This appliance consisted of wire elements, which were familiar because of their use in the labiolingual technique with molar bands. More precisely, the appliance was formed of a labial arch wire in the upper dental arch and a lingual arch wire in the lower arch. The only difference was that these wires were no longer fixed to the teeth, but to each other by small acrylic wings palatal to the upper buccal segments. The wires fitted the dentition in occlusion with the molars in a Class I relationship, thus enforcing a transitory repositioning of the mandible. With the dental arches apart, the device floated freely in the mouth.

The patient was supposed to treat himself under the supervision of the orthodontist and was encouraged to pick up the appliance from his models and to place it in his mouth by himself, right from the very beginning. He was instructed to wear it all day and night except during mealtime hours and while actively participating in rough sports.

Within four to six months, normal occlusion was observed in the cases in the eight- to twelve-year age group. During the retention period that followed, the same appliances were used instead of other retainers.

These encouraging results were the starting point of a new era of removable appliances, which differed distinctly from the Hawley type plates or bimaxillary blocks. In the English literature, these elastic bimaxillary wire appliances are generally known as "Bimler" appliances, so the author should be allowed to refer to them also under this name as a *terminus technicus*. The original name used in the first German paper was "Gebissformer," and, later, "oral adaptor" in some of the early English publications.

In the meantime, more than 25 years of clinical experience with this method have passed. The first clinical observations have been substantiated by thousands of model series and headplate sequences. They have revealed that only certain types of cases show such favorable results, since others need longer periods of time, and a certain number end up with unsatisfactory results. To recognize the factors that determine fast or slow reaction, success or failure, special methods of surveying the dental arch development and new points of view in cephalometric headplate evaluation had to be developed.

BIMLER CEPHALOMETRIC ANALYSIS

Our first concern became the definition of the various structures of the normal human face. For this project we could rely, in addition to our own work, on head plates taken in my father's office since 1937. The study of the human face in orthodontics was based originally on photographs; therefore, only external features such as the profile angulation were studied. This procedure was later transferred to x-ray cephalometrics, which still is centered on profile and incisor angulation and neglects linear measurements. This was understandable before a standardized target distance was generally accepted. Now it is no longer sufficient. We have profited from the work that has been done in anthropology in the past 100 years and have pursued the methods used in this basic science.

Facial Indices

In anthropology, facial types were assessed in the frontal aspect by the facial index (total) of Kollmann since 1897. He related facial width to facial height and differentiated between euryprosopic (broad faces), mesoprosopic (medium faces), and leptoprosopic (long faces). In the lateral aspect no such index existed, so we introduced in 1957 for x-ray cephalometrics a suborbital facial index (Bimler) relating suborbital facial height to facial depth. We differentiated between dolichoprosopic (deep faces), mesoprosopic (medium faces), leptoprosopic (long faces). As is the standard procedure in anthropology, we used the Frankfort horizontal as a reference line. A vertical through the pterygomaxillary fissure completes it to an orthogonal reference system. As anterior and posterior limits of the face, subspinale or point A (Downs) and capitulare or point C (Bimler—center of the head of the condyle) were

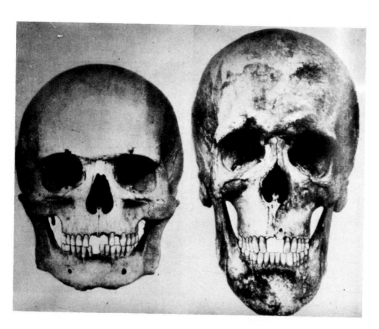

Figure 13–1. Extreme variations of Caucasian skulls.

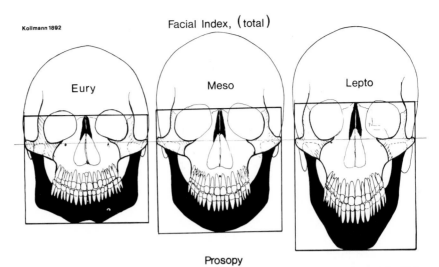

Figure 13-2. Facial index (total) proposed by Kollman in 1892. Facial width is related to facial height. Greek nomenclature: euryprosopic = broad face; mesoprosopic = medium face; leptoprosopic = long face.

selected. The suborbital facial height is defined as the distance between the Frankfort horizontal and point M (menton). Facial depth is defined as the distance between the anterior vertical through point A and the posterior vertical through point C. This index can easily be established by measuring the anterior suborbital height with a caliper and transferring it to the Frankfort horizontal. If the intersection is in front of the C vertical, the facial depth is larger and the facial type is D, dolicho or deep face. If the intersection is behind the clivus, facial height is greater and the type is L, lepto or long face. If the intersection is between point C and the clivus, the type is M, meso or medium face.

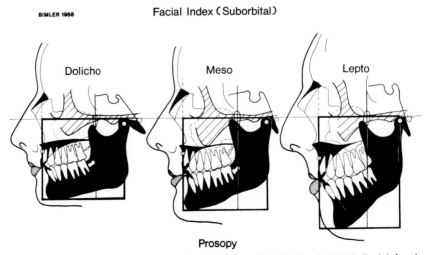

Figure 13-3. Facial index (suborbital) proposed by Bimler in 1958. Facial depth is related to facial height. Greek nomenclature: dolichoprosopic = deep face; mesoprosopic = medium face; leptoprosopic = long face.

Orthogonial Reference System

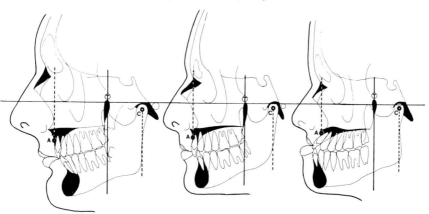

Frankfort Horizontal / A-T-C Verticals

Figure 13-4. The basis of our cephalometric analysis is an orthogonial reference system consisting of the Frankfort horizontal and the T vertical, a tangent to the most posterior part of the maxilla (tuberositas maxillae). Two additional verticals through points A and C build the anterior limits of the face as defined for this analysis.

Facial Angles

To define a face more precisely, the index alone is not sufficient. Since 1765 the profile angle has been used to describe characteristics of a face. An appropriate point of definition for the facial profile in orthodontic cephalometrics is the angle NAB (Fig. 13–10). In our analysis it is measured as the supplementary angle to 180 degrees. As a counterpart of the anterior profile angle, on lateral head plates a posterior profile angle can also be established. This

Facial Index suborbital (Height / Depth)

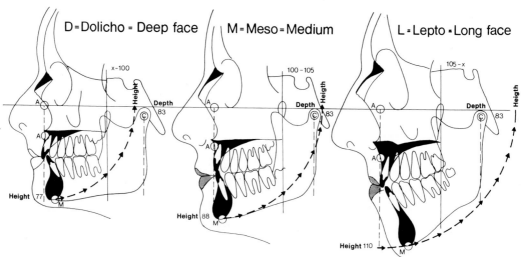

Figure 13-5. The facial index can easily be established by means of a caliper. Take the anterior suborbital height A′M on a caliper and draw a circle (dotted line) around A′. If the intersection with the Frankfort horizontal is in front of C, depth exceeds height, i.e., deep face. If the intersection is significantly behind the clivus, height exceeds depth, i.e., long face.

angle is formed by the tangents to the clivus and the lower border of the mandible. The clivus-mandibular plane angle is called in our analysis the basic angle of the face. The basic angle corresponds to the facial type in that the deeper the face, the more acute the angle, and the longer the face, the more obtuse the angle. There is a high correlation between facial type and basic angle in harmonious faces, whereas in clinical orthodontics, disharmonious faces must be considered. The study of the upper and the lower components of the total basic angle has proved to be more indicative of facial harmony or disharmony than the overall basic angle.

UPPER BASIC ANGLE

The upper basic angle is formed by a tangent to the clivus and the palatal plane. It is called the clivomaxillary angle. Between the extreme facial forms it has a range of variation of about 30 degrees. This allows division of the total into three equal parts of 10 degrees each. There is a range of 50 to 60 degrees in dolichoprosopic faces. To this range is assigned the capital letter D for dolicho or deep. The letter M stands for mesoprosopic or medium face, and the range is 60 to 70 degrees. The letter L indicates a leptoprosopic variation in the range of 70 to 80 degrees.

LOWER BASIC ANGLE

The lower basic angle between the palatal and mandibular plane is called the maxillomandibular angle and has a total range of 45 degrees. Corre-

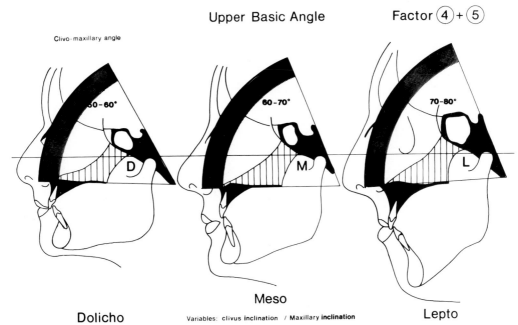

Figure 13–6. Upper basic angle = clivomaxillary angle. ANS-PNS to tangent of clivus; range of variation: 50 to 80 degrees. Dolichoprosopic or deep face range: 50 to 60 degrees (D). Mesoprosopic or medium face range: 60 to 70 degrees (M). Leptoprosopic or long face range: 70 to 80 degrees (L).

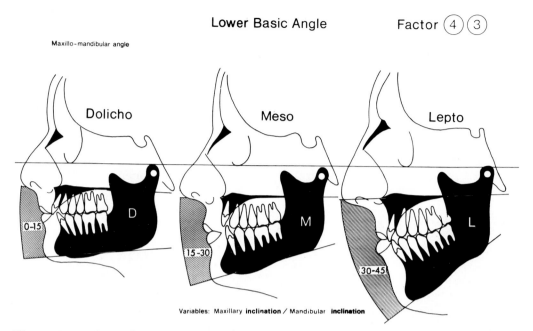

Figure 13–7. Lower basic angle = maxillomandibular angle. ANS-PNS to tangent to mandibular body, posteriorly from Menton (mandibular plane); range of variation: 0 to 45 degrees. Dolichoprosopic or deep face range: 0 to 15 degrees (D). Mesoprosopic or medium face range: 15 to 30 degrees (M). Leptoprosopic or long face range: 30 to 45 degrees (L).

sponding to the upper basic angle, the total range has been divided into three equal parts of 15 degrees each. The range of 0 to 15 degrees belongs to the dolicho or deep face and is expressed by the capital letter D. The range of 15 to 30 degrees is marked M, and the range from 30 to 45 degrees is L.

Facial Formula

This procedure allows us to define the general characteristics of a face by a facial formula consisting of the profile angle, the relation of the upper to the lower facial basic angles, and the facial index.

In harmonious faces one may expect that the upper and lower basic angles fall into the same range of variation corresponding to the facial index type, e.g., D/D, dolicho; M/M, meso; or L/L, lepto, as we see in our examples of normal faces. In disharmonious clinical cases, all sorts of combinations may occur, e.g., as most extreme D/L lepto, a combination typical for severe open bite cases (Fig. 13–9).

For about 20 years we have been using this facial formula to file the case histories of our finished patients according to their facial structure. This gave us the means by which to study on a long-range basis the influence of facial structure on the results of a uniform therapeutic approach. We will refer to our findings in this regard later in the chapter.

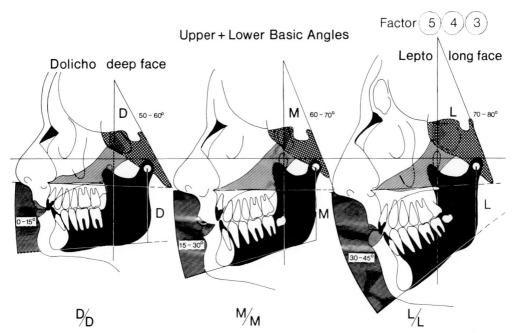

Figure 13-8. Relation of upper to lower basic angles. In harmonious faces the upper and lower basic angles belong to the corresponding ranges of variation, so the relation of the upper to the lower part of the face can be expressed by the code capital letters as follows: D/D, M/M, L/L (see Figs. 13-6 and 13-7).

Facial Polygon and Factor Analysis

To simplify the approach to the facial structure by angular measurements, facial polygons are used. They are constructed by drawing straight lines between selected points in the facial skeleton. The angles between the sides of the

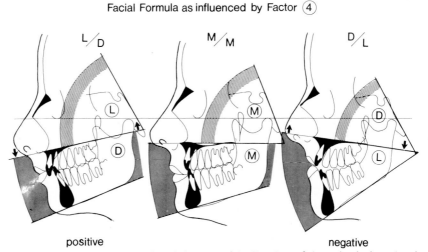

Figure 13-9. By a forward and downward inclination of the palatal plane (positive Factor 4), the upper basic angle will be increased and the lower decreased, resulting in an M/D or L/D relationship. A negative Factor 4 (downward and backward palatal plane inclination) will change the harmonious relations to M/L or D/L. The latter is very characteristic of open bite cases.

Facial Formula

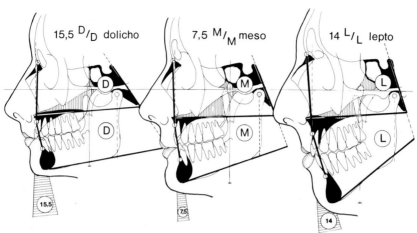

Figure 13–10. To define a given facial structure, a facial formula has been proposed. It consists of the profile angle NAB (15.5, 7.5, 14) expressed as the supplementary angle to 180 degrees, the relation of upper to lower basic angles represented by the ranges of variation (D/D, M/M, L/L), and the suborbital facial index (dolicho-, meso-, lepto-).

polygon are measured. This has been useful in constructing mean value polygons for certain populations. For individual longitudinal investigations we have to note that each side of the polygon is a variable, so that in the case of a change in the angulation between two variables, it cannot be determined whether the change is due to one or the other or both variables. To overcome this ambiguity we instituted the factor analysis. We no longer measured the angulation of the sides of the polygon to each other, but rather to an orthogonal reference system, and called the inclination of each side to the system a factor. Ten factors have been defined.

Factor 1 NA line	= Upper profile angle
Factor 2 AB line	= Lower profile angle
Factor 3 MNo line	= Mandibular plane
Factor 4 ANS-PNS	= Palatal plane
Factor 5 Cls-Cli	= Clivus tangent
Factor 6 Radius in spherical reference system	
Factor 7 NS line	= Anterior cranial base
Factor 8 CGo line	= Posterior border of ramus
Factor 9 Ethmoidal line ⎱ Factor 10 Nasal line ⎰	descriptive only

By means of factor analysis, we studied the behavior of single components of the face and learned to understand the meaning of typical deviations from their normal positions in establishing systematic growth deficiencies. It became necessary to assess growth increments, to demonstrate regions of growth deficiencies, and to check our angular measurements by the introduction of a series of linear measurements.

Orthogonial Reference System

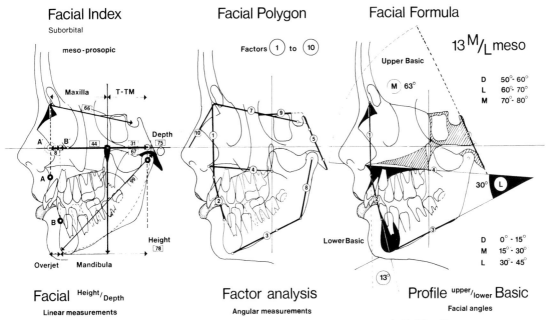

Figure 13–11. *Left,* Linear and angular measurements on Blue Boy (see p. 429). The linear measurements for the depth of the maxilla (44) and the T-TM distance (31), or temporal position, add up to the facial depth (75). The projected overjet between A and B (8) and the effective length of the mandible (67) projected on FH also add up to (75). The suborbital facial height (78) exceeds the facial depth, resulting in a mesoprosopic value for the facial index. *Center,* The angular measurements are performed on the facial polygon. The inclination of each side of the polygon is measured separately against the reference system. The factors have been numbered in essentially a counterclockwise fashion. *Right,* The facial profile angle, the relation of upper to lower basic angles, and the facial index build together our facial formula to define the facial structure. 13 M/L meso for Blue Boy indicates that the upper basic angle is relatively small and the lower too large, as evidenced by the negative downward and backward inclination of ANS-PNS or Factor 4. Note also the ranges for the upper and lower basic angles.

LINEAR MEASUREMENTS

For routine clinical purposes we use four measurements in the sagittal plane. The distances of the projected points A and C on the Frankfort horizontal are known as maxillary depth and temporal position, or T-TM distance. The two together represent the facial depth. The projection of point B on the Frankfort horizontal allows us to measure the effective length of the mandible and the basal bone overjet. Together they also give the facial depth, which allows us to double-check the measurements. The projection of M horizontally on to the tuber (T) vertical gives the suborbital facial height. By comparing facial height to facial depth, one may double-check the graphically established facial index. In addition, two direct measurements are taken, the diagonal length of the mandible and the distance NS, representing the length of the anterior cranial base. With both measurements the growth increments can easily be assessed.

BIMLER 1961

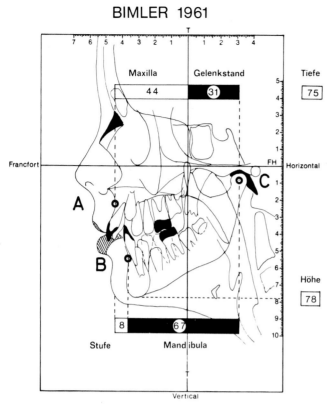

Figure 13–12. Linear measurements. The author proposed in 1961 to project points A, B, and C on the Frankfort horizontal and to measure in this way the depth of the maxilla (44), the position of the TM joints (31), the basal bone overjet (8), and the effective length of the mandible (67).

Figure 13–13. Following the recording of the linear measurements (Fig. 13–12), the ranges of variation for the maxilla (40 to 60 mm.) and the T-TM distance (20 to 40 mm.) were established. As the effective length of the mandible depends on various circumstances, ranges were given for the diagonal length of the mandible (99), representing better the skeletal pattern of the patient. Additionally, the NS distance for the length of the anterior cranial base is measured (66). The easiest way to read the growth increments is to compare these measurements at different stages of the development.

Korrelationsanalyse

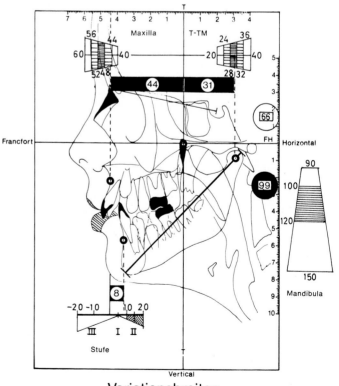

Variationsbreiten

GNATHIC INDEX FORMULA

The two most indicative measurements, linear and angular, have been selected to constitute the gnathic index formula. We chose the basal bone overjet and the T-TM distance, and the relationship of Factor 4, maxillary inclination, to Factor 8, mandibular flexion (Fig. 13–14 *left*). The linear measurements refer to sagittal problems and the angular to vertical problems. Details will be explained in the Blue Boy case later in this chapter.

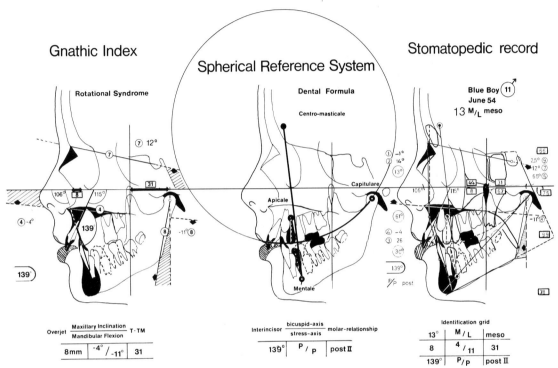

Figure 13–14. Further details of our stomatopedic recording methods are explained using Blue Boy (see p. 428 for full discussion of his case). In the center of the spherical reference system is the stress axis in a postnormal (retruded) position corresponding to the Class II molar relationship. The stress axis is further used to demonstrate a forward or backward inclination of the longitudinal axes of the cuspids and bicuspids. In Class II, Division 1 cases with crowding, bicuspids are usually inclined mesially. In Division 2 cases, it is characteristic that the incisors are very upright and the bicuspids are inclined distally. In Blue Boy, the upper and lower first bicuspids are proclined (tipped mesially), which is noted in the dental formula as P/P, besides the interincisor angle of 139 degrees and the *post*normal position of the stress axis and the Angle Class II relationship. The longitudinal axes of the incisors form a triangle with the Frankfort horizontal, as seen on the left. The outer angles of a triangle always add up to 360 degrees. We use this fact to double check our measurements on incisor angulation. 106 degrees for the lower incisors, 115 degrees for the upper incisors, and 139 degrees for the interincisor angulation must equal 360 degrees. Theoretical mean values are 115 degrees for the upper and lower incisor angulation against the Frankfort horizontal and 130 degrees for the interincisor angulation. Note further the rotational syndrome of micro-rhinic dysplasia (see Fig. 13–20) with a negative maxillary inclination of −4 degrees of Factor 4, a mandibular flexion of −11 degrees of Factor 8, and an increased slant of 12 degrees of Factor 7. Compared with harmonious faces, all three factors are rotated clockwise with regard to the reference system. Two linear measurements, the basal bone overjet of 8 mm. and the T-TM distance, were selected to represent the sagittal situation, and two angular measurements, Factors 4 and 8, to represent the vertical situation of the face in our gnathic index formula. It appears on the left side and on the right side on the second line of the stomatopedic identification grid. This grid combines the facial formula, the gnathic formula, and the dental formula as a condensed source of cephalometric information.

Spherical Reference System

For the swinging functional system of the masticatory muscles, the temporomandibular joints, and the lower dental arch related to the upper dental arch, a spherical reference system has proved to be most adequate. Empirically, it was determined that the curve of Spee could be represented on lateral head plates by a segment of an arc going through the masticatory surfaces of the buccal segments and through the center point of the head of the condyle (Fig. 13–15). The hypothetical center of the curve of Spee is called "centro-masticale," and the inner chin point is named "mentale." It coincides with the anthropologic point of gonion. The points CM (centro-masticale), Me (mentale), C (capitulare), and Ap (apicale) as the apex of the first premolars are the reference points of this system. The radius going through mentale is called the stress axis of the dentition, and with regard to point Ap it serves as an important indicator of gnathodental relations.[31]

Dental Formula

As a condensed record of our findings with regard to the dentition and the curve of Spee we use a dental formula (Fig. 13–14 *center*). It consists of the incisor angulation (139 degrees), the premolar relationship of the proclined

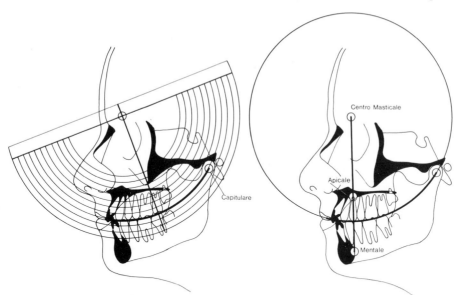

Figure 13–15. Spherical reference system. With a template consisting of a series of concentric semicircles, one can establish the center point of the curve of Spee by selecting the arc that fits the buccal segments of the dental arches and passes at the same time through point C (*capitulare*), the center of the head of the condyle. The center point of the curve of Spee is regarded as the virtual center of mastication and as a reference point called *centro masticale*. The radius from centro masticale to the inner chin point (*mentale*) will coincide in harmonious faces with the longitudinal axes of the upper first premolars and is therefore named the stress axis of the dentition, or Factor 6 in our analysis. As a third reference point representing the position of the maxilla, the apices of the upper first premolars were selected and the point called *apicale*. Deviations from balanced harmony in the dentition and the facial structure will indicate themselves by a pre- or postnormal (mesial or distal) position of the stress axis with regard to the reference point *apicale*. This system can be used to supplement the Angle classification.

upper and lower first premolars (P/P) with regard to the stress axis, and the postnormal position (post) of the stress axis with regard to reference point apicale and the Angle Class II relationship.

Stomatopedic Records

For an advanced understanding of the orthodontic problems, we must consider more detailed information, which must always be available when we see a patient. Its constant availability is necessary, since we should be able to check a certain question or problem when it arises. For this purpose we have selected a limited number of correlated angular and linear measurements and put them together in our cephalometric analysis (Fig. 13–14 *right*). The tracings as well as the measurements are routinely done by staff members. The facial and intraoral photographs are always added to the analysis sheet, which is placed on the front page of our case history.

Harmony Versus Norms

Usually in orthodontic cephalometrics the data established are compared with norms. But what is behind these norms? Statistical analyses performed on limited selected groups, are most questionable in their value for the individual. We therefore dropped most of the so-called norms and mean values, replacing them with ranges of variability, and tried to visualize the difference between harmony in its various forms and disharmony as we found it during the decades of our systematic recording.

KEY SYMPTOMS OF DISHARMONY IN THE FACIAL STRUCTURE

Four features aroused our interest as morphologic keys for typical deviations from balanced structures, which became for us indicators of systemic growth deficiencies. The first symptom is the maxillary inclination, as indicated by our Factor 4. In harmonious cases the nasal floor is more or less parallel to the Frankfort horizontal. In a few cases, associated mostly with a closed bite, the palatal plane is inclined forward and downward. It is also referred to as positive Factor 4. On the other hand, a forward and upward inclined nasal floor, or negative Factor 4, is the most common symptom of underdevelopment of the middle part of the face. It occurs in about 50 per cent of our patients.

The second symptom is the amount of *mandibular flexion* or rotation. In the harmonious cases in our collection, the posterior border of the ramus is more or less perpendicular to the Frankfort horizontal. Any reduction in the vertical dimension of the middle part of the face or complete loss of teeth leads to an overclosure of the mandible. This can be readily observed in aged edentulous persons. This overclosure is called *hyperflexion*, in comparison with the flexion movement of the forearm. By itself a secondary symptom, it is clinically an excellent guide to the primary lesion. The contrary, an incomplete closing due to premature occlusal contact, is called *hypoflexion* or deflexion. We express the degree of mandibular flexion by our Factor 8. In hyperflexion, Factor 8 is inclined forward and in hypoflexion it is inclined backward.

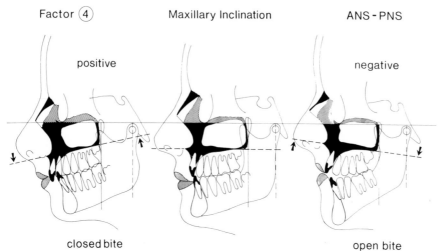

Figure 13-16. Maxillary inclination, the primary symptom for an increased or decreased vertical development of the middle part of the face. A forward and downward inclination or positive Factor 4 is mostly associated with Class II, Division 2 or Class III closed bite cases. Downward and backward inclination of ANS-PNS or negative Factor 4 is found in Class II, Division 1 or Class III open bite cases.

The third symptom is the *temporal position.* As mentioned before, we check the position of the temporomandibular joints (TMJ) by measuring the T-TM distance between the vertical tuber and point C as representative of the temporomandibular joint. Our experience has demonstrated that a Class II or Class III malocclusion depends not only on the depth of the maxilla or the length of the mandible but also, especially in extreme cases, on the position of the temporomandibular joints.

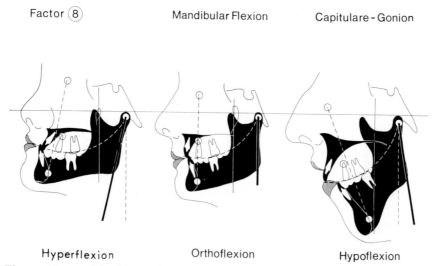

Figure 13-17. Mandibular flexion, a secondary symptom of reduced midfacial height (hyperflexion, overclosure of mandible), measured as forward inclination of Factor 8 of more than 8 degrees. Premature blockage of closing movement due to high alveolar processes and negative Factor 4 expresses itself as a backward inclined Factor 8 or hypoflexion.

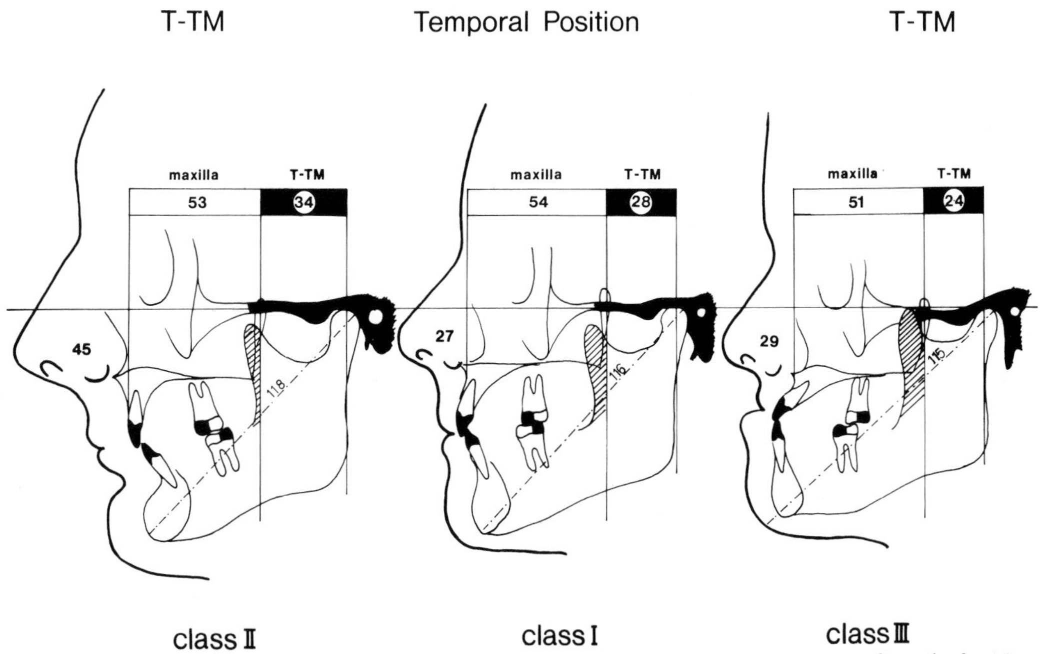

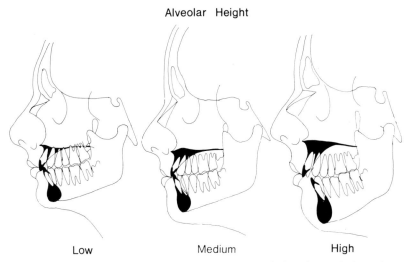

T-TM Temporal Position T-TM

maxilla	T-TM
53	③④

45

118

class II

maxilla	T-TM
54	②⑧

27

class I

maxilla	T-TM
51	②④

29

class III

Figure 13–18. Temporal fossa position. In the literature, very often Class II cases are described with a large maxilla or a small mandible. Conversely, Class III cases are supposed to have either small maxillae or excessively large mandibles. Note that the main difference is not the depth of the maxilla or the length of the mandible. On the contrary, the mandible in the Class II case may be even longer (118 mm.) than in the Class III case (115 mm.), and the difference in the maxillae is only 2 mm. The difference in the T-TM distance or the temporal position (10 mm.) is the decisive factor for the malocclusion. This is likewise demonstrated by the position of the anterior margin of the ramus, either near the vertical through the pterygomaxillary fissure or far in front of the vertical in the Class III case with the short T-TM distance (24 mm.).

The fourth symptom is the *alveolar height*. Besides the maxillary inclination for the occurrence of a closed or open bite, the vertical development of the alveolar processes, which is probably genetically determined, is a very important factor.

Alveolar Height

Low Medium High

Figure 13–19. The height of the alveolar process differs distinctly in various facial types and is apparently genetically predetermined.

Mechanism of Growth Disturbances

Starting from the three types of harmonious faces with a well-balanced structure and the knowledge of the primary symptoms for a disturbed facial development, we later came to define three standard mechanisms which apparently govern the growth disturbances of the human face. We differentiated between the micro-rhinic, the microtic, and the leptoid dysplasias. They can be found singly or in any possible combination.

The first to be described (1965) was the *micro-rhinic dysplasia.* Its name derived from the external features of the involved face. There is a small saddle nose, with an upward tilted base showing the nostrils, an incompetent upper lip, no oral seal, and an anterior open bite. These characteristics are occasionally accompanied by an antimongoloid slant of the eyelids and desisting ears. This characteristic picture is known in otolaryngology as an "adenoid face" and has been associated with enlarged tonsils and adenoids. The skeletal deviations, can, of course, be detected only by x-ray cephalometrics. They can be described as the rotational syndrome, if the Frankfort horizontal is used as a reference. In our analysis, Factors 4, 7, and 8 are rotated clockwise (Fig. 13–22); in other words, we see a negative maxillary inclination, a mandibular overclosure, and a flattening of the cranial base. This syndrome had been found in so many of our cases that we were looking for some common cause. We found in embryology a theoretical key to the understanding of this phenomenon. Starck of Frankfurt has claimed that for the differentiation of the rhino-encephalon and the nasal capsule, an anterior "head organizer" is responsible.[35] If any disturbance, such as a virus infection or simply lack of oxygen, occurs in the third week of pregnancy, a typical malformation of the face can be observed. As

Growth Disturbances

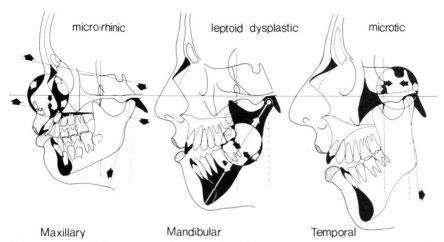

Maxillary   Mandibular   Temporal

Figure 13–20. Three types of growth disturbances. *Left,* In the micro-rhinic dysplasia, predominantly the maxilla is involved. It is supposedly caused by a disturbance in the anterior head organizer (Starck) in the third week of pregnancy. *Center,* The leptoid dysplasia involves the mandible, which is elongated but weakened in its structure. The gonial angle is flattened. The malformation is most common in Class III cases, but it is also associated with skeletal open bite. *Right,* A disturbance in the posterior head organizer apparently retards the development in the temporal region and involves mainly the position of the temporomandibular joints.

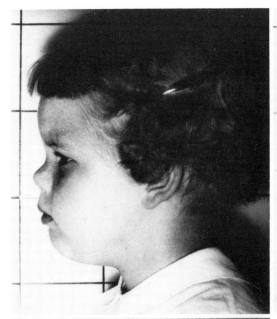

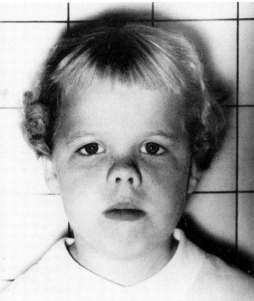

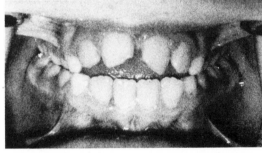

Figure 13–21. The term *micro-rhinic dysplasia* is derived from the external view of the patient. A small saddle-nose showing the nostrils is the most striking feature. Note also the anti-mongoloid slant of the eyes.

Starck described also a posterior head organizer, which induces the development of the rhomboencephalon, we screened our material on dysplastic patients and found corresponding malformations in the otic area.

The *microtic dysplasia* leads to an underdevelopment in the posterior region of the cranial base and in the adjacent parts of the temporal bones, especially the petrous bones. The position of the temporomandibular joints is influenced by the latter. Owing to the high degree of natural variability in the structure of the human face, all statistical group mean values are of limited importance in the evaluation of a given malformation. In our experience one can best compare the patient with other members of the same generation of his family. Our patient suffered from craniofacial dysostosis or pseudo-Crouzon's disease. He had a repaired cleft lip and deformed ears, but was of normal intelligence. In addition to a small nose, he showed the full rotational syndrome of micro-rhinic dysplasia. The length of the mandible and the anterior cranial base, as well as the depth of the maxilla, were not reduced. The changes in the posterior part of the cranial base and the otic region were not limited to single bones, but the whole region was involved. Note the shortened and uprighted clivus and the accompanying forward and upward inclination of the foramen magnum. By the reduction of the T-TM distance, the mandible is carried forward, as can be seen by the Class III relationship of the molars and the position of the an-

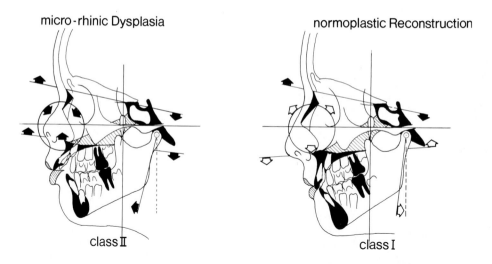

micro-rhinic Dysplasia

normoplastic Reconstruction

class II

class I

Effect of maxillary rotation

Figure 13-22. The lasting effect of the temporary disturbance in the development of the middle face can be described as a forward and upward rotation of the maxilla. To reconstruct or normalize such a face graphically, one has only to rotate the palatal plane in a forward and downward direction and to insert a bigger nose. With the same contours of maxilla and mandible, a face is created in which all the symptoms of the malocclusion have disappeared.

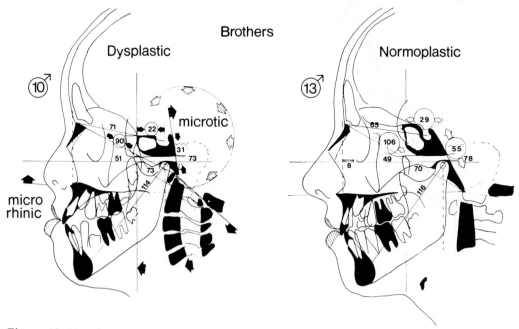

Brothers

Dysplastic

Normoplastic

Figure 13-23. A patient with dysostosis craniofacialis (pseudo-Crouzon's disease) is compared with his normoplastic brother at about the same age. The dysplastic brother shows symptoms of the micro-rhinic and microtic mechanisms. Note the reduction of the linear measurements in the posterior region of the cranial base and the change in the angulation of the clivus and of the foramen magnum. The length of the mandible apparently is not affected.

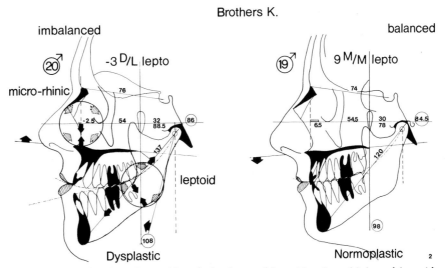

Figure 13-24. A patient with a skeletal open bite with micro-rhinic and leptoid dysplastic symptoms is compared with his normoplastic brother. Note the reduction in the vertical dimension of the anterior part of the middle face as demonstrated by the upward inclined palatal plane. The mandible is elongated and the gonial angle flattened. Body and ramus appear weakened and reduced in width. The open bite is due to the high and resisting alveolar processes. Compare with Figure 13-25 *center,* where low and yielding alveolar processes lead to a Class III closed bite malocclusion.

terior border of the ramus in front of the vertical tuber. The comparison of the evaluated tracings of the two brothers can better demonstrate the differences between normal and abnormal than can any verbal description.

Leptoid Dysplasia. While the micro-rhinic and the microtic dysplasias show locally hypoplastic areas, the *leptoid dysplasia* is of a more generalized nature. It involves the whole facial structure but is most obvious in the mandible. The sagittal facial development, i.e., the facial depth, is often diminished, while the facial height and facial width are increased. The mandible shows a flattened gonial angle and weakened structure but increased length from chin to condyle. Whether a Class III malocclusion, an open bite, or a combination of both develops depends on the height of the alveolar processes.

In the pair of brothers, the normoplastic brother shows a balanced structure with a formula M/M lepto, while the dysplastic one demonstrates a combination of micro-rhinic and leptoid deformation. By the negative Factor 4, the facial formula is changed: the upper basic angle is reduced while the lower is increased, resulting in a D/L lepto formula. This is due to the reduced anterior height of the middle part of the face. The facial depth is not involved, but the patient's facial height exceeds that of his brother by 10 mm. This difference is partly due to an excess in mandibular length of 17 mm. compared with the brother and partly due to high alveolar processes in the maxilla. Note that at the same time the alveolar height in the mandible is not increased and the structure of the mandible in the region of the gonial angle is weak by comparison with the brother's. Compare with Figure 13-25 *center* and *right* to understand the influence of alveolar height on the degree of flexion of the mandible.

Prenatal extrinsic factors are presumed to be responsible for these growth disturbances. They can occur in any genetically determined facial type and in

Growth Deficiencies

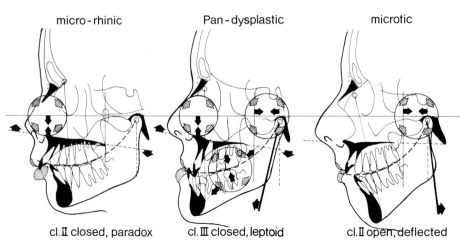

micro-rhinic   Pan-dysplastic   microtic

cl.Ⅱ closed, paradox   cl.Ⅲ closed, leptoid   cl.Ⅱ open, deflected

Figure 13-25. *Left,* In certain cases with low or deficient alveolar height, the rotation of the maxilla along the curve of Spee will result in a Class II closed bite. Note the undisturbed position of the mandible, with the posterior margin of the ramus perpendicular to the Frankfort horizontal. *Center,* A pan-dysplastic case, which combines symptoms of all three mechanisms. This offers the biggest problem for treatment and often ends up as a severe Class III open bite malocclusion. Compare with Figure 13-17. Surgical intervention can be recommended only after growth comes to a complete standstill. *Right,* A mandible with a well-formed gonial angle and a broad but rather short ramus is deflected to an open bite associated with a microtic reduction of the T-TM distance. Mandibular plane inclination is steep, also.

any combination. There are examples of micro-rhinic Class II, Division 1 closed bite cases as microtic open bite cases, in which we see a rather short ramus in addition to a short T-TM distance, but with an excellent gonial angle. Associated with high alveolar processes, this produces a deflection of the mandible that has hardly any influence at all.

In severe dysplastic cases, the natural forces derived from muscular actions are no longer sufficient to correct the morphologic discrepancies. Here we have to rely on orthopedic and/or surgical intervention, including tooth extraction. Despite these limitations, we are able adequately to handle 85 per cent of all our cases with the three types of Bimler appliance. This reduces the chair time needed for the bulk of our patient load, and gives us plenty of time to concentrate on the few problem cases that require more time-consuming orthodontic methods.

DENTAL ARCH SURVEY

The cephalometric study of the facial structures and their disturbances gives us the background for the understanding of dental malocclusions on a higher level. The working area in which to establish our treatment plan and to supervise its realization is the dental arches. In stomatopedics we use two correlated procedures for a reliable survey: first, a dental arch analysis comprising a graphic dental arch predetermination and appliance prescription, and second, treatment check curves established by continuous dental arch measurements.

Dental Arch Analysis

In the graphic dental arch analysis we took up the ideas of Stanton of New York and Pont of France and developed them into a diagnostic procedure, which was first published in a thesis in 1943. The method was refined and is now the basis of our treatment planning, which results finally in the appliance prescription.

Pont Index

In Europe, dental arch measurements are almost always performed according to the proposals of Pont. At the beginning of this century Pont had published an anthropologic index relating the sum of the mesiodistal diameters of the upper incisors (SI) to the anterior and posterior dental arch width:

$$x = \frac{(SI) \times 100}{\text{Dental arch width}} \qquad \begin{array}{l} x \text{ for molars } = 64 \\ x \text{ for premolars} = 80 \end{array}$$

This formula by itself does not make a specific statement but simply expresses the sum of the incisors as a percentage of the dental arch width. Using this formula, statistical investigations were performed by different authors or various populations, establishing only slightly differing mean values for th dental arch width. Usually they are in the form of numerical tables. We prefer them as graphic scales.

SUM OF INCISORS (SI)

The Pont index expresses the dental arch width with regard to the mesiodistal diameters of the upper incisors. Therefore, these measurements

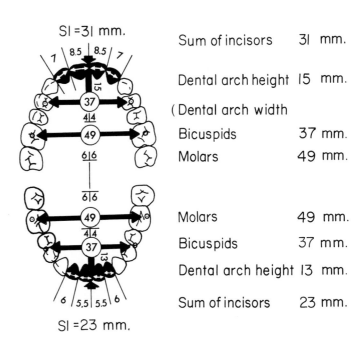

Figure 13–26. The Pont index.

Sum of incisors	31 mm.
Dental arch height	15 mm.
(Dental arch width	
Bicuspids	37 mm.
Molars	49 mm.
Molars	49 mm.
Bicuspids	37 mm.
Dental arch height	13 mm.
Sum of incisors	23 mm.

have to be taken first with calipers and transferred to any millimeter grid. In our example, the sum of the upper incisors is 7 + 8.5 + 8.5 + 7 mm. = (SI) = 31 mm. (Fig. 13–26). To check the undisturbed correlation of upper and lower incisors, the SI of the lower arch is measured: 6 + 5.5 + 5.5 + 6 mm. = (SI) = 23 mm.

DENTAL ARCH WIDTH

According to Pont, the dental arch width is measured between the first molars and the first premolars. The measuring points coincide in the occluding arches. For the posterior width they are defined by Pont as the central fossa of the upper molars and the distobuccal cusps of the lower molars. In the example the posterior width is 49 mm. For the anterior width, we measure the center points of the first premolars in the upper arch, and the buccal interproximal embrasure of the first and second premolars in the lower arch. The distance is 37 mm.

DENTAL ARCH HEIGHT

Korkhaus defined the dental arch height as the distance between the connecting line of the anterior measuring points and the labial aspects of the central incisors. In the example, upper height is 15 mm. and lower height is 13 mm.

Dental Arch Analysis Sheet

Our treatment planning is based on a graphic dental arch analysis and results in the appliance prescription. All this work is nowadays delegated to specially trained auxiliary personnel. Therefore, a printed analysis sheet has been developed, which automatically guides the one who performs the analysis from one step to the next.

First, the name of the patient, the date of the analysis, and the name of the responsible orthodontist are inserted on the top line. The main feature of the analysis sheet is the double cross of reference for the orientation of the projected upper and lower dental arches. The sagittal line should coincide with the midline of the dental arches. The horizontal lines should correspond to the anterior measuring points for the Pont index.

To simplify the comparison of any dental arch traced on the analysis sheet with the Pont mean values, a special scale has been developed. The Pont values for the dental arch width and height are represented by light and heavy lines printed symmetrically on the double cross of reference. Heavy and light lines are arranged in an alternating sequence, each line representing a certain Pont value. In the upper left corner of the analysis sheet a table is printed, indicating which symbol, consisting of a heavy line or a pair of light lines, belongs to a certain SI (sum of incisors). As the values are rather close together, only every second one is mentioned. The values for the others are found in between.

Because of the growing mesiodistal diameters of the buccal teeth, the symbols for the molars had to be arranged on oblique lines. The values for the height of the arches are on the sagittal line, the ones for the lower being 2 mm.

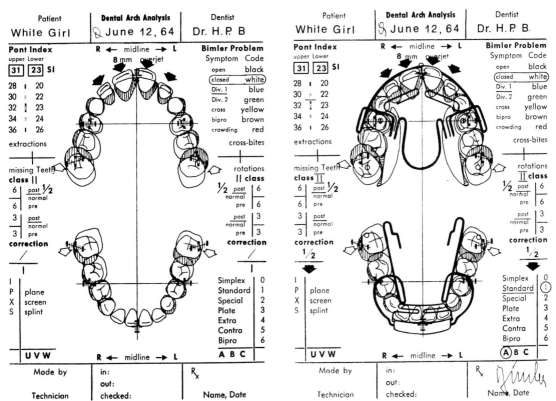

Figure 13-27. Dental arch analysis sheet with projected upper and lower dental arches. *Left,* Dental arch predetermination and, *right,* appliance prescription.

shorter than those for the upper. The two brackets beside SI are provided for the figures of the actual measurements of the sum of the upper and lower incisors.

Below the Pont index table a small cross is printed to register any extracted or missing teeth. On the right side there is a similar place, where cross bites or rotated teeth can be noted. Deviations of the midlines in the upper and lower arches can be marked by encircling the respective arrows and capital letters R and L for right and left above and below the cross of reference. The intermaxillary relationship will be marked as the amount of overjet (in millimeters) in the same place. On both sides in the middle of the sheet the pre- or postnormal relations of the molars and canines are registered. Likewise, the Angle Class I, II, or III will be inserted. Under the headline of "correction," orders are written to the technician concerning how much the occlusion should be corrected in the articulator. In addition to the the graphic appliance prescription, a printed recapitulation of the prescription is provided. In the lower part of the sheet on the right side the appliance type and variation by name and number should be circled. On the left side any additional parts, such as interdental springs **(I),** a bite plane **(P),** a screen **(X),** or a splint **(S),** should be marked. When the analysis is finished, Bimler classification of the problem should be made in the upper right corner. Usually the staff member who performs the analysis and prescribes the appliance will put his initials beside the date. The prescription will become valid only after it has been signed by the responsible dentist in the lower right corner. No prescriptions will be accepted in our laboratory without this signature. The technician making the appliance has to sign on the left side. The date when the order is given to the laboratory, when the appliance is delivered, and by whom it was checked are inserted in the middle of the last line.

Stomatopedic Treatment Sheet

The stomatopedic treatment sheet is the principal record of information in our case histories. On its top line it bears the name of the patient, his age and birthday, the start of the treatment, the name of the responsible orthodontist, and a case number. Then space is provided for the diagnosis, a written treatment plan, and the prognosis. The rest of the sheet is for the dental arch analysis and the individual reaction curves.

Continuous Dental Arch Measurements

For effective and rational treatment procedures, it is absolutely necessary that the orthodontist is at all times fully informed about the extent to which his treatment plan has been realized and what is left to be done. The best way we know of to keep full control is to measure the dental arches routinely at each appointment, and to record the treatment progress graphically. We adopted this method from the pulse and temperature charts in general medicine, and instituted individual reaction curves of the dental development with regard to arch width and arch height.

To register these measurements, we use a chart with a millimeter grid. It is divided by a heavy midline into an upper and a lower part for the measured distances in the maxillary and mandibular arches, respectively. The time is marked from left to right along the midline, reserving 1 cm. for each quarter of a year in the actual treatment time, and half of that space for the following years of retention and supervision. A vertical line signifies the start of treatment. We utilize green base lines, parallel to the midline, which represent statistical mean values based on the Pont index, for the purpose of comparison only. The mean values can simply be taken from a scale on the left side of the chart. For a detailed description see page 404 in the White Girl case concerning preparation of the reaction curve chart.

TWO-DIMENSIONAL CALIPER

To facilitate measurements in the mouth of the patient, a precision instrument (Fig. 13–30) has been developed by which the dental arch width and the dental arch height can be taken simultaneously and immediately transferred to the graph paper of our record chart (see Fig. 13–28).

AUTOMATIC SELF-LIMITATION OF REFLEX-CONTROLLED EXPANSION

The most important finding we discovered from this recording method was the revelation that arch expansions resulting from reactions to the wearing

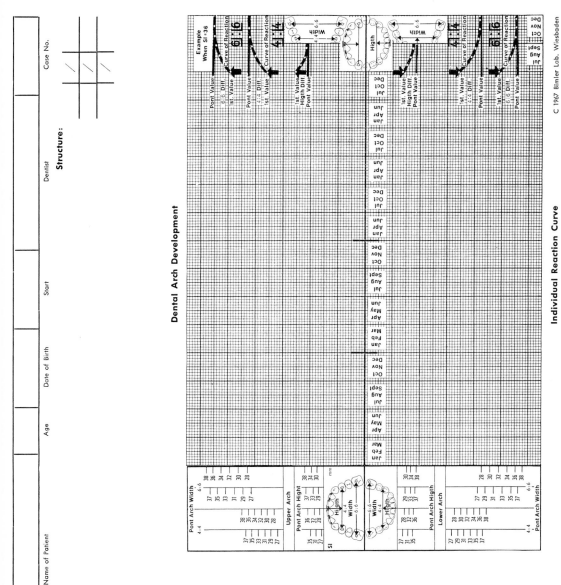

Figure 13–28. Bimler Stomatopedic Treatment Sheet.

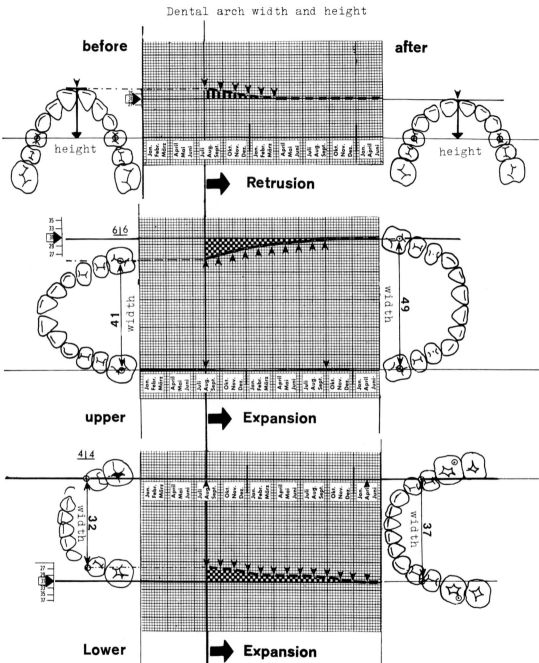

Figure 13–29. *Left,* The retrusion of the upper front teeth as measured by the two-dimensional caliper (Fig. 13–30) demonstrates itself as a declining line toward the mean value line. *Center,* Molar expansion in the upper arch presented by a climbing line of consecutive measuring points. Mean values are reached after 13 months. *Below,* Expansion of lower buccal segments occurs slowly but steadily, simultaneously with space opening and tooth eruption. (See discussion of Blue Boy, p. 436).

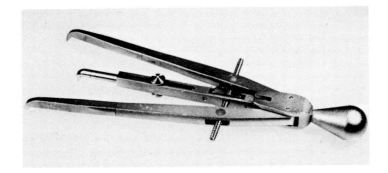

Figure 13-30. Bimler two-dimensional caliper. The caliper consists of two arms, which are moved by winding the wheel on the center pole. Also on the center pole is a sliding rod that can be moved sagittally. It is designed to allow one to measure both the height and the width of the dental arch.

of a floating elastic appliance slow down after a while so that they eventually level out with the base lines (Fig. 13-31). This occurs without any deactivating adjustment of the appliance. A renewed expansion while the appliance is worn as a retainer, or a spontaneous increase in arch width without any appliance, has been observed during puberty or even later. Once this individual bor-

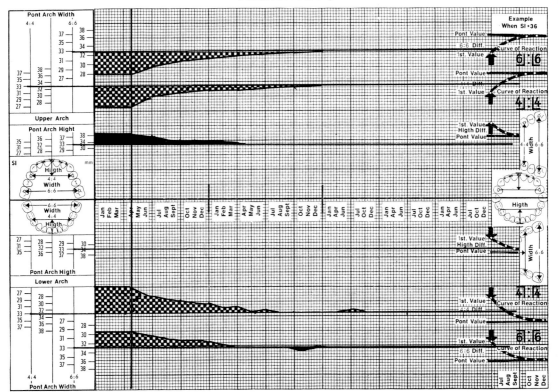

Figure 13-31. Typical curve of patient reacting well to a floating bimaxillary appliance. Onset of expansion with about 1 mm. per month on all measuring points. Simultaneously the incisor protrusion is reduced. The expansion slows down in the second year and finally comes to a complete standstill, coinciding with the Pont mean values. This coincidence can be observed in about 50 per cent of our patients. Later, no reaction can be seen in this particular patient, even though the unchanged appliance has been worn as a retainer. The amount of expansion is limited automatically to correspond to the physiological borderline of adaptability. The reduction of the arch height has to be controlled by the anterior springs, counteracting the labial arch as soon as the base line is reached.

derline of arch expansion has been established, it has to be respected. If it is exceeded by means of any active plate or fixed orthodontic appliance, relapses are usually observed afterward.

THE PHYSIOLOGICAL BORDERLINE OF ADAPTABILITY

Contrary to the automatic self-limitation of expansion using reflex-controlled floating appliances, in all cases with any sort of fixed wire appliance or plate the physiological borderline will establish itself by relapse. In our example case (Fig. 13–32) with a narrow upper arch and ectopic canines, the parents had adamantly refused the indicated extractions, so we had to treat the case on a nonextraction basis. As we saw little or no chance to develop the upper arch with a floating appliance alone, we used simultaneously a fixed lingual arch wire with redoubling free ends as palatal bars. The initial effect seemed to disprove our skepticism, for the arch was expanded up to the Pont mean values. At this point we removed the fixed arch wire and used the floating appliance as a retainer. A relapse could not be prevented. As the parents still refused extractions, we tried a Schwarz-type expansion plate, which worked against the alveolar processes. Again expansion was achieved, but the sad experience of the first attempt was only repeated. As a last effort we used a fixed palatal plate for a rapid expansion. An extraordinary overexpansion took place. The occlusion was temporarily disturbed, but another relapse could not be prevented. It should be noted that the relapses on all three occasions went down to the same level (Fig. 13–32E). This unusual experience proves dramatically that each patient has his individual physiologic borderline of adaptability. It is the epoch-making quality of the reflex-controlled floating appliances that they respect automatically this physiologic borderline.

REMARKS ON DENTAL ARCH EXPANSION

In Europe, arch expansion has always been practiced as the standard approach to crowding problems, despite the fact that relapse has often been observed. In the United States, expansion has been practically abandoned for the last 30 years. Based on the overwhelming evidence of successfully treated expansion cases, we are convinced that arch expansion cannot simply be denied; on the other hand, we are aware that the inherent danger of relapse should not be neglected either. So the question arises how much expansion can be tolerated by the individual case. For the reflex-controlled functional therapy, the problem has been definitely solved. The amount of tolerable dental arch expansion is established individually in the initial test period of the treatment and documents itself automatically in the leveling out of the reaction curve. When the borderline of adaptability is reached, the curves will remain parallel to the reference line, which represents the Pont and Korkhaus mean values. Retrospectively, after 20 years of clinical experience we may state that in about 50 per cent of the cases, the individual adaptability will finally coincide with the Pont mean values; in other cases it will even surpass the mean; and in those cases in which extractions are indicated, the curves will constantly fall short of the mean.

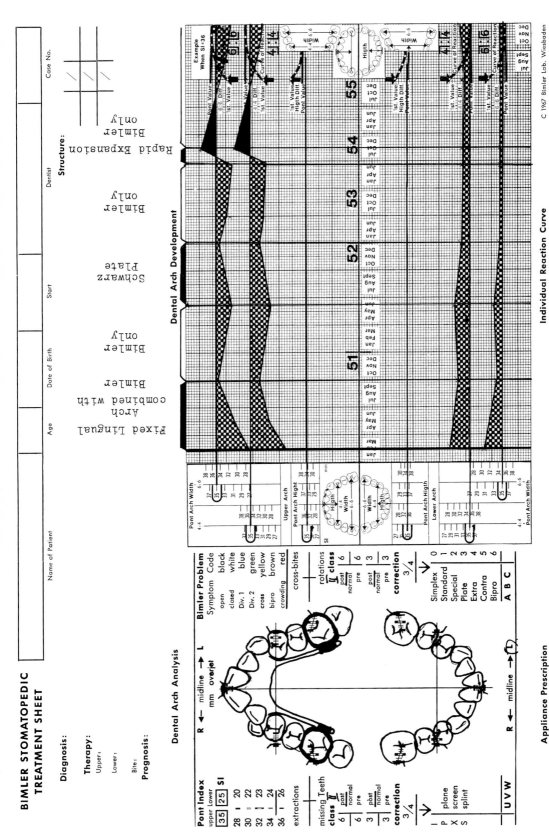

Figure 13–32. Stomatopedic treatment sheet of a patient whose parents did not agree to the planned extractions. After each active treatment period, there was a relapse of the occlusion almost to the original malocclusion.

Dental Arch Development

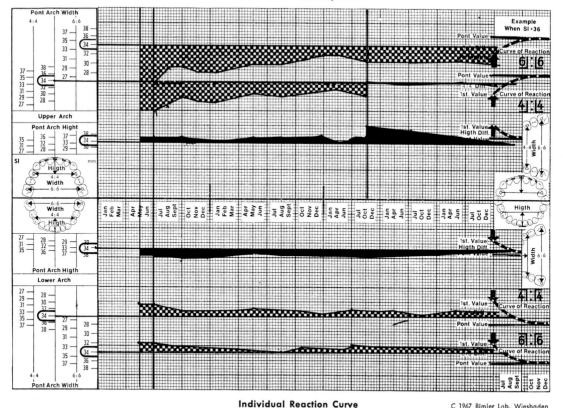

Individual Reaction Curve

C 1967 Bimler Lab. Wiesbaden

Figure 13–33. Indication for extraction. If a patient shows a big deficiency on his measurement chart at the beginning and no continuous reaction or even repeated slight relapses in his curve, this will be regarded as an indication for extraction. Afterwards, the anterior arch width and the arch height will be measured from the second premolars. The decrease of these two measurements will demonstrate the progress in space closing. The molar curve reacts only little or not at all to the anterior extraction. More about the treatment planning in extraction cases is found in the discussion of Red Girl (p. 452).

INCISOR CLASSIFICATION

Appliance Typing

In the time of Edward H. Angle, factory-made arch wires were used in all sorts of malocclusions. The main difference in the therapy was the placement of the intermaxillary elastics. For this purpose the Angle molar classification gave a clear directive. With bimaxillary appliances the intermaxillary relationship is taken care of automatically. It is no longer the main criterion for the selection of the therapeutic device.

By contrast, the indications for Bimler appliances depend on the incisor relationship, which was described by Angle as Division 1 for protrusive and Division 2 for retrusive incisors. The reversed incisor relationship in Class III cases was not particularly considered by Angle.

In 1950 the author proposed a classification of three types of malocclusions according to the incisor relationship: Type A for protrusive incisors, Type B for retrusive incisors, and Type C for reversed incisors. For each of these groups a special type of appliance was developed and named correspondingly.

THE A APPLIANCE

To correct protrusive incisors, an upper labial arch wire is necessary. In addition, the **A** appliance consists of other elements from the labiolingual fixed appliance technique. The labial arch in the upper and a labiolingual arch in the lower are connected by two palatal acrylic wings. They are complemented by two frontal springs on the lingual side in the upper and a frontal loop in the lower part of the appliance.

THE B APPLIANCE

The cases with retrusive incisors offer different problems. The dental arches have to be stretched, and the incisors need uprighting. For this purpose a stretching arch was devised, which works in the upper against the palatal aspects of the incisors. It is fixed in an upper palatal plate, which offers the necessary anchorage for the sagittal action of the arch wire. An additional support is provided by interdental springs, which work against the upper laterals and canines. Molar supports in the lower dental arch serve the same purpose.

THE C APPLIANCE

The **C** appliance is designed to correct any sort of anterior crossbites. It has occlusal wires upholstered with rubber tubing to block the occlusion and to open the bite. The labial arch originates in the upper wings and is bent down to work against the lower incisors. It is counteracted by upper frontal springs, which protrude the upper incisors. In the lower arch, the divided linguolabial arch wires are not connected on the labial side as in the **A** and **B** types, but lingually with an undulate bar **W.**

Appliance Variations

In addition to the main characteristics of a malocclusion as defined by the types A, B, and C according to the incisor classification, the therapeutic task in each individual case depends on a number of accompanying features, such as a minor or major degree of crowding, incisor rotations, blocked-out teeth, diastemas, or crossbites. For these additional problems, about six variations of the three main types of appliance have been developed.

The main parts of all the appliances are always the same. The variations consist only of additional items that can be eliminated at any time, reducing the variation to the standard form again. In Figure 13–35 16 appliances are arranged in three horizontal lines according to the three types and in six vertical columns for the variations, which have the same characteristics for all three types. They are further divided into two groups—on the left side for crowded cases with space-creating appliances and on the right side with space-closing appliances for cases with or without extractions.

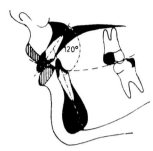

Protrusive Incisors

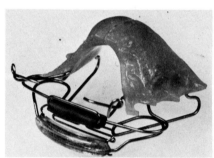

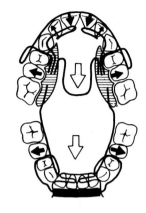

Class II, Division I

A

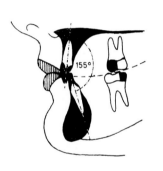

Retrusive Incisors

B

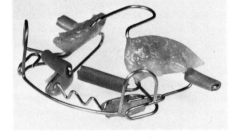

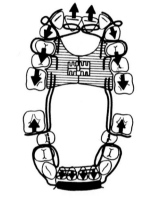

Class II, Division 2

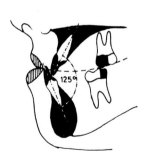

Reversed Incisors

C

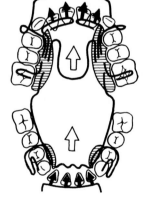

Class III

Figure 13-34. The three basic types of Bimler appliances.

VARIATION 1: STANDARD

The idea is that the indication for these variations starts on the far left, with the standard form for more or less normal arches with only minor occurrence of crowding, where the interarch malrelationship is our greatest concern.

VARIATION 2: SPECIAL

In the majority of our cases the normal development of the dental arches is either delayed or, more often, disturbed, owing to an underdevelopment in the bony structures and/or the functional matrix. The symptoms within the arches are rotated anterior teeth or blocked-out teeth in the buccal segments. It is our clinical experience that a lot can be done toward a normalizing development by attacking these symptoms in the mixed dentition by means of a series of interdental springs. As these interdental springs have been devised for special tasks within the general problem, variation 2 has been named "special." The numerous possibilities of the interdental springs enable us to finish our cases with the functional appliance, whereas many clinicians using other modifications of the activator are still obliged to use fixed techniques for rotations, space closing, or space opening.

VARIATION 3: HYPO

Cases with a hypoplastic development in the middle part of the face very often show a narrow dental arch and a high palated vault with uni- or bilateral open bites. Here we are looking for sutural apposition through a direct attack on the alveolar processes. An anteriorly cutout palatal plate with a jackscrew serves this purpose best. The A_3 and C_3 variations have proved so effective that they have completely replaced any rapid expansion procedures in our office. In crossbite cases the upper expansion can be complemented by lower contraction by means of crossbite springs. In later stages of the treatment the jackscrew and the central part of the plate are usually cut away and replaced by a Coffin spring.

VARIATION 4: EXTRA

In cases with an even higher degree of crowding due to basal bone hypoplasia or macrodontia, the extraction of first premolars may be indicated. Tooth alignment and space closing are performed with a variation that resembles variation 2, with the exception that the upper **A** or **C** labial arches have oblique crossover wires. They span the extraction gaps from the mesial aspects of the second premolars to the distal aspects of the canines.

VARIATION 5: CONTRA

In cases with telescoped bite, the upper arch has to be contracted while the lower is expanded. This can be performed only if the bite is blocked to prevent continuous relapse. In reliable patients with excellent cooperation, we can use the A_5 variation with I_6 interdental springs and/or bite planes **P** to separate the arches. The upper will be contracted by means of buccal springs I_5, with a double Coffin spring **R** in the Types **A** and **C** or an open jackscrew in the **B** type.

Crowding

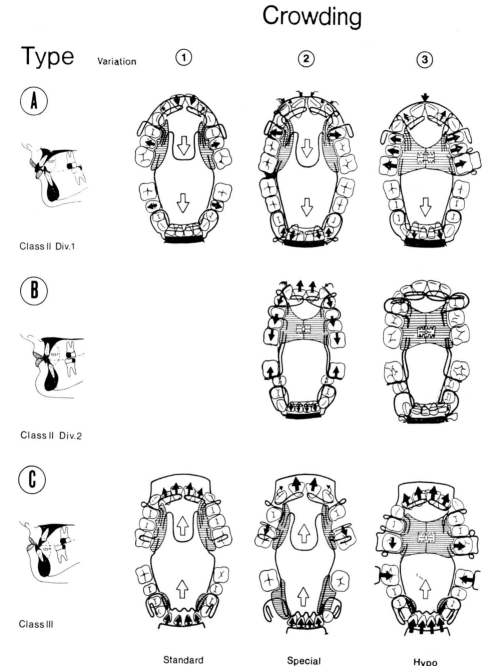

Figure 13–35. Systematic chart of the three types and six variations of the Bimler appliances.

Spacing

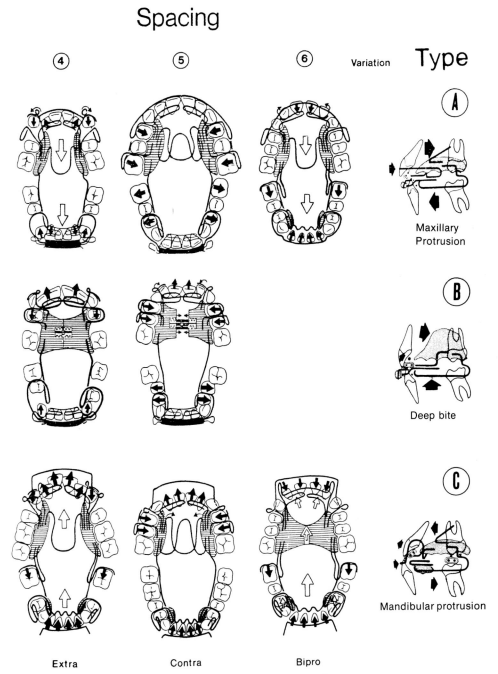

Figure 13-35 *Continued.*

VARIATION 6: BIPRO

Cases with bimaxillary dental protrusion and spacing of the anteriors usually do not need any expansion but do need sagittal tooth movements. In the mesial direction we may count on spontaneous drifting. By careful grinding of the upper wings, we can ensure that these movements are not impeded. For the uprighting of the lower incisors especially, we need a good sagittal support. Two little acrylic wings kept apart by an undulated bar **W** will provide this support. If this is not sufficient, additional mesial supports can be fixed with oval tubes to the anterior recurved loops of the sleds. These supports rest distal to the premolars. Also, reversed molar supports **M** can be used to accelerate space closing in the buccal segments. In the C_6 variation, an additional upper arch can be used for torquing.

BIMLER PROBLEM GROUPING AND COLOR

Assigning a certain appliance type and variation to a case includes a condensed diagnosis and treatment plan. In our office we will refer to a certain case with regard to the therapy simply by calling it an A2 or C3 case. This is based mostly on the findings seen on the models. It does not say anything about the prognosis, which depends far more on the anatomic facial structure and its deficiencies. To classify a patient according to his predominant symptoms with regard to the prognosis, so-called problem groups have been established and each group has been given a special code color.

Predominant Symptom	Code Color
Open bite	Black
Closed bite	White
Class II, Division 1	Blue
Class II, Division 2	Green
Class III	Yellow
Bimaxillary protrusion with spacing	Brown
Hypoplasia with crowding	Red

Symptoms and code colors are printed on our analysis sheet and the grouping is an integrated part of our diagnostic and prognostic procedure. The folders of our case histories are also color-coded, so the clinician can see from the color which sort of problem the patient offers. Later, after treatment has been finished, the folders will be filed according to their color. Within their problem group they are subdivided according to their facial formula and the appliance used. Over the years we have assembled a large number of cases, which has allowed us to compare the influence of certain facial features with regard to the prognosis and to evaluate the experiences of previous cases to enable us to handle later ones even better.

Clinical experience of 25 years has taught us that dolichoprosopic or deep faces have in general a bad prognosis in the green group, but a good prognosis in the yellow and black groups. Leptoprosopic or long faces, however, have a bad prognosis in the black and yellow groups but a good prognosis in the green group.

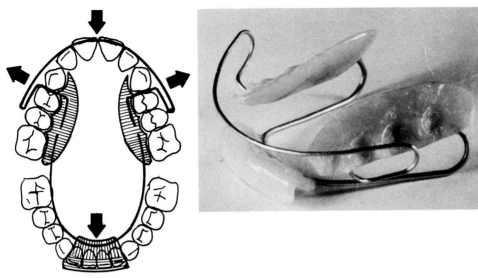

Figure 13-36. Bimler primary appliance (1948).

Indication: Class II, Division 1 cases, mixed and permanent dentitions.

Possibilities: Upper expansion
Anterior retrusion
Repositioning of lower arch.

Advantages (compared with the activator):
Daytime wearing
Adjustability of lower part in sagittal direction
Independent transverse adaptability of upper part

Shortcomings: Solid cap interferes with upper incisors during last stages of retrusion
No transverse adaptability from lingual
Arch wire in lower cuspid area

Appliance Evolution

Our work was aimed from the very beginning toward a synthesis of the American wire techniques and the European functional methods. It could be realized only by disregarding traditional opinions held by both of these competing methods. It was based on a completely open mind and the pursuit of one constructive idea.

The earliest form of the Bimler appliance was a simple circular arrangement of an upper labial arch wire combined with a lower lingual arch wire, connected by two acrylic palatal wings and completed by a lower acrylic cap (Fig. 13–36). In this prototype the main characteristics of the later Bimler wire parts, the redoubling U-shaped loops, were used for the first time in the upper labial arch. Instead of vertical loops used in the Hawley appliance for adjustment, the distal portion of the labial arch was brought back in two redoubling loops in a posteroanterior direction. This arrangement has a number of advantages. First, the labial arch wire is simplified and kept in one plane of space, the horizontal. Second, the adjustment loops are arranged in a plane perpendicular to the main arch, in the vertical. This is an important point for mechanical stability. Third, the redoubling loop serves as a compensating element for the lateral movements of the mandible while the appliance is in place. Fourth, the U-shaped loop allows dimensional and positional changes, precisely lengthening and shortening or raising and lowering the arch without changing its form.

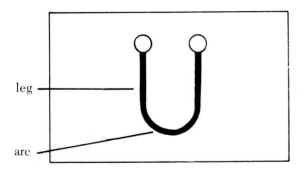

leg

arc

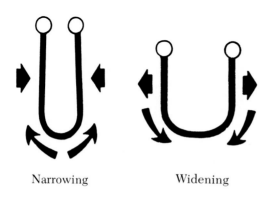

Narrowing   Widening

Figure 13-37. The redoubling **U** loop: exclusive adjustment element. What looked in the beginning like just a modification of an adjustment loop became the fundamental constructive element for all dimensional changes in the Bimler appliances. The recurved loops were strategically placed all over the appliance to allow adjustments in all three planes of space. They all consist of a semicircular arc and two parallel legs. These **U** loops can be widened, resulting in a bigger arc and shorter legs, or narrowed, resulting in a smaller arc but longer legs. Principally, these maneuvers serve to transfer wire material from the legs to the arc or vice versa. When material is transferred first from one leg to the arc and then from the arc to the other leg, the first leg will become shorter and the other leg longer.

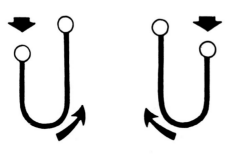

Shortening   Lengthening

Similar redoubling loops in the vertical plane build the connection of the lingual arch with the upper part, allowing for the first time a continuous anteroposterior adjustment of a bimaxillary appliance.

With this possibility for adjustment we were able to overcome one of the main reasons why bimaxillary appliances are lost at night. Only a certain amount of forward positioning of the mandible will be tolerated by the child. If the first correction in the wax bite for an activator is too much, the appliance is unconsciously removed. Whenever this occurs with a Bimler appliance, the forward position of the lower part of the appliance can easily be reduced and later increased again.

Mechanical Stability

In a bimaxillary three-dimensional wire appliance, the first concern has to be stability, to prevent mechanical distortion. In the Bimler appliance, this stability has been achieved by a continuous change from one plane of space to another in the arrangement of the elements of the appliance. To illustrate, we will analyze the elements of the appliance and their positions in space (Fig. 13–38). Beginning with the upper labial arch, we notice that it is placed in the horizontal plane. The connecting elements, the lateral adjustment loops, are found at right angles to the upper labial arch, in the vertical plane. From the vertical loops, the wires cross the dental arches in the horizontal plane, to end up in the acrylic wings, which are more or less in the vertical plane once again.

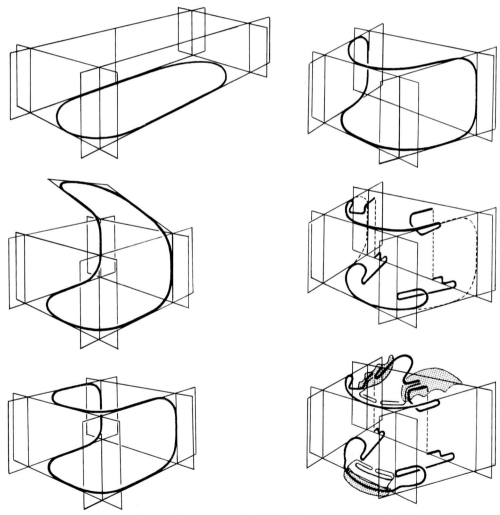

Figure 13-38. The Bimler appliance as a redoubled ellipse. We believe that it is very important for the successful application of this therapy to understand first the general aspects of the appliances. As mentioned before, they are circular arrangements of prefabricated parts that can be reduced theoretically to an ellipse. We have to image the ellipse folded back onto itself, forming a double U-shaped loop diverging toward the rear. The main arches of the appliance and the acrylic wings that unite the two to the full circle fit into this theoretical framework of the redoubling ellipse.

The lingual arch originates in the posterior end of the acrylic wings. From there it forms the so-called sleds, with two loops in the molar and two more in the canine region. The loops are oriented in the vertical plane. The arch wire continues to the labial side of the dental arch, forming two large loops in the horizontal plane. Finally, in the frontal aspect, the labial part has a depression which is imbedded in the acrylic of the frontal shield. This can be regarded as in the vertical plane again. This continually changing arrangement of the constructive elements of the appliance results in remarkable stability of the whole structure, averting the possibility of permanent distortion while allowing temporary elastic deformation.

THE DEVELOPMENT OF ORTHODONTIC ARCH WIRES

In addition to the abilities of the operator, the result of any mechanotherapy depends, to a certain degree, on the efficiency of the appliances used. To handle the problems offered by more complicated cases, we have taken advantage of the progress that has been achieved in the development of fixed wire appliances. It will be useful to briefly summarize this development.

Like the dental arch wire, all labial and lingual arch wires are of ellipsoid form and are therefore subject to the geometric laws of the ellipse. This means that if one diameter of the ellipse is enlarged—for example, the width—the other diameter, the length, will automatically become smaller. In other words, if the lateral segments of the dental arch are expanded, the anterior segment will become flattened and retruded. Furthermore, the canines are in a sort of neutral zone, moving neither buccally nor lingually. With the expansion arch of Angle (Fig. 13–39*A*), molars could be moved buccally while the incisors were retracted. To move both canines and premolars, ligation was necessary. Very soon, attempts were made to replace these ligatures. In the appliance of Simon (Berlin) (Fig. 13–39*B*), the expanding forces of the labial arch wire were transferred by means of the palatal bars to the lingual aspects of the canines and premolars. Unfortunately, the disadvantage resulting from this design was molar rotation. The idea of Ainsworth (Fig. 13–39*C*) to use a shortened labial arch with a tube-and-pin stress-breaker attached to a premolar band, in combination with palatal bars, brought two more advantages: the forces of the labial arch became most effective in the canine-premolar region, and any rotational effect was eliminated. The same principle is used in the upper part of the Bimler appliance (Fig. 13–39*D*). The redoubled U-shaped adjustment loops replace the stress-breakers, and the crossover wires are inserted in front of the premolars in the palatal acrylic wings. In this design, the neutral zone of the labial arch has been placed between the laterals and the canines. This is the physiologic border between premaxilla and maxilla. As will be seen later, we are taking advantage of the neutral zone to cross the dental arch in this place with our interdental springs. Frontal springs have been introduced to influence the incisor teeth from the lingual aspect.

In the lower arch wires, we can find a corresponding development. With the simple lingual arch (Fig. 13–16*E*), only the molars could be more or less influenced without the help of ligation. Therefore, the soldered auxiliary springs, introduced by Mershon (Fig. 13–16*F*), were regarded as a progressive

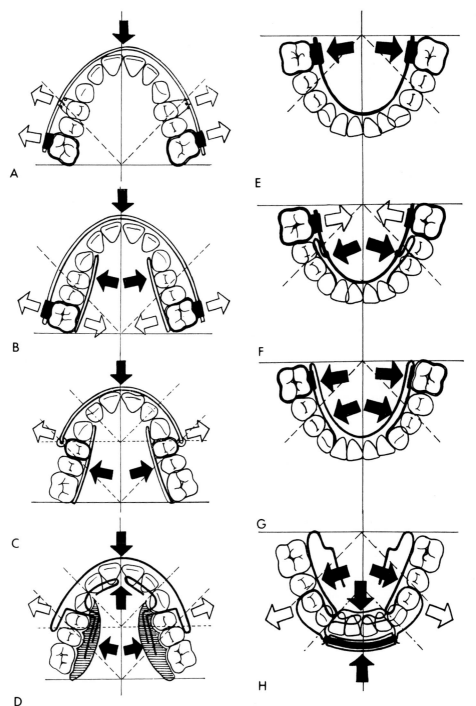

Figure 13-39. The development of orthodontic arch wires. Lower arches: *A*, Primitive labial arch wire with ligatures. Expansion in the buccal segments and retrusion in the anterior segment (Angle). *B*, Palatal bars transfer expanding forces as pressure to palatal aspects of buccal segments (Simon). *C*, Shortened labial arch is most effective in the canine region. Note stress-breaking pin and tube attachment (Ainsworth). *D*, Same arrangement of shortened labial arch in free-floating version with additional frontal springs. The redoubled loop of the labial arch replaces the stress-breaker (Bimler). *E*, Simple lingual arch wire with molar bands. Expansion only in the molar region (Lefoulon). *F*, Lingual arch wire with soldered auxiliary springs. Good expansion in premolar and canine regions, but not always correlated with molar expansion (Mershon). *G*, Redoubled ends of lingual arch with molar bands. Good expansion of total buccal segment (Coffin, Herbst). *H*, Combination of shortened labial arch with two lingual sleds and frontal loop controls expansion of buccal segments and alignment of anteriors (Bimler).

development. Using the elastic springs and a rather rigid main arch, very often one could observe that the premolars were moved but the molars stayed. After stainless steel and lighter wires were introduced, the redoubled free ends of the main lingual arch wire were used to obtain a balanced expansion of the whole buccal segment (Fig. 13–16*G*). Early attempts by the author to use free-ending lingual bars failed in removable devices. The breakthrough in the lower arch wire design came only after the lingual arch was turned around with the recurved loops to the anterior and the free-ending parts to the posterior (Fig. 13–16*H*). The free ends were bent upward and then were fixed in the palatal wings. In this manner, they formed a sort of sled that could be kept stable even in removable appliances. The former anterior lingual part was generously enlarged and was bent back onto itself in two vertical loops. By means of two horizontal loops, it was then carried to the vestibule. There it constitutes the labial portion analogous to the shortened upper labial arch wire. This labiolingual lower arch became the standard form of nearly all Bimler appliances. It was later completed by a lower anterior loop to align the incisor teeth. Because they incorporate the use of the most progressive currently developed arch forms, the Bimler wire parts represent the experience of half a century of labiolingual wire technique, along with the advantages of the reflex-controlled action of the free-floating functional appliance.

PREFABRICATED PARTS

Code Letters and Colors

The effectiveness of the Bimler appliance depends a great deal on well-balanced relationships between the single parts and components. In order to secure a uniform look and effect of the devices throughout the world, prefabricated parts have been developed and are available in different sizes (Fig. 13–40). They are made of a special alloy of consistent quality and are carefully bent with special tools or by hand, to reduce the risk of breakage to a minimum. The appliances are nowadays simply assembled in dental laboratories from the matching parts selected according to an individual prescription. In case of a necessary repair, all soldering has been discontinued and the broken parts are always replaced by spare parts of the same size.

All the prefabs are identified by code letters and numbers indicating their form and size. These code letters are used to order the parts from the manufacturer or to refer to them in case histories, repair orders, and published descriptions.

Preservation of Shape

For balanced action of the appliance, it is absolutely necessary to preserve its original shape as a whole by maintaining the position and form of the individual components. For guidance, it should be noted that the main arches must always be kept parallel in the horizontal plane. Likewise within the components, the legs of the recurved U-loops should always be kept parallel and the same distance from each other. Experience has taught us that this precondition

TABLE 13-1. BIMLER PREFABRICATED PARTS

Upper Arches

A	Upper labial arch
B	Stretching arch
C	Bimaxillary arch
D	Labial arch

Lower Arches

UV	Lower arch
U	Lower arch (divided)
M	Molar supports (push-back)
UC	Lower arch (Class III)
W	Lower connecting bar

Accessories

I		Interdental springs
	I$_1$	Cuspid support
	I$_2$	Cuspid support with mesial extension, incisor rotation
	I$_3$	Cuspid support with distal extension, cuspid rotation
	I$_4$	Vertical loop (push-back)
	I$_5$	Buccal spring, bicuspids
	I$_6$	Horizontal loop, bite opening
K		Crossbite spring
F		Frontal springs
R		Coffin spring
L		Lower frontal loop
S		Lower frontal splint
E		Lower cuspid support
P		Equiplane (bite block)
X		Frontal shield (bumper)

to success is endangered chiefly by iatrogenic distortion. The mistakes made by dentists in misguided attempts to adjust the appliances create more difficulties than anything else. It is therefore our advice to beginners to observe the action of the appliance for the first four weeks and then to use only their fingers for adjustment. Later, the adjustments are restricted to special areas, the recurved loops. Beginners should follow the programmed handling instructions without introducing any personal variations. In general, the circular arrangement of the main wires requires strictly symmetrical activation of equal amount and at homologous places.

TOOLS AND RULES: A SYSTEMATIC HANDLING PROGRAM

Standardized Tools. Programmed adjustment procedures require standardized tools. Two special pairs of pliers matching the size and shape of the prefabricated wire parts are used exclusively, for fabrication and adjustment.

One pair of pliers has two flat jaws and the other has one round and one concave jaw. The two are opposite in their effect and are used alternatively. In the instructions for our adjustment program, these two pairs of pliers will be referred to as FLAT-(beak) and ROUND-(beak) in capital letters (Fig. 13–41).

Text continued on page 383

PREFAB UPPER ARCHES

A Upper Labial Arches   0,9 mm = .036"
for class I and II

order No.	color	sum of upper incisors
A 00	black	primaries small
A 0	white	primaries large
A 1	yellow	27 – 29 mm
A 2	red	30 – 32 mm
A 3	green	33 – 35 mm
A 4	blue	36 – 38 mm

for extraction cases

Aa 2	red	30 – 32 mm
Aa 3	green	33 – 35 mm
Aa 4	blue	36 – 38 mm

Bipro cases

Ad 2	red	30 – 32 mm
Ad 3	green	33 – 35 mm
Ad 4	blue	36 – 38 mm

B Stretching Arches   0,9 mm = .036"
for Div. 2 cases

order No.	color	sum of upper incisors
Bb 1	yellow	27 – 32 mm
Bb 2	red	33 – 38 mm
B 1	yellow	27 – 29 mm
B 2	red	30 – 32 mm
B 3	green	33 – 35 mm
B 4	blue	36 – 38 mm

C Bimaxillary Arches   0,9 mm = 036"
for class III and pseudo class III

order No.	color	sum of upper incisors
C 00	black	primaries small
C 0	white	primaries large
C 1	yellow	27 – 29 mm
C 2	red	30 – 32 mm
C 3	green	33 – 35 mm
C 4	blue	36 – 38 mm

D Labial Arches   0,8 mm   .032"
   0,7 mm   .028"
for retainers and simple plates

order No.	color	sum of upper incisors
D 00	black	primaries small
D 0	white	primaries large
D 1	yellow	27 – 29 mm
D 2	red	30 – 32 mm
D 3	green	33 – 35 mm
D 4	blue	36 – 38 mm

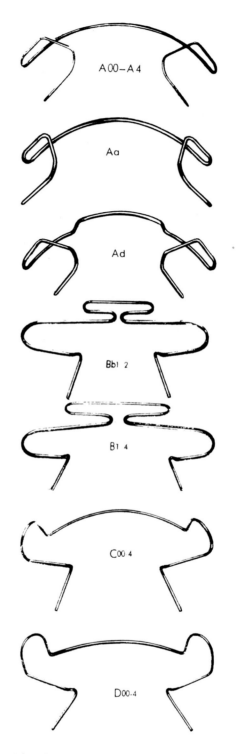

A 00 – A 4

Aa

Ad

Bb1 2

B1 4

C00 4

D00-4

Figure 13-40. Prefabricated parts available for the Bimler appliances.

Illustration continued on opposite page

PREFAB LOWER ARCHES

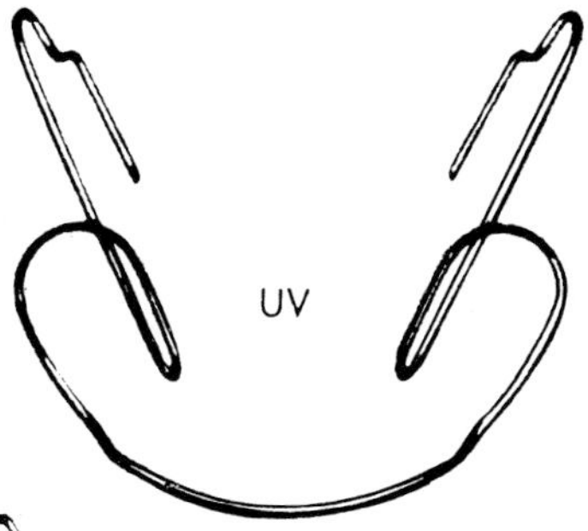

Lower Arches   0,9 mm = .036   **UV**

order No.	color	sum of upper incisors
UV 0	white	primaries
UV 1	yellow	27 – 29 mm
UV 2	red	30 – 32 mm
UV 3	green	33 – 35 mm
UV 4	blue	36 – 38 mm

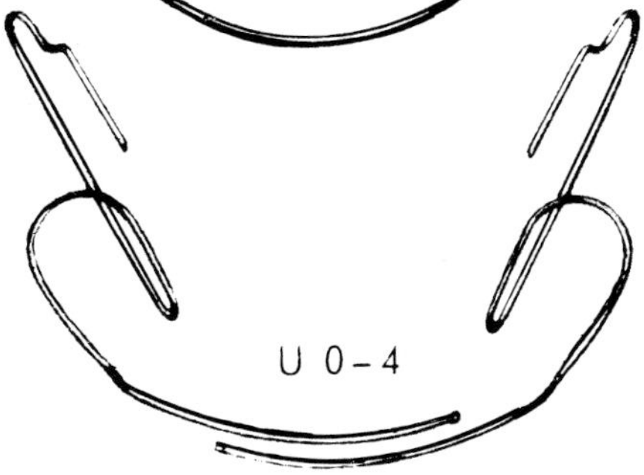

Lower Arches (divided)   0,9 mm = .036 " r+l   **U**

order No.	color	sum of upper incisors
U 0	white	primaries
U 1	yellow	27 – 29 mm
U 2	red	30 – 32 mm
U 3	green	33 – 35 mm
U 4	blue	36 – 38 mm

M molar-supports
(push back) 0,8 mm = .032" (r+l)   **M**

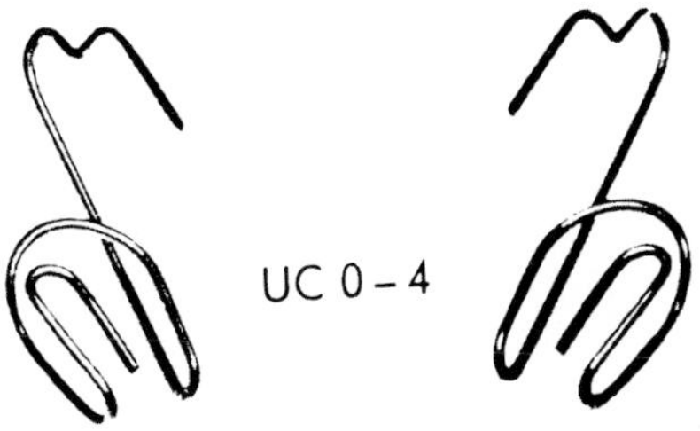

Lower Arches (class III) 0,9 mm = .036 " r+l   **UC**

order No.	color	sum of upper incisors
UC 0	white	primaries
UC 1	yellow	27 – 31 mm
UC 2	red	32 – 34 mm
UC 3	green	33 – 35 mm
UC 4	blue	36 – 38 mm

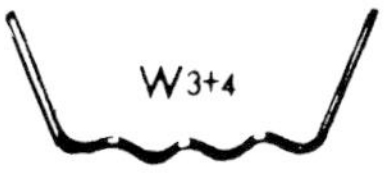

Lower Connecting Bars 0,8 mm = .032"   **W**

order No.	description
W	3 loops

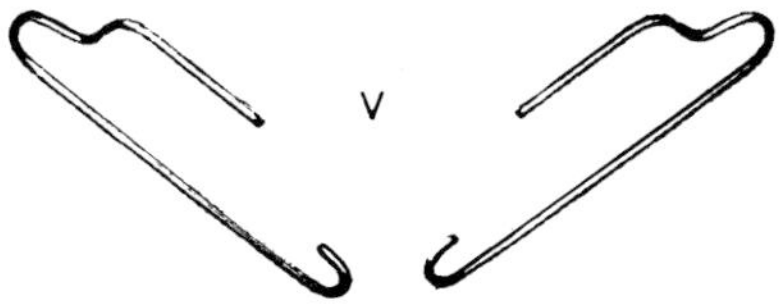

Connecting Springs for double plates 0,9 mm   **V**

order Nr.	description
V	Connecting spring

Figure 13–40   *Continued.*

Illustration continued on following page

PREFAB ACCESSORIES

I **Interdental springs** 0,8 mm .032″ (r+l)

order No.	description
I 1	Cuspid support
I 2	Cuspid support with mesial extension, incisor rotation
I 3	Cuspid support with distal extension, cuspid rotation
I 5	Buccal spring, Bicuspids
I 4	Vertical Loop, push back
I 6	Horizontal Loop, bite opening

K K   cross-bite-spring 0,8 mm =.032″ (r+l)

F **Frontal Springs**   0,8 mm = .032″ (r+l)

order No.	color	sum of upper incisors
F 0	white	plain
F 1	yellow	27—30 mm
F 2	red	30—35 mm
F 3	blue	36—38 mm
Ff1	yellow	27—30 mm
Ff2	red	30—35 mm
Ff3	blue	36—38 mm

R R   Coffinsprings 0,9 mm =.036″

L **Lower Frontal Loops**   0,6 mm = .024″

order No.	color	sum of upper incisors
L 1	yellow	27—30 mm
L 2	red	31—34 mm
L 3	blue	35—38 mm

S **Lower Frontal Splints**

order No.	description
S	with attachments

E **Lower Cuspid Supports**   0,7 mm = .028″

order No.	color	sum of upper incisors
E 1	yellew	27—30 mm
E 2	red	31—34 mm
E 3	blue	35—38 mm

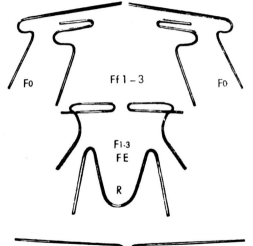

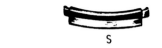

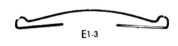

Figure 13–40   *Continued.*

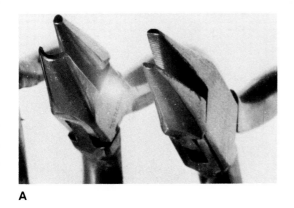

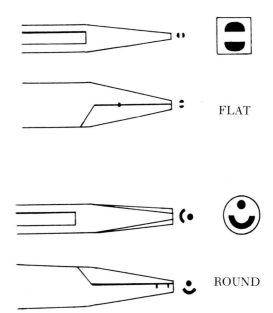

Figure 13–41. *A*, Round (*left*) and flat (*right*) pliers. *B*, Flat-beak pliers (*top*) and round- and concave-beak pliers (*bottom*).

Standardized Objects. Generally speaking, we have to work with only two forms of wires—straight and curved. The straight wires will be referred to in this text as "flat" and the curved wire parts as "round" (in lower case letters) (Fig. 13–45*B*). Practically speaking, the flat wires are identical to the legs and the curved ones to the arcs of the U-shaped loops.

Three-Point Attack. To preserve the original form of the appliance, the operator should be able to foresee clearly the effect of each adjustment he makes. He must be able to correct or to reverse his action immediately, if necessary. This can easily be achieved by the alternating use of the two standard pairs of pliers, provided we restrict our maneuvers to a simple closing of the pliers around a wire of incongruent shape. That means we use the FLAT-(beak) pliers on a curved piece of wire and the ROUND-(beak) pliers on a straight wire. The different shape of tool and material leads to a "three-point attack" by which the deforming force and the retaining force are potential powers in the same tool (Fig. 13–45*C*). With each pressure of the pliers, only a limited amount of deformation will occur. The effect has to be checked immediately to be either intensified by a second grip or reversed by the use of the other pliers.

Programmed Instructions. To simplify the handling, we have established short instructions using the abbreviations we mentioned before—"FLAT" and "ROUND" for the two pairs of pliers, and "flat" and "round" for the two forms of wires. The instruction "FLAT on round" consequently means to use the FLAT-(beak) pliers on a curved piece of wire, and "ROUND on flat" means to use the ROUND-(concave-beak) pliers on a straight piece of wire.

Basic Rules. With the use of the FLAT-(beak) pliers on a curved piece of wire, the wire will not only be straightened but lengthened at the same time (Fig. 13–45*D*). We formulate this in our first rule:

FLAT GIVES

In the opposite case, with the use of the ROUND-(beak) pliers on a straight wire, the wire will not only be bent, but shortened at the same time. We express this in our second rule:

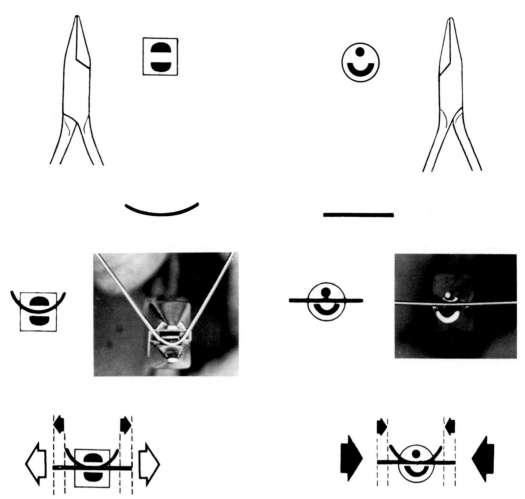

Figure 13-42. Standardized tools and their uses in the fabrication of wires for the Bimler appliances.

ROUND TAKES

We have only two alternatives in the handling of the appliance anyway: either the FLAT-(beak) or the ROUND-(beak) pliers. Habitually we start with the FLAT-(beak) tool. To decide where to place it, follow the basic rule, FLAT gives, and put the pliers on the part that will profit.

Exceptions. As mentioned before, the basis for our whole program of controlled pliers action is the incongruence of tool (contour of pliers' beaks) and material (shape of wire). If you drop this condition, using FLAT-(beak) pliers on a flat wire, nothing happens, of course (Fig. 13–43). Your action would have to be based on the exceptions of our program, employing the technique of pulling and twisting a wire part while the whole appliance is firmly held by the other hand. Always be aware that these manipulations are exceptions and that you should have the necessary experience with the appliance and its equilibrium before employing them.

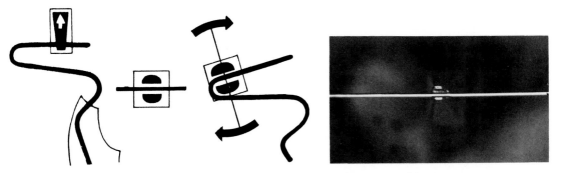

Figure 13-43. When flat-beak pliers are used on flat wire, nothing happens.

BIMLER TRAINING PROGRAM

Before anyone starts to adjust an appliance, he should perform systematic exercises to become familiar with the action of his pliers and the reaction of the single wire parts and the appliance as a whole. As mentioned before, the U-shaped redoubling loops are generally the only places where adjustments

Text continued on page 389

Figure 13-44. Bimler training program: U loop for basic exercise. *A*, FLAT on round. *B*, Loop opens. *C*, ROUND on flat. *D*, Loop closes.
Objective: Opening and closing of legs
Tools: Flat-beak and round-beak pliers
Instruction: FLAT on round
Result: Legs diverge, loop opens: FLAT gives
Instruction: ROUND on flat
Result: Legs converge, loop closes: ROUND takes
Comments: For initial exercises in the adjustment of the appliance, it is recommended that the operator make his own U-shaped training loops with two little eyelets at the ends of the legs. In all wire bending, it is most important to use the pliers in a position perpendicular to the plane of the looped wires. The simplest exercise is the narrowing and widening of the U-shaped training loop. Place the pliers perpendicular to the loop and press gently. The legs will converge or diverge according to the pliers used. With each closure of the pliers, only a limited amount of change in form will occur. By alternating the opposite pliers, the bending can easily be reversed.

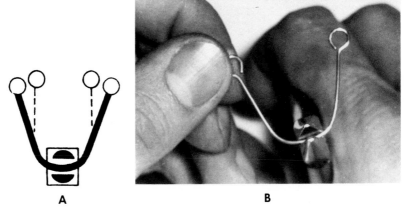

A

B

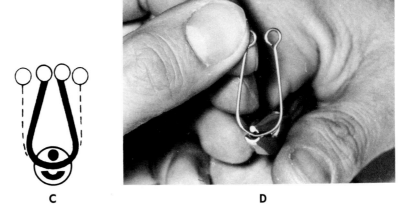

C

D

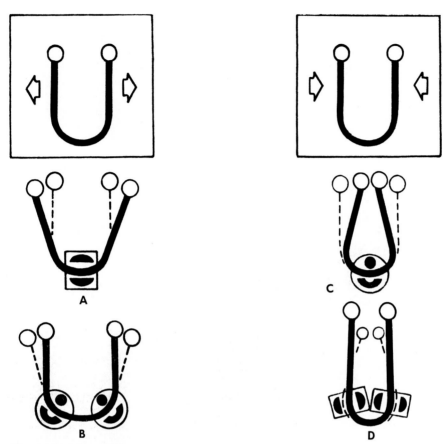

Figure 13-45. Bimler training program: U loop for basic exercises. *A,* FLAT on round. *B,* ROUND on flat. *C,* ROUND on round. *D,* FLAT on round.

    Objective: Parallel widening of loop
    Tools: Flat-beak and round-beak pliers
    Instructions: FLAT on round—center
                 ROUND on flat—both sides
    Result: Diverged legs are brought back into a parallel position, loop widened
    Objective: Parallel narrowing of loop
    Instructions: ROUND on flat—center
                 FLAT on round—both sides
    Result: Converged legs are brought back into parallel position, loop narrowed
    Comments: As a second exercise, one can try to widen and then narrow the loop so that the parallel position of the legs is maintained. We start with FLAT on round, using the flat-beak pliers in the middle of the arc. When the pliers are closed, the legs spread and the loop is widened according to the rule "FLAT gives." Now we change pliers and, following the instruction ROUND on flat, we use the round-beak pliers on both sides of the loop, where the straight parts of the legs adjoin the arc. According to the rule "ROUND takes," the arc of the loop is enlarged by taking wire from the flat legs. It may be necessary to use the pliers several times alternately before the maneuver results in a widened loop with exactly parallel but shortened legs. The reverse effect of a narrowed loop with lengthened legs will be obtained by using the round-beak pliers in the middle of the arc and then FLAT on round two times to move material from the arc to the legs.

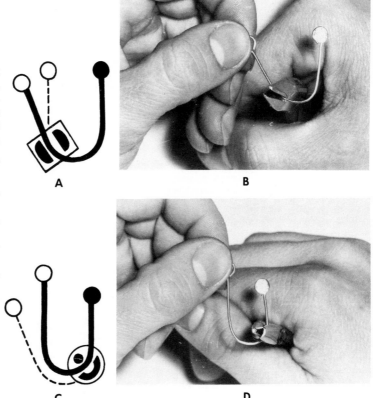

Figure 13-46. Bimler U loop: Training wire for basic exercises. *A,* FLAT on round, on empty circle leg. *B,* Give to empty circle leg. *C,* ROUND on flat, on filled circle leg. *D,* Take from filled circle leg.

    Objective: Lengthening of empty circle leg

    Tools: Flat-beak and round-beak pliers

    Instruction: FLAT on round, on empty circle leg

    Result: Empty circle leg diverges

    Instruction: ROUND on flat, on filled circle leg

    Result: Filled circle leg becomes parallel and shorter

Figure 13-47. Bimler U loop: Sagittal adjustments. *A,* FLAT on round, on filled circle leg. *B,* ROUND on flat, on empty circle leg.

    Objective: Shortening of empty circle leg

    Instructions: FLAT on round, on filled circle leg, gives to filled circle leg; ROUND on flat, on empty circle leg, takes from empty circle leg

    Result: Empty circle leg is shortened; both legs are parallel again.

    Comments: Just as important as the transverse changes in the loops are the sagittal changes, meaning the lengthening and shortening of the legs with regard to each other. Rules and tools are the same. Following the rule "FLAT gives," take the flat-beak pliers and use them on the leg that should increase in length (empty circle). Since the instructions are FLAT on round, we put the pliers on the part of the arc adjoining the empty circle leg, and press. The empty circle leg will diverge from its parallel position. At once we change the pliers and put the round-beak ones on a flat part of the filled circle leg and press until the legs are parallel again. "ROUND takes" material from the filled circle leg and transfers it to the arc. For the reverse action, start with the flat-beak pliers on the filled circle legs, as described above. With this approach we are able to alter the size and relative position of all parts of the Bimler appliance.

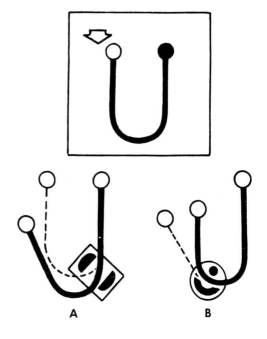

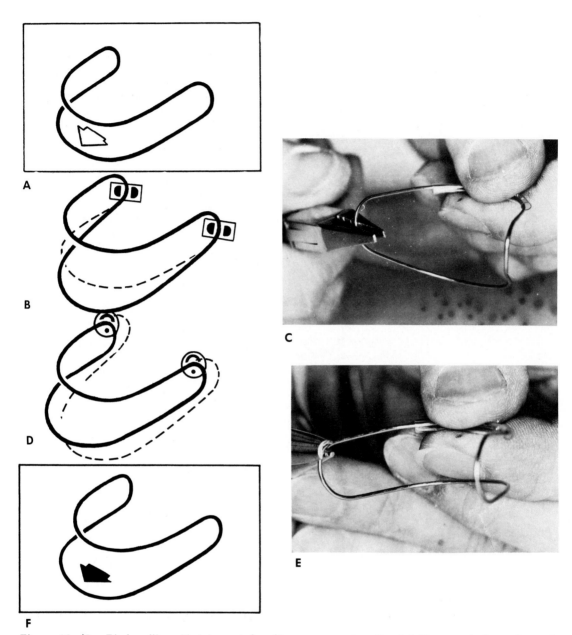

Figure 13–48.   Bimler ellipse: Training unit for adjustment exercises. *B* and *C*, To move the lower forward, give to lower by FLAT on round on lower legs. *D*, ROUND on flat on upper legs takes from the upper part (*E*).

    Objective: Move lower arch forward (give to lower) (*A*)
    Instruction: FLAT on round on lower legs
               ROUND on flat on upper legs
    Result: Lower arch moved forward (*F*)

Figure 13–49. Bimler ellipse: Sagittal adjustments. *A* and *B*, To move lower backward, give to upper by FLAT on round on upper legs. *C*, ROUND on flat on lower legs takes from lower part and moves it backward (*D*).

    Objective: Move lower arch backward (give to upper)
    Instructions: FLAT on round on upper legs
                ROUND on flat on lower legs
    Result: Lower arch moved backward

    Comments: For training purposes, the Bimler appliance can be reduced to a simplified model in the form of an ellipse. We recommend that each operator learn to form the properly shaped ellipse by practicing with a length of 0.36 inch wire. It should be kept together by a small piece of plastic tubing, as this best allows the study of undue tensions occurring during the adjustment and, at the same time, permits application of the method of preventing these tensions. Before anything else is made with this model, the operator can acquaint himself with the probably unexpected resistance against mechanical deformation by pressing the model in his hands in various directions. The reason for this sort of resilient stability can be seen in the fact that each of the consecutive loops of this model is in a plane perpendicular to the preceding and following ones. This is exactly the construction principle used in all types of Bimler appliances and their parts. Our next objective with the training ellipse is to perform the forward or backward adjustment of the lower part of any Bimler appliance, as they all have in common two U-shaped posterior connecting loops. First we want to bring the lower part forward; in other words, the lower part has to gain. Since the basic rule says "FLAT gives, ROUND takes," we begin with the flat-beak pliers on the arc nearest the lower leg that should gain. Pressure on both sides will bring the lower part downward. The next step is ROUND on flat on the upper leg. The round-beak pliers will take some wire material from the upper leg and incorporate it into the arc. With adequate pressure on both sides, the lower arc will come upward again, and forward at the same time. At the end of the maneuver, the arc must appear unchanged—the legs must be parallel again—but the lower arch should be forward in comparison to the upper.

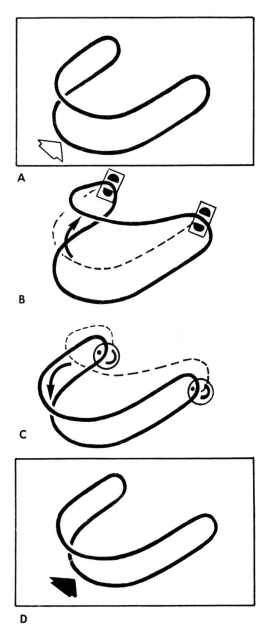

A

B

C

D

should be made. It is hard to believe, but if someone has learned to control completely our simple training object, the U loop, he will be able to handle all types and variations of our appliances simply by performing the same standard procedures. With widening and narrowing, lengthening and shortening of recurved loops, the appliances can be adapted in all three planes of space. The behavior of a circular set-up, as the Bimler appliances are, can best be studied by the training ellipse. Furthermore, direct hints on how to use the pliers in a specific situation will be given throughout the chapter following the presentation of each new part.

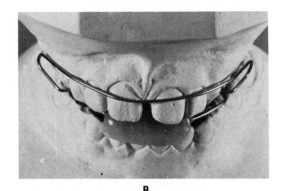

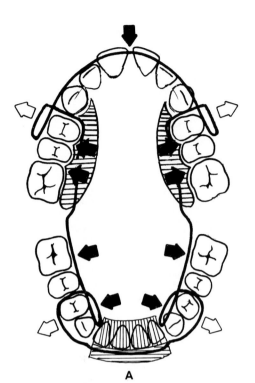

A   **C**

Figure 13–50. Bimler Prestandard (1949), Type **A**: Experimental expansion appliance.
  Indications: Class I and Class II, Division 1 cases, mixed and permanent dentitions
  Possibilities: Upper and lower expansion
              Upper anterior (frontal) retrusion
              Lower anterior (frontal) protrusion
              Repositioning of lower arch
  Advantages (compared with basic appliance):
              Expansion also possible in anterior section of lower arch
              Horizontal guiding plane as support between upper and lower parts
  Shortcomings: Solid cap, as in primary appliance

THE DEVELOPMENT OF THE
LOWER ARCH WIRE

The prestandard variation of the Type **A** appliance is a transitory stage in the development from the primitive version to the later standard form. It is no longer used, but is mentioned here to facilitate explanation of the form and function of the basic components of a Bimler appliance. It differs from the primary form (1948) mainly in the further development of the lower arch.

The breakthrough in the lower arch design was the combination of a shortened labial arch with two lingual sleds. The labial arch crosses the dental arches in the occlusal plane with two large loops between the first and second premolars. The wire is carried forward to the mesial of the canines, where it turns downward in a 180 degree curve, forming lingual wires running along the gingival border. Again, the remarkable stability of the appliance is achieved by the fact that the set of loops mentioned first is in the horizontal plane and the second set of loops is vertical. The formerly free-ending bars now form two symmetrical sleds attached posteriorly in the palatal wings and are kept in position anteriorly by the labial portion. Furthermore, the labial arch adds its forces to the lingual sleds for expansion in the critical zone of the canines.

A gliding surface is provided for the crossover wires of the upper labial arch by the horizontal loops in the occlusal plane. To prevent breakage of the posterior connecting loops, it is essential that the labial arch always be kept in gliding contact with the horizontal loops of the lingual arch.

In treating Class II, Division 1 cases, the solid lower cap prevents the final closure of the dental overjet, so it has to be cut away in the last stages of treatment and a depression bent into the anterior part of the labial segment of the lower arch. Now the upper incisors can be moved backwards to contact the lower anteriors. With the cut-away lower cap, the appliance is currently used as a retainer called A_0 or Simplex.

THE DEVELOPMENT OF THE UPPER PART

Frontal (Anterior) Springs, Coffin Spring

A further development towards the later standard appliance was accomplished by modification of the maxillary part of the appliance. Experiences in the first half of 1948 had shown that for better control of the upper anterior teeth, frontal springs **F** are essential (Fig. 13–51). These frontal springs follow the basic construction principle of changing from one plane of space into a perpendicular one between the individual elements. They consist of an anchored stem, two generously dimensioned adjustment bows in the *horizontal* plane, and two recurved working loops in the *vertical* plane. These springs are comparable in their adaptability to the human arms and their joints. Therefore, the parts that emerge from the acrylic wings are called the shoulders (Fig. 13–52), the lateral extremes of the horizontal adjustment bows are the elbows, and the vertical working loops are analogous to the hands. Any interdental extensions bent out of the free legs of the working loops are called fingers. In addition, a Coffin spring **R** for stabilization of the whole appliance was introduced and became an integral part of the appliance, as are the frontal springs.

The simplest Bimler appliance consists of only five wire parts and their acrylic wings. It is an ideal retainer after any kind of treatment in any age group. It is worn mainly at night and allows, on the one hand, the natural post-treatment adaptations into individual stability; but, on the other hand, minor corrections, especially of formerly rotated incisors, can still be performed.

Besides its usefulness in the post-treatment period, the appliance is just as effective in the early age groups for interception of expected crowding in the deciduous and early mixed dentitions. Its effect in this age group is primarily a coordinated expansion in the upper and lower arches, while simultaneously it can be used as a tongue guard and/or space maintainer in the buccal segments.

Text continued on page 395

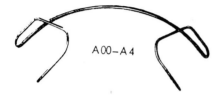

A00—A4

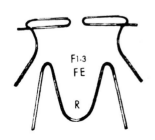

Ff 1—3

F1-3
FE

R

UV

A

Figure 13–51. Bimler Simplex, Type **A₀**: Interceptive appliance and retainer. *A,* Schematic drawing of the parts of the appliance. *B,* Schematic view of the appliance in place. *C,* Two views of the appliance.

Components: Prefabricated parts **A, F, R,** and **UV**

Indications: Class I and Class II, Division 1 cases, early mixed dentition

Bimaxillary dental protrusion

Finished cases, permanent dentition

Advantages: Frontal springs for control of upper incisors

Coffin spring (**R**) for more stability

No solid cap to interfere with upper incisors

Shortcomings: No control of lower anteriors from the lingual side

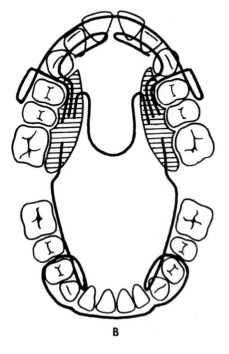

B

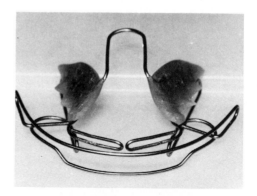

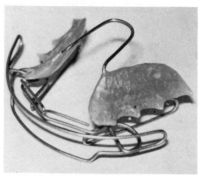

C

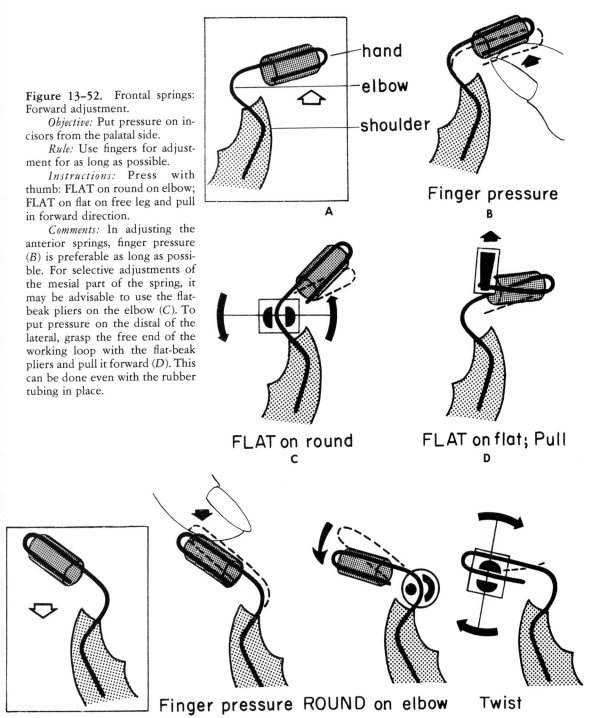

Figure 13–52. Frontal springs: Forward adjustment.

Objective: Put pressure on incisors from the palatal side.

Rule: Use fingers for adjustment for as long as possible.

Instructions: Press with thumb: FLAT on round on elbow; FLAT on flat on free leg and pull in forward direction.

Comments: In adjusting the anterior springs, finger pressure (B) is preferable as long as possible. For selective adjustments of the mesial part of the spring, it may be advisable to use the flat-beak pliers on the elbow (C). To put pressure on the distal of the lateral, grasp the free end of the working loop with the flat-beak pliers and pull it forward (D). This can be done even with the rubber tubing in place.

Figure 13–53. Frontal springs: Backward adjustment.

Objective: Relieve pressure on incisors.

Rule: Use fingers first.

Instructions: Press with forefinger, or ROUND on round on elbow; twist wrist to free arm.

Comments: The ordinary backward adjustment will always be performed by simple finger pressure. If the placement of the spring, e.g., for the rotation of a lateral incisor, has to be very precise, the alternating use of flat-beak and round-beak pliers is recommended. By flattening and accentuating the "elbow" angle, the position of the springs can be accurately corrected. Simple pressure with three-point attack can be supplemented by selective bends produced by twisting the hand from the wrist.

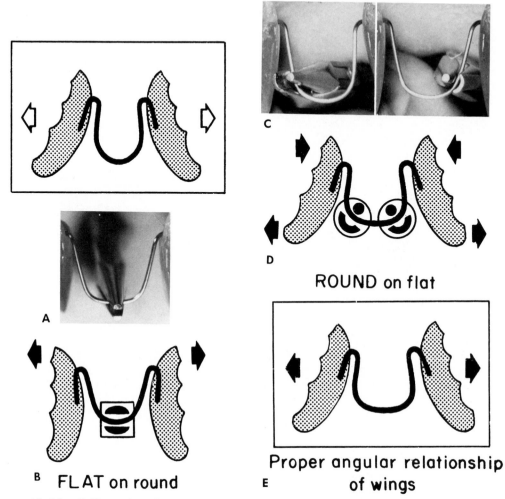

Figure 13-54. Coffin spring: Connecting element for stabilization, active element for expansion, and transverse adjustment.

Objective: Anterior widening (*A* and *B*)

Rule: FLAT gives

Tools: Flat-beak pliers

Instruction: FLAT on round

Comment: The widening of the appliance should be done primarily by finger pressure. If an accentuated widening effect in the cuspid region is necessary, the pliers can be used. Working with the flat-beak pliers on the arc of the Coffin spring will open the wings.

Objective: Anterior narrowing and posterior widening (*C* and *D*)

Rule: ROUND takes

Tools: Round-beak pliers

Instruction: ROUND on flat

Comment: In the long run, the anterior widening has to be compensated for by countering actions with the round-beak pliers, which will narrow the wings anteriorly and widen them posteriorly until the wings are back in the proper angular relationship (*E*).

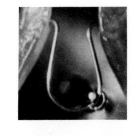

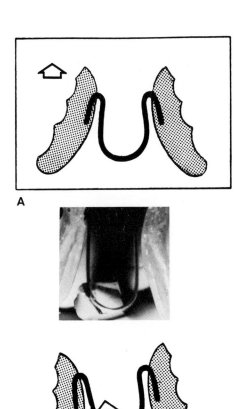

A

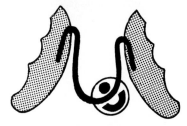

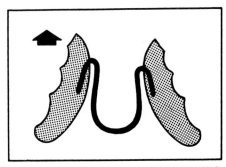

C   **ROUND on flat**

B   **FLAT on round**

D   **Proper angular relationship of wings**

Figure 13-55. Coffin spring: Sagittal adjustment.

Objective: Bring left side forward

Rule: FLAT gives

Instructions: FLAT on round on left side

ROUND on flat on right side

Comments: The need for sagittal adjustments will be rather rare but may occur in special situations. Following the rule "FLAT gives," start with flat-beak pliers on the leg that should gain—in our example the left leg (*B*). The left wing will diverge. By means of the round-beak pliers on the right leg, the right wing will swing into a position corresponding to the left one, but more posteriorly (*C*). At the end of this maneuver, the arc of the Coffin spring should have the same form as at the beginning, and the wings should have the same angular relationship (*D*).

THE DEVELOPMENT OF THE LOWER ANTERIOR SECTION

Originally, the early appliances had a rather solid plastic cap which served as guidance for the lower jaw (Fig. 13–56*A*). The top of this cap was sometimes used as a flat bite plane or as an inclined plane to protrude the upper incisors in crossbite cases. During the course of treatment, the cap usually had to be cut down to a small anterior shield. Its function as a bite plane was taken over by

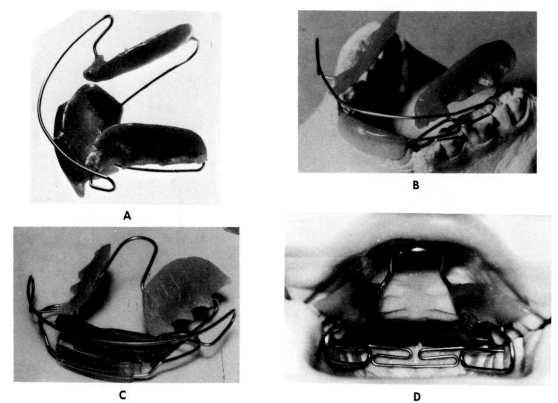

Figure 13-56. *A*, Primary appliance with very large lower cap. *B*, Prestandard appliance with small plastic cap. *C*, Early standard appliance, with small metal band with vertical tubes as attachments for the anterior loop. *D*, Posterior view of C in place on a study cast.

rubber tubings on the upper anterior springs. In time, we learned that the use of adjustable wire springs offered significantly greater possibilities of influencing the upper incisors than did inclined planes. Consequently, similar wire loops were tried for alignment of crowded lower incisors. Instead of two separate springs, one continuous double loop was used tentatively. The free ends were fixed in the anterior plastic shield, which was what remained of the former lower anterior cap (Fig. 13–56*B*). From past experience it was established that a 0.024 inch wire was most appropriate for the lower incisors, to prevent any soreness of the teeth. In the next step, a small metal band with two vertical tubes was incorporated into the anterior plastic shield. It has now been further developed into an all-metal lower frontal splint **S** (Fig. 13–57). It consists of a U-shaped metal trough which follows the contours of the lower anterior arch. On both sides, it has two vertical tubes as attachments for the free ends of the wire loop. The excess wires have only to be bent back on themselves to attach the wire loop. The anterior loop can be exchanged very quickly if it should break.

The divided lower arch was developed out of experiences acquired while repairing unilaterally broken lower sleds. Initially, the broken lower arch wire was cut off where it inserted into the anterior plastic shield, and only half was replaced. The second labial portion was placed on top of the first one in a renewed plastic shield. The metal trough of the newly developed anterior splint invited the use of divided arches from the very beginning. It proved to be easier to place the lower arch without any tension if it was composed of two halves.

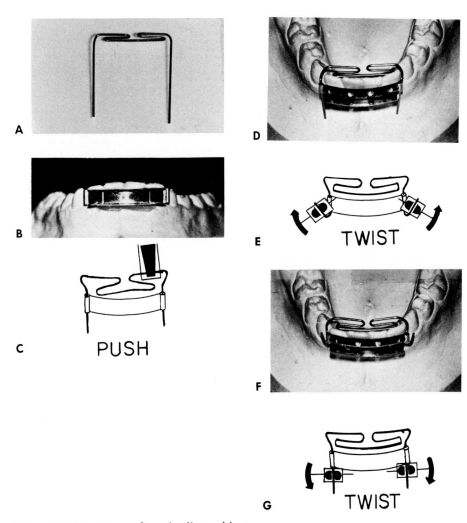

Figure 13–57. Lower frontal splint and loop.

Objective: Placement of lower frontal loop (*A*)

Tools: Round-beak and flat-beak pliers

Comments: The lower frontal loop wires are available in three different sizes. The matching size is selected by comparing with the model. The free ends are bent in the horizontal plane to cross the dental arch between the laterals and the canines (*B*). Then another right-angle bend is made in the vertical plane so that the free ends are parallel to the tubes and can be inserted without difficulty. The free ends are inserted as far as they can go into the tubing and the ends bent back 180 degrees (*C*). The excess is removed with a wire cutter.

Objective: Removal of lower frontal loop (*D*).

Tools: Flat-beak pliers

Comments: To remove, grasp the free end with the flat-beak pliers and bend until the wire is straight (*E*). Do this on both sides and pull the entire loop out of the tubing (*G*).

The standard model represents the fully developed basic form of the Type **A** line. It has all the essential parts for a bimaxillary coordinated arch expansion and the control of the anterior teeth from the labial and the lingual sides. The lower frontal splint (Fig. 13–58*C*) and loop (Fig. 13–58*B*) provide good guidance of the lower arch in the corrected forward position, but most of the forward-pushing forces in the lower arch are directed against the buccal seg-

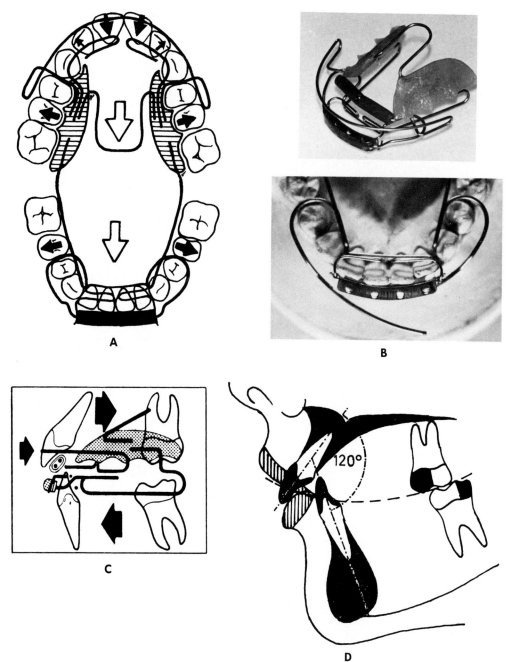

Figure 13–58. Bimler standard appliance, Type A_1: Basic appliance. *A*, Schematic drawing of the design of the appliance. *B*, Two views of the appliance. *C*, Forces exerted by the appliance. *D*, Pretreatment occlusion tracing.

Components: Prefabricated parts **U**, **L**, and **S** (see Fig. 13–40).

Indications: Class I and Class II cases, mixed and permanent dentitions

Possibilities: Upper and lower expansion
Upper anterior retrusion and alignment
Lower anterior protrusion and alignment
Bite opening
Repositioning lower arch

ments by means of the two sleds. By addition of auxiliary springs and supports, the standard appliance can be transformed into a number of variations, each for a special purpose. They will be described in detail in the following sections. In addition, these variations can be reduced at any time to the standard form by cutting away the auxiliaries after they have fulfilled their special tasks. Even the A_3 variation with the palatal plate and screw is usually reshaped to the standard form after a while, to be used as a retainer. The middle part of the plate, including the screw, is simply cut away and the remaining parts are remodeled into the form of the palatal wings and completed with a Coffin spring.

PRESENTATION OF APPLIANCE

In stomatopedics, the patient is supposed to treat himself under the supervision of the orthodontist. It is very important that he realize this from the very beginning of therapy. Therefore, we never put an appliance into the mouth of the patient, but present it to him on the models (Fig. 13–59A). He is asked to pick it up and to take it between his forefinger and thumb (Fig. 13–59B). The lateral redoubling loops of the labial arch offer themselves as handles. Then the patient is encouraged to place the appliance in his mouth. The younger the patient, the easier this will work. Next, the patient is asked some questions to which he cannot reply "yes" or "no," e.g., "Where do you live?" or "What is the name of your teacher?" and so on. In this manner he experiences for the first time how to speak with the appliance. He is told that within a few days his tongue will become adjusted to its new surroundings, and no one will notice that he has something in his mouth.

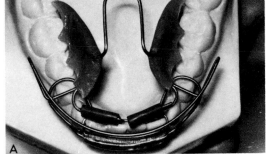

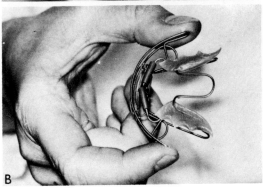

Figure 13–59. The Bimler appliance as (A) shown to and (B) held by the patient.

FORWARD POSITIONING OF MANDIBLE

The immediate effect of the placing of a bimaxillary appliance, in all Class II cases, is a change in the intermaxillary relationship of the dental arches. The lower jaw is brought forward into a Class I molar relationship and held there as long as the appliance is worn (Fig. 13–60). In this position, the retractor muscles will be stretched and, as a reaction, they will try to pull the lower jaw back into its former position. These backward-directed forces will be transferred by the appliance to the upper dental arch, especially against the protruded anteriors. The same amount of force is, of course, directed against the lower arch in a forward direction (Fig. 13–58). The objective of our treatment planning must be to predetermine which teeth should be exposed to these forces or protected from them by auxiliary springs or supports.

This forward positioning of the mandible is a temporary therapeutic one and *not* identical with the permanent position at the end of the treatment, when the dental arches are found in Class I occlusion, but with the head of the condyle back in the fossa. Generally speaking, the muscle action is comparable to that of cervical headgear pull: the mandible acts as the outer bow of the headgear, while the labial arch wire can be compared with the inner bow.

LATERAL MOVEMENTS OF THE MANDIBLE

The dental arch expansion observed after the placement of a Bimler appliance results from the activity of the internal pterygoid muscles. In a chain of neuromuscular reactions, the elastic appliance has a sort of trigger function. It acts like a foreign body for the proprioceptive nerve endings in the periodontal membrane. It provokes chewing and similar movements by stimulating re-

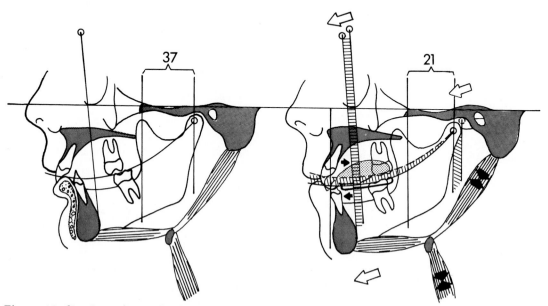

Figure 13–60. Immediate effect of placing a bimaxillary appliance in a Class II patient. The mandible is moved into a Class I molar relationship and held there as long as the appliance is in place.

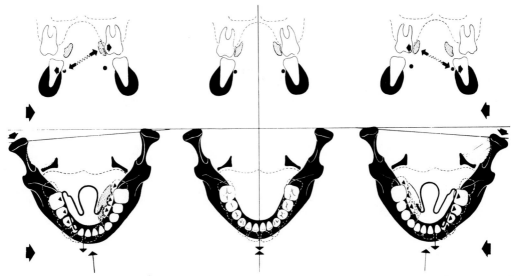

Figure 13-61. The pterygoid contraction creates reciprocal pressures in contralateral segments of the upper and lower jaws.

peated lateral displacements of the mandible. The resilient appliance offers an elastic resistance against these movements. The pterygoid contraction, necessary to overcome this resistance, creates reciprocal pressures against contralateral segments of the upper and lower jaws (Fig. 13-61). This intermittent action changes continuously from one side to the other. It occurs completely unconsciously and works also when the patient is asleep. Therefore, it is unnecessary to ask the patient to do any exercises. Contrary to experiences with the activator, no vertical displacement of the mandible, as obtained by bite-opening "working bites," is necessary to make the appliance effective. The use of such a "working bite," with all its implications, has therefore been completely abandoned. It is also no longer advisable or worthwhile to replace an appliance after six to eight months for better results.

MECHANISM OF ARCH EXPANSION

To study the mechanism of arch expansion, we take an appliance seated in a Bimler articulator (Fig. 13-62). There we can easily observe the actions of the appliance from the rear (Fig. 13-62C, F, and I). In centric occlusion, the acrylic wings of the appliance will just touch the buccal segments, and the lower sleds will contact the lower buccal segments. No mechanical forces are exerted in this position (Fig. 13-62E and F). When the mandible is moved to the left side, the right lower buccal segment meets the resistance of the right sled and an expanding force is exerted on these teeth (Fig. 13-62B and C). The same pressure is directed against the left upper buccal segment as the appliance is temporarily compressed. This can be seen from the distances between the left sled and the left lower molars as well as from the distance between the right upper wing and the right upper teeth (Fig. 13-62B and C). The reverse action takes place when the mandible is moved to the right side (Fig. 13-62H and I).

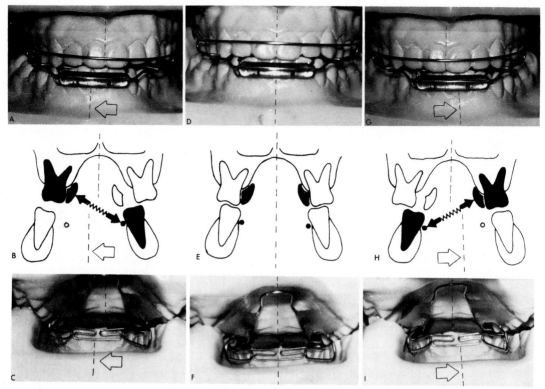

Figure 13–62. The mechanism of arch expansion. See text for discussion.

VERTICAL MOVEMENTS OF THE MANDIBLE

For space opening and tooth rotation, special springs must be used. Since the appliance has no anchorage on the teeth, any spring action has to be counteracted by some sort of support either through the acrylic parts or through some wire supports placed strategically opposite the acting springs. This spring action of the floating appliance depends on the system of inclined planes, provided by the anatomy of the teeth. In closing the jaw around the appliance, the springs initially glide along the inclined planes of the crowns and single cusps and gradually become activated. The moment the pressure becomes too heavy, the muscles relax by reflex action, and the next moment, this interplay is repeated. By selectively adapting the diameter of the wire parts to the clinical effect, we finally produced an appliance that never creates any sore teeth or pathologic gum reactions. Root resorption is absolutely unknown in this treatment. We are not concerned about relapses, as experienced with clasp-anchored plates or any other sort of fixed appliances. If the patient fails to wear the appliance for a while during sickness or vacation, it can be used afterward without any difficulty.

THE WHITE GIRL CASE

We will present an uncomplicated case in the mixed dentition to explain the stomatopedic methods of diagnosis and rational treatment planning. White Girl

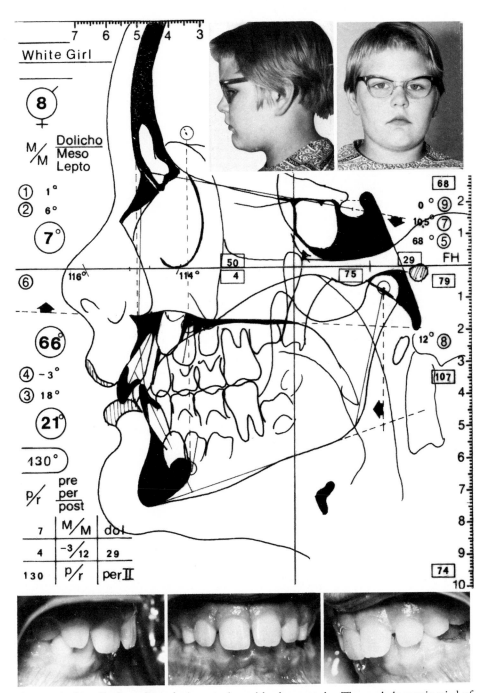

Figure 13-63. Evaluated head plate tracing with photographs. The cephalometric triad of negative maxillary inclination (Factor 4 = −3 degrees), mandibular hyperflexion (Factor 8 = 12 degrees), and a flattened cranial base (Factor 7 = 10.5 degrees) confirms the diagnosis of micro-rhinic dysplasia, which could have been predicted from the small nose seen in the facial photographs. The dolichoprosopic facial index (deep face) and the low alveolar process indicate that the predominant treatment problem would be to reduce the closed bite.

was an eight-year-old patient who had a Class II, Division 1 closed bite malocclusion with upper spacing. The dental anomaly was due to the vertical underdevelopment of the middle part of the face, as seen by the forward-upward rotation of the maxilla and the overclosure of the mandible (Fig. 13–63). Together with a rather high slant of the anterior cranial base, we find the full triad of micro-rhinic dysplasia. Factor 4 was 3 degrees; Factor 7, 10.5 degrees; and Factor 8, 12 degrees. Her facial formula, 7 M/M dolicho, was fairly well balanced, and the discrepancy between the M/M basic relation and the dolicho facial type can easily be understood as the consequence of the deficiency in the vertical development and the low alveolar processes. The profile angulation with only 7 degrees for the NAB angle and 4 mm. of basal bone overjet was very light, so no problems with the Class II relationship were expected. Consequently, the situation was regarded as predominantly a closed bite case and grouped as a Bimler White problem.

Preparation of Records

In order to formulate a definite diagnosis and treatment plan, a complete set of records had to be taken. These records consist of (1) head plate of diagnostic quality, (2) study models, (3) Panorex film, and (4) photographs of profile, full face, and intraoral views. For their evaluation we need (1) tracing of the head plate on the cephalometric analysis sheet, (2) tracing of the occlusal view on the dental arch analysis sheet, (3) stomatopedic treatment sheet with mean value scale and millimeter grid, and (4) translucent three-leaf folder for visualized case history.

Cephalometric Analysis

We have tried to explain the fundamental ideas of our cephalometric analysis on pages 338 to 356. For further details we refer to V. A. Nord.[31]

Stomatopedic Treatment Sheet

As mentioned before under Dental Arch Survey, a graphic dental arch analysis and treatment check curves represent our treatment plan and indicate how far it has been realized. They are both attached to the stomatopedic treatment sheet. Our assistants mark the two forms with the name of White Girl and further details. Then the dental arches are projected and drawn on the translucent analysis sheet. The next step is to establish the sum of the incisors (SI = 31 mm.) and to mark the corresponding mean values on the printed scales on both sheets.

PREPARATION OF REACTION CURVE CHART

On the stomatopedic treatment sheet (Fig. 13–65) we find a mean value scale in the middle. In its center the occlusal view of the two dental arches is printed with the measuring points in the upper and lower jaws. On the upper and lower parts of the scale four columns of figures are to be seen. The two on

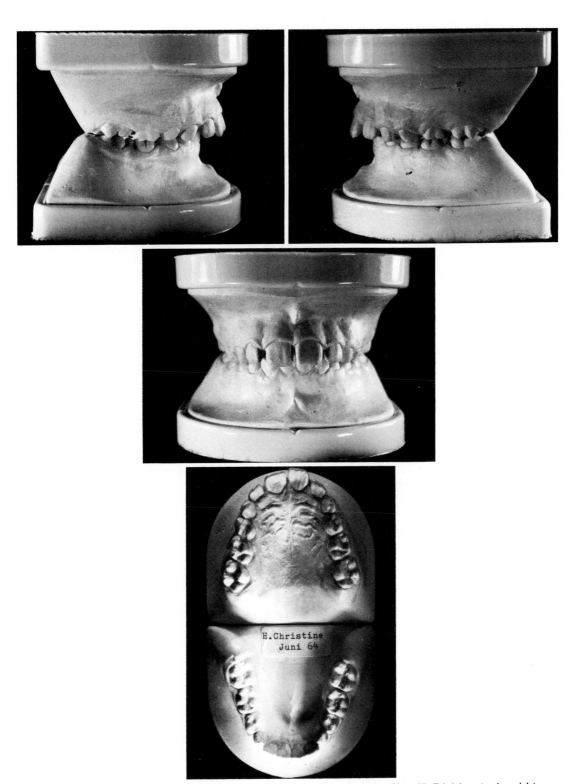

Figure 13-64. White Girl case, maldeveloping phase. Age, 8 years. Class II, Division 1, closed bite.

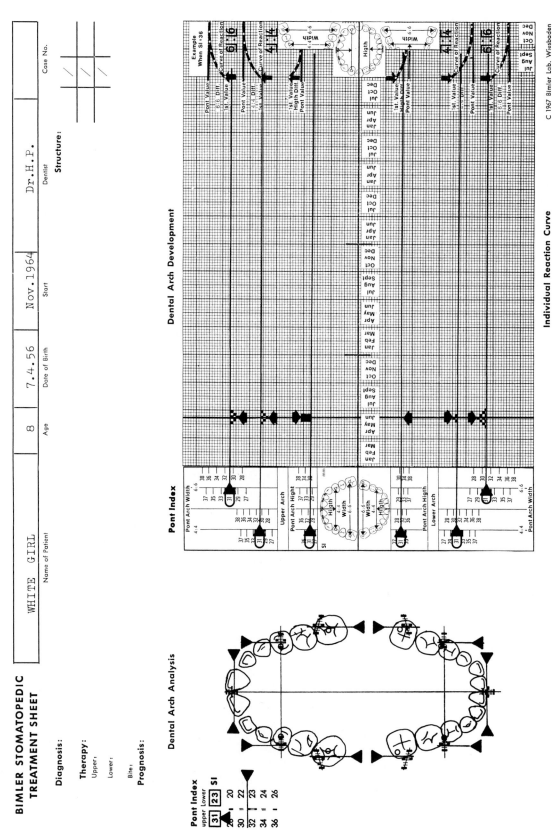

Figure 13–65. Stomatopedic treatment sheet for White Girl.

the left are for the premolars, and the two on the right are for the molars. The little lines to the right of the figures represent graphically the mean values for the anterior and posterior dental arch width. The corresponding figures for the dental arch height are on the scales nearer to the midline.

We have already encircled the figure 31 on the scale while establishing the SI for the arch analysis. From the little lines beside 31, base lines are drawn in green which are parallel to the center line. They represent the statistical means for the whole course of treatment but should not be misinterpreted as the individual treatment goal. With the two-dimensional caliper the distances between the measuring points are taken from the casts and transferred to the millimeter grid from midline on up and down, under the date on which the analysis is performed. These starting points are accentuated by small red arrowheads (black in print) pointed toward the green mean value lines. The distance between red and green is colored in yellow (checked in print) and visualizes the deficiency in the dental arch development. The surplus in dental arch height is colored in red (black in print).

DENTAL ARCH PREDETERMINATION

For our dental arch predetermination, a graphic set-up is performed. The tracing of the occlusal view of the dental arches, which has been done before in a special projector, serves as a base. First, with calipers, the widths of the upper centrals and laterals are transferred to any millimeter grid. We prefer to use the one on the chart for the individual reaction curve (Fig. 13–65). The sum of the incisors (SI) in the upper is 31 mm. We put it down in its bracket in the left corner of the analysis sheet. At the same time we circle the number 31 in the Pont index table of the stomatopedic treatment sheet. The same is done with the lower incisors. Their SI is 23 mm. and we put 23 in the respective bracket. As this value is fairly well correlated to 31 mm. in the upper, no further attention has to be given to this finding. With the calipers we now take from the models the widths of each individual tooth and transfer them to the tracing of the arches by starting at the midline and proceeding distally. We start on the midline for the planned position of the centrals about 2 mm. behind the symbol for 31, which should later coincide with the labial aspect of the contours of the centrals. In the case of White Girl, where there is not a permanent canine erupted, a measurement of 9/10 of the upper central will suffice. In a mixed dentition case the diameter of the premolars is estimated by x-ray interpolation. The diameters of all the teeth are arranged along the line of contact points. The contours of the permanent teeth, in the positions we expect them to occupy, are now drawn in (Fig. 13–66). Note that in White Girl, the deciduous teeth have a greater mesiodistal width than their permanent successors, providing a leeway that will allow the molars to move mesially in both arches. These expected spontaneous movements are indicated on the drawing by green arrows, whereas the planned movements, to be achieved by the appliance, are indicated by red arrows (white and black in print). As there are no extractions, missing teeth, crossbites, or rotations, the respective crosses are neglected. There are no midline deviations. The overjet is 8 mm. According to Angle we see a Class II: the molar relationship is ½ postnormal and the canines occlude fully postnormal. For the problem grouping (Fig. 13–66 *center*) we have to consider two symptoms, the Class II, Division 1 occlusion as a Blue problem and the closed bite as a White problem. Judging primarily from the head plate, the distal

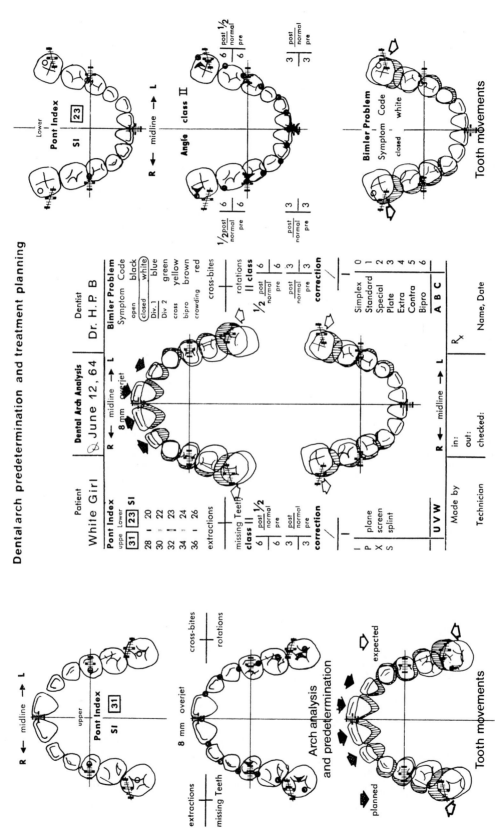

Figure 13-66. Dental arch predetermination and treatment planning for White Girl.

occlusion is not regarded as very serious, but owing to the reduced midfacial height, the overrotated mandible, and the low alveolar processes, the closed bite component was regarded as the predominant symptom and the case classified as a White problem, expressed by the code name of White Girl.

APPLIANCE PRESCRIPTION

So far we have on our dental arch analysis sheet the arch predetermination with the expected and planned tooth movements. Now this plan has to be transferred into therapeutic reality and the appliance has to be individually constructed out of the parts that will serve this purpose best. For the retrusion of the incisors we need a labial arch wire **A**. For the alignment and probably slight rotation and torque of the upper anteriors, we choose the frontal springs **F**. For expansion and stabilization, the Coffin spring **R** is indicated. The three are kept together by the acrylic wings.

In the lower we start with the frontal splint **S** as a connective element and add the lower frontal loop **L** for proper guidance of the lower arch and alignment of the incisors. The divided lower arches **U** will complete the lower part. We next have to advise the technician how much to correct the bite in the articulator, and according to the occlusal situation we prescribe a correction of half a premolar's width in the anterior direction. Finally, the graphic prescription is confirmed by a printed one, and we circle in the right lower corner Type **A** and variation 1, Standard. When the planning and prescription are performed by an assistant, the proposal is presented to the orthodontist for final approval. By his signature he takes over full responsibility.

In the dental arch predetermination we anticipated a mesial drift of the molars. In the lower arch this is no problem at all. The lingual sleds have been constructed to allow slight sagittal movements of the appliance along the buccal segments during lateral movements of the mandible in order to reduce breakage. But they also allow the mesial drift of the molars after the shedding of the deciduous teeth. In the upper arch, for this purpose the orthodontist has to interfere in time and has to grind the acrylic spurs fitting into the interdental embrasures in front of the molars. To remind him to do so, there are little shaded areas distal to the wings.

Construction of the Appliance

Models and the prescription sheet, in a transparent cover, are given to the laboratory. Following the prescription, the chief technician will select the parts out of his stock and check them with regard to size on the models. The models are mounted in the Bimler articulator by a junior trainee. This is a special construction which allows the anteroposterior adjustment of the upper and lower casts and gives free access to the lingual aspect of the dental arches from the rear. Working models are fixed in the habitual occlusion by plaster. For study models in plastic bases we use a special mounting device. Models will not be damaged during fabrication. For the construction of the appliance, the upper cast fixed to the metal bow has to be separated again from the rest of the articulator by compressing the bow, and put aside. The assembly starts in the lower arch, where the frontal splint **S** is fixed with sticky wax in a vertical position in front of the lower incisors. Next, the lower frontal loop **L** is adapted to

Text continued on page 413

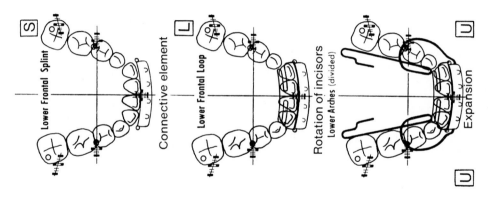

S — Lower Frontal Splint

L — Connective element / Lower Frontal Loop

U — Rotation of incisors / Lower Arches (divided)

U — Expansion

Appliance Prescription

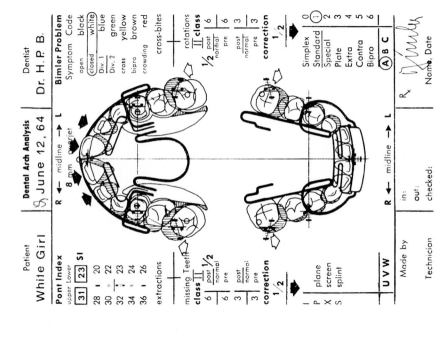

Patient	Dental Arch Analysis	Dentist
White Girl	♀ June 12, 64	Dr. H. P. B.

Pont Index

upper Lower

| 31 | 23 | SI |

R ◄— midline —► L

8 mm overjet

28	▪	20
30	▪	22
32	▪	23
34	▪	24
36	▪	26

extractions

missing Teeth

class II

6	post 1/2
	normal
6	pre
3	post
	normal
3	pre

correction 1/2

I	plane
P	screen
X	splint
S	

U V W

R ◄— midline —► L

in:
out:
checked:

Made by

Technician

Bimler Problem

Symptom Code

open	black
closed	white
Div. 1	blue
Div. 2	green
cross	yellow
bipro	brown
crowding	red

cross-bites

rotations

II class

6	post	6
	normal	
6	pre	6
3	post	3
	normal	
3	pre	3

correction 1/2

Simplex	0	①
Standard		2
Special		3
Plate		4
Extra		5
Contra		6
Bipro		

Ⓐ B C

Name, Date

Figure 13–67. Appliance prescription for White Girl.

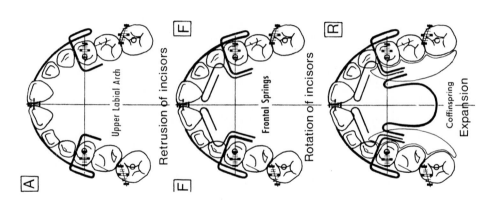

A — Upper Labial Arch

F — Retrusion of incisors / Frontal Springs

R — Rotation of incisors / Coffinspring / Expansion

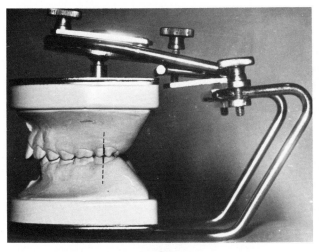

A

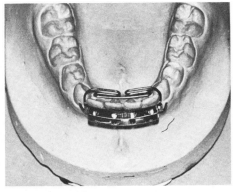

B

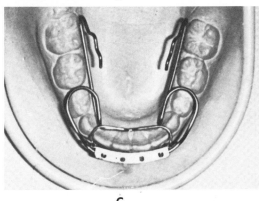

C

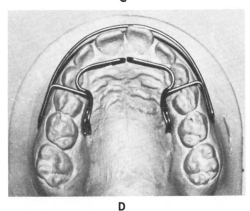

D

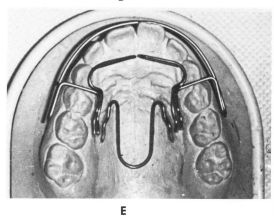

E

Dental Arch Analysis

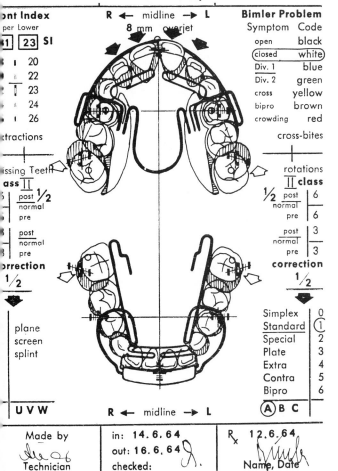

ont Index	R ← midline → L
per Lower	8 mm overjet
1 23 SI	

I	20	
II	22	
	23	
II	24	
	26	

tractions

issing Teeth

ass II

	post	1/2
	normal	
	pre	

	post	
	normal	
	pre	

rrection

1/2

plane
screen
splint

U V W

R ← midline → L

Bimler Problem

Symptom Code

open	black
closed	white
Div. 1	blue
Div. 2	green
cross	yellow
bipro	brown
crowding	red

cross-bites

rotations

II class

1/2	post		6
	normal		
	pre		6

	post		3
	normal		
	pre		3

correction

1/2

Simplex	0
Standard	1
Special	2
Plate	3
Extra	4
Contra	5
Bipro	6

A B C

Made by	in: 14. 6. 64	Rx 12. 6. 64
Technician	out: 16. 6. 64	
	checked:	Name, Date

F

Figure 13–68. White Girl case. A_1 appliance construction. *A,* Models are mounted in the original Class II malocclusion. *B,* Lower frontal loop. *C,* Lower arches (divided). *D,* Frontal springs. *E,* Coffin spring.

Illustration continued on following page

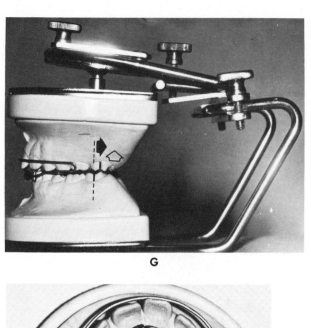

G

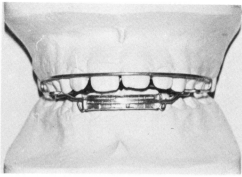

J

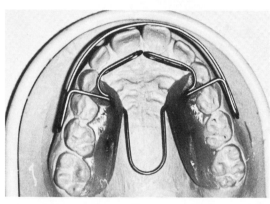

H

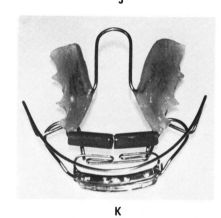

K

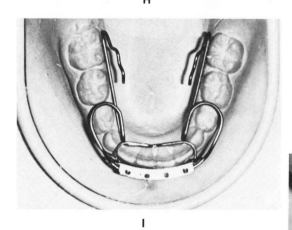

I

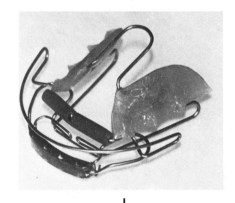

L

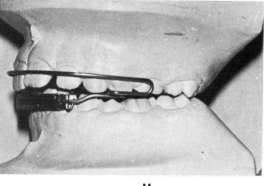

M

Figure 13–68 *Continued.* Following the appliance prescription (*F*), the technician will correct the occlusion in the articulator (*G*) by pushing back the upper cast and fixing it in a Class I relationship (black arrow). The bite will be raised by turning the screw provided (white arrow). *H* to *M,* Various views of the finished appliance.

the anterior teeth. The free ends are inserted into the tubes of the splint **S** and fixed by bending them up. Now the two halves of the divided lower arch **U** are adapted and fixed with wax to the lingual side of the buccal teeth. The free ends of the labial parts of the lower arch have to sit in the trough of the lower frontal splint without any tension. Then the lower cast is put aside and the assembling continues in the upper. First, the labial arch wire **A** is placed. The free ends are undulated by means of the ROUND pliers and kept about 1 mm. off the palate. The arch is fixed with wax on the labial side, leaving the undulated ends free. Next the frontal springs **F** are adapted and fixed to the anterior part of the palate. A small strip of wax is placed in the vault of the palate and the adapted Coffin spring **R** pressed into it. The undulated free ends of the Coffin spring, labial arch, and frontal springs are supposed to lie next to each other, but without direct contact, about 1 mm. off the surface of the model. The contours of the palatal wings can be drawn with a pencil on the palate. Then these parts are covered with cold-curing acrylic, imbedding the undulated ends of the wires. The wings are molded to their final form while the acrylic is setting. Simultaneously, the trough of the frontal splint is filled with acrylic too, fixing the divided lower arches. After the acrylic is set, the wings and the splint are finished and polished. Then two grooves are cut into the posterior part of the wings to receive the free ends of the lower arch. For final adaptation of these ends the upper cast has to be inserted into the articulator again. Now the bite correction has to be performed and the upper cast is pushed back after the fixing nuts have been released. In the new position the nuts are fixed again and the free ends of the lower arch fitted into the grooves of the wings. When they fit without any tension, they are fixed with acrylic and the wings are given a final polish.

Evaluation of Long-Term Observation in White Girl

White Girl has been observed over a period of 11 years. Growth and development and the dental axial angulation have been followed by lateral head plates and photographs. Dental positions and occlusal changes were documented by models and the behavior of dental arch width and height by means of the reaction curves. Composite tracings of the dental arches correlated to the main facial structures further helped us to understand the interdependence of skeletal growth and tooth movements.

We have to realize that White Girl at the age of eight years was still in an early stage of the mixed dentition. A rather short period of reacting to the therapeutic influence of the appliance was followed by a long rest period during which tooth eruption took place. It is characteristic of the stomatopedic approach that the therapeutic device allows an undisturbed natural development of the dentition with all the sagittal and vertical adjustments of the teeth, but at the same time is always ready to provide the necessary guides to influence this development if it deviates from harmony.

The arch expansion, as the first reaction to the appliance, took place for only two to three months. Then it discontinued automatically. Some time later, during the eruption of the premolars, in the upper arch the values measured were temporarily above the mean. Most likely this was due to the appliance, which was worn as a retainer during this time. The values normalized in 1968, when the appliance was discontinued. In 1975 a further reduction of the arch

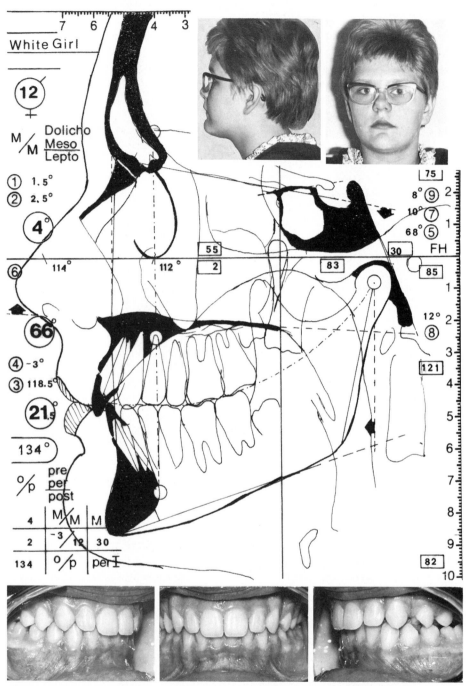

Figure 13–69. Compare with Figure 13–63. Angular measurements in circles. (Small circles = factors; large circles = profile and basic angles.) Note that the profile angle was reduced from 7 to 4 degrees, owing to reduction of Factor 2 by 3.5 degrees and increase of Factor 1 by 0.5 degree. Linear measurements are in rectangular brackets. Maxillary depth increased by 5 mm., mandibular length by 14 mm., and T-TM distance by 1 mm., and bony overjet (apical base discrepancy) reduced from 4 to 2 mm.

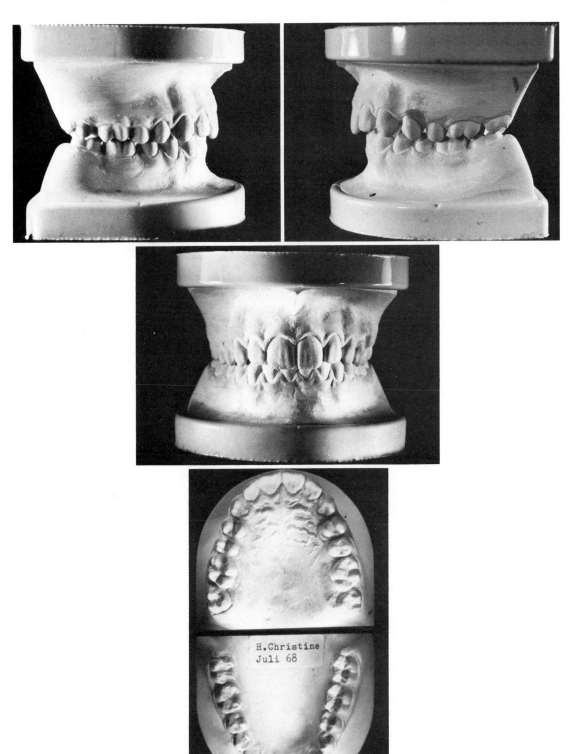

Figure 13–70. White Girl case. Age, 12 years. Normal Class I occlusion.

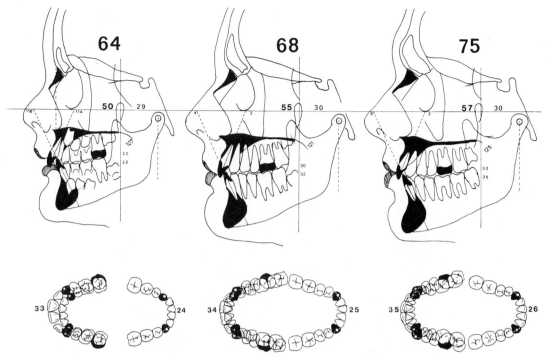

Figure 13–71. Comparison of linear measurements of the depth of the maxilla, the length of mandible, and the temporal position (T-TM). Note that the joint was carried backward by synchondrosis growth in the cranial base, while the dental occlusion changed from Class II to Class I. The intercanine distance increased 1 mm. each in the treatment period and in the observation period afterward. The patient is apparently still in the constructive phase of her dentition.

width at the Pont measuring points was found, apparently due to the mesial shift of the dentition. It is remarkable to see that at the same time the intercanine distance increased by a total of 2 mm. in both arches. No secondary crowding occurred in the lower anterior. This finding is related to her facial type.

In comparing the growth increments in Figure 13–71 we can state that the depth of the maxilla increased 5 mm. in the first four years and 2 mm. more in the following seven years. Simultaneously, the diagonal length of the mandible increased by 14 mm. Note that the distance from the first molars to the vertical tuber increased 8 mm. in the upper and 10 mm. in the lower arch in the first four years. This demonstrates an alveolar mesial drift of the molars of 3 mm. The participation of skeletal growth and tooth drifting in establishing a normal occlusion differs from patient to patient and cannot be predicted on the basis of our current knowledge.

AUTOMATIC EFFECTS AND COMPENSATING MANIPULATIONS

For the upper part, remember the law of the ellipse. If one diameter of an ellipse is increased, the other will decrease. Owing to this law of the ellipse, the labial arches of all Type **A** appliances will automatically retrude if the appliance is expanded (Fig. 13–74*A*). As long as the upper incisors are protruded, this is a welcome coordinated action. But usually the retrusion has to be stopped

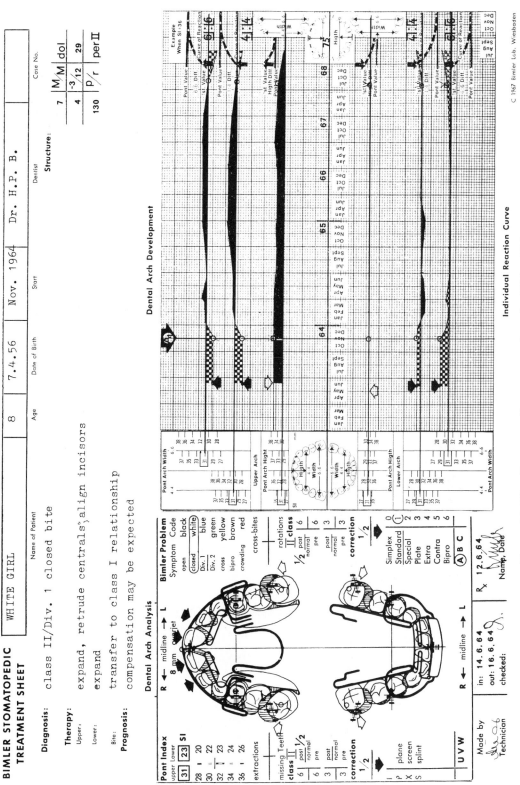

Figure 13–72. Stomatopedic treatment sheet for White Girl.

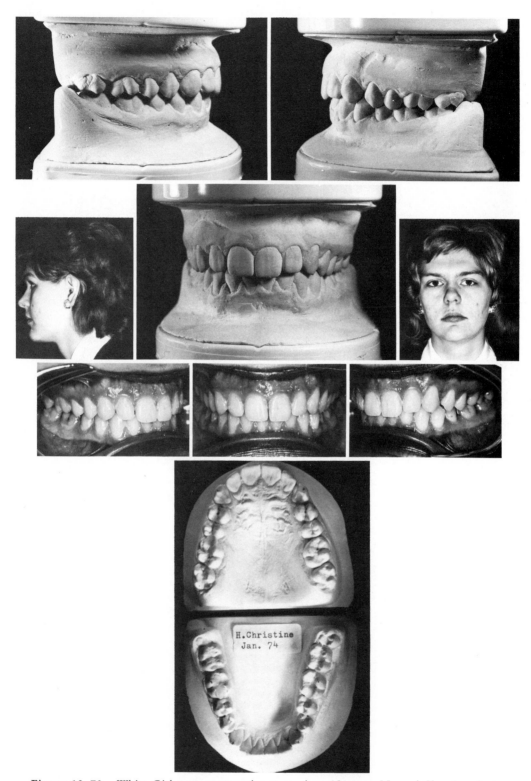

Figure 13-73. White Girl case, constructive stage. Age, 19 years. Normal Class I occlusion.

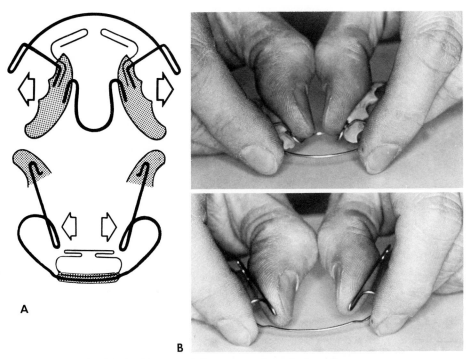

Figure 13-74.   Bimler Type **A**: Adjustment of standard appliance.
   Objective: Lateral reactivation of upper and lower parts for expansion of arches
   Tools: Fingers
   Instructions: Thumbs against wings or sleds; knuckles against knuckles; press gently
   Result: More tension in appliance
   Comments: The Bimler appliance should be kept in slight tension in the mouth. Within three to four weeks this tension disappears either by increase in the width of the arches or by weakening of the appliance. Children will remark that the appliance feels loose. Therefore, it has to be activated routinely at each appointment. This is best done by slight finger pressure.

before the expansion ends. Therefore, we insist that both tooth movements be regularly checked and recorded. The measurements can be performed by the caliper, and the reading transferred to the reaction curves. The moment the proper position of the incisors is achieved, the labial arch has to be lengthened with each lateral activation.

For the lower part, the sleds are narrowed. Owing to the constant lateral movements of the mandible, the sleds of the lower part are narrowed and the appliance loses its effectiveness in the lower canine region. To compensate for this unavoidable side effect, the orthodontist has to reactivate the lower part by simple finger pressure every two to three weeks. For this purpose, the terminal phalanges of the thumbs are placed against the lower sleds while the knuckles support each other (Fig. 13-74*B*). This can even be taught to the patients, so that they can do it themselves. Sometimes the widening is overdone, and in this case, there will be some interference in the closure of the arches. Simply press the fingers slightly toward the lingual to correct this problem (Fig. 13-74*C*).

In cases with extreme dental and basal bone overjet (Fig. 13-64), the muscular forces evoked by the forward positioning of the mandible may become so heavy that the lower anterior loops will break rather often. It would be unwise to use a heavier wire for the frontal loop, because then no warning would be given if there were too much pressure on the lower incisors. Consequently, they would become labially proclined, as is very often seen in

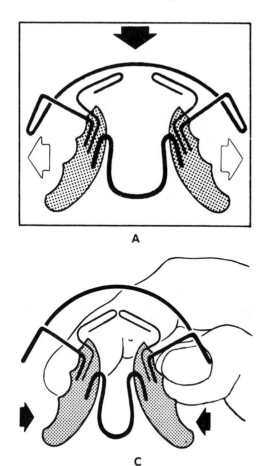

A

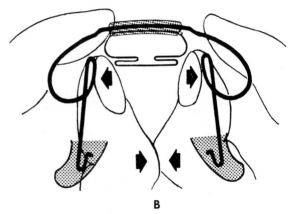

B

C

Figure 13–75. *A*, Expansion automatically causes retrusion of the upper anterior teeth. *D*, Direction of finger pressure to expand. *C*, Direction of finger pressure to contract.

cases treated with rigid activators. Instead, we maintain the light wire loop as a safety device, but add a lip bumper that relieves the pressure against the incisors from the lingual and directs it against the lower lip. The backward-directed counterpressure of the lower lip against the bumper is transferred through the appliance and, finally, is directed by the upper labial arch against the protruded upper incisors, exactly where we need it. The bumper is adjustable, fixed into the frontal splint by a wire similar to the upper labial arch. For the forward or backward adjustment of the bumper, the same instructions apply as for the Type **A** labial arch.

There is a special group of Class II, Division 1 cases with closed bite, overjet, and the lower lip between the upper and lower incisors. The upper incisors are more or less protruded, and the lower incisors are very upright and elongated. Owing to this condition, the second premolars are either impacted or erupt lingually. If they have to be treated by a nonextraction procedure, the A_{1M} variation is indicated. The standard appliance is complemented with two arms in front of the molars, the so-called "molar supports," for the purpose of stretching the lower arch. By adjusting these supports in a backward direction, the distance between the frontal loop lingual to the incisors and the supports mesial to the molars is increased. This causes the anterior loop to ride up higher on the cinguli of the lower incisors. The patient, closing his teeth on the appliance, makes the loop glide downward and backward, and the pressure is

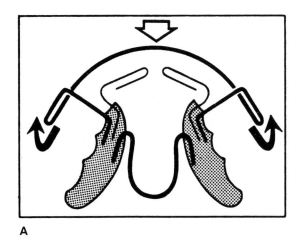

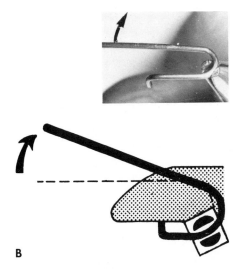

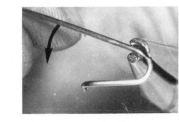

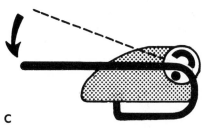

Figure 13-76. Bimler Type **A**: Labial arch adjustment.
    Objective: Retrusion of incisors by shortening labial arch (*A*)
    Rule: To shorten, start on short leg
    Tools: Flat-beak and round-beak pliers
    Instructions: FLAT on round on short leg
                 ROUND on flat on long leg
    Result: Upper arch is first lifted upward and then brought down in a retruded position.
    Comments: The main point to keep in mind is the basic rule: to shorten, start with the short leg. The next steps are always the same. Start with the flat-beak pliers on both sides of the short legs (*B*). Then change to the round-beak pliers and work on the opposite legs on both sides (*C*). Be careful to use the same amount of pressure so that the legs of the adjustment loops are accurately parallel again.

transferred by the appliance to the molars in a backward direction. The same amount of pressure is, of course, directed against the lower incisors in a forward direction. The case of Blue Boy will demonstrate in detail how we arrive at our treatment goal with this mechanism.

THE BLUE BOY CASE

With Blue Boy we present a more complex case, in which mesiodistal tooth movements and the question of anterior bite opening are involved. We will further use the case to demonstrate that far more sophisticated methods in cephalometrics are necessary to take advantage of the very differentiated processes of growth and development.

Blue Boy was an 11-year-old patient in the last stage of the mixed dentition, with a Class II, Division 1 closed bite malocclusion. The left lower premolar was completely blocked out. The lower incisors were very upright and appeared to be elongated.

Text continued on page 427

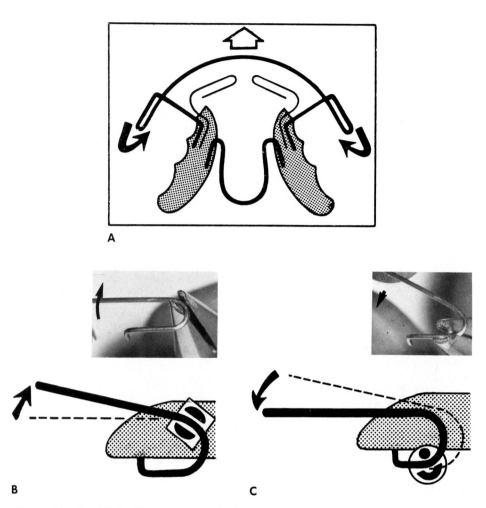

Figure 13-77. Bimler Type **A**: Forward adjustment of labial arch.
 Objective: To lengthen labial arch (**A**)
 Rule: To lengthen, start on long leg
 Tools: Flat-beak and round-beak pliers
 Instructions: FLAT on round on long leg
      ROUND on flat on short leg
 Result: FLAT gives to long leg
    ROUND takes from short leg
 Comments: The lengthening of the labial arch becomes necessary as soon as the anteriors are correctly positioned (sufficiently retruded). This is continually checked by periodic dental arch measurements, which are transferred to the reaction curves. In Class II, Division 2 and in many Class I crowded cases, anteriors even have to be protruded. In such cases it is most important to keep the labial arch off the incisors. The rule, "To lengthen, start on long leg," helps to put the flat-beak pliers at the right place on the long leg of the adjustment loops on both sides (*B*). As usual, the next step is ROUND on flat on the short leg (*C*). By this maneuver, wire material is first taken from the arc and added to the long legs and in the second step this material is again incorporated into the arch and taken away from the short leg.

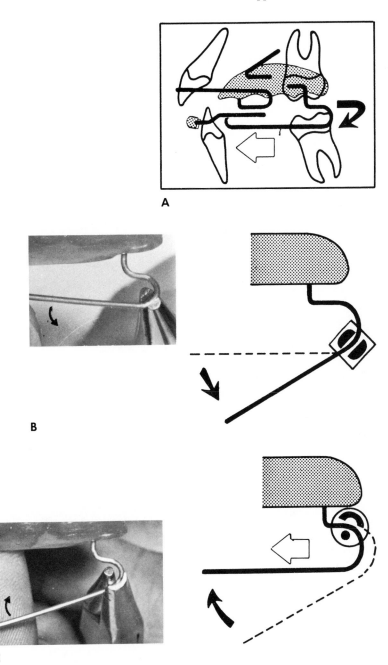

Figure 13-78. Lower arch wire: Forward adjustment of posterior connecting loops.

    Objective: Bring lower part forward (*A*)

    Rule: To lengthen (bring forward), start on long leg

    Instructions: FLAT on round on long leg (*B*)

                 ROUND on flat on short leg (*C*)

    Result: Lower part comes forward

    Comments: Whenever it is necessary, the position of the lower arch can be corrected to a more forward position. Overcorrection with an edge-to-edge bite, as with the activator, is not done with the Bimler appliance. This is a major advantage, in view of the fact that overcorrection of the mandibular position has to be regarded as the main reason for losing a removable appliance at night, as well as for losing anchorage.

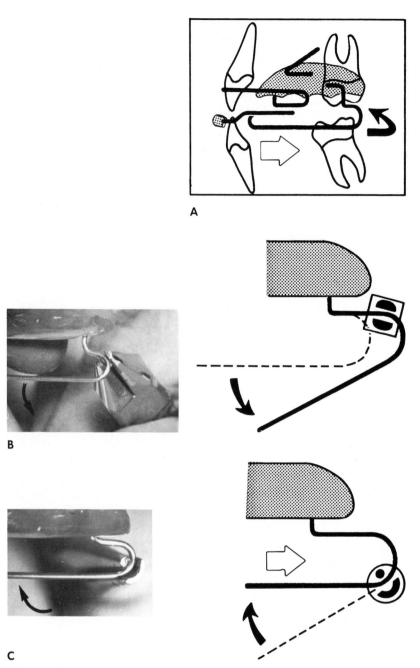

A

B

C

Figure 13-79.   Lower arch wire: Backward adjustment of posterior connecting loops.

    Objective: Bring lower part backward (*A*)

    Rule: To shorten, start on short leg

    Instructions: FLAT on round on short leg (*B*)

                 ROUND on flat on long leg (*C*)

    Result: Lower part moves backward

    Comments: If the appliance is lost at night in severe Class II, Division 1 cases, it is most likely that the bite correction was overdone. It is wise to follow the hint of nature and reduce the forward positioning of the mandible by taking the lower part back. In most cases, the appliance will thereafter not be lost at night. This is true for all functional appliances (activator, Bionator, Fränkel, etc.) except that the latter cannot be adapted once they have been constructed in the wrong position.

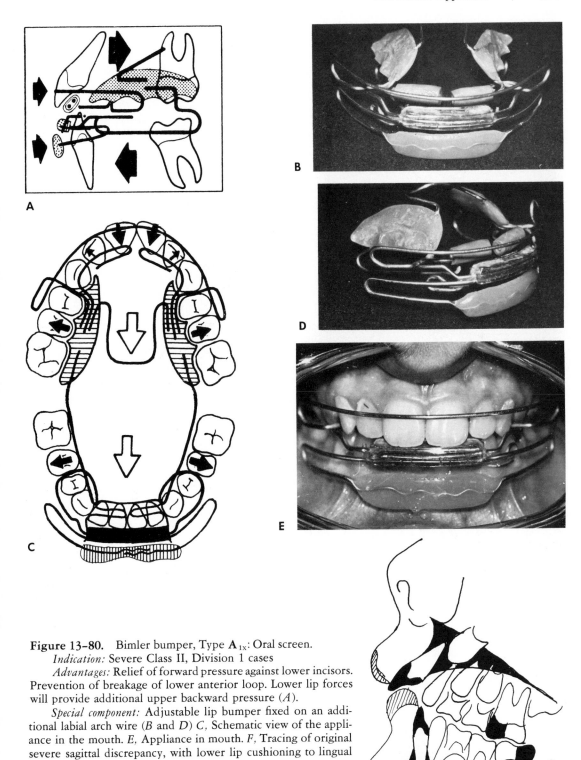

Figure 13-80. Bimler bumper, Type A_{1x}: Oral screen.

Indication: Severe Class II, Division 1 cases

Advantages: Relief of forward pressure against lower incisors. Prevention of breakage of lower anterior loop. Lower lip forces will provide additional upper backward pressure (*A*).

Special component: Adjustable lip bumper fixed on an additional labial arch wire (*B* and *D*) *C*, Schematic view of the appliance in the mouth. *E*, Appliance in mouth. *F*, Tracing of original severe sagittal discrepancy, with lower lip cushioning to lingual of upper incisors.

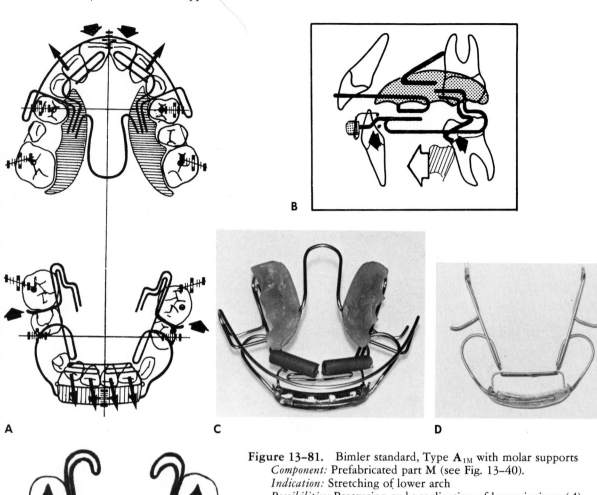

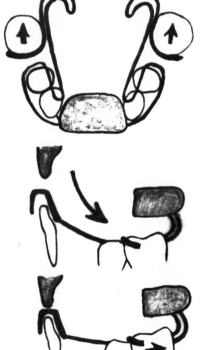

Figure 13–81. Bimler standard, Type $\mathbf{A}_{1M}$ with molar supports
   Component: Prefabricated part M (see Fig. 13–40).
   Indication: Stretching of lower arch
   Possibilities: Protrusion and proclination of lower incisors (*A*)
           Opening of spaces for second premolars
           Bite opening
   Additional component: Lower molar supports (*E*)

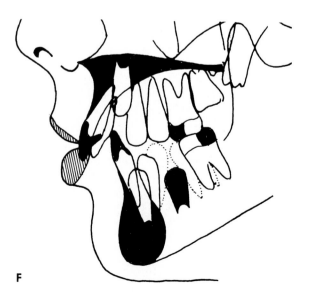

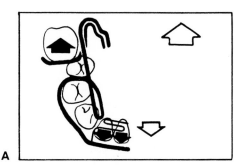

A

Figure 13–82. Molar supports

> *Objective:* Opening of space in front of molars (*A*)
>   Push incisors forward
>
> *Tools:* Flat-beak and round-beak pliers
>
> *Instructions:* FLAT on flat and twist (*B*)
>   FLAT on round (*C*) gives to free leg
>   ROUND on flat (*D*) takes from fixed leg
>
> *Result:* Space opened in front of molar (*E*)
>
> *Comments:* The adjustment of the molar supports is somehow characteristic for the activation of the floating appliances in general. If you are trying to get too much, you will not achieve anything. The moment the activation is overdone, the effectiveness is completely lost. Each adjustment of the molar supports must be checked immediately in the mouth of the patient to see if the supports are still in front of the molars or on top of them. If they are on top, we have overactivated and no result can be expected. To deactivate them, twisting the free leg in the forward direction will usually be sufficient. In our experience, the eruption of the premolars is not impeded by the supports, which lie partially on top of them.

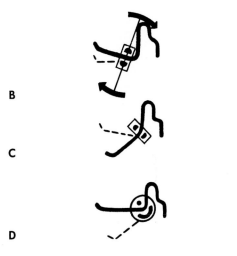

B

C

D

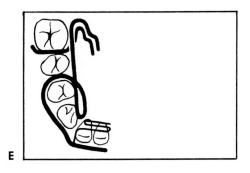

E

The cephalometric background of the malocclusion is again a micro-rhinic dysplasia with the typical triad of maxillary inclination, mandibular overclosure, and increased tilt of the anterior cranial base (Fig. 13–83). The photographs show the slant of the eyelids, the incompetent lips, and the prominent ears (Fig. 13–84). The primary disturbance is seen in the reduced midfacial height. Clinically one can observe an excessive freeway space, when the mandible is in the rest position. In the head plate we find under these conditions the ramus more in the vertical. This picture invites theoretical speculation: if the primary cause is a deficiency in vertical height, the ideal compensation would be to enlarge the midfacial height and bring Factor 4 into a positive inclination. This has been done in the graphic facial reconstruction. Only by this maxillary rotation does the malocclusion disappear. This is the concept of the headgear

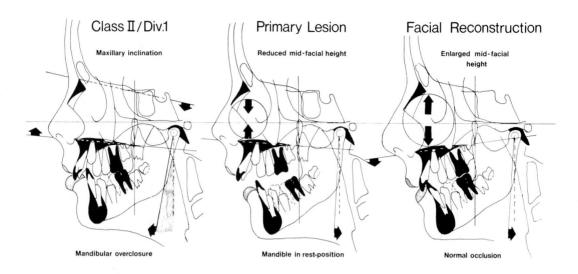

Micro-rhinic Dysplasia

Class II / Div.1	Primary Lesion	Facial Reconstruction
Maxillary inclination	Reduced mid-facial height	Enlarged mid-facial height
Mandibular overclosure	Mandible in rest-position	Normal occlusion
Rotational Syndrome	Excessive Free Way Space	Ideal compensation

Figure 13–83. A maxillary forward and upward inclination (Factor 4), a mandibular hyperflexion (Factor 8), and the increased tilt of the anterior cranial base (Factor 7) form the cephalometric triad of micro-rhinic dysplasia. The primary lesion is located in the anterior part of the middle face. The deficiency in the vertical dimension becomes obvious when the mandible is in the rest position, with an excessive amount of freeway space. Theoretically, a forward and downward rotation of the nasal floor would correct the malocclusion by eliminating the primary cause.

treatment of Class II cases with orthopedic forces. The reaction to a floating appliance is largely different.

The usual diagnostic procedures were performed. Within the dental arches a reopening of the lost space and a proclination of the lower incisors were anticipated. The graphic appliance prescription was completed according to this plan. We used an A_{1M} Standard appliance with molar supports (Fig. 13–86). The arch measurements on the reaction curve chart disclosed an arch width deficiency of about 5 mm. and an arch length deficiency of a similar amount (Fig. 13–88).

Stomatopedic Treatment Sheet, Reaction Curves, and Head Plates

The curves demonstrate in the initial period of the treatment an arch expansion of a little less than 1 mm. per month, so that after eight months the green base lines were reached. At the same time the reduced lower arch height was corrected. We could follow this change on the head plates by a proclination of the lower incisors. The steep position of 106 degrees to the Frankfort horizontal normalized itself to 115 degrees measured anteriorly, which corresponds to the 65 degrees of Tweed measured posteriorly (Fig. 13–89). Measured within the dental arch, the upper incisors were kept in position. From the uprighting of their longitudinal axis on the head plate, the torquing effect of

Text continued on page 432

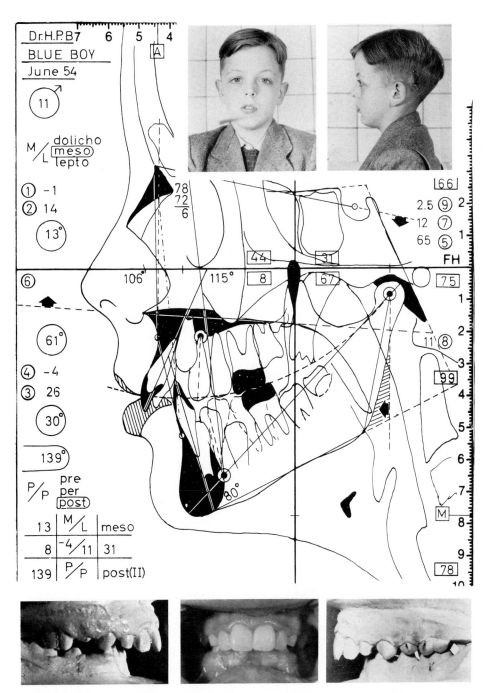

Figure 13–84. Blue Boy case. Age, 11 years. Class II, Division 1, closed bite. Note that in addition to the cephalometric micro-rhinic triad (Factors 4, 7, and 8) he has the matching external features of slanting eyes, prominent ears, and missing oral seal. Lingually inclined lower incisors are associated with the abnormal lower lip posture and function. With regard to the closed bite, the relation of the upper incisors to the curve of Spee is normal. The incisal edges of the lower incisors are 5 mm. above the curve of Spee.

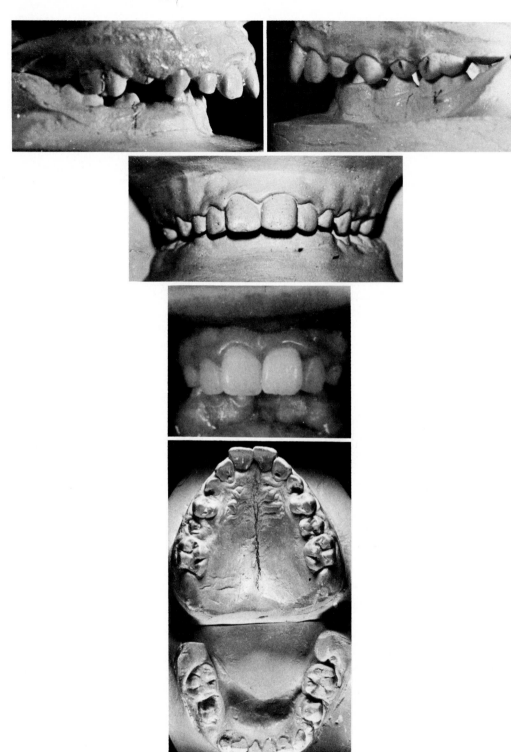

Figure 13-85. Maldeveloping stage in the Blue Boy case. Note the amount of distal occlusion, overjet, and overbite. The left lower second premolar is completely blocked out. Space for the upper canines is reduced and the centrals are protruded.

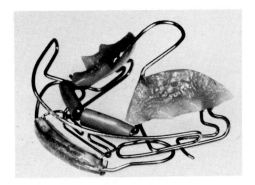
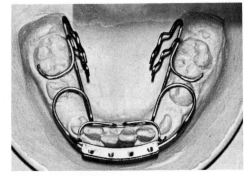

Appliance Prescription

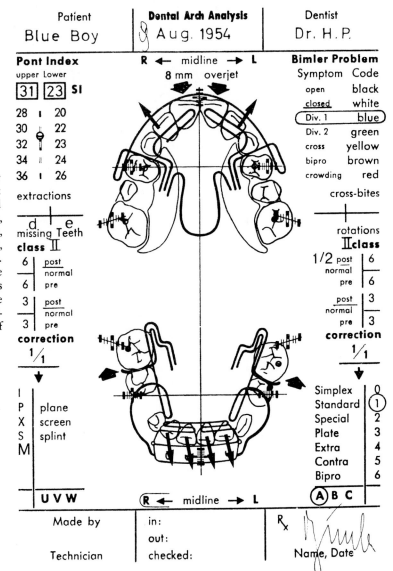

	Dental Arch Analysis	
Patient	⅏ Aug. 1954	Dentist
Blue Boy		**Dr. H.P.**

Pont Index

upper Lower

31	23	SI
28	ı	20
30		22
32	⊕	23
34	ıı	24
36	ı	26

extractions

d	e

missing Teeth

class Ⅱ

6	post
	normal
6	pre
3	post
	normal
3	pre

correction

$\frac{1}{1}$

↓

I	
P	plane
X	screen
S	splint
M	

U V W

R ← midline → L

8 mm overjet

Bimler Problem

Symptom Code

open	black
closed	white
Div. 1	blue
Div. 2	green
cross	yellow
bipro	brown
crowding	red

cross-bites

rotations

Ⅱclass

1/2	post	6
	normal	
	pre	6
	post	3
	normal	
	pre	3

correction

$\frac{1}{1}$

↓

Simplex	0
Standard	1
Special	2
Plate	3
Extra	4
Contra	5
Bipro	6

A B C

R ← midline → L

Made by	in:	Rx
	out:	
Technician	checked:	Name, Date

Figure 13-86. Blue Boy case. Appliance prescription: Bimler Type **A**₁M. Standard appliance for upper expansion, retrusion of upper centrals, alignment of upper anteriors, and space opening for canines. Molar supports are used in the lower arch to protrude incisors against the resistance of the molars. *Upper left*, **A**₁M appliance. *Upper right*, Position of molar supports.

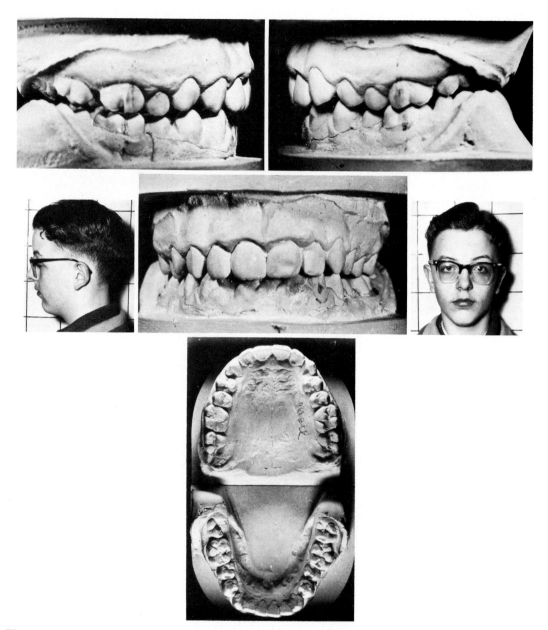

Figure 13-87. Blue Boy case. Age, 13 years. Provisional results after two years (corrective stage). Distal occlusion is nearly corrected, dental overjet and overbite are reduced, and space for blocked out bicuspid has been reopened.

the appliance between labial arch and frontal springs can be demonstrated (compare Figs. 13–84 and 13–89). The Class II relationship and the closed bite disappeared within two years. How the normalization occurs can only be assessed retrospectively. It differs from case to case. The floating appliance apparently sets only a certain frame and leaves it to the individual potential of growth and adaptability, by which mechanism the goal of normal occlusion is achieved.

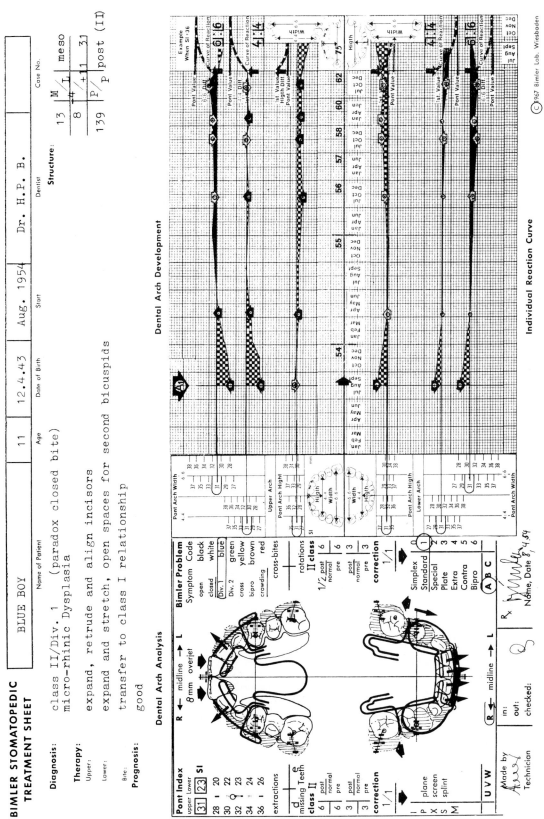

Figure 13-88. Stomatopedic treatment sheet for Blue Boy.

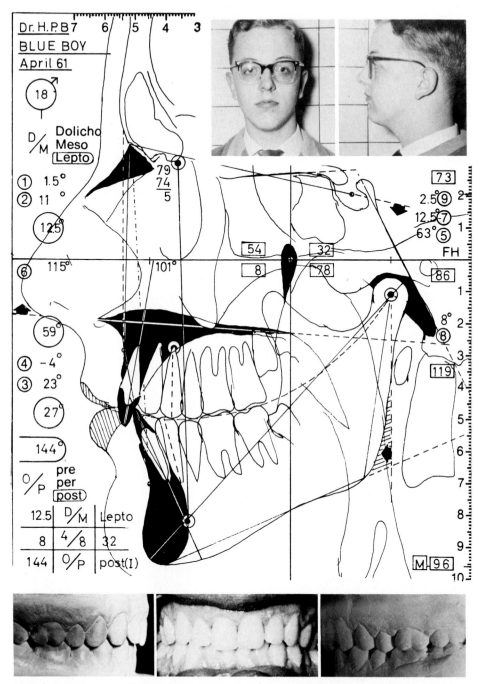

Figure 13–89. Blue Boy case. Age, 18 years. Class I normal occlusion (constructive stage). There was a 10 mm. growth of the maxilla and 20 mm. of the mandible. Bony overjet remained unchanged at 8 mm. The lower profile angle (Factor 2) was reduced by 3 degrees owing to vertical facial growth. Note that the angular measurements are not reliable to express AB relationship. The bite opening was due partly to an increase in alveolar height and partly to proclination of the lower incisors. Further development of the third molars should be supervised.

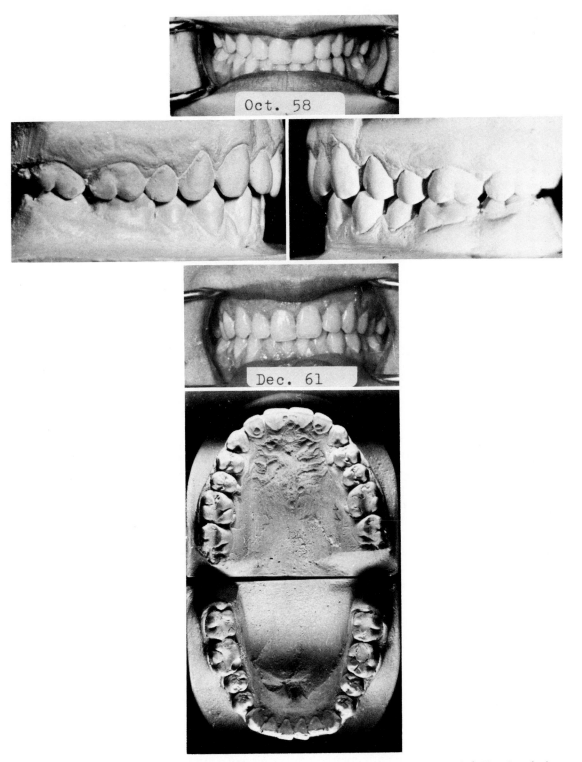

Figure 13–90. Blue Boy case, three years out of retention. There is a completely settled Class I occlusion with normal overjet and overbite. Note the further bite opening in the post-treatment period from 1958 to 1961.

class II / Div.1   micro-rhinic dysplasia

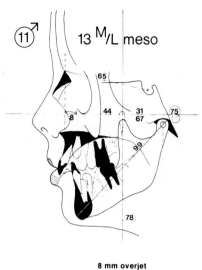

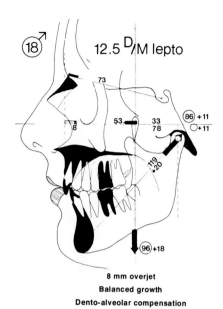

8 mm overjet

Maxillary inclination

Mandibular hyperflexion

8 mm overjet

Balanced growth

Dento-alveolar compensation

Figure 13-91. Class II correction by dentoalveolar adaptation. There was balanced growth of the maxilla, mandible, and T-TM distance. The maxillary inclination and basal bone overjet were unchanged. Mandibular hyperflexion was reduced by tooth eruption in the buccal segments.

We will use all the evidence to follow the development of Blue Boy through the different stages of his dentition. In Figure 13–91 we find the linear measurements separately to study the growth increments. Table 13–2 gives us a good guide for this purpose. At age 11 the facial formula was 13 M/L meso; at age 18, 12.5 D/M lepto, a change in the facial type from meso to lepto. This is explained by a vertical growth of 18 mm. against a sagittal growth of 11 mm. The upper basic angle changed from M to D. The reason can be attributed to a flattening of the clivus by Factor 5, which changed from 65 to 63 degrees. Factor 4, the maxillary inclination, stayed unchanged at −4 degrees, and the upper basic angle changed from 61 to 59 degrees, or from M to D. In Blue Boy, as in the majority of our patients, an orthopedic effect on the tilt of the maxilla did not occur. The lower basic angle, or Frankfort-mandibular angle, was reduced from 26 to 23 degrees. This is often interpreted as a forward rotation of the mandible. We do not accept this opinion. That Factor 8 was at the same time reduced from 11 to 8 degrees would indicate the contrary, a backward rotation. Both changes have to be understood as remodeling procedures during growth.

The facial profile angle is nearly the same, but analyzing it precisely, the upper profile angle, Factor 1, changed from −1 to + 1.5 degrees, from slightly retrognathic to slightly prognathic. This can be confirmed by linear measurements: the distance NS increased by only 8 mm., the distance A to T vertical by 9 mm. Consequently, point A has to be more forward with regard to point N. The correction of the Class II relationship was apparently not due to a retrusion of point A.

The lower profile angle, Factor 2, was reduced from 14 to 11 degrees. This looks like a forward movement of point B. The SNA-SNB difference seems to

TABLE 13–2.   COMPARISON OF 20 FEATURES IN BLUE BOY

No.	Feature	Factor	Age 11	Age 18	Comments
1	NA upper profile angle	1	−1°	+1.5°	A grew more forward than N
2	AB lower profile angle	2	14°	11°	Vertical distance A to B became bigger
3	NAB profile angle	A	13°	12.5°	Nearly unchanged by compensatory changes of Nos. 1 and 2
4	ANS-PNS maxillary inclination	4	−4°	−4°	Due to unchanged micro-rhinic dysplasia
5	FMPA	3	26°	23°	Usual finding in growing children
6	Lower basic angle	B	30°(L)	27°(M)	Due to reduced Factor (3)
7	N-S versus FH	7	12°	12.5°	Slight change is NS tilt
8	Clivus inclination	5	65°	63°	Flattening of clivus by growth
9	Upper basic angle	C	61°(M)	59°(D)	Due to clivus flattening
10	Mandibular flexion	8	11°	8°	Reduced by vertical growth in alveolar region
11	Maxillary depth	A-T	44 mm.	54 mm.	10 mm. increase
12	Temporal position	T-TM	31 mm.	32 mm.	Backward growth of fossa
13	Facial depth	A-TM	75 mm.	86 mm.	11 mm. increase as sum of maxillary depth and T-TM distance
14	Facial height	FH-M	78 mm.	96 mm.	18 mm. increase due to vertical growth tendency in leptoprosopic faces
15	Mandibular length — projected	B-TM	67 mm.	78 mm.	11 mm. increase as horizontal vector of No. 16
16	Mandibular length — diagonal	gn-cd	99 mm.	119 mm.	20 mm. increase
17	A-B horizontal overjet	A-B	8 mm.	8 mm.	Unchanged owing to balanced growth of Nos. 11 and 16
18	Lower incisors/FH		106°	115°	Due to protrusion. Note bite opening relative to curve of Spee
19	Upper incisors/FH		115°	101°	Due to uprighting
20	Interincisal angle		139°	144°	Increase due to upper uprighting

confirm this, as it changed from 6 to 5 degrees. Unfortunately, both findings cannot be corroborated by linear measurements. The projected overjet of A and B to the Frankfort horizontal is still 8 mm. The reduction of the angles is due to the vertical growth of the face. These findings prove that angular measurements alone are no longer sufficient and have to be checked by linear ones.

class II / Div.1   delayed mandibular growth

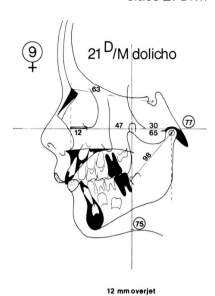

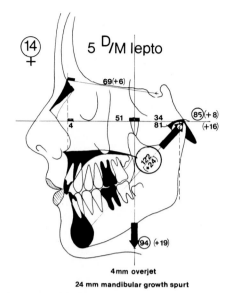

12 mm overjet   24 mm mandibular growth spurt

Figure 13-92. Class II, Division 1 correction by large mandibular growth. The basal bone overjet was reduced by 8 mm., or two thirds of the original overjet. The mandibular growth spurt was independent of appliance wearing, as there was very poor cooperation.

Blue Boy, with his balanced growth, seems to prove the former American point of view, that the skeletal pattern cannot be changed. To the contrary, the next case seems to prove the wishful thinking of certain European groups that one can cause growth of a mandible with functional appliances. By a large growth spurt of the mandible, the basal bone overjet A-B was reduced drastically and a correction of the Class II relationship achieved. Fortunately for the understanding of the real causes in such cases, the child was very uncooperative and moved out of town for a while. We left her the appliance, as it is practically fool-proof and can do no harm. After two years a happy mother appeared again and presented her daughter with a very acceptable result. An unexpected and unpredictable growth spurt of the mandible had solved the problem even without better cooperation from the patient herself.

Our next example (Fig. 13-93) shows a Class II, Division 1 case with a formula of 26.5 D/L meso. The profile angle NAB is rather high, and Factor 4 is negative. After four years the formula is 21.5 M/M lepto. The profile angle is reduced by 5 degrees, corresponding to a reduction of the overjet of 2 mm. The relation of upper basic angle to lower basic angle changed from D/L to M/M owing to a spontaneous rotation of the maxilla. Factor 4 is positive at age 13. This happened without any extraoral forces, but this is a very rare finding. The index changed from meso to lepto owing to a vertical increase of 10 mm., against only 5 mm. in the sagittal direction. Of this 5 mm. increase in facial depth, only 2 mm. was in the maxilla, with 3 mm. in the T-TM distance.

In the early days of functional therapy in Europe, some authors believed that the TM joints would be transferred in a forward direction. This was a mistake. We have never found it. Whenever we have found a reduced T-TM distance, we have also found a dual bite with the condyle no longer in the fossa. In our example, growth in the sutures of the cranial base carried the petrous

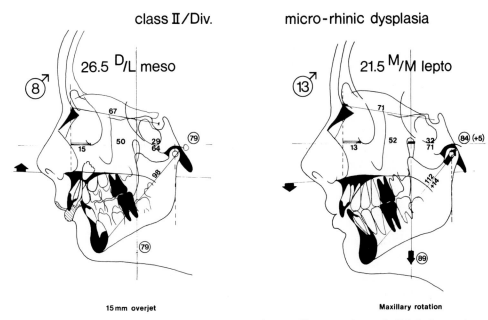

Figure 13-93. Class II, Division 1 correction by maxillary rotation and slightly larger than expected mandibular growth. No extraoral forces were applied.

bones, including the fossae, away from the maxilla by 3 mm. The diagonal growth of the mandible of 14 mm. resulted in an increase of 7 mm. in the effective length of the lower jaw as measured on Frankfort horizontal, reducing the overjet by 2 mm.

Our last case in the Blue group (Fig. 13-94) shows still another mechanism by which a Class II relationship can be compensated. Here we find total cessa-

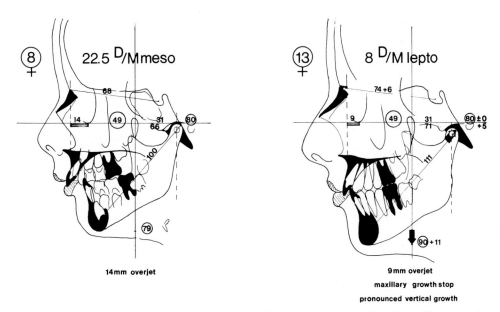

Figure 13-94. Class II, Division 1 correction by a complete cessation of maxillary growth coupled with normal mandibular growth. Overjet was reduced by 5 mm. No extraoral forces were used.

tion of growth in the maxilla between 8 and 13 years of age in a girl. No extraoral forces were applied, but the maxilla stayed at 49 mm. At the same time, the mandible grew 11 mm. in the diagonal, the facial height increased by 11 mm., and the anterior cranial base, represented by the distance NS, increased by 6 mm.

It is our experience, based on thousands of fully documented cases, that nearly every case will react differently and we do not dare to predict according to which of the presented mechanisms or combinations of them an individual case will react. We follow individual development with our reaction curves and head plate sequences, always ready to correct our treatment plan if a satisfying effect cannot be noted.

Long-term Observations on Blue Boy

Usually in the literature reports on cases five years out of retention are used to demonstrate the stability of the therapeutic results. This may lead to illusory ideas. Blue Boy at age 18, five years after the intensive period of treatment, was at the peak of the constructive stage of his dentition. Even if his teeth had been aligned five years ago, the bite had improved until recently and the occlusion was settled in a perfect Class I molar relationship. To believe this will last forever is unrealistic. The teeth are ready to move all through life. The moment one or more of the factors which keep the dentition in balance are lost, the dentition will start to change immediately. The releasing factor may be a different muscle tonus or simply a loss of teeth. Only a small percentage of patients are seen in later years, and nearly never are findings published. As we have never discarded any models or other documents in 25 years, we are now able to study the cases of our own after longer periods of time. So we found Blue Boy at age 33. His physiognomy had changed so much that we would not have recognized him on the street. The intraoral finding was a bit disappointing, too. Clinically the dentition looked like a Division 2 case with rather steep incisors and a closed bite again. Remember that he had started as a Class II, Division 1 malocclusion 22 years earlier. The Class I molar relationship achieved 20 years ago by our treatment had not changed at all. Comparing the projected occlusal views of the models showed that the upper centrals were a bit retruded and the lower incisors were tilted backward by 3 mm. and elongated by 1 to 2 mm. A key factor in these changes was the loss of the right lower first molar. As we know from other cases, the loss of vertical support makes the tip of the lower canine move up to the margin of the upper canine. By this development the lower canine distance is reduced and the lower incisors present a secondary crowding. This mechanism let us understand that extraction of first premolars and removal of wisdom teeth cannot always prevent the crowding. It is interesting to note that this process took place unilaterally in Blue Boy. The right lower canine moved mesially by 2 mm. and pushed the incisors to the left side. The left lower canine, which looks protruded, is still in place but the incisors have moved lingually. Because two more molars have been lost on the right side, the lowering of the bite will probably proceed. Blue Boy has come into the destructive stages of his dentition, and we are not sure if he will follow our advice and get himself the necessary restorative work.

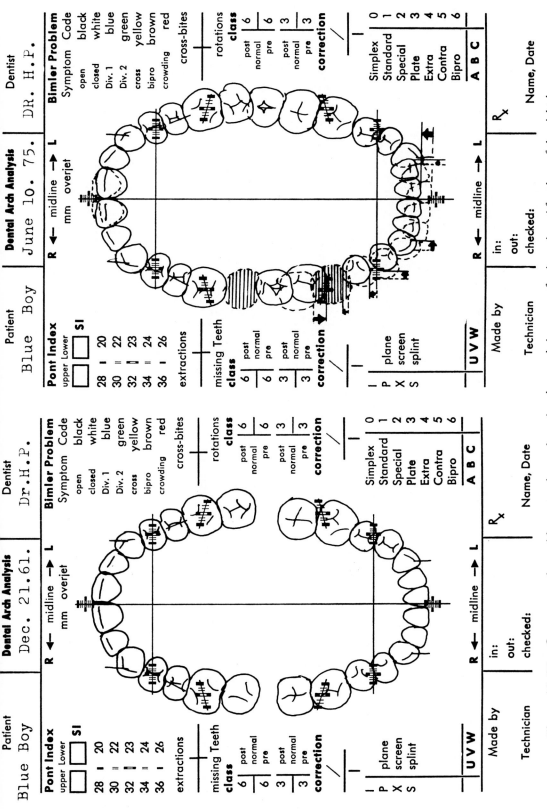

Figure 13–95. Compare tracings with mean value scales printed around the cross of orientation. After loss of the right lower first molar, note the mesial drift of the second and third molars and the distolingual drift of the first and second premolars. The right lower canine has tilted lingually, and the incisors are pushed to the left and retruded behind the left lower canine, which has not moved.

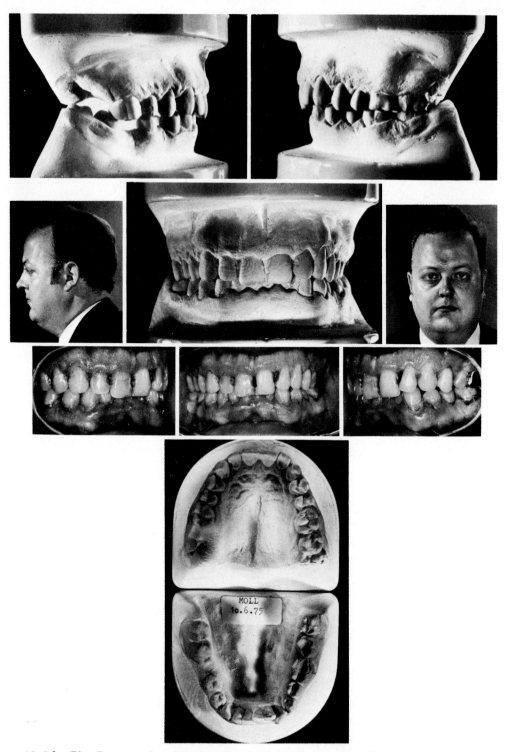

Figure 13-96. Blue Boy case. Age, 33 years. Class I, Division 2 signs, closed bite and mutilated arches, following 15 years without any treatment (destructive stage). The June, 1975, models show that Blue Boy had lost his right lower first molar a considerable time ago, and recently lost the right upper second and third molars. The effect of the loss of the lower molar was a forward drift of the second and third molars and a lingual and distal drift of the premolars. As we know from other cases, it is the loss of vertical support that makes the lower canine move lingually and pushes the incisors to the opposite side. At the same time, the incisors were tilted lingually. Note the same mentalis fold on the facial photographs that was seen at age 11. The apparently protruded position of the lower left canine proved by superimposition to be the same as on the 1961 models, but the incisors have been retruded.

442

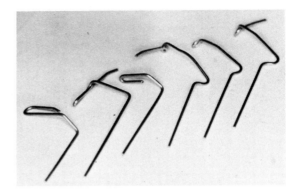

Figure 13-97. Interdental springs for Bimler appliances.

INTERDENTAL SPRINGS

The main problem with auxiliary springs in floating appliances is, again, stability and resistance to mechanical deformation. Both problems have been adequately solved by imitating nature's examples. The stability of stems of grass or bamboo is derived from the joints that divide the whole stem into sections. Likewise, our interdental springs have joints or knots in the form of little loops vertical to the stem of the spring (Fig. 13-97). We mentioned before that the orthodontic elliptic arches have a neutral zone in the canine region; in the Bimler appliance, the neutral spot is between the laterals and the canines. Therefore, the I_1, I_2, and I_3 springs cross the dental arch exactly at this place (Fig. 13-98). While the anterior springs contact the lingual from the midline to the distal of the lateral incisor, the I_2 spring utilizes its mesial extension to control rotations from the labial (Fig. 13-98B). The I_3 spring controls canine rota-

Figure 13-98. Interdental springs. *A*, I_1 Upper canine support. *Objective:* Retrusion of upper canines in extraction cases; support to counteract pushing of frontal spring F. (see Fig. 13-40). *B*, I_2 Upper canine support with mesial extension. *Objective:* Rotation of laterals; can be effective only when used with frontal spring (*F*) rotating the distal of the lateral forward, or with stretching arch (*B*). *C*, I_3 Upper canine support with distal extension. *Objective:* Rotation of canines, in severe cases counteract with palatal finger spring. *D*, I_4 Vertical support for buccal segment. *Objective:* Push back first premolars to open spaces for canines; support for forward pushing of frontal springs; can be used anywhere in the buccal segment. *E*, I_5 Buccal spring for premolars. *Objective:* Move one or two teeth from the outer side for palatal movement or rotation. Used in A_5 appliance to contract the whole upper arch while the lower is expanding. *F*, I_6 Interocclusal horizontal support. *Objective:* Placed in an interocclusal space as a bite block to open the bite in cross-bite cases and to stabilize Type **B** appliances in very deep bite cases.

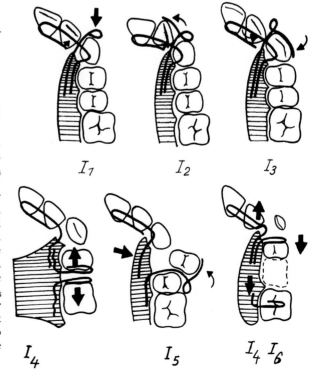

I_1 I_2 I_3

I_4 I_5 $I_4 I_6$

tion from the buccal aspect (Fig. 13–98*C*). The pressure of the free end of the extension is countered by pressure against the mesial of the palatal aspect from a strategically placed finger spring. By means of the aforementioned little loops, the direction of the wire changes three times: first, by 90 degrees into the vertical plane, and then, by 180 degrees vertically, going to the distal first and coming around the loop to the mesial. In the I_3 version it is the opposite. In the I_5 buccal spring, the loop can be elongated to cover the adjacent premolar or molar (Fig. 13–98*E*). Recurving loops in the vertical plane of the I_4 spring allow the teeth in the buccal segment to push forward or backward to open or close spaces (Fig. 13–98*D*). The I_6 spring is placed in the horizontal plane between the molars to block the bite. It is used in crossbite cases.

Bimler Special Type A_2

The particular problems arising from rotated or ectopic teeth are attacked in the Bimler method at the same time as the general ones, such as crowding, open or closed bite, and the Class II malrelationship. For this purpose, the standard version can be complemented with a number of interdental springs and/or the lower canine supports (Fig. 13–99). It has been observed that rotated teeth, corrected while they are erupting, show far less tendency to relapse. The rotation is performed by a labiolingual approach. The action of lingually placed anterior springs is counteracted by the labial extensions of the interdental springs. Vertical loops I_4 keep spaces open or reopen them in connection with anterior springs or another vertical loop. Furthermore, the A_2 version has proved to be especially beneficial in treating the Class II, Division 2 cases in the early mixed dentition, so that the Type **B** appliances are now reserved for the Division 2 cases in the permanent dentition.

In all kinds of crossbite cases, some sort of bite blocking is necessary to separate the overlapping teeth. The simplest means for achieving this purpose are represented by the I_6 interocclusal springs placed in the molar region.

Another highly effective device is the so-called Equiplane. This is a small metal sheet fixed on top of the anterior splint. It separates the incisor teeth and helps to intrude any of them that have been elongated in the crossbite occlusion (Fig. 13–102).

In cases with more severe midfacial hypoplasia with unilateral or bilateral crossbites, better results have been achieved when pressure is brought to bear directly on the alveolar processes by means of a palatal plate and jackscrew (Fig. 13–103). It can be assumed that this will create bone apposition in the midpalatal suture. Thus, transverse expansion can be achieved, in many cases correcting the lateral crossbites. In the long run, we are getting the same results as in rapid palatal suture splitting, but without the relapse tendency. It must be kept in mind that the midfacial hypoplasia affects the maxilla in all three dimensions of space, and that the vertical and sagittal dimensions are not influenced by transverse expansion. This explains why expansion cannot always solve the problem, and that in certain cases, extraction cannot be avoided. The advantage of slow suture widening with functionally controlled appliances has to be acknowledged in view of the fact that expansion will decrease and finally stop when the borderline of individual adaptability is reached.

Text continued on page 448

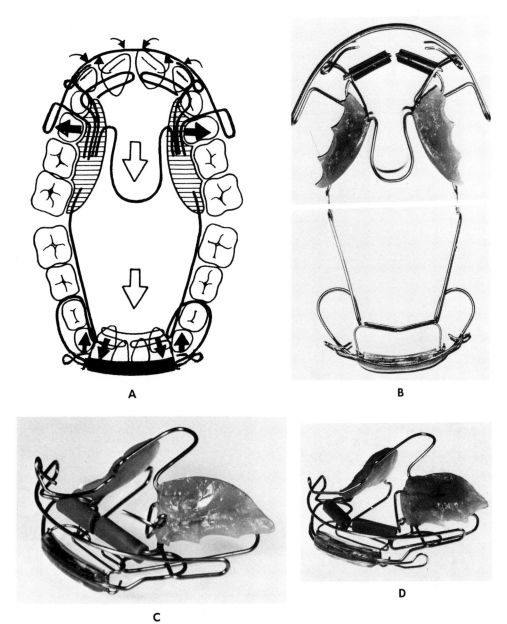

A

B

C

D

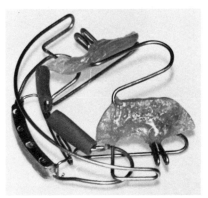

E

Figure 13-99. Bimler special, Type **A**ₐ for special tooth movements.

Components: 0.8 mm. (0.32 inch) interdental springs (see Figs. 13-40 and 13-97).

Indications: Class I, Class II, Division 1, mixed and permanent dentitions; Class II, Division 2, mixed dentition; anterior crowding with rotations; buccal crowding with blocked-out teeth. *C,* **A**₂ version with **I**₂ springs for the rotation of laterals. This type is especially indicated for Class II, Division 2 cases in the mixed dentition. *D,* **A**₂ version with **I**₁ and **E** supports to align ectopic canines. *E,* **A**₂ version with double **I**₄ springs to open spaces for second premolars.

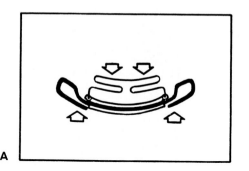

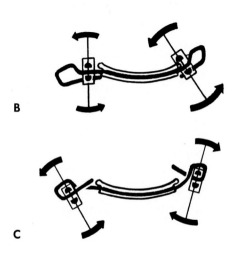

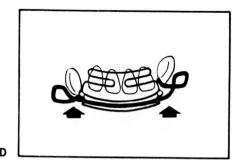

Figure 13–100. Lower canine supports (**E**) for sagittal movements.

Objective: Move canines backward or incisors forward

Instructions: FLAT on flat and twist

Comments: Ordinarily the pressure of the anterior loop on the lateral incisors will be counteracted by the frontal splint that is placed on the labial of the central incisors. In cases in which all the lower incisors are too far back, it is necessary to use the buccal segments for counteraction. The lower canine supports, which are anchored in the frontal splint, are used for this purpose. The canine supports are always used in pairs and consist of a continuous wire following the direction of the labial part of the lower arch (*B*). In the area of the canines, a U loop is formed which is open at the front and has a free leg engaging the canine on the mesial. The adjustment range of the free-ending canine supports is much greater than the adjustment range of the lingual frontal loop. Therefore, it is not necessary to change the frontal loop itself in order to influence the entire lower anterior area. Just activate the lower canine supports and the counterpressure will take over. The fixed leg of the canine support can be used to move the free leg into position for the best action available, in cases where the canines erupt mesially or distally. Place the flat-beak pliers on the fixed leg or stem, and twist the wrist (*B*). In order to increase the pressure on the canines and automatically put pressure labially on the front teeth, activate the supports by twisting motions on the free legs (*C*).

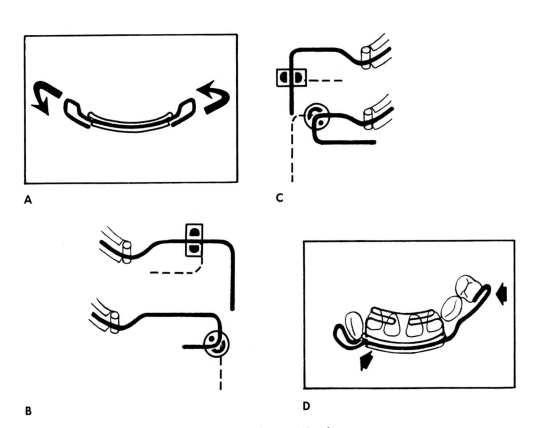

A

B

C

D

Figure 13–101. Lower canine supports (**E**) for special tasks.

> *Objective:* Elongate the stem (*B*)
> *Instructions:* FLAT on round on fixed leg
> ROUND on flat on free leg
> *Objective:* Elongate free leg (*C*)
> *Instructions:* FLAT on round on free leg
> ROUND on flat on fixed leg

Comments: If the primary canine was lost prematurely in the mixed dentition, the canine supports can be placed against the primary first molar, and later against the first premolar, to open space for the lower canines. This versatile spring can also be used to lingually move a buccally placed premolar. To reach far enough back, have the stem of the spring as long as possible. First, open up the spring stem angle with flat-beak pliers and then use the round-beak pliers on the free-leg material to create a new angle (*B*). In this way, the **E** spring can reach sufficiently to the distal and can influence a buccally placed premolar toward the lingual. The free leg of the **U** loop must be long enough to engage a canine that has erupted mesially. Straighten out the angle at the free leg with the flat-beak pliers and create a new angle with the round-beak pliers in the area of the spring stem or at the fixed leg (*C*). This gives the free leg a greater mesial reach.

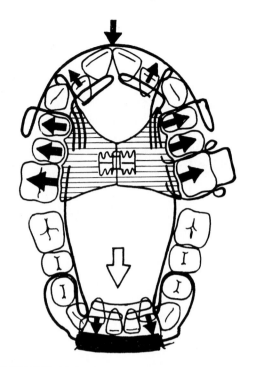

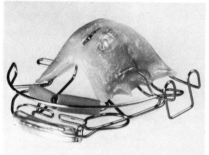
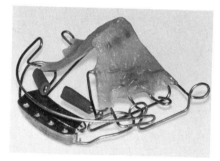

Figure 13–102. Bimler Hypo, Type A_3: Palatal plate and screw.
   Indication: Hypoplastic cases of Class I and Class II, Division 1 with unilateral and bilateral crossbites, mixed and permanent dentitions.
   Special components: Palatal plate with jackscrew
                    0.8 mm. crossbite spring (**K**) (see Fig. 13–40)
                    Equiplane metal platform for anterior crossbite (**P**)

INDICATION FOR EXTRACTION

In all borderline cases with lack of space for all the teeth, we explore the individual limit of adaptability by a conservative test-treatment. If our check curves tell us after some time, by leveling out with the base lines, that no more expansion can be expected, extraction will be considered. The teeth to be pulled do not always have to be the first premolars. Second premolars or molars can also be selected, depending on the individual facial structure. This procedure is often recommended in Europe. Treatment usually starts in the mixed dentition, when it is too early for a definite decision anyway. We do extract first premolars when the canines break through and it is obvious that other procedures will not succeed in aligning these teeth properly.

Figure 13–103. Cross bite springs (**K**): Expansion plate with jackscrew.

Objective: Correct crossbite by expanding upper and contracting lower (*A* and *B*)

Instructions: FLAT on joint and twist (*B*)

Objective: Prevent blockage of lower contraction (*D*)

Instructions: FLAT on sled and twist (*C*)

Comments: With the **A**$_3$ appliance, the cross bite is attacked in two different ways. First, the expansion of the upper arch will occur owing to the action of the plate and screw. On the lower arch, a second contracting force will be directed against the lower molars lingually (*A*). To increase this pressure, place the flat-beak pliers at the loops of the crossbite springs and use a twisting motion to adjust them (*B*). Keep in mind that with the opening of the expansion screw the crossbite springs are carried away from the lower teeth, while the lingual sleds are carried toward the lower buccal segments. The former action decreases the pressure on the buccal surfaces, and the latter may block any contraction of the lower arch. Both facts must be taken into consideration when the **A**$_3$ is adjusted. The lower sleds can be bent lingually by a similar twisting movement with the flat-beak pliers (*C*).

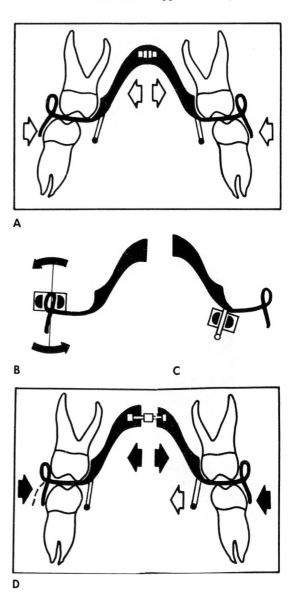

It is a common belief that closing up spaces after premolar extraction requires fixed appliances to prevent severe tipping of the neighboring teeth. Therefore, it may be surprising for many to discover the contrary. In extraction cases we have to differentiate between one group in which the apex of the canine is above the first premolar and the canine only has to be uprighted by backward tilting into the extraction space, and a second group in which the canine and premolar have parallel roots and a wide apical base. Our indication for extraction, with a few exceptions, is more or less limited to extremely crowded cases with a short maxilla in the anteroposterior direction. They belong to the group mentioned first. Here, the **A**$_4$ variation proves to be a very simple and convenient way to align the anteriors and to close the spaces without forward tilting of the teeth distal to the extraction site. Space-closing takes place usually two thirds from the mesial and one third from the distal. The reason we see this favorable reaction seems to be a headgear-like action of

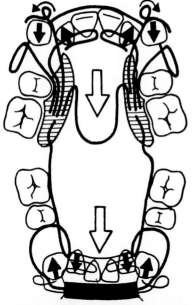

Figure 13–104. Bimler extra, Type **A**$_4$: First premolar extraction cases.

Indication: Extraction cases of Class I and Class II, Division 1, permanent dentition only.

Special components: Upper labial arches **Aa,** interdental springs **I,** and lower cuspid supports **E** (see Fig. 13–40)

Comments: As we have mentioned before, for the equilibrium of the appliance, a well-balanced relationship of the dimensions of the single components is very important. In extraction cases, the upper labial arch has to be anchored in the palatal wings on the level of the second premolars. This would mean elongating the middle part of the labial arch at the start of treatment and shortening it in favor of the adjustment loops later. This results in disturbance of the balanced dimensions. Further, the cross-over wires tend to fall behind the horizontal loops in the lower arch and the necessary vertical support is lost. To remedy this, we introduced a special variation **Aa** with oblique cross-over wires. The frontal springs (**F**), the interdental springs, and the Coffin springs (**R**) also have to be inserted at the level of the second premolars. In the lower arch, it must be decided individually if the horizontal loops will be placed in front of the second premolar or in front of the molar or somewhere in between.

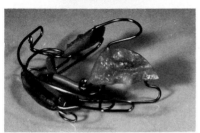

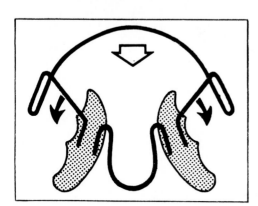

A

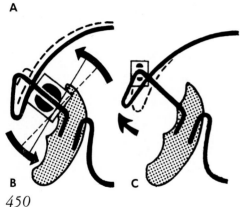

B　　　　C

Figure 13–105. Labial arch **Aa**; Premolar extraction cases.

First objective: Swing back cross-over wires (*A*)
Instructions: FLAT on flat and twist (*B*)
Second objective: Disengage loop from buccal teeth
Instructions: FLAT on round (*C*)

Comments: Generally speaking, all form changes on appliances should be done on the U bows and no other parts should be touched. The exception to this rule is where the upper first premolars were extracted and where the cross-over arms of the labial arch do not cross the arches in front of the upper first premolars at a right angle, as seen in the usual case. The cross-over arms run diagonally across the extraction spaces to support the upper appliance parts against the lower part (*A*). Leaving its anchored position in the palatal wings, the wire runs diagonally across the extraction spaces and turns behind the canines into the lateral adjustment bows. The desired result of therapy in extraction cases is that the extraction spaces close during the course of treatment. At the end of the treatment period, the distal surfaces of the canines should contact the mesial surfaces of the second premolars. To bring this about, the labial arch should slowly be brought back by adjustment of the wires that run diagonally across the extraction spaces. The cross-over arms will finally appear as seen in the standard Type **A** appliance and will cross the arches at a right angle. After achieving closure of the spaces, the appliance has not only aligned the teeth, but it has gradually been guided back into its standard form. While holding the appliance steadily in one hand, turn distally or twist the cross-over arm with the flat-beak pliers (*B*). The distal twisting of the cross-over arms carries the adjustment bows of the labial arch against the teeth. To remedy this, the buccal angle should be enlarged with the tip of the flat-beak pliers to bend the bow away from the teeth (*C*).

Figure 13–106. Labial arch **Aa:** Premolar extraction cases.

    Objective: Shorten crossover wires *(A)*

    Instructions: FLAT on round gives to short leg of U loop
                 ROUND on flat takes from crossover wires

    Comments: Because the diagonal radius of the cross-over arm of the **Aa** arch is longer than its counterpart in the **A** arch, it becomes necessary to shorten this length while distal movement is being accomplished. To do this, material from the cross-over arm is transferred to the short leg of the **U** bow of the labial arch. Use the flat-beak pliers to open the buccal angle on both sides *(B)*. Then, with the round-beak pliers, form a new angle from the material that originally belonged to the crossover arm *(C)*. From the handling of the normal labial arch, it was determined that a lengthening of the short leg of the adjustment bow goes hand-in-hand with the shortening of the overall arch. In the foregoing procedure, shortening of the arch was accomplished by distally twisting the cross-over arms. Thus, the labial arch may become too short with two maneuvers in the same backward direction. In this case, the labial arch must be lengthened.

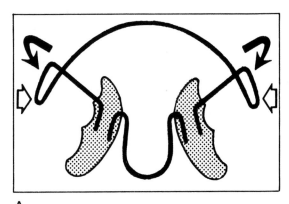
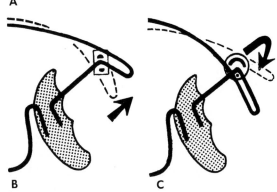

the retractor muscles, activated by the forward positioning of the mandible through the bimaxillary appliance (Fig. 13–104). Secondly, the floating device exerts only extremely light, interrupted forces, moving the canines quickly by direct resorption.

Figure 13–107. Frontal springs **(F):** Premolar extraction cases.

    Objective: Adjust backward in elbow

    Instructions: FLAT on flat on shoulder and twist
                 ROUND on round on elbow

    Comments: The anterior springs are inserted in the palatal wings farther back, as are the labial arch and the Coffin spring. They are positioned more distally to leave more space between their free ends. When the oblique arms are twisted back, the anterior springs will follow in a similar manner. For this purpose, twist them with the flat-beak pliers in the shoulder region backward and outward *(B)*. Then make a more acute elbow with the round-beak pliers *(C)*. After the extraction spaces are closed, the anterior springs should be positioned as in the standard appliance, nearly touchdng at the midline.

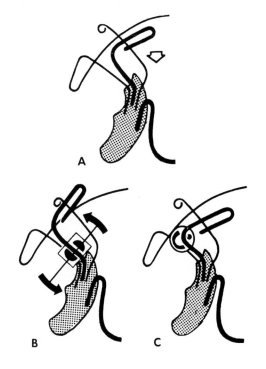

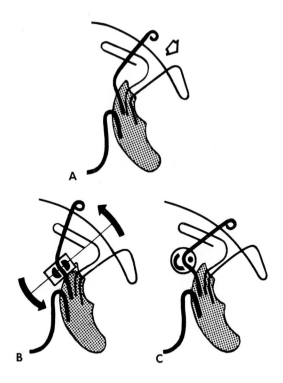

Figure 13–108. Upper canine supports (**I**): Premolar extraction cases

Objective: Shorten canine retraction spring

Instructions: FLAT on flat on shoulder and twist toward midline.

ROUND on flat and form "anti-elbow" to consume excess wire

Comments: The activation of the canine retraction spring in extraction cases requires special handling. To prevent this spring from extending buccally into the cheek tissue, form an "anti-elbow" *(B)*. This is done by twisting the spring stem at the shoulder toward the midline and then, using the round-beak pliers, forming the anti-elbow *(C)*.

THE RED GIRL CASE

Red Girl was 20 years of age, with a severe crowding in a Class I bimaxillary dental protrusion (Figs. 13–109 and 13–110). The ectopic upper canines had their apices above the first premolars. There was no doubt about the need for extraction. The case belonged to the group where we can expect the canines to swing around their apices into the extraction sites. Owing to a rotation of the right lower canine, the right lower lateral would be the tooth to be sacrificed to allow the canine this movement (Fig. 13–111). With regard to the age of the patient, one could assume that the correction had to be achieved by alveolar tooth movements only. We were able to follow the case for 15 years, and the result is an example that the floating approach can be as successful in adults as in growing children. The main movements were performed within nine months. The quick result was favored by the fact that the patient could wear the appliance day and night. On the other hand, she could take it off during meals and for social events, which is, no doubt, a big advantage in adults.

DENTAL ARCH PREDETERMINATION

Choice of Teeth to Extract

In extraction cases the second premolars have to replace the first premolars in the corrected arch. Consequently the cross of reference is oriented on the second premolars in the upper and on the interproximal embrasures of second premolars and molars in the lower. The symbols for dental arch height can then

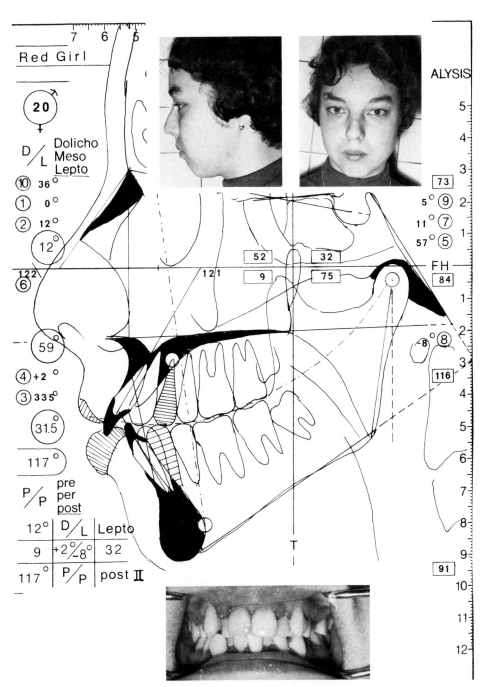

Figure 13–109. Red Girl case. Age, 20 years. Class I, severe anterior crowding. A bimaxillary proclination of canines and premolars combined with anterior crowding is a clear indication for immediate extraction of first premolars. Note blocked-out lower third molars.

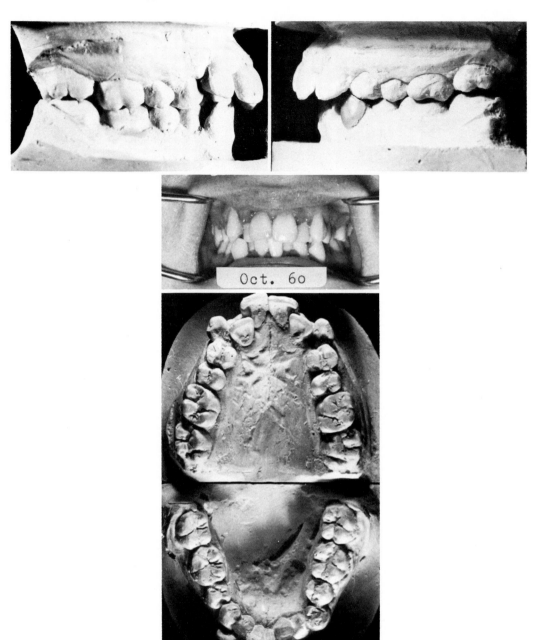

Figure 13-110. Red Girl case. Age, 20 years. Class I bimaxillary dental protrusion.

be used as in nonextraction cases. The SI is established and noted in the brackets. The wide upper centrals of Red Girl may be responsible for the fact that the upper and lower incisor widths are not fully correlated. The diameters of the anterior teeth are taken into the divider and transferred along the line of contact points to the tracing of the dental arches. An additional arch expansion is not considered. The contours of the teeth in the new position are drawn in and colored in yellow (shaded in print). The resulting tooth movements are marked by red arrows (black in print). The fact that the buccal segments may

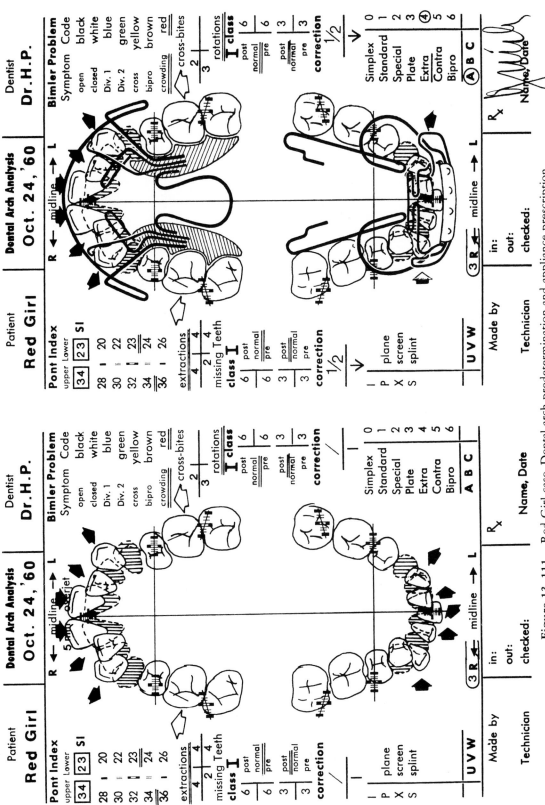

Figure 13–111. Red Girl case. Dental arch predetermination and appliance prescription.

move forward is neglected, and the movements of the anterior teeth are shown relative to the second premolars. In the lower arch we selected the right lateral for extraction. Our motive in doing so is our principle of tilting a tooth around its apex whenever possible. This best prevents any root resorption. Besides the fact that the right lower canine is laterally inclined, it further presents its buccal aspect in the anterior plane. By extracting the lateral, the canine can easily be uprighted and aligned in the row of the incisors. The result 10 years out of retention has supported this concept. The buccal cusp of the right lower first premolar has completely taken over the role of the canine without any periodontal reaction. The analysis sheet is completed by mentioning the extractions and crossbites. We noted a Class I occlusion and a Bimler Red problem.

Appliance Prescription

According to the tooth movements planned graphically, the wire parts are drawn in. Note that the anterior springs **F** leave a free space in the midline. The springs will come closer together when the whole appliance moves forward, together with the upper buccal segments. This forward movement can easily be observed by an increasing distance between the middle part of the labial arch **Aa** and the labial aspects of the centrals. It has to be compensated by swinging back the crossover wires. Note that with this forward movement the lower part of the appliance is also carried forward. This has to be compensated, too, by a backward adjustment of the lower arch. For the planned mesial tilt of the right lower canine, the lower canine support **E** has to get a rather long stem on the right side and a long free leg on the other side to engage the mesially inclined left lower canine. For the headgear-like action, the laboratory is advised to bring the lower part half a unit forward even if there is a Class I occlusion.

Appliance Construction

The prefabs are selected according to the prescription and adapted to the individual situation. Note that the acrylic wings are shorter than usual. It may even be advisable to grind the anterior parts a bit when the canines are moving in. Sometimes the interdental springs have to pass between the legs of the anterior springs as long as the canines are so far forward. In the lower the horizontal loops are placed behind the second bicuspids. Consequently the anterior vertical loops of the sleds end on the level of the right lower first premolar, which is supposed to take the place of the canine. Note the form of the lower anterior loop **L** and the position of the lower canine supports **E** (Fig. 13–112). In the articulator the casts are corrected toward a Class III molar relationship. Note that the upper oblique crossover wires have to have gliding contact with the lower horizontal loops.

Individual Reaction Curve

In adult extraction cases no arch expansion is intended or expected. To avoid the impression of a constant arch width deficiency in the reaction curves,

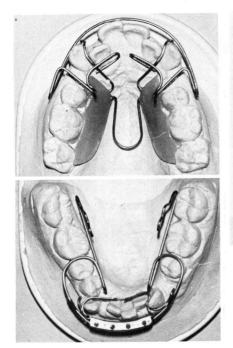

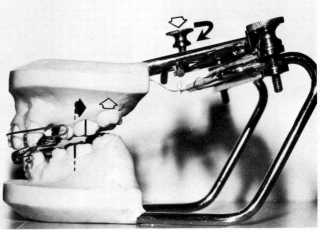

Figure 13-112. *Left,* Upper and lower parts of the appliance before being put together in the articulator. *Right,* To achieve a headgear-like action of the retractor muscles, the casts are overcorrected in extraction cases toward a Class III molar relationship. There is a relative forward positioning of the mandible (black arrow) and a raising of the bite (white arrows).

the base lines are individually altered to reasonable values, in Red Girl corresponding with SI = 31. The measuring points are likewise transferred to 7:7 and 5:5. The arch height is measured from the second premolars and compared with the means of the actual SI of 34. It shows a surplus of 5 mm., which is reduced to zero in the course of the space closing and uprighting of the centrals (Fig. 13-115). The decreasing curve for the arch height illustrates the effect of the appliance.

Long-term Observation

We had the chance to reinvestigate the case 10 years after we had finished the treatment (Fig. 13-116). As the curves demonstrate, the arch width and height remained nearly the same. Only the width between the second molars increased a bit. Because in the United States the main interest with regard to changes in the width of dental arches is focused on the intercanine distance, we compared these measurements with those at the Pont measuring points in our long-term observations. It seems that the different opinions on arch expansion are based on the choice of the measuring points. Often we observed changes in the intercanine distance while the premolars and the molars showed only little or no change. In Red Girl we have an upper intercanine distance of 34 mm. in 1960, of 37 mm. in 1963, and of 36 mm. in 1974. This means that the distance between the upper canines increased while they were moved backward and they remained more or less in this position. The lower intercanine distance was 23 mm. in 1960, 21 mm. in 1963 after the extraction of the right lower lateral, and 21 mm. in 1974. The distance between the left lower canine and the right lower first premolar, which took the place of the canine, was 24 mm., 1 mm.

Text continued on page 461

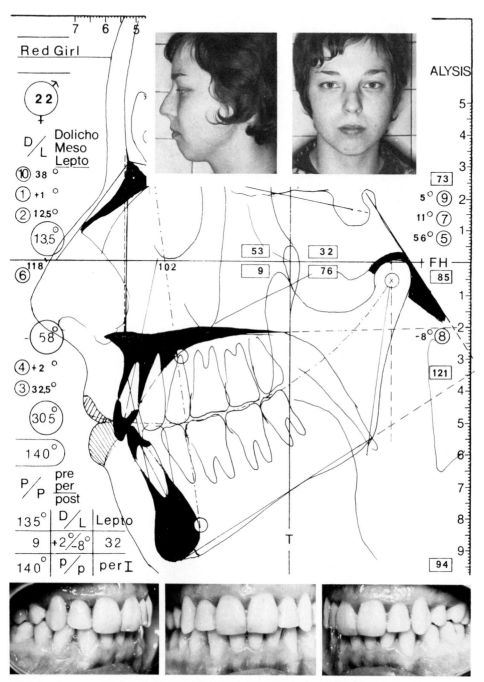

Figure 13–113. Red Girl case. Age, 22 years. Balanced occlusion after extractions. Note uprighting of incisors and canines. Third molars have erupted.

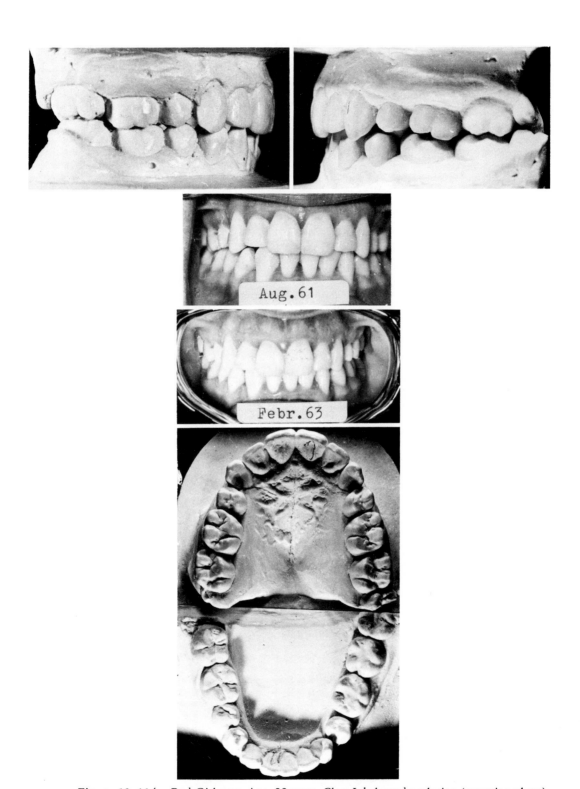

Figure 13-114. Red Girl case. Age, 22 years. Class I, balanced occlusion (retention phase).

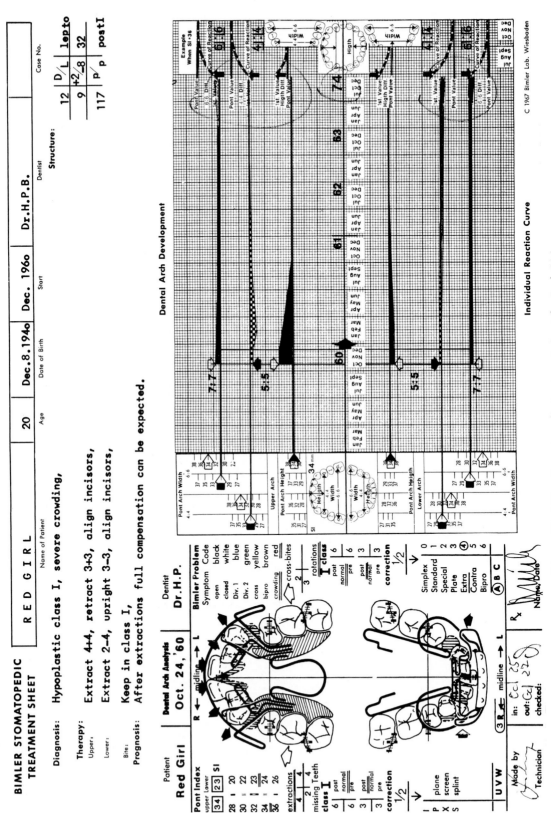

Figure 13–115. Stomatopedic treatment sheet for Red Girl.

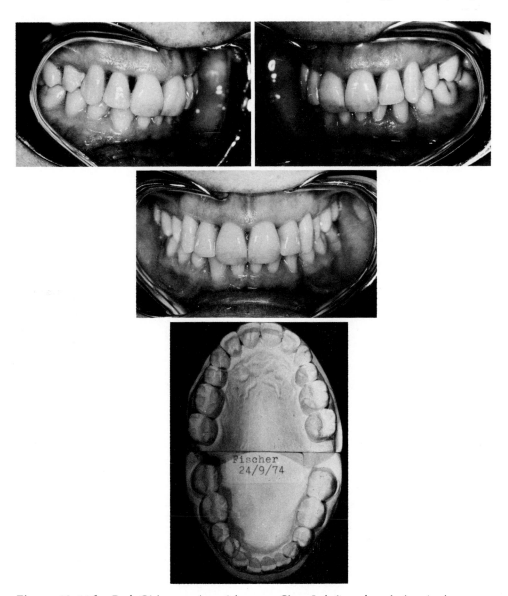

Figure 13-116. Red Girl case. Age, 34 years. Class I, balanced occlusion (maintenance phase).

more than in 1960. In following the changes in the axial inclination on the lateral head plates, we see the uprighting of the upper centrals from 121 to 102 degrees in 1963. In 1974 the inclination is 100 degrees. The buccal segments moved forward 2 mm. in both jaws and no changes were found in 1974. Note that the lower third molar uprighted itself after the extraction of the premolars. The intraoral views from 1974 show a nicely balanced occlusion and no irritation of the gum, in contrast to the initial picture of 1960. It may be added that no root resorption could be seen in the intraoral x-rays in 1963 and that the case was published for the first time in 1965.

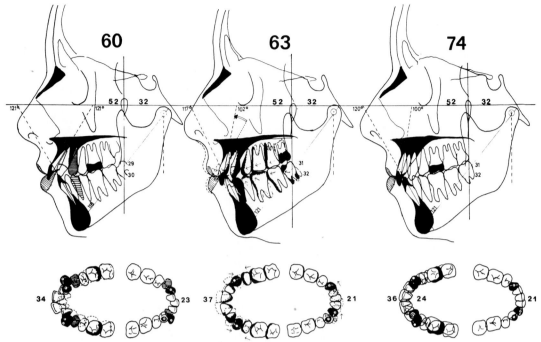

Figure 13–117.   Red Girl case. Note uprighting of the upper incisors and canines. Space closed two-thirds from the mesial and approximately 2 mm. from the distal. There was spontaneous uprighting of the lower third molars after premolar extraction. There is a permanent increase of intercanine distance. The right lower premolar took over the function of the canine after extraction of the right lower lateral incisor.

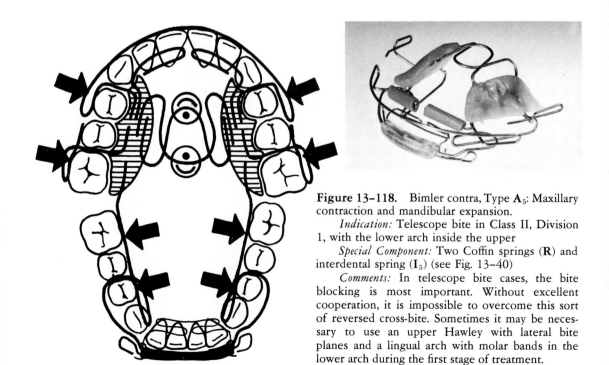

Figure 13–118.   Bimler contra, Type A_5: Maxillary contraction and mandibular expansion.

Indication: Telescope bite in Class II, Division 1, with the lower arch inside the upper

Special Component: Two Coffin springs (**R**) and interdental spring (I_5) (see Fig. 13–40)

Comments: In telescope bite cases, the bite blocking is most important. Without excellent cooperation, it is impossible to overcome this sort of reversed cross-bite. Sometimes it may be necessary to use an upper Hawley with lateral bite planes and a lingual arch with molar bands in the lower arch during the first stage of treatment.

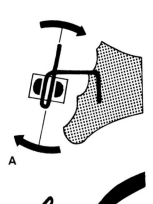

Figure 13–119. *Objective:* More molars and premolars lingually
Instructions: FLAT on joint and twist (*A*)
ROUND on stem and press (*B*)
Comments: The adjustment of the buccal springs requires some common sense and dexterity to place them as near to the marginal ridge as possible without interfering with the gums.

Bimler Bipro A_0

The Bimler A_0 (Simplex) (Fig. 13–51) and A_6 (Bipro) (Fig. 13–120) have in common the undivided lower labiolingual arch wire without any cap. The A_6 variation is indicated in all cases with sufficient or excess room for the teeth (Fig. 13–121), and is recommended independently if the space is due to small teeth,

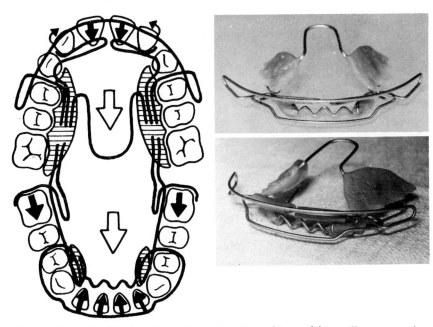

Figure 13–120. Bimler Bipro, Type A_6: Open bite and bimaxillary protrusion cases
Components: Frontal springs (**F**), lower connecting bars (**W**), and molar supports (**M**) (see Fig. 13–40).
Indications: Class I and Class II, Division 1 cases, mixed and permanent dentitions
Bimaxillary dental protrusion
Anterior spacing
Tongue thrust
Special features: Horizontal anterior springs
Interdental extensions for space closing (fingers)
Rubber tubes as bite planes
Lower connecting bar for stabilization
Lateral support wings
Vertical anterior springs with broadened working loop as tongue guard

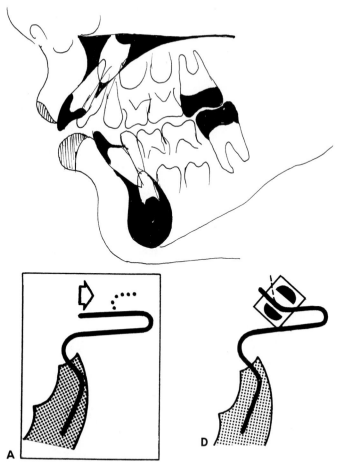

Figure 13–121. Type of case with space adequacy, with bimaxillary protrusion tendency, where Bipro A_6 appliance is indicated.

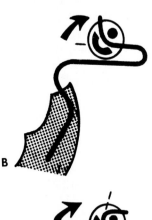

Figure 13–122. Frontal springs with horizontal loop (**Ff**): Interdental extensions (fingers for central incisors)

Objective: Close midline diastema

Tool: Round-beak pliers

Instructions: ROUND on flat on free leg

Comments: In the early mixed dentition, the central incisors often erupt with a relatively wide diastema. This can easily be closed by means of the frontal springs, provided there is no elastic fibrous tissue between the teeth. In the latter case, the tissue must be removed by frenectomy. To produce an interdental extension distal from the central incisors, the round-beak pliers are placed on the free legs and a 90 degree finger is bent into each leg (*B*). To increase the pressure and to keep the centrals moving, the finger extensions are slowly rolled toward the midline by repeated pliers actions (*C*). It is preferable not to cut away the excess wire, as we may need the material later to repeat the entire procedure on the laterals. For this purpose, the extension has to be rolled back to its original position, parallel to the fixed leg, using the flat-beak pliers (*D*). To reverse, FLAT on round on free leg. The use of fingers on the frontal springs affords the practitioner considerable dexterity. Recently we found that the additional use of plain interdental springs (I_0) can ease the procedure. They are similar to the I_1 cuspid support, but without an anterior loop.

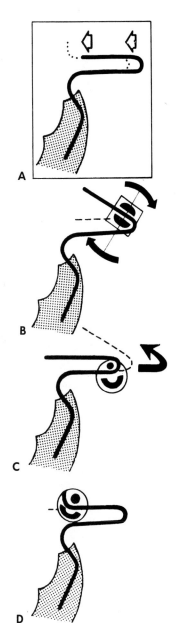

Figure 13-123. Frontal springs (**Ff**): Interdental extensions (finger springs for lateral incisors)

Objective: More lateral incisors toward the midline (*A*)

Tools: Flat-beak and round-beak pliers

Rules: FLAT gives; ROUND takes.

Instructions: Step 1. To elongate free leg, use flat on flat with a twist to open the loop (*B*). Use flat on round in the arc (FLAT gives). Then use round on flat on the fixed leg (ROUND takes) and bring the free leg back in parallel position (*C*). Repeat until free leg exceeds the distal of the lateral incisor. *Step 2.* Use round-beak pliers to bend in a finger (*D*).

Comments: It is typical of the Bimler appliance that with the use of shortening and elongation of the recurved loops, the standard parts can be used for many purposes. After finger springs have fulfilled their task, they are not cut away, but are rebent into their original form. The same I_0 interdental springs can be used after the midline diastema has been closed.

big arches, or temporarily unbalanced muscles. For uprighting of proclined incisors, a labial arch wire and a palatal fulcrum, as well as some buccal support, are necessary. In the upper arch, the anterior springs serve as a fulcrum, and buccal support is given by the palatal wings. In the lower arch, the lingual sleds do not provide such anchorage. Therefore, in the A_6 variation, two small lingual wings serve as anteroposterior support. To prevent loss of this support by narrowing of the sleds, an undulated bar has been devised. It keeps the sleds apart and stabilizes the lower part of the appliance. Usually, the cases with bimaxillary dental protrusion will show spacing, so that the elastic expansion qualities are not required.

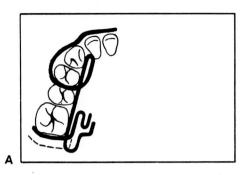

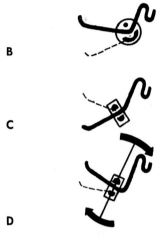

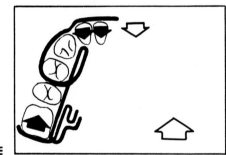

Figure 13–124. Molar supports (**M**) (reversed)

Objective: Move molars forward; counteract up-righting of incisors

Tools: Flat-beak and round-beak pliers

Note: Do not overactivate so that supports rest on molars instead of behind them.

Comments: The forward activation can be performed in several ways. The simplest at the beginning restricts itself to a forward twist of the free leg using FLAT on flat (*B*). This can be done only one or two times. For the next step, the fixed leg of the support has to be shortened, an action that will lengthen the free leg. Start with the flat-beak pliers on the right angle (round), opening the angle (*C*). Continue with ROUND on flat on the fixed leg, which will take from this section and add to the horizontal cross-over part (*D*). If the cross-over part becomes too long, it can be shortened with a wire cutter, since there will be no further uses for the excess wire material. Do not forget to make the end of the wire smooth.

The anterior springs in the **A₆** have horizontal working loops **Ff** (Fig. 13–122). Extensions of the free legs around the distal of the laterals, called interdental finger springs, can be additionally employed to close the diastema. Rubber tubing on the anterior springs **Ff** may serve as a bite-opening device.

THE DEVELOPMENT OF THE B APPLIANCE

The idea of the primary version of Class II, Division 2 appliances was to block the bite anteriorly to allow the buccal segments to erupt. Therefore, the anterior teeth were covered with an acrylic cap. In those days we did not know yet that the eruption of buccal segments is genetically predetermined and can only

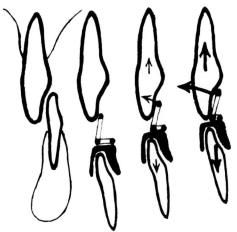

Figure 13-125. The vertical loop rests initially at the incisal edge of the upper centrals. When the patient closes his jaws, the vertical loop glides up the inclined lingual aspects of the incisors and the redoubling horizontal loops are more and more compressed. The resulting forces are split into forward- and backward-directed vectors.

be expected in leptoprosopic faces. The bite blocking by itself will show no effect in a dolichoprosopic face. More important for the Green problem group apparently are the sagittal forces to stretch the arches. For this purpose the rigid connecting arch of the upper wings was given two large horizontal loops. These loops encircle the first premolars from the lingual to the buccal and back to the lingual side. In the front, the arch was given a vertical working loop to protrude the incisors. The redoubling horizontal loops were gliding on the platform of the lower cap. Following the standardization of the lower part, the compact cap was abandoned. A rubber tube placed on the horizontal loops served to provide a bite plate action for the lower incisors. According to the law of the ellipse, the activation of the **B** arch induces a narrowing of the palatal wings. To prevent this, we tentatively used a rigid bar posteriorly. As Class II, Division 2 cases show a transverse expansion of the upper arch by the push-back action of the **B** arch, we found it better to use a palatal plate with a jackscrew. We were thus able to follow the expansion by turning the screw and did not lose any more of our anchorage. To secure further a good sagittal support for the stretching arch, I_1 to I_3 interdental springs are used in the upper and **M** molar supports in the lower part of the appliance.

Bimler Class II, Division 2, Type B

The Type **B** appliances have been constructed according to the special requirements of Division 2 cases—very upright or retrusive incisors in the upper jaw, and blocked-out premolars in the lower jaw (Fig. 13–126). Owing to other facial features, such as low mandibular plane angle and low alveolar processes, we try to avoid extractions, because, in our experience, this has resulted in a better chance for a long-lasting bite-opening effect. Fortunately, most of these cases can be expanded beyond statistical mean values, and buccal segments can be pushed backward against the slowly yielding resistance of the retrusive incisors. The typical Class II, Division 2 case, with protruded lateral and retruded central incisors, can be aligned in a short period of time with the forward action of the stretching arch and the counteraction of the I_2 springs.

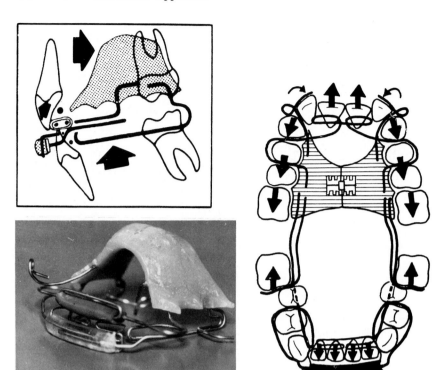

Figure 13–126.   Bimler Type **B**₂ for Class II, Division 2 cases.
Components: Stretching arches **B** and interdental springs **I** (see Fig. 13–40)
Indication: Class II, Division 2 cases, permanent dentition only

The stretching arch can be described as a pair of oversized anterior springs connected in the middle. Again we find the principle of constructive elements situated in planes perpendicular to each other. The two lateral horizontal loops of the **B** arch cross the dental arch from the palatal side, in front of the second premolars, to turn around the first premolars and come back to the lingual side between canine and premolar. The arch continues, forming two small horizontal loops that serve as a bite plane for the lower incisors. The arch is finally united in the middle in a vertical loop, which glides on the inclined planes built by the palatal aspects of the incisors. When the stretching arch is activated, initially it will touch the upper incisor near the incisal edge. The more the patient bites down, the more the upper wire of the vertical loop is forced upward and backward, activating the stretching arch even more. The moment the patient opens up, the arch will automatically glide down the inclined plane and relieve the pressure. This interrupted form of pressure application entirely prevents any sort of root resorption. This should be kept in mind by all who have accepted root resorption as inevitable.

Rules of the Ellipse

In Type **A** appliances, buccal expansion and anterior retrusion are nicely coordinated by virtue of the elliptical arch wire construction and principle. Both tooth movements occur automatically when the appliance is activated.

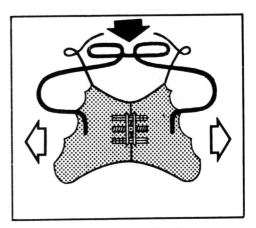

Figure 13-127. Expansion automatically causes retrusion of the upper anterior arch.

Figure 13-128. Bimler Type **B**: Stretching arch

Objective: Expansion and extension: Bring arch forward while plate is expanded (*A*)

Instructions: FLAT on round on long legs of elbow (*B*)

ROUND on flat on short legs of elbow (*C*)

Comments: At the beginning of the treatment, it will be sufficient to simply use the flat-beak pliers on the long legs to reinforce the pressure against the incisors. In the long run, the opening of the jackscrew carries the anchored ends of the **B** arch laterally, and undue tension develops in the arch. To prevent breakage, take material from the short legs (*C*) and transfer it via the arc to the long legs to compensate for the widening of the plate (*B*). To deactivate the stretching arch, simply press it back with your thumb (*D*).

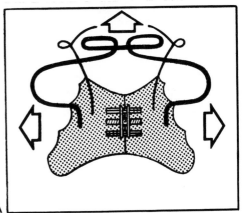

A

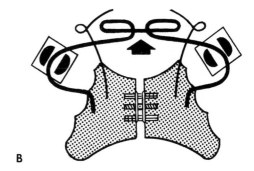

B

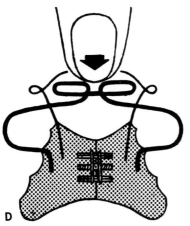

D

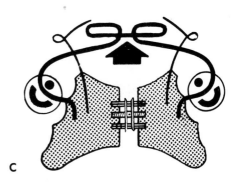

C

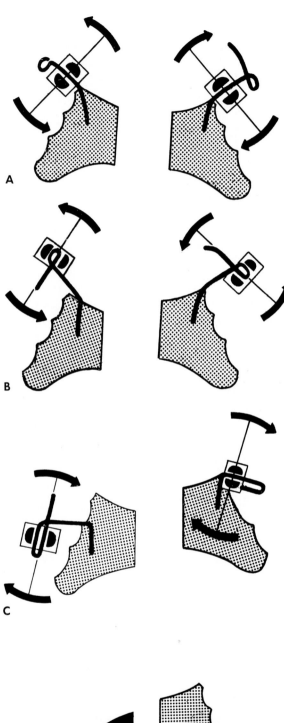

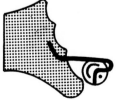

Figure 13–129. Interdental springs, I_1 to I_6. *A,* I_1 and I_2: Canine support with mesial extension. *Objective:* Push canine back. *Instructions:* Twist backward. *Note:* Check position of spring immediately in the mouth of the patient. Overactivation will have the reverse effect of what is intended. *B,* I_3 and I_2: Canine support with distal (I_3) or mesial (I_2) extension. *Objective:* Rotate canine or lateral. *Instructions:* FLAT on joint and twist (*B*). *Note:* For laterals, counteract with anterior springs (*F*); for canines, use short finger spring (*C*). *C,* I_4: Vertical loop. *Objective:* Push back premolars. *Instructions:* FLAT on stem or free leg and twist backward (*B*); I_5: Buccal spring. *Objective:* Move premolar lingually. *Instructions:* FLAT on joint and twist; ROUND on stem and press. *D,* I_6: Horizontal loop. *Objective:* Bend in occlusal rest. *Instructions:* Press.

This is exactly opposite in the Class II, Division 2 Type **B** appliances. The stretching arch of the Type **B** appliance is under the influence of the same geometric law of the ellipse, but the treatment goal in the anterior region is the opposite, and we can no longer expect an automatically coupled action. On the contrary, opening up of the jackscrew of the upper plate will retrude the stretching arch (Fig. 13–127). This unfavorable effect has to be compensated for continuously with the corresponding activation by the dentist (Figs. 13–128 and 13–129).

THE GREEN GIRL CASE

With Green Girl we selected a 12-year-old borderline case of a Class II, Division 2 malocclusion with severe upper crowding and a rather deep closed bite. The central incisors were inverted, but the first premolars proclined with regard to the stress axis. The molar relationship was a full Class II with the lower dental arch fairly well developed. The alveolar processes were rather low, but the facial formula of 28.5 L/M lepto promised further vertical development. As the symptoms were rather contradictory and our general experience with Division 2 cases indicated that the closed bite is very hard to influence if extractions are performed, we planned a conservative test-treatment first.

The dental arch predetermination and appliance prescription were based on a full complement of teeth with lateral expansion and sagittal extension. The I_2 interdental springs with mesial extensions were indicated for the rotation of the laterals. In order to concentrate the forward pushing forces on the centrals, we selected a **Bb** stretching arch with a small vertical loop. As usual in **B** appliances, a palatal plate with a jackscrew provided sagittal support and strong expansion facilities (Figs. 13–130 to 13–133).

The initial effect was amazing. Within two months we registered 6 mm. of arch expansion, and the intraoral photograph documents the changes in the front. The central incisors tilted forward 3 mm. at the incisal edges and later we had to realize on the head plates that the buccal segments had moved distally 1 to 2 mm. We were a bit skeptical about the long-lasting effect of such a quick rearrangement of teeth, but we observed the case for several years without seeing noticeable relapse. The patient wore the appliance every night as a retainer, as she was afraid her left upper lateral would come forward again. The mandible grew 6 mm. in the first nine months and 7 mm. more within the next five years. This brought the lower dental arch into a full Class I relationship, but the projected overjet was reduced by only 1 mm. Along with the bite opening, the Frankfort-mandibular plane angle opened up 1 degree, but only temporarily. Also, the dental arch width went up to 2 mm. above the mean and came down later to 2 mm. below the mean. I gave her a second **B** appliance as a retainer. Then I lost contact with the patient (Figs. 13–134 to 13–137).

It was only 15 years later that we succeeded in calling her back to the office. All records were taken. The Class I relationship and the overbite were as before, but upper and lower incisors were crowded again. The upper laterals were slightly rotated. We checked the inclination of the centrals and found 85 degrees at the beginning, 88 degrees after nine months, 94 degrees after five years, and 93 degrees after 20 years. It was interesting to see that in the meantime she had lost the second and third molars in the upper arch. She had fixed bridges in the rest of her buccal segments, including the canines. In the lower

Text continued on page 475

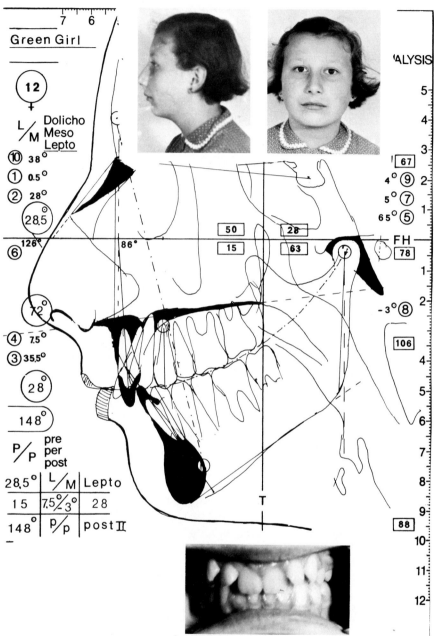

Figure 13-130. Green Girl case. Age, 12 years. Class II, Division 2, closed bite. Note the downward and forward inclination of the nasal floor (Factor 4 = 7.5 degrees) and the retruded upper centrals (86 degrees). The proclined canines and premolars with regard to the stress axis indicate a strong hypoplastic component. The sagittal relations are characterized by the high profile angulation of 15 degrees, the basal bone overjet (apical base dysplasia) of 15 mm., and the Class II molar relationship.

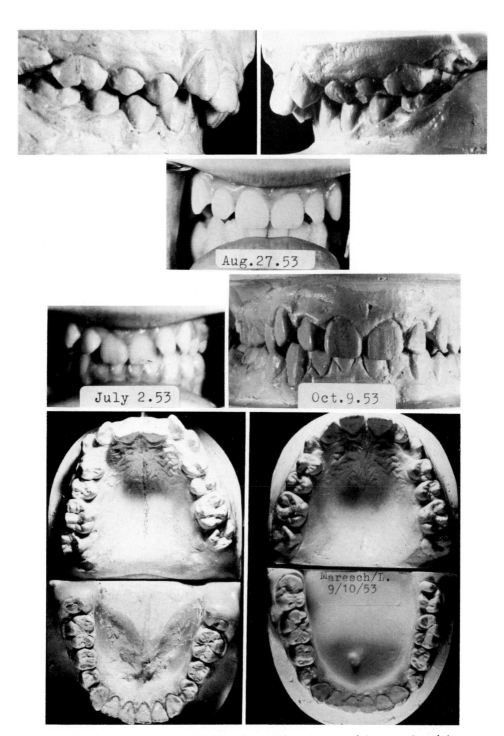

Figure 13-131. Green Girl case. Note the rapid protrusion of the centrals and the opening of the bite under Bimler appliance guidance over a three-month period.

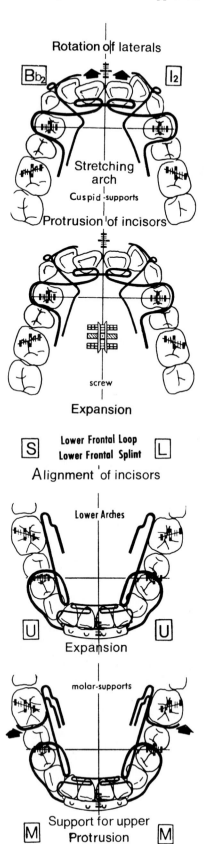

Rotation of laterals

B_{b_2} I_2

Stretching arch

Cuspid-supports

Protrusion of incisors

screw

Expansion

S Lower Frontal Loop

Lower Frontal Splint L

Alignment of incisors

Lower Arches

U Expansion U

molar-supports

M Support for upper M

Protrusion

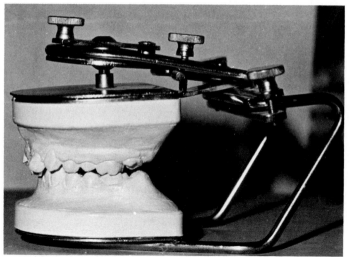

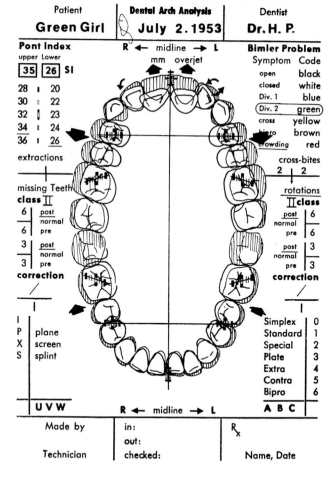

Patient	Dental Arch Analysis	Dentist
Green Girl	**July 2.1953**	**Dr. H. P.**

Pont Index

upper	Lower	
35	**26**	**SI**
28	I	20
30	II	22
32	III	23
34	II	24
36	I	26

R ← midline → L

mm overjet

Bimler Problem

Symptom	Code
open	black
closed	white
Div. 1	blue
Div. 2	green
cross	yellow
bipro	brown
crowding	red

extractions

cross-bites

2 | 2

missing Teeth

rotations

class II

6	post
	normal
6	pre
3	post
	normal
3	pre
correction	
/	
	I

II class

post	6
normal	
pre	6
post	3
normal	
pre	3
correction	
	/
I	

I	P	X	S	plane screen splint

Simplex	0
Standard	1
Special	2
Plate	3
Extra	4
Contra	5
Bipro	6

U V W R ← midline → L **A B C**

Made by	in:	R_x
	out:	
Technician	checked:	Name, Date

Figure 13–132. Green Girl case: Appliance prescription. Owing to the initial retruded upper incisors, the lower arch is blocked in a Class II molar relationship on the articulator.

she had lost the left first and third molars. On the right side the second molar was lost and the first deeply destroyed. No exact information was available about when these losses had occurred. As the continuity of the buccal segments apparently was broken rather early, pressure of the third molars did not seem to be very important in this case. So we checked the intercanine distances. At the beginning of the treatment they were 39 mm. in the upper and 29 in the lower in Class II relationship (Fig. 13–138). Under these conditions the lower incisors were in a well-rounded arch. Ten months later the upper canine distance was 41 mm. and the lower 31 mm. in Class I relationship with no crowding of the incisors. Five years later the upper canine distance was back to the initial 39 mm. and the lower back to 29 mm. but now in Class I relationship.

Text continued on page 479

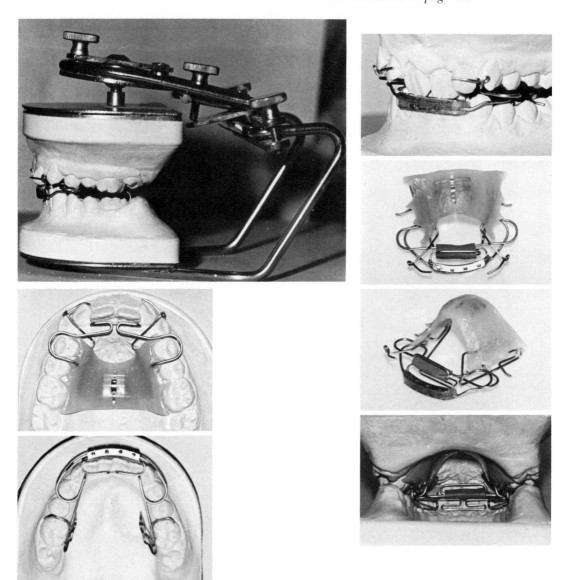

Figure 13–133. Green Girl case: Appliance construction. The bite correction in the articulator is restricted to a bite raising. The Class II correction will be performed by the clinician during the treatment corresponding with the progress in upper central incisor protrusion and alignment.

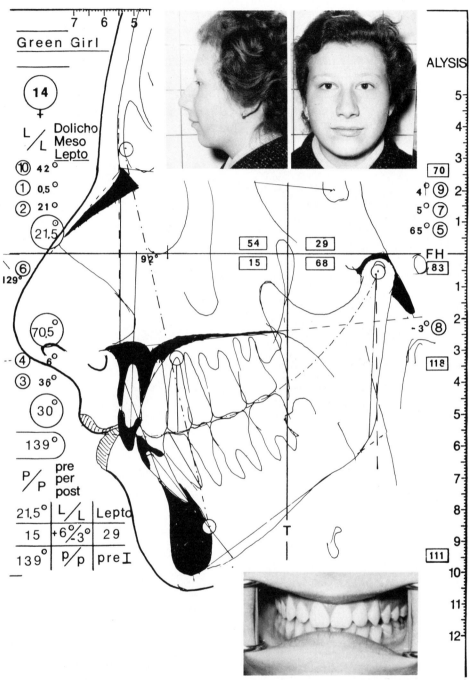

Figure 13–134. Green Girl case. Age, 14 years. Class II, Division 2, normal occlusion. Profile angle NAB was reduced by 7 degrees through vertical growth. Basal bone overjet was unchanged at 15 mm. Maxillary depth increased by 4 mm. and mandibular growth by 12 mm.

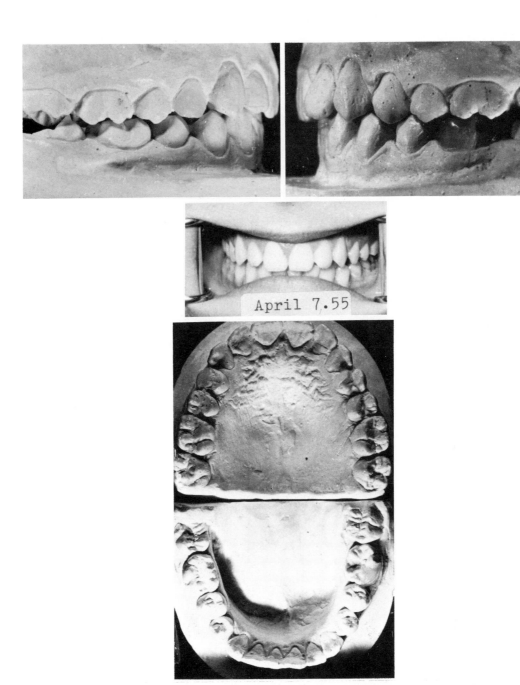

Figure 13-135. Green Girl case, same stage as in Figure 13-134. At this stage the patient was asked to leave out the appliance for a while. We told her that owing to the hypoplastic component in her dentition, we would consider extraction if a relapse occurred. The patient was not seen for six months but wore the appliance as a retainer each night. She was happy with the result and did not agree to extractions.

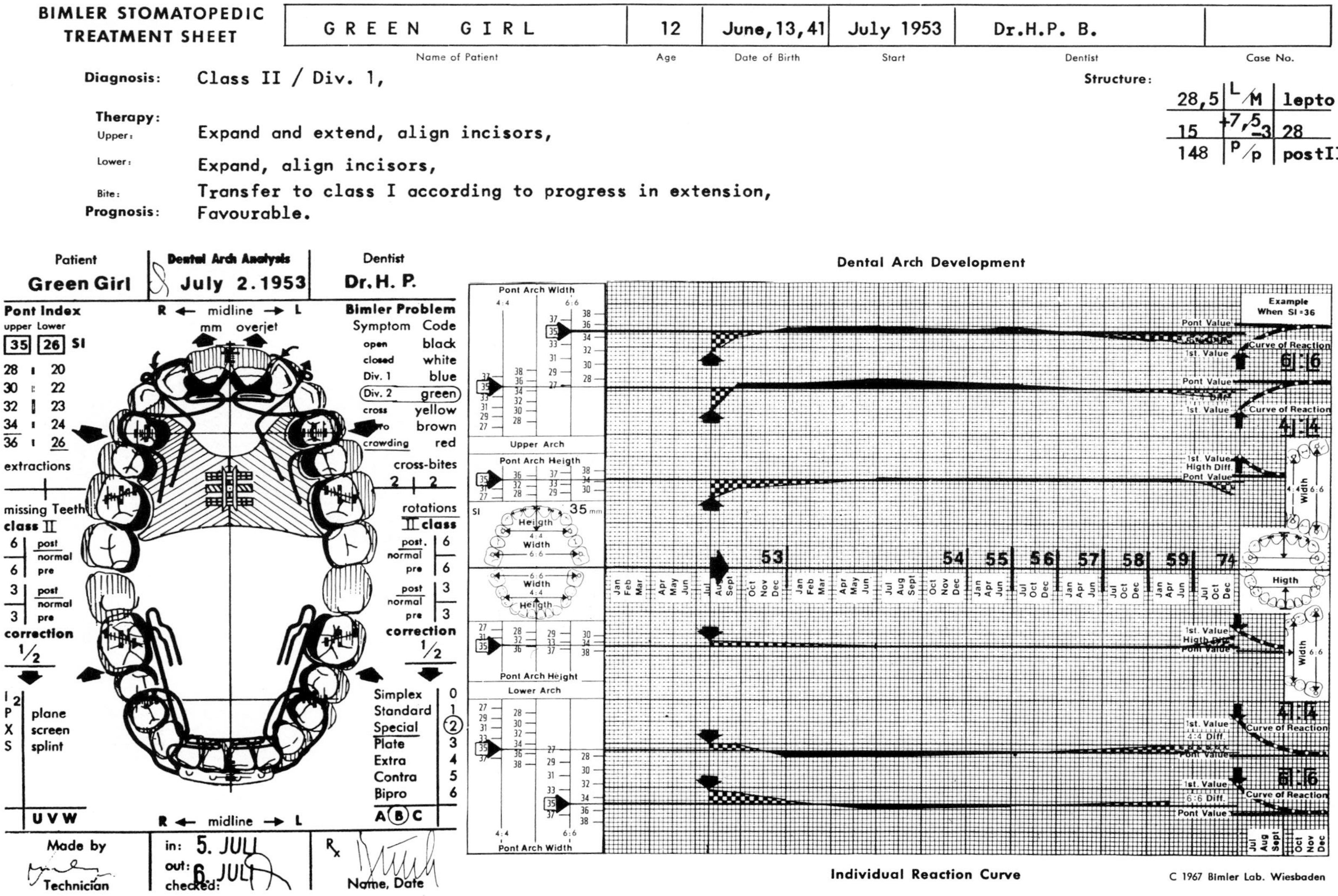
BIMLER STOMATOPEDIC TREATMENT SHEET

GREEN GIRL	12	June,13,41	July 1953	Dr.H.P. B.	
Name of Patient	Age	Date of Birth	Start	Dentist	Case No.

Diagnosis: Class II / Div. 1,

Therapy:
Upper: Expand and extend, align incisors,
Lower: Expand, align incisors,
Bite: Transfer to class I according to progress in extension,
Prognosis: Favourable.

Structure:

28,5	L/M	lepto
15	+7,5/-3	28
148	P/p	postII

Figure 13–136. Stomatopedic treatment sheet for Green Girl.

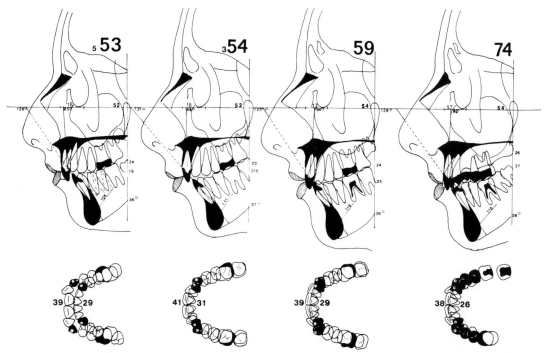

Figure 13–137. Occlusal views correlated to head plate tracings of Green Girl from 1953 to 1974. Compare depth of maxilla (52), inclination of upper incisors (85), overjet (18), inclination of lower incisors (126), distance of upper and lower molars to T-vertical (24, 19), length of mandible (105), and FMP angle (36). Values in parentheses are for 1953. Note the change in the intercanine distance (39, 29).

One could notice the onset of crowding of the anteriors in both arches. Another 15 years later the upper distance was 38 mm., 1 mm. below the pretreatment value and the lower down to 26 mm., with distinct crowding. As usual in these situations, the tips of the lower canines are found at the marginal ridge of the upper canines. It should be noted that the upper canines had halfcrowns with bigger contours than the natural teeth. The patient herself was happy about the condition (Fig. 13–138).

THE DEVELOPMENT OF THE TYPE C APPLIANCE

A reversed appliance for the reversed bite would be the simplest definition for the earliest steps in the development of the later Type **C** appliance. Tentatively we turned our primary appliance of 1948 upside down, cut the anterior part of the cap away, and used it as an adjustable inclined plane against the upper incisors. At the same time the labial arch worked against lower incisors. Soon we dropped the **A** labial wire in favor of a bimaxillary wire that originated in the upper wings and worked against the lower incisors. Simultaneously the rigid anterior inclined plane was replaced by elastic frontal springs. To improve the mechanical qualities of the bimaxillary arch, it was given generously dimensioned vertical adjustment loops. In our efforts to standardize the appliances, the upper part of the Type **C** became identical with the upper part of the **A** type, except for the **C** bimaxillary arch.

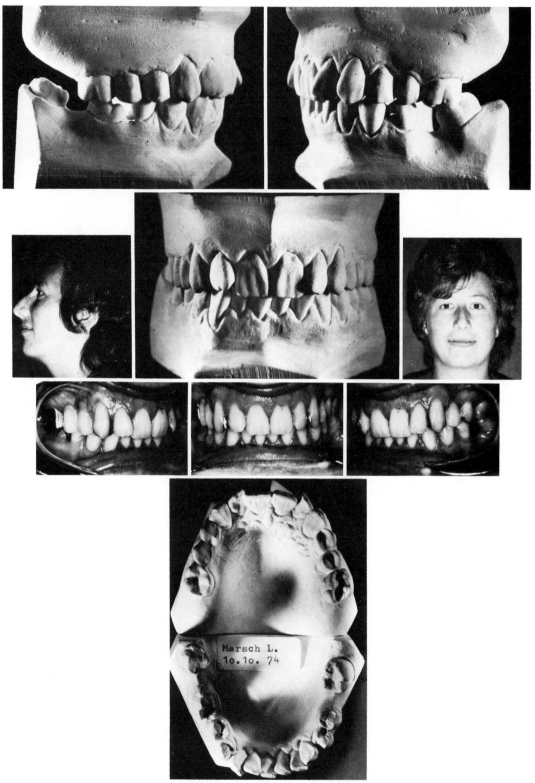

Figure 13–138. Green Girl case. Age, 33 years. Class II, Division 2, mutilated arches, partly restored (destructive stage). Predominance of morphogenetic pattern is apparent.

The matching counterpart in the lower was developed out of the A_6 variation with the lower connecting bar **W.** As the labial parts of the divided lower arch **U** would interfere with the upper **C** arch, they are bent back first in a vertical loop and afterwards in another redoubling horizontal loop. These horizontal loops provide the gliding surface for the upper crossover wires of the **C** arch. The I_6 horizontal loops block the bite as long as necessary.

MECHANICS IN TYPE C APPLIANCES

The anomalies in the facial structure of Class III cases include in part a deficiency in the vertical development of the midfacial region. This results in a rotating overclosure movement of the mandible in order to get occlusal contact. The same is seen in edentulous old people. The chin is thrown forward by this overclosure. In the stomatopedic therapy of Class III cases, the first step is to open up the bite and so to reduce the overclosure. In simpler cases this will be enough to bring the anteriors to an edge-to-edge bite. The elastic rubber tubing on the I_6 springs for bite blocking provoke contractions of the masseter and temporalis muscles. At the inclined posterior aspects of the upper incisors, the upward-directed forces are split up into forward- and backward-directed vectors. With the *forward-directed* part of the forces, the *upper* incisors are protruded. The *backward-directed* part is transferred by means of the maxillomandibular labial arch against the *lower* incisors, so that they are uprighted backwards. Using these mechanics, anterior crossbites are usually corrected with a Bimler Type **C** within a period of three days to three weeks, provided the patient wears the appliance day and night as prescribed. It is our clinical experience that patients with a crossbite cooperate very well. Once the therapy has started, the patient feels more comfortable with the appliance than without it. In true Class III cases with severe deviations in the facial structure, func-

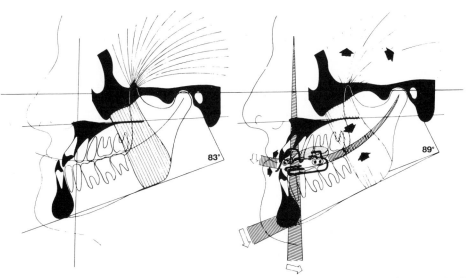

Figure 13–139. Masseter and temporalis muscles are activated to reflex-controlled contractions through the bite-blocking interocclusal springs (I_6) encased in rubber tubes. (For similar use of rubber tubing, see Chapter 14.)

tional adjustments in the alveolar region may not suffice to compensate for the underlying dysmorphosis, and surgical interventions are necessary (Fig. 13–139).

Bimler Type C for Class III Malocclusion

With the Type **C** appliances, the mode of action is the reverse of that in the Type **A.** The forces created by the closing movements of the mandible against the resilient resistance of the elastic appliance are directed forward in the upper and backward in the lower arch (Fig. 13–140). By proper activation, the resistance of the appliance can be increased and will provoke heavier muscular forces. Owing to lack of any anchorage to the teeth, the mechanism is fool-proof. The overactivated appliance interferes with the occlusion and prevents any action.

While the Type **A** appliance is constructed in a corrected Class I position for the lower part, the Type **C** appliance has to be made in the abnormal mesio-occlusion, except for raising the bite. This, of course, is dependent upon the fact that the mandible cannot be pushed back in the joint any considerable amount. Nevertheless, it is possible to change the relation of the upper part to

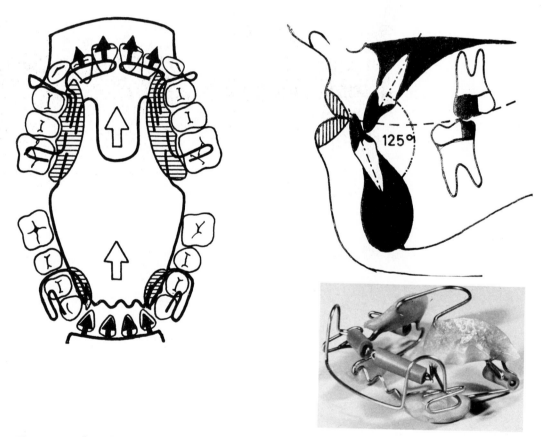

Figure 13–140.   Bimler Type C appliance for Class III malocclusion.
Indications: All anterior cross-bites in Class I, pseudo Class III, and Class III cases; deciduous, mixed, and permanent dentitions.
Special components: Bimaxillary arches (**C**), interdental springs (**I**), lower arches (**UC**), and lower connecting bars (**W**) (see Fig. 13–40).

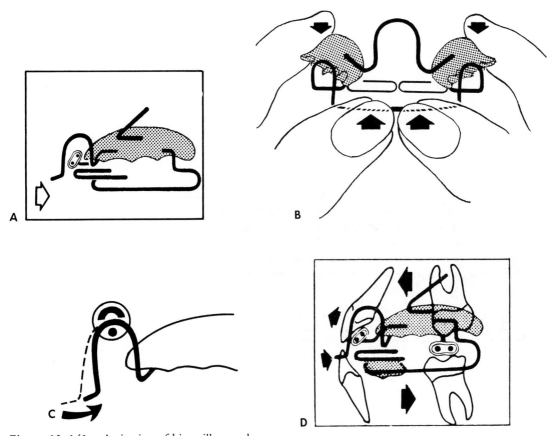

Figure 13–141. Activation of bimaxillary arch.
  Objective: Push lower anterior teeth lingually (*A*)
  Instructions: Finger pressure for intensive action
          ROUND on round on both sides
  Comments: The maxillomandibular labial arch of the Type **C** or Class III appliance puts backward pressure on the lower anterior teeth (*D*) and, through them, on the entire mandible. The simplest way to activate the bimaxillary arch is by pressure of the thumbs of both hands (*B*). If this simple method of adjustment is not sufficient, then the use of round on round pliers at the top of the arc will produce backward activation (*C*). Adjustment with the pliers also permits a different amount of pressure to be placed on either side.

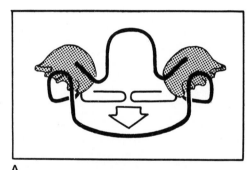

A

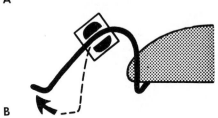

B

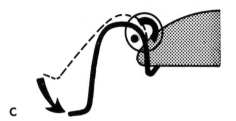

C

Figure 13-142. Vertical adjustment of the bimaxillary arch.

Objective: Lowering of the **C** arch

Instructions: FLAT on round on long legs
ROUND on flat on short legs

Comments: The vertical adjustments of the bimaxillary arch are performed in the **U** loop as the lengthening of the labial arch. To lower, as in lengthening, start on the long legs. Apply the same amount of pressure on both sides. Flat gives to the long legs (*B*), and round takes from the short legs (*C*).

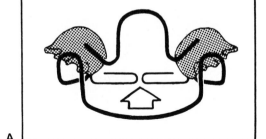

Figure 13-143. Vertical adjustment of the bimaxillary arch.

A

Objective: Raising of the **C** arch

Instructions: FLAT on round on short legs
ROUND on flat on long legs

Comments: The reverse procedure will raise the labial bar of the arch. In cases where the anterior crossbite has been corrected and some rotation of the upper incisors still has to be achieved, the bimaxillary arch can be raised high enough for it to become a maxillary arch and work against the upper incisors.

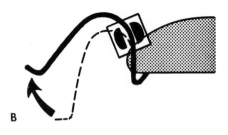

B

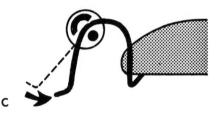

C

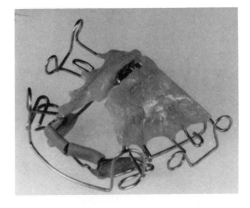

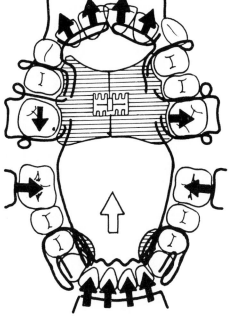

Figure 13–144. Bimler Type **C₃** for Class III malocclusion.
Indications: Cleft palate cases; maxillary underdevelopment. True Class III and total Class III cross-bite cases.
Special components: Upper plate with jackscrew
Cross-bite spring (**K**) (see Fig. 13–40)
Comments: See discussion of **A₃** for the use and adjustment of the cross-bite springs. Keep in mind that lower sleds may block lower arch contraction.

the lower part of the appliance very slowly during the course of treatment, corresponding to the forward displacement of the upper arch and the downward and backward shifting of the lower. The adjustment is described in Figure 13–141, and is absolutely the same as for the Type **A** appliance. Once the anterior crossbite is corrected, the bite-opening **I₆** springs are removed to allow the lateral open bite to close (Figs. 13–142 to 13–145).

THE DIFFERENT TYPES OF CLASS III MALOCCLUSIONS

The three mechanisms of general growth disturbances of the facial structure produce under certain conditions three different types of Class III malocclusion. Easiest to understand is the Class III due to a reduced T-TM distance. If the position of the fossa articularis in the petrous bone is closer to the tuber vertical, the mandible as a whole is carried forward and a Class III molar relationship is established. Form and length of the mandible may appear quite normal. The gonial angle is obtuse and the ramus well developed. Only the anterior margin of the ramus is far in front of the fissura pterygomaxillaris, indicating that the whole mandible is displaced forward. The case shown in Figure 13–146 on the right was never treated but somehow compensated itself by proclining not only the incisors but the buccal segments as well. The same result will be achieved by treating such cases orthopedically. In the facial profile the accentuated lower lip and the negative NAB angle will always produce an unfavorable impression, even if the incisor relationship has been corrected. As the position of the fossa in the petrous bone cannot be influenced, the only way to a better cosmetic result is surgical intervention. A reduced T-TM distance in a Class III case can be regarded in general as a symptom with a poor prognosis (Fig. 13–146).

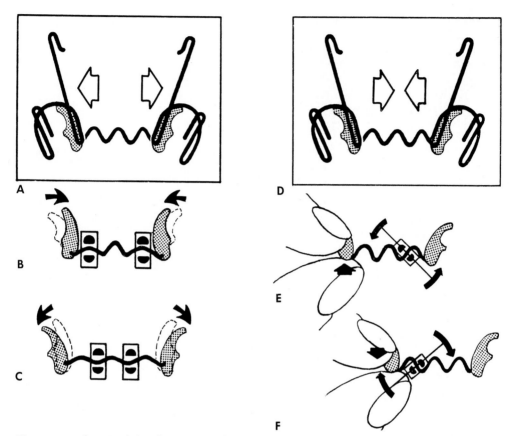

Figure 13–145. Undulated connecting bar.

Objective: Lengthening or shortening of undulated bar

Tools: Flat-beak pliers

Comments: Besides being used in the **A**₆ variation, the connecting bar is also used in the Type **C** appliances. The continuous lower lingual arch of the **A**₆ variation, as well as the divided arch of the Type **C** appliances, are connected in the anterior area by an undulated bar, which is attached on both sides in two small acrylic wings. An increase or decrease in the length of the bridge is possible only through the use of the pliers. The flat-beak pliers are used on both tops, causing a slight flattening of the bar (*B*). A distortion of the lower parts occurs, so an equal amount of compensatory flattening must be done with the flat-beak pliers on the bottom of two valleys or waves (*C*). This allows the labiolingual arches to return to their original horizontal positions, but wider apart. The adjustment can be made several times, but always remember to bring the horizontal compensation bows back to their original horizontal positions. To avoid internal tension and subsequent breakage, always stick meticulously to the original shape of the appliance. To bring the undulations or waves closer together, the vertical distance between the wave tops and bottoms has to be made longer or deeper. The simplest method of accomplishing this is to place the tip of the flat-beak pliers at the connecting part between the top and the bottom of the wave (*E*). Through reversed twisting motions, the top and bottom angles are made more acute. This will bring the two lingual arch parts closer together. Hold the connection bridge firmly with the thumb and forefinger of the stationary hand while making this adjustment.

CLASS III
Growth Deficiencies

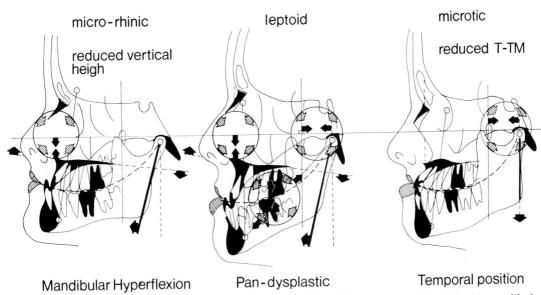

micro-rhinic

reduced vertical heigh

leptoid

microtic

reduced T-TM

Mandibular Hyperflexion   Pan-dysplastic   Temporal position

Figure 13–146.   Three types of Class III cases. On the left is a dolichoprosopic Class III with mandibular hyperflexion due to a reduced midfacial height. There is usually a good prognosis, with compensation by eruption of buccal segments after a quick correction of the anterior cross-bite. On the right is an externally similar dolichoprosopic Class III caused by a reduced T-TM distance or antepositioned joints. There is a rather poor prognosis, as the position of the joints cannot be influenced. Compensation by protrusion of the upper incisors is cosmetically disappointing. Surgical intervention is indicated. *Center,* Pan-dysplastic leptoprosopic "true" Class III with nearly always a poor prognosis. There is a combination of micro-rhinic, microtic, and leptoid symptoms.

It is important to know this association, as more often we see dolichoprosopic (deep face) Class III cases, which look very much alike externally but which will react most favorably to stomatopedic treatment. Again the ramus of the mandible is well developed and the gonial angle rather low. Clinically a deep reversed overbite impresses parents and inexperienced clinicians, but the proclined posterior margin of the ramus, metrically expressed by a high value for Factor 8, indicates an overclosure rotation of the mandible. This of course is only a secondary symptom based on a reduced vertical dimension of the middle part of the face owing to micro-rhinic dysplasia. Long before these associations were understood, there existed a clinical rule of thumb that Class III cases with a deep bite have a better prognosis than those with a tendency toward open bite. This is correct as far as square dolichoprosopic faces are concerned. A deep overbite in a long leptoprosopic face does not mean a good prognosis at all, especially when symptoms of leptoid dysplasia can be recognized. As mentioned before, the leptoid dysplasia is characterized by an elongated but weakly developed mandible with a flat gonial angle. The sagittal dimensions of the face are usually reduced, including the T-TM distance. The unfavorable effect of a forward position of the petrous bone with the fossa has been mentioned before. The position has to be regarded as even more serious if additionally symptoms of the micro-rhinic mechanism can be observed. Very often, in the younger years, only by the negative tilt of the nasal floor can the relative reduction of the height of the middle part of the face be detected in an otherwise long leptoprosopic face. The hyperflexion of the mandible (high Factor 8) again may be helpful as a guiding secondary symptom. In all pandysplastic cases with micro-rhinic, microtic, and leptoid symptoms the prognosis is always poor. The decision for a surgical intervention should be postponed into the twenties. Earlier surgical intervention cannot be recommended, as the danger of relapse is considerable. These cases are identical with the so-called "true" Class III cases with "bad" mandibles (high Frankfort-mandibular plane angles).

The Yellow Girl Case

Yellow Girl had a severe anterior crossbite and came from a family with hereditary Class III malocclusions. She was 10 years of age with a mutilated mixed dentition (Figs. 13-147 to 13-154). Her molars were still in Class I relationship. Her head plate disclosed that she belonged to the dolichoprosopic, square-faced type with low mandibular plane angle. The distance between maxilla and TM joint was at the margin of normal values (28 mm.), so that despite the clinical picture, the prognosis was good. The dental arch analysis showed that the upper incisors had to be brought forward, whereas the lower incisors had to be uprighted. A Bimler Type C_1 was prescribed and fabricated. The bite was blocked by two I_6 horizontal loops with rubber tubing. The correction of the incisors took three weeks to reach an edge-to-edge bite. Then the **I** springs were removed and the lateral open bite was closed within some months. In the permanent dentition, she had a perfect occlusion that was completely self-retaining. The control head plate showed that this case could be explained as a delayed maxillary development, because after the correction of the malocclusion, the maxilla caught up in growth in all three dimensions. Hypoplastic and true Class III cases will fall short of this ideal result.

Good Prognosis in Class III Cases

In general the dolichoprosopic, square-faced patients with mandibular hyperflexion have the best prognosis in Class III cases. In trying to compensate a vertical and sagittal underdevelopment, they protrude the mandible in function mostly asymmetrically (Fig. 13-154 *left*). The amount of the vertical deficiency can be seen from the freeway space in rest position. With the lowered mandible the negative overjet is automatically reduced. This corresponds to our therapeutic approach first to open the bite by interocclusal springs I_6. By means of the **C** appliance the upper incisors are easily proclined. Initially it was surprising for us to see that these teeth can be tilted by several degrees in a few days or even within a few hours. This takes place without any irritation of the gum or soreness of the teeth. Nowadays we usually expect to see an edge-to-edge bite on the second visit. This can be after only three days, and usually within the first week. The parents are instructed to present the children for photographic documentation immediately after a slight overbite is achieved. The lateral open bite, of course, will induce the patients to protrude the mandible for chewing. It is therefore very important to attain this transitional period as soon as possible. It seems to be the decisive advantage of the **C**

Text continued on page 497

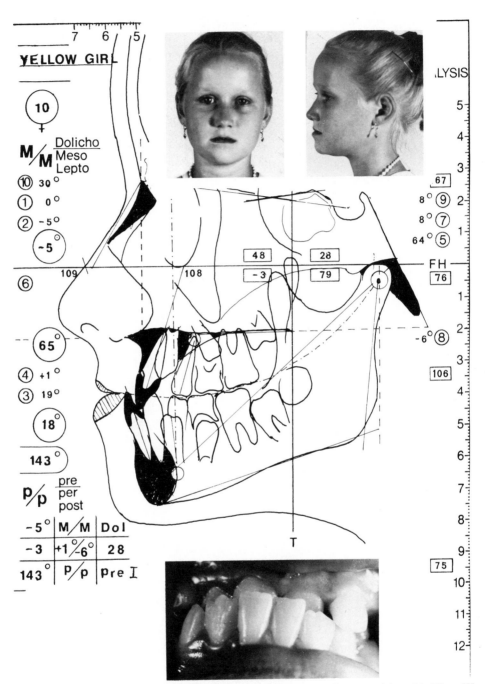

Figure 13–147. Yellow Girl case. Age, 10 years. Reversed deep overbite with Class III tendency (maldeveloping stage). Owing to maxillary underdevelopment in all three planes of space, the mandibular overclosure with hyperflexion, anterior cross-bite, and a tendency toward a Class III molar relationship occurred.

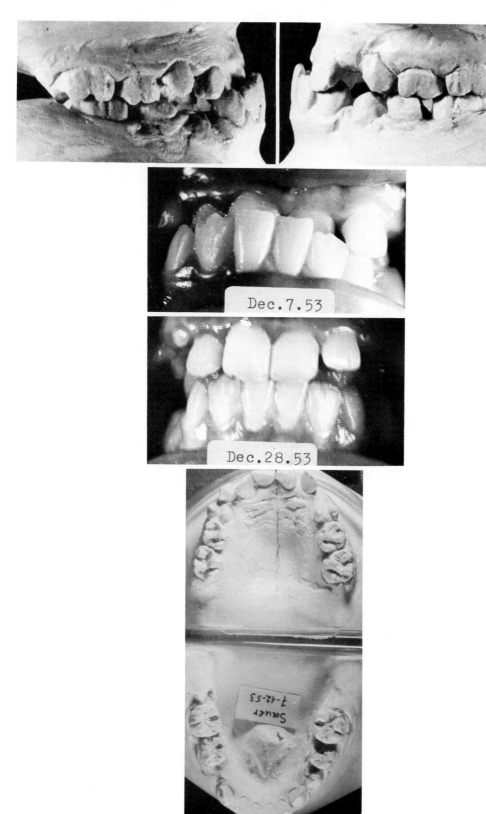

Figure 13-148. Yellow Girl case. Age, 10 years. Reversed deep overbite with Class III tendency (corrective stage).

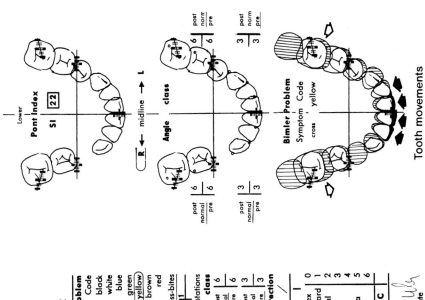

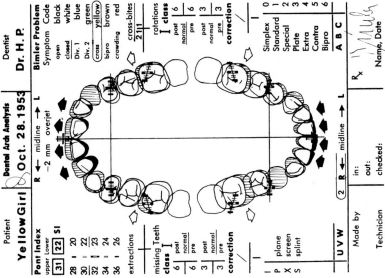

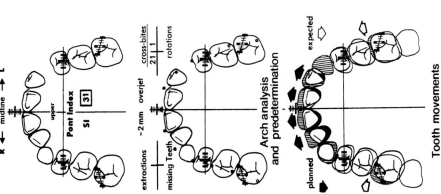

Figure 13–149. Dental arch predetermination and treatment planning for Yellow Girl.

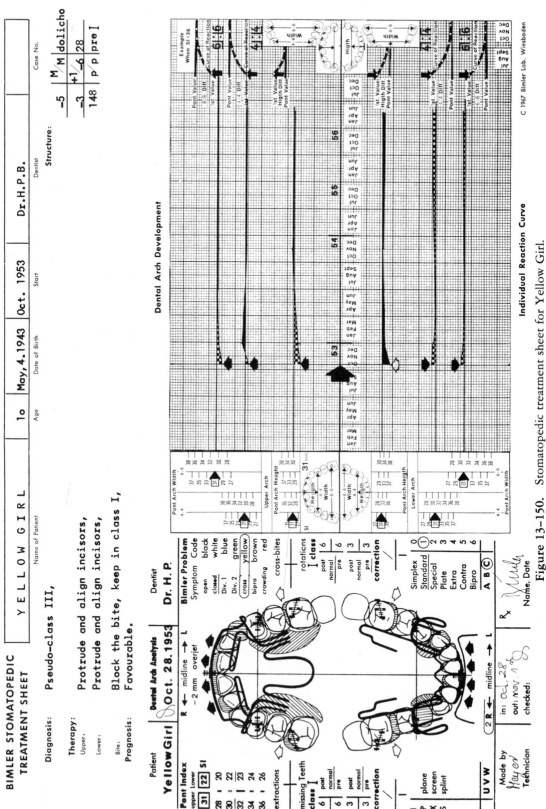

Figure 13–150. Stomatopedic treatment sheet for Yellow Girl.

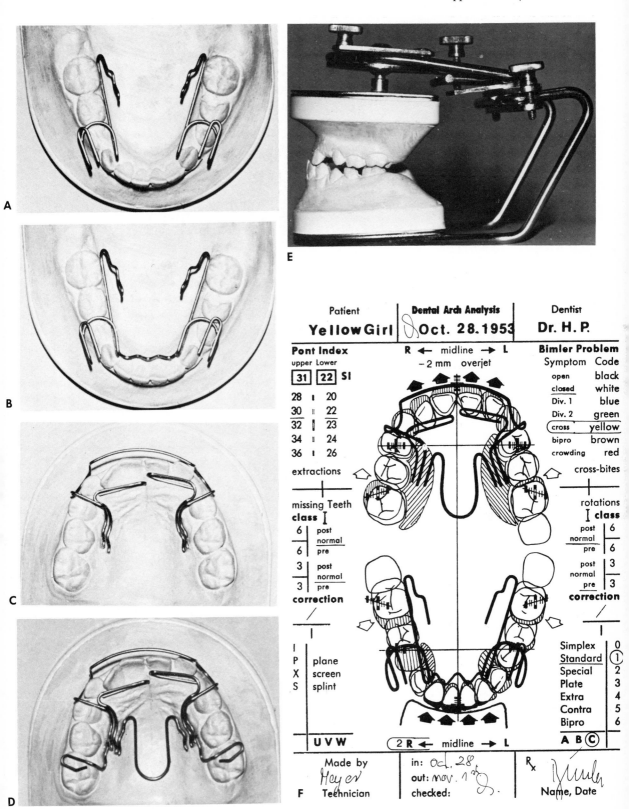

Figure 13–151. Yellow Girl case: Appliance construction. *A,* Lower arches. *B,* Lower connecting bar. *C,* Frontal springs. *D,* Horizontal loop, bite opening, Coffin spring. *E,* Original malocclusion: arches in reversed overbite. *F,* Appliance prescription.

Illustration continued on following page

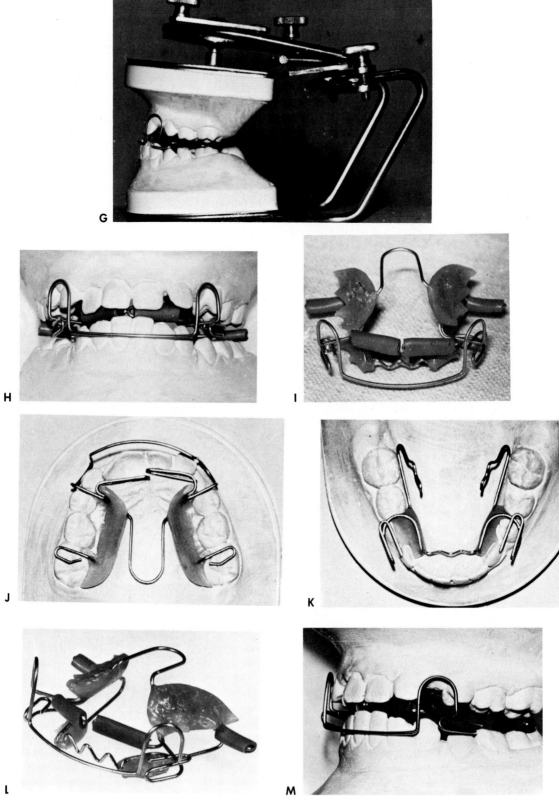

Figure 13–151 *Continued.* *G*, Bite raising. *H* to *M*, Final appliance and results.

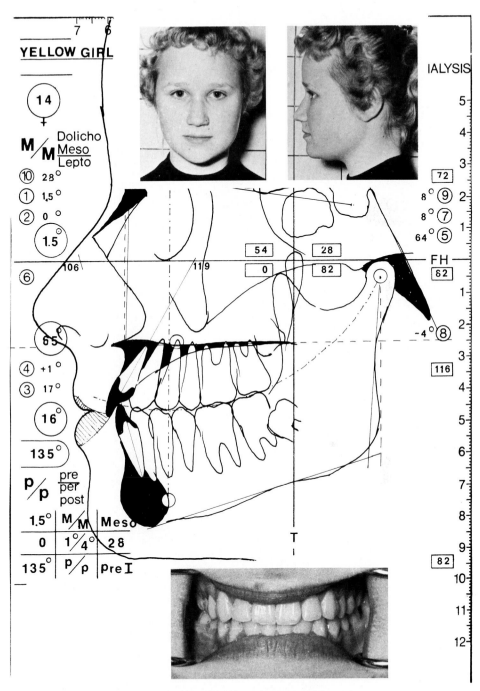

Figure 13–152. Yellow Girl case. Age, 14 years. Class I normal occlusion (constructive stage). Compare with Figure 13–147. Note the increase of 6 mm. in the maxillary depth. The growth in the diagonal length of the mandible of 10 mm. was actually only an effective change of 3 mm. in the length of B-TTM, thus reducing the negative skeletal overjet B-A to zero. The negative profile angulation of −5 degrees became positive, to 1.5 degrees. There was a 7 mm. increase in the suborbital facial height.

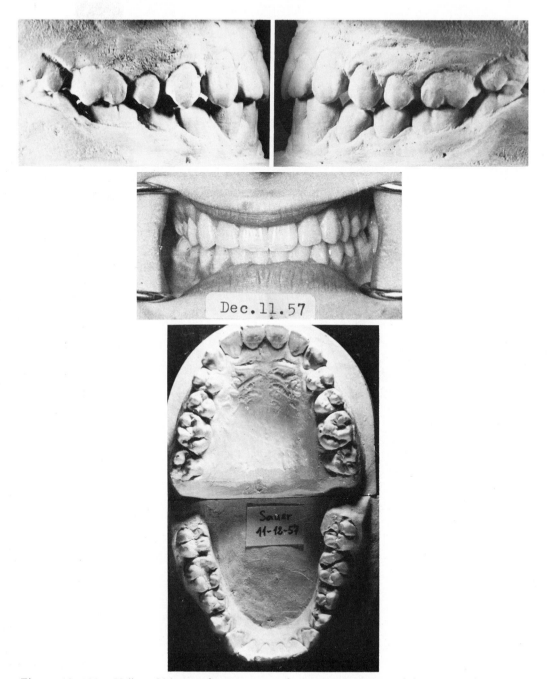

Figure 13–153. Yellow Girl case after two years of treatment in the mixed dentition and two years of self-retention in the permanent dentition.

CLASS III
Micro-rhinic Dysplasia

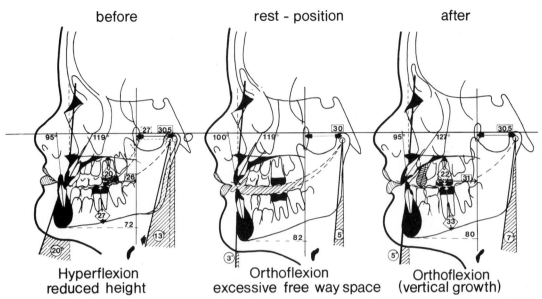

Figure 13–154. Note the asymmetrical position of the condyles in left tracing (27 to 30.5 mm. T-TM). There is a profile angle of −20 degrees and a Factor 8 of 13 degrees. The upper alveolar height is 20 mm. and the lower 27 mm. In the center tracing in rest position, we find a large freeway space and the Factor 8 reduced to 5 degrees. The condyle position is now symmetrical and the suborbital facial height is 10 mm. larger. The anterior cross-bite was compensated by proclination of the upper incisors. The upper molars moved forward 5 mm. The patient discontinued cooperation after the correction of the anterior relationship. Lack of space for the upper canines will necessitate the extraction of the upper first premolars later and result in a Class II molar relationship. The initial posterior open bite was closed by the eruption of the buccal segments of 2 mm. in the upper and 6 mm. in the lower. The corresponding increase of suborbital facial height is 8 mm.

appliances that they can be worn day and night. The patients report that the temporary relapse into the old position during meals provokes a certain discomfort in the joint region, which disappears immediately when the appliance is reinserted. So the extraordinarily good cooperation of Class III patients is to be understood. As soon as the overbite is secured, the I_6 springs are removed.

The same initial **C** appliance is used for the rest of the treatment time, which may last for years. Arch expansion occurs still in the mixed dentition. Tooth rotations or space opening is performed by different interdental springs I_1 to I_5. As the Class III growth tendencies will last until the midtwenties, it is advisable in certain cases to use the appliance as a sort of retainer up to this age. The appliance has to be regarded as an additional factor in the functional matrix transposing muscle forces in a forward direction to the upper arch and a backward pressure against the lower incisors and the mandible as a whole. So sometimes even unfavorable cases can be kept in an acceptable balance.

Poor Prognosis in Class III Cases

The final results to be achieved in Class III cases do not depend so much on the therapeutic methods as on the facial structure and the character of the

LEPTOPROSOPY
Facial Growth and Tooth Eruption

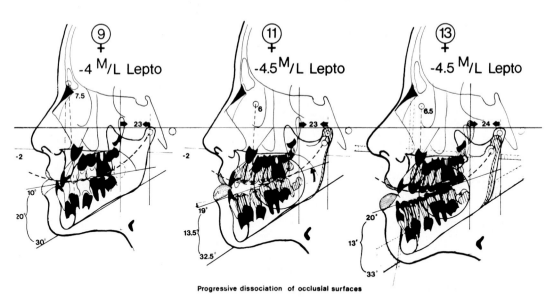

Progressive dissociation of occlusial surfaces

Figure 13-155. Leptoprosopic Class III case with developing open bite. Note the accentuated curve of Spee in the upper and the flat occlusal plane in the lower. The increasing tilt of the occlusal plane caused by eruption of the lower molars opens the bite anteriorly. This eruption takes place against the functional forces of mastication, which are often concentrated on one pair of molars. Depression of molars by extra-oral forces will bring only temporary relief. Surgical intervention is likely to relapse.

growth deficiencies. Of course, with certain removable appliances the work will be easier for the orthodontist and the treatment more comfortable for the patient. On the other hand, fixed techniques may offer advantages in other cases to solve special problems at the cost of more chair time for the orthodontist and more inconvenience for the patient. But all kinds of therapy will find their limitations in unfavorable growth tendencies, which cannot be controlled by either orthodontic or orthopedic intervention. As an example, a leptoprosopic patient is presented who had an inherited pandysplastic Class III malocclusion. Clinically the deep reversed overbite did not disclose the poor prognosis. The lateral head plate gave an early warning by the very short T-M distance of only 23 mm. A lepto facial index at the age of 9 let us expect more vertical growth. At this time low alveolar processes still allowed a balanced Class III occlusion, but soon the bite opened anteriorly by the irresistible eruption of the lower molars. Such cases show a rather accentuated curve of Spee in the maxilla, while in the lower a flat occlusal plane develops. By the eruption of the molars this occlusal plane is tilted upward posteriorly and consequently the bite opens anteriorly. Some times molar extraction can be helpful, but if it is done in the wrong case or at the wrong time the second molars will take the place of the first ones and reopen the bite again. Also, surgical intervention has sometimes had an unfavorable result. We are becoming aware that all our therapeutic endeavors have their definite limitations (Fig. 13-155).

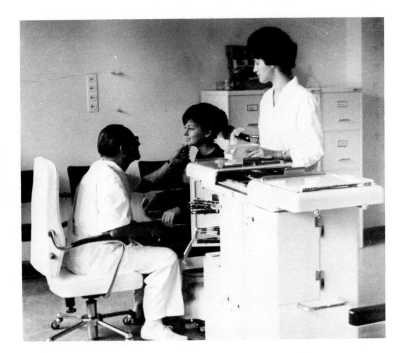

Figure 13–156. Position for dentist when he delivers appliance to patient. Operator sits in front and hands appliance to patient, who must insert it unaided.

ASPECTS FOR THE DENTIST

Working with removable appliances not only has its advantages for the patient, but has just as important conveniences for the dentist. Dental work in general obliges the dentist to assume positions which usually cause strain and fatigue in the practitioner's back and feet. This has been partly overcome by having the dentist sit down to work while the patient rests in a horizontal position. In stomatopedics, we rarely have to work on the patient himself. The adjustment of the appliance is done outside the mouth. What must be done on the patient is limited to controlling the position and action of the appliance, inspecting the teeth, and measuring the arches. For these purposes, the best relative position of dentist to patient is the one that has always been practiced in otolaryngology, with the patient sitting between the knees of the doctor, facing him (Fig. 13–156). From this position the dentist can easily view the dental arches, as well as the oral cavity, from all sides, without bending his own back. While the doctor remains stationary in his chair, the patient is moved up and down in a motor-driven chair to the most favorable position. The necessary pliers and calipers are placed to the operator's right, so that they are easily accessible. Models and case histories are displayed on top of the cabinet.

References

1. Bimler, H. P.: Die elastischen Gebissformer. Zahnärztl. Welt, *19*:499–503, 1949.
2. Bimler, H. P.: Die Behandlung des Deckbisses mit den Gebissformern. Zahnärztl. Welt, *11*:315–319, 1950.
3. Bimler, H. P.: Handhabung der elastischen Gebissformer. Zahnärztl. Welt, 5:119–125, 1952.
4. Bimler, H. P.: Die Behandlung der Progenien mit Gebissformern. Zahnärztl. Welt, *24*:549–555, 1952.
5. Bimler, H. P.: Kieferorthopädie mit Gebissformern. Dtsch. Zahnärztl. Z., *16/17*:811–817, 865–872, 1953.

6. Bimler, H. P.: Die graphische Gebissanalyse. Zahnärztekalender Hanserverlag, 118–130, 1954.
7. Bimler, H. P.: Fernröntgenstudien über Zahnwanderungen während der Gebissentwicklung. Fortschr. Kieferorthop., *19*:119–129, 1958.
8. Bimler, H. P.: Die Bedeutung des Fernröntgenbildes. Fortschr. Kieferorthop., *20*:256–273, 1959.
9. Bimler, H. P.: Indikation der Gebissformer. Frotschr. Kieferorthop., *25*:121–144, 1964.
10. Bimler, H. P.: Photo- und Fernröntgentechnik in der zahnärztlichen Praxis. Zahnärztl. Z., *11*:1025–1036, 1964.
11. Bimler, H. P.: Über die microrhine Dysplasie. Fortschr. Kieferorthop., *26*:417–434, 1965.
12. Bimler, H. P.: Indikation zur Extraktionstherapie auf Grund des Fernröntgenbilder. Fortschr. Kieferorthop., *28*:459–470, 1967.
13. Bimler, H. P.: Untersuchungen über die Spee'sche Kurve. Scritti medici in Onore di O. Hoffer, 19–31 clinica odonto-iatrica milano, 1967.
14. Bimler, H. P.: Unterschiedliche Gebisstypen im Fernröntgenbild. Fortschr. Kieferorthop., *31*:261–274, 1971.
15. Bimler, H. P.: Neue Gesichtspunkte zur Ätiologie der Progenie. Zum 60. Geburtstag Prof. Hauser. Fortschr. Kieferorthop., *32*:169–185, 1970.
18. Bimler, H. P.: Appareils fonctionels élastiques. Orthod. Franc., Vol. 24, 1953.
19. Bimler, H. P.: Traitement du cas de la classe II div. 1 avec l'appareil d'orthodontie. Rev. Franc. Odontostomatol., *12*:568–577, 1964.
16. Bimler, H. P.: Indicazioni del modellatore del morso. Minerva Stomat., *17*:820–840, 1968.
17. Bimler, H. P.: Indicaciones del Modelador Elastico. Buenos Aires, Editorial Mundi, 1966.
18. Bimler, H. P.: Appareils fonctionels élastiques. Orthod. Frac., 1953.
19. Bimler, H. P.: Traitement du cas de las classe II div. 1 avec l'appareil d'orthodontie. Rev. Franc. Odontostomatol., *12*:568–577, 1964.
20. Bimler, H. P.: Rapport préliminaire sur une formule d'identification dento-maxillaire. Orthod. Franc., *39*:119–124, 1968.
21. Bimler, H. P.: Kephalometrische Methoden zur Erfassung des Gebisses im Verhaltnis zum Gesichtsschädel. Fortschr. Kieferorthop., *33*:257–276, 1972.
22. Brink, H.: Indikation zur Extraktionstherapie auf Grand des Fernröntgenbildes. Fortschr. Kieferorthop., *28*:471–477, 1967.
23. Schilla, G.: Die Durchführung der Extraktionstherapie mit den Gebissformern. Fortschr. Kieferorthop., *29*:181–192, 1968.
24. Bimler, H. P.: Possibilities and limitations of treatment in Class II cases. Trans. Eur. Orthod. Soc., 1956, pp. 55–67.
25. Bimler, H. P.: A roentgenoscopic method of analysing the facial correlations. Trans. Eur. Orthod. Soc., 1957, pp. 241–253.
26. Bimler, H. P.: Facial pattern formula. Trans. Eur. Orthod. Soc., 1960, pp. 224–236.
27. Bimler, H. P.: Prefabricated parts for oral adaptors. Trans. Eur. Orthod. Soc., 1960, pp. 355–358.
28. Bimler, H. P.: Information for ordering prefabs. Wiebaden, Bimler-Laboratorien, 1965.
29. Bimler, H. P.: Stomatopedics in theory and practice. Int. J. Orthod., *2*:5–20, 1965.
30. Bimler, H. P.: The Bimler Appliance: Construction and Adjustment. Great Falls, Montana, V. A. Nord, 1966.
31. Bimler, H. P.: The Bimler Cephalometric Analysis. Great Falls, Montana, V. A. Nord, 1969.
32. Bimler, H. P.: Some etiologic factors of the Class III malocclusion. Trans. Eur. Orthod. Soc., 1970, pp. 115–129.
33. Bimler, H. P.: A review on my approach. Unpublished manuscript.
34. Bimler, H. P.: Les troubles de la croissance faciale de causes générales et leur rapport avec les malocclusions. Chir. Dent. Franc., 1974, pp. 63–72.
35. Bimler, H. P.: Lineare Messungen am Fernröntgenbild. Fortschr. Kieferorothop., *36*:34–45, 1975.
36. Martin-Saller: Lehrbuch der Anthropologie. Stuttgart, G. Fischer Verlag, 1957.
37. Starck, D.: Embryologie. Stuttgart, G. Thieme Verlag, 1965.
38. Blechschmidt, E.: The Stages of Human Development Before Birth. Basel/New York, S. Karger Verlag, 1960.

CHAPTER 14

The Kinetor

The Kinetor, an ingenious combination of active and myofunctional treatment methods, was first described in orthodontic literature in 1951 by Dr. Hugo Stockfisch.* A skillful blending of his own principles and experiences with details of construction taken from other appliances has gradually improved the Kinetor. Muscular forces derived from the mandibular dislocation are joined with the active operation of screws and springs. Wire and plastic prefabricated parts were introduced, as well as detachable rubber tubes.

As with other functional appliances, treatment should be started in time to take advantage of mandibular growth during the mixed dentition period. Complete correction of the malocclusion is achieved in 2 to 4 years if the appliance is worn regularly at night. During the first 12 to 18 months, it also must be worn for 2 to 3 hours during the day. Additional daytime hours of wear are desirable for open bite, Class II, Division 2, Class III, and some cases of more severe Class II, Division 1 malocclusions with strong distorting lip habits. Short interruptions during the hours of daytime wear are permissible, however.

The Kinetor consists essentially of two active plates, each with a screw for transverse expansion. The plates are joined by two prefabricated, detachable vestibular loops anchored in the plastic prefabs (Fig. 14–1). The resulting bimaxillary appliance provides simultaneous force application in the maxillary and the mandibular plates and is combined with functional elements. The vestibular loops keep the plates in a correct Class I relationship; the detachable rubber tubes, placed between the upper and lower plate, enlarge the freeway space and impede contact between upper and lower dentitions (Fig. 14–2).

The resulting construction thus provides force application in all three dimensions—horizontal, sagittal, and vertical. The intrinsic force of screws and springs is intensified by the functional pressure of the rubber tubes on the plates. Extrinsic functional impulses, originating from tongue and other muscular movements and transmitted to the jaw, teeth, and supporting structures, are directed and strengthened by the active components.

Since the plates are pressed against teeth and jaws by the rubber tubes, no clasps for retention are used with the Kinetor. The wires contacting the molars or canines are designed to stabilize the appliance simultaneously, enhancing the effect of the expansion. The three-dimensional efficiency of the Kinetor is quite apparent when the appliance is on the plaster cast, but even more so when in-

---

*This chapter is based on personal communication with Dr. Hugo Stockfisch of Stuttgart, F. R. G., who also furnished all the illustrations.

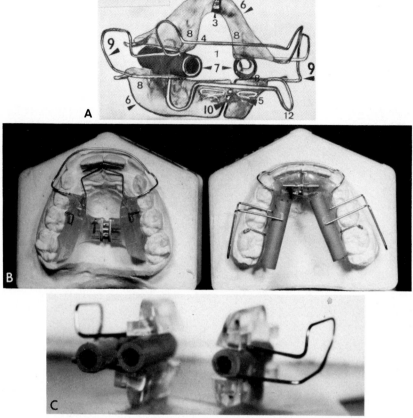

Figure 14-1. The Kinetor developed by Stockfisch. *A,* Upper and lower plate, both with expansion screws, are movably joined by prefabricated detachable vestibular wire loops. **1,** Freeway space for the tongue. **3** and **10,** Expansion screws in the upper and lower plates (**6**). **4,** Upper arch wire. **5,** Springs. **7,** Prefabricated rubber tubes. **8,** Ready-made parts of plastic for the (changeable) fixation of the tubes (**7**) and the prefabricated vestibular loops (**9**). *B,* A single rubber tube is locked between the plates lingual to occlusal surfaces, leaving posterior teeth free to erupt. The maxillary plate does not cover the anterior part of the plate. *C,* Two types of rubber tube assembly for treatment with the Kinetor. The twin rubber tube is used for closing the bite, i.e., in Class III and anterior open bite cases and is interposed between occlusal surface of posterior teeth. The single tube is used in opening the bite (stimulating eruption), as in Class II malocclusions.

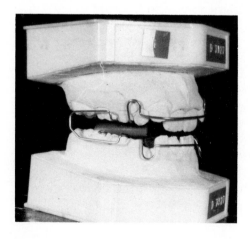

Figure 14-2. Contact between the maxillary and mandibular dentitions is prevented by the Kinetor (rubber tube interposed). Vestibular wire loops serve as buccal shields, holding the cheeks away from the posterior teeth. The single rubber tube is lingual to the occlusal surfaces, leaving teeth free to erupt. Finger springs on the lingual of maxillary central incisors move them labially and are anchored in palatal acrylic (see Fig. 14-1). The mandible is automatically brought into a Class I position. The model shows the appliance used for treatment of Case 1 (Fig. 14-3).

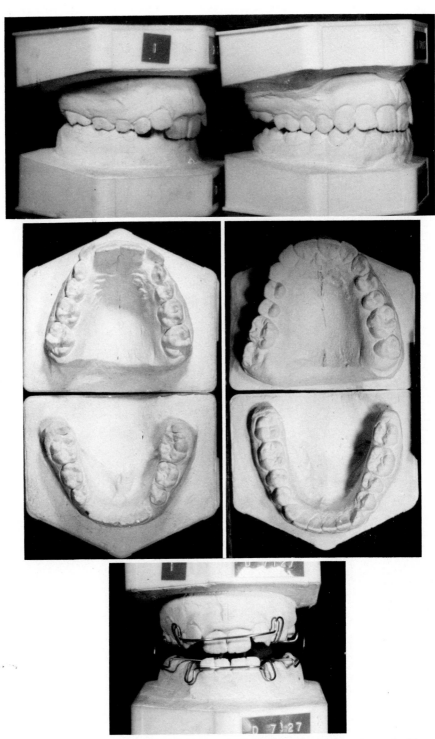

Figure 14-3. Case 1. Class II, Division 2 malocclusion. Age 9 years, 4 months. Treatment with one Kinetor. The appliance used is shown in Figure 14–2. *Right,* Corrected occlusion shown at 15 years, two years out of retention.

serted in the mouth. This is illustrated by the result of treatment obtained with two patients, about 10 years of age (Cases 1 and 2). For each of them, one Kinetor was sufficient to correct their Class II, Division 2 malocclusion. Crowding was relieved, and vertical, transverse, and sagittal irregularities were successfully treated. Space was gained for the erupting premolars and canines, the bite was leveled and normal intermaxillary relations were established. After 12 months, the patients were already unable to get the mandible into the previous posterior occlusion (Figs. 14–3 to 14–6).

The Kinetor is interposed into the buccinator mechanism (Brodie) (Figs. 14–7 and 14–8). Its mobile and elastic forces take part in the interplay of muscular forces. The vestibular loops (e.g., providing the mobile connection between the maxillary and mandibular plate) are kept at a distance of 3 mm. from the teeth. They counterbalance the transverse pressure of the buccinator muscle and create space for the widening of both dental arches. An expansion of 5 to 7 mm. is effected by the combined action of the screws inserted in the plates and the muscles of mastication. Thus, according to Stockfisch, correction is achieved in much less time than by functional appliances without active parts.

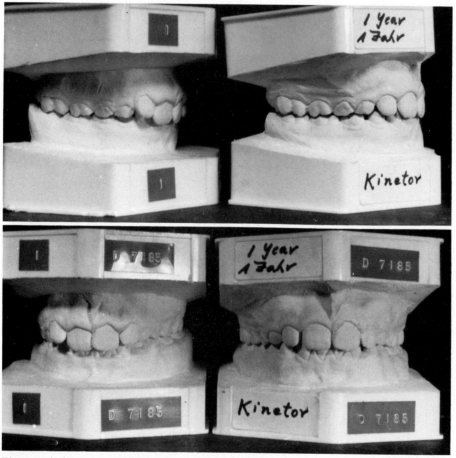

Figure 14–4. Case 2 (Th. M.). Age 9 years. Class II, Division 2 malocclusion. Treatment with Kinetor at the optimum time. Correction after one year, followed by retention and controls during the changing of the dentition. For retention, a Kinetor or an anteriorly open (palate-free) activator may be used.

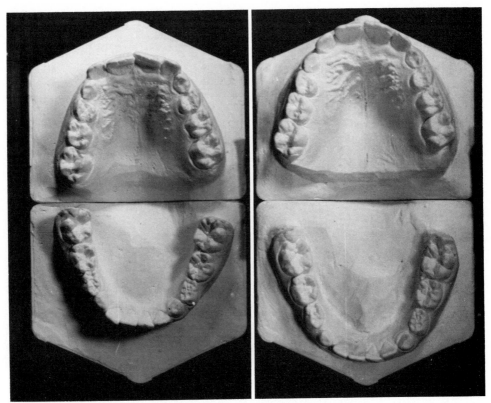

Figure 14-5. Case 2 (see Fig. 14-4). Transverse and sagittal expansion after one year of treatment.

The treatment objective of the vestibular loops, to relieve the adverse muscular pressure of the cheeks, is complemented by the concurrent use of rubber tubes impeding the contact between upper and lower teeth. The single and twin tubes supplied serve different purposes. The single tubes (one third of the original size is used on each side) are locked between the plates. The occlusal surfaces remain free. The twin tubes extend over the occlusal surfaces of all lateral teeth. They are longer because it is imperative that the second molar be covered if it has erupted. Any excess length is cut off.

It is well known that chewing gum stimulates muscular activity. The rubber tube of the Kinetor works similarly. As soon as the appliance is inserted, the patient will quite involuntarily start to "chew" it. Because of this muscular action, the patient is hardly conscious that both plates of the Kinetor are pressed into the narrow dental arches like a double cone (Fig. 14-9). In this manner, continuous sagittal, vertical, and transverse impulses are produced and amplified, as indicated previously, by the concurrent action of the screw. Figure 14-10 illustrates the expansion achieved. The single rubber tube impeding the contact between upper and lower teeth favors their eruption. The subsequent leveling of the bite is shown in Figs. 14-2 to 14-6. For this purpose, all buccal segment occlusal surfaces remain free when the single rubber tube is used. They are entirely covered by the twin rubber tube, which is used for Class III malocclusion, open bite, crossbite and cases with a very slight incisor overbite. This design element is to prevent undesirable vertical growth in these cases. Stockfisch does

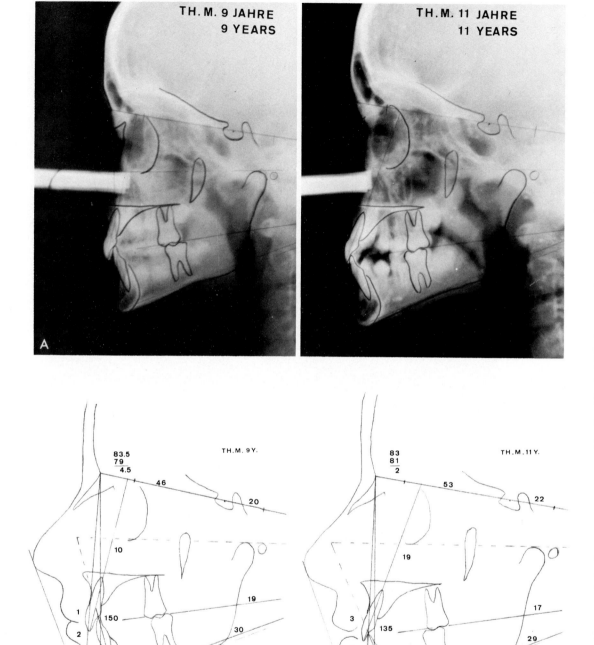

Figure 14-6. Head plates and cephalometric tracings of Case 2 (Figs. 14–4 and 14–5). Premolars and canines are now expected to erupt into their correct positions. ANB angle has been reduced 2.5 degrees.

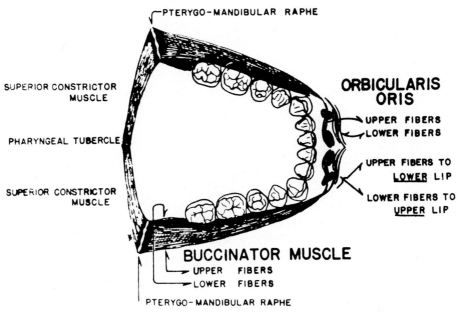

Figure 14-7. The buccinator mechanism. (From Graber, T. M.: Orthodontics, Principles and Practice, 3rd Ed. Philadelphia, W. B. Saunders Company, 1972.)

not think it unlikely that under the load of the twin rubber tubes, posterior teeth are actually depressed (see Fig. 14–12).

In the 10-year-old patient in Case 3 (Figs. 14–10 to 14–12), a Class III malocclusion with a crossbite was corrected in 11 months (Fig. 14–11A). In addition to the sagittal and transverse expansion of the maxillary arch, the first molars were moved posteriorly by distal screws. For that kind of tooth movement, a headgear is generally deemed necessary. Yet it was accomplished by the Kinetor in a simpler and more convenient way for the patient. However, a headgear may be used in conjunction with the Kinetor. Such a case is described and illustrated in Figure 16–28.

Figure 14-8. The Kinetor, interposed into the buccinator mechanism. Vestibular loops and anterior wires keep muscular pressure away from upper and lower jaw. According to Winders, the pressure of the cheeks is about 3.3 grams per sq. cm., lip pressure 6.6 to 11.6 grams per sq. cm. See the Fränkel appliance for similar use of labial and buccal shields.

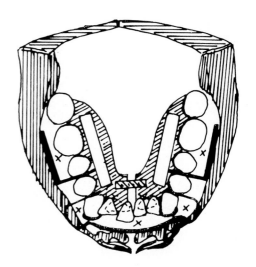

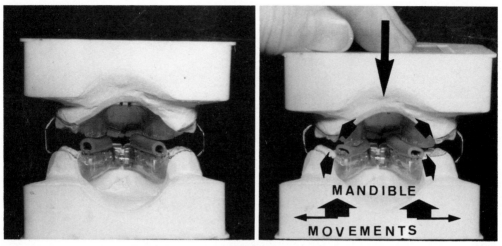

Figure 14–9. *Left,* The Kinetor on the models, showing its mode of action in the mouth. The bite is opened about 5 mm., thus providing functional stimuli. *Right,* Further functional stimuli originate through mandibular movements in a vertical, transverse, and sagittal direction. The rubber tube, compressed between the plates, again presses the plates against the dental arches, which are constricted in most cases. The result will be tooth movements in all three directions. Both upper and lower acrylic portions also have expansions screws, which are opened as needed.

It should be emphasized that the posterior movement by the screw was regarded as appropriate for this particular case. Stockfisch does not regard the distal screw as a possibility to replace the headgear in its many indications. The lower right first molar of this patient was also moved posteriorly by a distal screw (Fig. 14–11*B*). The extent of the distal displacement of both the upper and the lower right molars is visible in the lateral aspects of the models (Fig. 14–11*A*). The intraoral photograph of the patient, taken after 17 months of treatment, at the age of 11½ years, demonstrates the final correction of the irregularities (Fig. 14–12).

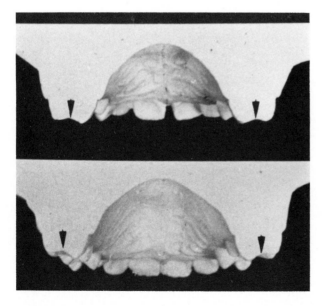

Figure 14–10. Case 3. Transverse expansion by the maxillary plate of the Kinetor. If treatment is initiated in time, the alveolar process and apical base, and even the medial palatal suture, will be widened. The casts are cut in the region of the first molars. The average expansion effected by the Kinetor is 6 mm., with a maximum of 12 mm.

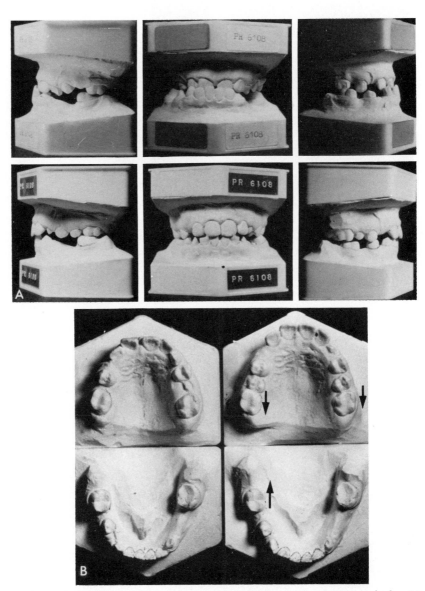

Figure 14-11. Case 3, age 9 years. Class III malocclusion before and after 11 months of treatment with the Kinetor. Upper first and lower right first molars have been moved distally, and inverted bite and bilateral crossbite have been corrected. The maxillary arch was expanded transversely and sagittally.

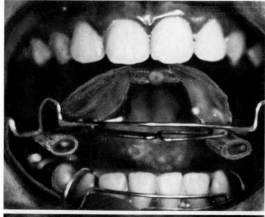

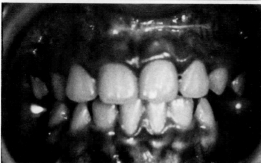

Figure 14–12. The Kinetor used for Case 3 in place in the mouth (see Figs. 14–10 and 14–11). The rubber tube is situated *on* the occlusal surfaces. This is to *prevent* eruption of posterior teeth.

With some cases of the Class III malocclusion, a faulty functional position of the tongue may be observed. Under these circumstances, it becomes necessary to stimulate the tongue to emerge from the lower dental arch and to redirect it upward and forward. This should happen under the influence of the Kinetor. There are cases of Class III malocclusion connected with an excessive growth of the tongue. His quite considerable clinical experience has con-

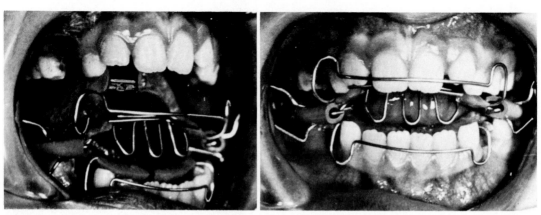

Figure 14–13. Case 4. Treatment of anterior open bite associated with tongue thrust, with the Kinetor. Maxillary expansion of 7 mm., already achieved, will posteriorly create more space for the tongue, now prevented from touching the incisors. The rubber tube is interposed between the occlusal surfaces, to prevent eruption or actually depress posterior teeth. A lingual tongue crib has been incorporated and is anchored in the palatal appliance acrylic.

vinced Stockfisch that success then depends on the surgical shortening of the tongue. This, of course, does not apply to patients with an habitual tongue thrust, associated with deglutition, speech, or laughter. This type of "functional" open bite, even if the tongue is at times oversized, does not require surgery. The task is to eliminate the unfavorable function of the tongue. Anterior open bite, however, corrected by usual orthodontic treatment, will all too frequently relapse. This may happen if the tongue has insufficient freedom of movement in a space diminished by incisor retraction. Functional treatment will often give more promise of success. The Kinetor, combined with a tongue crib and with twin rubber tubes extending over the occlusal surfaces, both aiding in the closing of the bite, is well suited to accomplish the task. The tongue, temporarily kept away from the anterior teeth, will not seem to miss the aperture now blocked by the appliance. This is because concurrent expansion of the dental arches will provide more tongue space in the posterior part of the dentition (Fig. 14–13). A permanent correction thus becomes more probable (Cases 4, 5, 6, Figs. 14–14 to 14–16).

The Kinetor provides a systematic and logical rationale for orthodontics. It is easy to understand its construction and handling. The important parts are prefabricated* and put together quickly without difficulty. The particular requirements of the case at hand are met by the addition of finger springs and

---

*The prefabricated parts are available in kits for 1, 3, 10, and more Kinetor appliances (Fig. 14–17). USA patent No. 3,454,001.

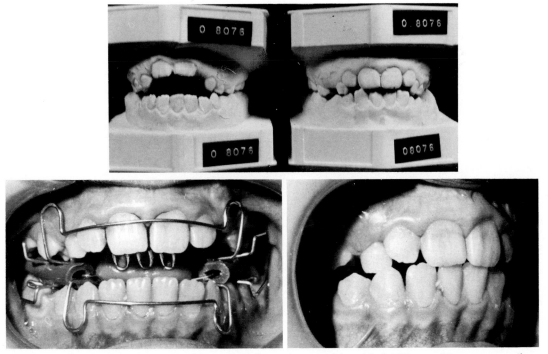

Figure 14–14. Case 5. Age 9 years. Treatment of anterior open bite with the Kinetor. Note tongue crib on lingual. Initial result after one year.

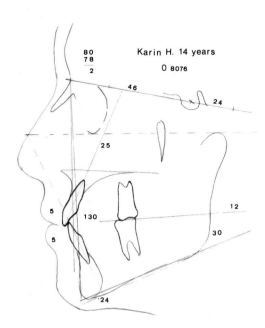

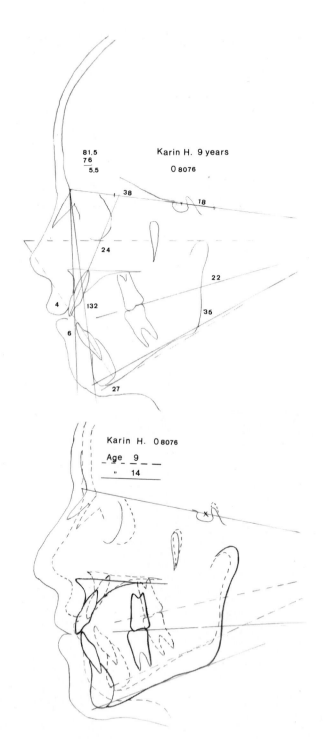

Figure 14–15. Same patient as Figure 14–14, with tracings at 9 and 14 years of age and a superimposition showing the stable effects of treatment. The open bite correction has held, and anterior face height is reduced to a smaller percentage. Retrusive effect of lower lip at time of original malocclusion has been eliminated and the mandibular growth direction is strongly horizontal, with a reduction of the mandibular plane angle.

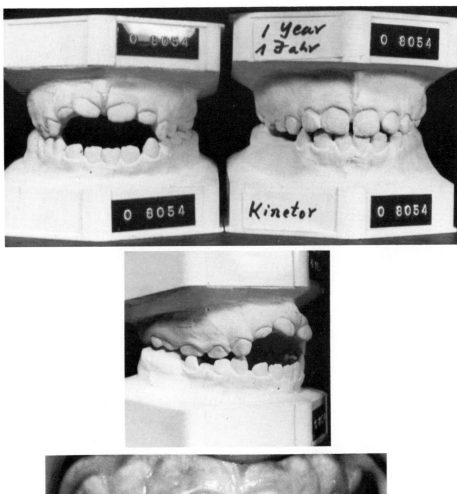

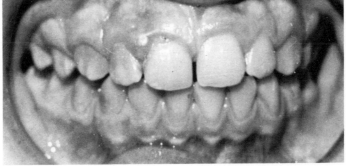

Figure 14–16. Case 6. Anterior open bite caused by tongue thrust. Result of treatment after one year. Oral photograph taken after three years out of retention.

sometimes by other appurtenances. For the protrusion of maxillary incisors, open springs are used, and closed springs aid in correction of the mandibular incisors, if necessary.

The Kinetor always needs stabilization to prevent sagittal displacement. This is provided by a clasplike short piece of 0.6 mm. wire placed anterior to the upper first molar, and sometimes also the lower first molar. Occasionally, premolars are used for spur placement. The treatment of crowding may demand additional stabilizing wires on the mesial surface of the lower canines

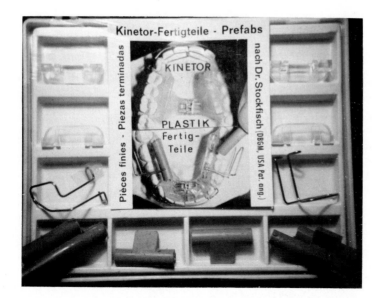

Figure 14-17. The prefabricated parts of the Kinetor. Assembly kits are available. Vestibular loops are prefabricated, but labial bows are usually bent for each case. Plastic and rubber tube parts (single and double) are easily assembled.

(Figs. 14-2, 14-8, and 14-21). Posteriorly directed screws may occasionally take the place of the stabilizing wires contacting the first molars. The spurs contacting the first molars will also serve to prevent their anterior movement after the shedding of the deciduous molars (Fig. 14-18).

Essentially, the construction of the Kinetor is the same for all kinds of treatment. It consists of an upper and a lower expansion plate. Two plastic

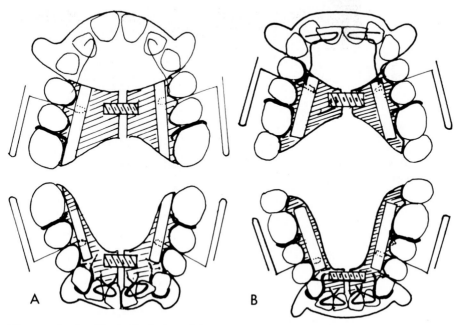

Figure 14-18. The basic design of the Kinetor is always the same: two plates with prefabricated plastic parts, two symmetrical prefabricated, detachable and exchangeable vestibular loops, upper and lower anterior wires (labial bows), and single or twin rubber tubes. The requirements of a particular case are met by screws and different springs, which are added.

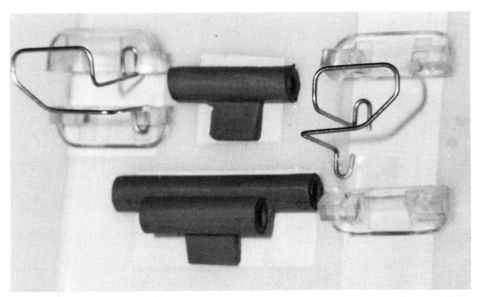

Figure 14–19. The plastic prefabricated parts are one size only. They are shown with the exchangeable rubber tubes and exchangeable prefabricated vestibular loops. The plastic portion is constructed with holes to receive the vestibular loop wires and slots for the rubber tube tabs. Tubes must be replaced every month or two.

prefabs are incorporated into each of these when the cold-curing acrylic is still in the molding stage. The removable prefabricated parts, the vestibular loops, and the rubber tubes are inserted into the prefabs (Fig. 14–19). The seat of the vestibular loops is secured by two small U bends. They fit precisely into holes in the plastic parts, where they are placed. The construction allows limited freedom of movement in the plastic for the U bend. Too rigid a connection could overload the wire by the pressure exerted on the appliance. The rubber tubes are provided with square extensions, fitting into openings of corresponding size in the plastic.

The Kinetor is constructed in the following manner: the plaster models are fixed on an articulator. If no construction bite is available, the bite is opened on the articulator to create an interocclusal space of 4 to 5 mm. Class II conditions are corrected by moving the lower cast forward on the articulator to establish a Class I relationship of the casts. However, a construction bite taken directly in the mouth, as with the activator, is preferable.

The upper and lower anterior wires and, if required, protrusion springs are adapted. For the anterior wires, 0.8 mm. hard spring wire is used. For the upper open protrusion springs, 0.7 mm. wire, and for the lower closed springs, 0.5 mm. wire is recommended. Ready-made labial wires and protrusion springs are available. Most technicians, however, prefer to bend them individually. Labial wires and springs are put in place and fixed with sticky wax in the usual manner. The tags remain free (Fig. 14–20).

The screws are set in a small amount of cold-cure acrylic, placed on the casts beforehand. The maxillary screw, kept at a distance of 3 mm. from the palate, is placed on a transverse line connecting the contact points of the first and second premolars or deciduous molars.

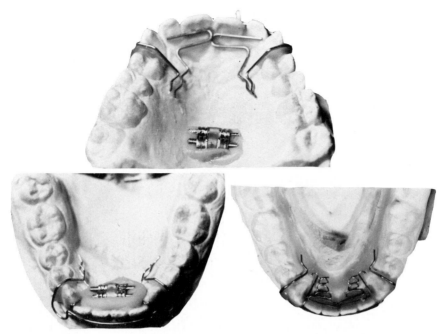

Figure 14–20. Anterior wires and protrusion springs waxed in place. The screws are put in place by a small amount of cold-curing acrylic. Protrusion springs are used only when indicated, as in Class II, Division 2 malocclusion.

THE CONSTRUCTION OF THE MANDIBULAR PLATE

The construction of the appliance proper begins with the mandibular plate. After wires and screw have been placed, a piece of cold-curing acrylic is put on the cast (Fig. 14–21). It is lightly smoothed and the mandibular plastic prefabs, having vestibular loops with single rubber tubes inserted, are set in the acrylic (Fig. 14–22). The longer leg of the loop is connected with the man-

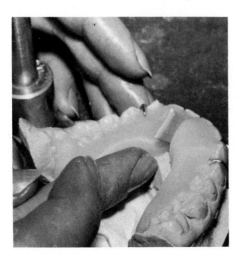

Figure 14–21. Cold-curing acrylic put on the lower cast, ready to receive prefabricated plastic portion.

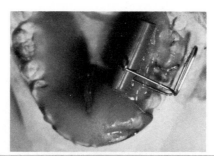

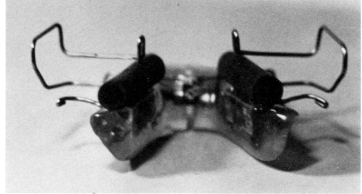

Figure 14–22. Insertion of the prefabricated plastic part into the soft acrylic. This is a precise maneuver, requiring parallelism of both upper and lower plastic prefabs.

dibular plate. According to the requirements of the particular case, the prefabricated plastic part may contact the lingual aspects of the teeth or may be a slight distance away. The precise position of the plastic part is determined by the inserted vestibular loop. The loop itself is kept at a distance of 3 mm. from the labial aspects of the teeth. The horizontal connecting part of the wire is invariably between the cusps of the first and second premolars or deciduous molars, if eruption must not be impeded. The single rubber tube is used, and the connecting wire is kept at a slight distance from the posterior occlusal aspects in deep bite cases and where buccal segment eruption is required (i.e., Class II, Division 2, or deep bite Class II, Division 1 malocclusions). If no further eruption is desired, the twin rubber tube may be employed, allowing the wire to contact the occlusal surfaces. The same principles apply to the connecting wire of the maxillary plate. The plastic prefabs have to be incorporated in a strictly horizontal position and precisely on the same level. They must not be tipped anteroposteriorly or lingually. Following these rules, the mandibular plate is constructed quickly. According to Stockfisch, it should not take more than 10 to 15 minutes.

CONSTRUCTION OF THE MAXILLARY PLATE

Before the construction of the maxillary plate is undertaken, an important detail must not be forgotten. Screws and wires are already in place. A short piece of 0.8 mm. wire is bent to represent the little U bend of the vestibular loop and its horizontal connecting piece. This wire is placed into the prefabricated plastic parts to be used for the maxillary plate. The vestibular loop and rubber tube are then withdrawn from the mandibular plate. Otherwise, they

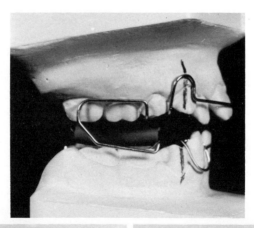

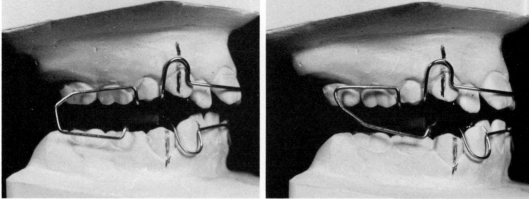

Figure 14–23. The prefabricated vestibular loop will keep the jaws in a Class I position and the cheek away as well. Generally, it will not be necessary to make individual adjustments. By bending the loop wires, however, it is possible at any time to change the relation of the two plates in an anterior or posterior direction. Note change in vestibular loop configuration as the mandible is advanced.

would interfere with the position of the maxillary plastic part when the two casts are joined on the articulator.

Now cold-curing acrylic is put on the maxillary cast to form the plate. Only the region of the molars and premolars is covered; the whole anterior part of the palate remains free. The two lateral parts are joined by a rather small acrylic "bridge" containing the screw, positioned as previously described. The prefabricated plastic parts are set on the soft acrylic. The square space, in which, in the mandibular plate, the extension of the rubber tube is seated, is filled with acrylic. Otherwise, the same rules apply as described with the construction of the mandibular plate. It is emphasized that the plastic parts have to be in the same plane, placed horizontally and not tilted in any direction. Equally valid are the instructions previously given for the placement of the wire representing the connecting part of the vestibular loops. It is also situated between the cusps of the first and second premolars.

The two casts are now joined on the articulator and are closely inspected before the acrylic of the upper plate hardens. The upper and lower plastic parts have to be parallel to each other. Any deviation must be corrected now.

The technical process is finished by smoothing and polishing the acrylic parts. The vestibular loops are put in place. They will keep the upper and lower dentitions in the relation determined by the plan of treatment. Changes, however, are made easily by adjustment of the loops (Fig. 14–23).

The Kinetor can be modified to meet particular demands of treatment. Screws exerting pressure on the first molars in a posterior direction may be easily inserted. However, they have to be restricted to one plate at a time. If their use is indicated with both plates, they are first inserted where more extensive tooth movement is required. A lateral mandibular screw may conflict with the square extension of the rubber tube. If that happens, the rubber tube has to be anchored in the maxillary plate instead. To place the screw, it is necessary to grind off part of the plastic prefab. The hole for the insertion of the U bends anchoring the vestibular loop has to remain intact, however. The use of small screws will facilitate technical procedures. Screws for anterior movement of the first molar are also practicable. They are inserted into the divided prefab.

The use of functional appliances is quite generally associated with the conviction that the period of the mixed dentition is the most favorable treatment time. Correction is obtained later only with considerably greater difficulty. Simultaneous significant spontaneous growth and adaptation will intensify the stimuli originating from the appliance. Stockfisch claims that the Kinetor, com-

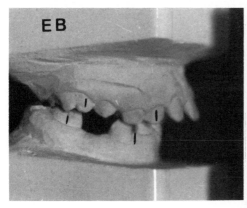
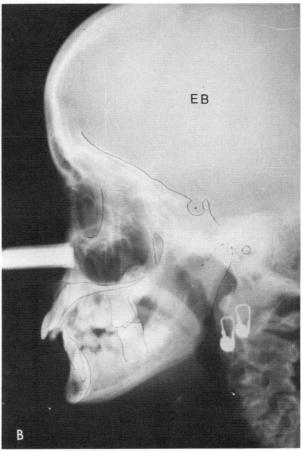

Figure 14–24. Case 7 (E. B.), age 9 years. Original casts and cephalogram, Class II, Division 1 malocclusion with excessive overbite, abnormal perioral function, mouth-breathing, etc. Overjet, 9 mm.

bining the advantages of functional and active components, makes the best use of that comparatively short period of time.

The 9-year-old girl in Case 7 (Fig. 14–24) has a typical Class II, Division 1 malocclusion, with spaced protrusion, an overjet of 10 mm., deep overbite, and narrow jaws, in addition to mouth breathing. Two years of treatment with one Kinetor and only 10 appointments during the first year produced the result shown by the headplate tracings (Fig. 14–25). Breathing and lip closure are now

Figure 14–25. Case 7 (see Fig. 14–24). Cephalometric tracings. *Upper,* At the beginning of treatment. *Lower left,* After two years of treatment with the Kinetor. *Lower right,* The tracings superimposed.

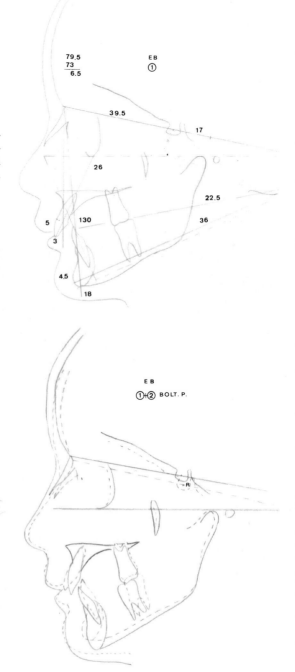

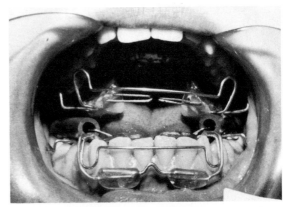

Figure 14-26. Exaggerated, functionally conditioned deforming pressure of the lower lip against the incisors is alleviated by a "lip bumper" kept at a distance from the incisors and the alveolar process. This offsets a hyperactive mentalis muscle activity. The lip bumper is quite similar to the lip shields of the Fränkel function corrector (FRI).

normal. The upper first molars were retained in their position without the use of a headgear. An open activator was used for retention.

Open bite cases often require the addition of a tongue crib to the Kinetor. It is easily inserted into the maxillary space (see Figs. 14–13 and 14–14). A lip bumper is another useful device occasionally utilized with the Kinetor (Fig. 14–26). It will counteract the pressure of the lower lip. It helped to bring about the considerable changes achieved within 18 months in a 9-year-old with a Class II, Division 1 malocclusion (Case 8, Fig. 14–27). The Class II condition is corrected and the bite leveled. Both arches are expanded. The mandibular incisor section is now well rounded after the elimination of lip pressure. At this stage, an open activator is inserted as a retainer and for subsequent desirable minor adjustments.

In the same manner, a maxillary lip bumper may prove useful in some Class III cases to further sagittal development of the anterior region. Fränkel uses this same philosophy with his lip pads on the function corrector.

The permanency of the results achieved by treatment with the Kinetor is proved by the many cases followed after active treatment. Treatment of Case 9 (Fig. 14–28) was initiated at the age of 9 years. The Kinetor was used for one year, followed by two years of additional treatment and retention with an activator. The intraoral photograph, 10 years after the removal of all appliances, shows the lasting result obtained without extractions.

Case 10 (Fig. 14–29), a girl 12 years old at the beginning of treatment, had one Kinetor for one year and an activator for one more year. Satisfied with the result, she had the treatment terminated, although the period of retention was not regarded as sufficient. Nevertheless, the result proved to be stable, as models, photographs, and headplate tracing show six years later.

Patients adapt quickly to the Kinetor. If the anterior displacement effected by the appliance is not tolerated well, it is easily lessened by adjustment of the vestibular loops. About three months after the beginning of treatment, improvement should be evident.

The screws are turned 90 degrees once a week; distal screws are turned every 10 to 15 days. The rubber tube has to be exchanged every month or two. A vestibular loop will break once in a while. It is under considerable strain because of the constant movement of the jaws. A spare part is easily inserted.

The patient cleans the Kinetor with a toothbrush and water. When not inserted, it is kept in a receptacle filled with water, to which a few drops of cleans-

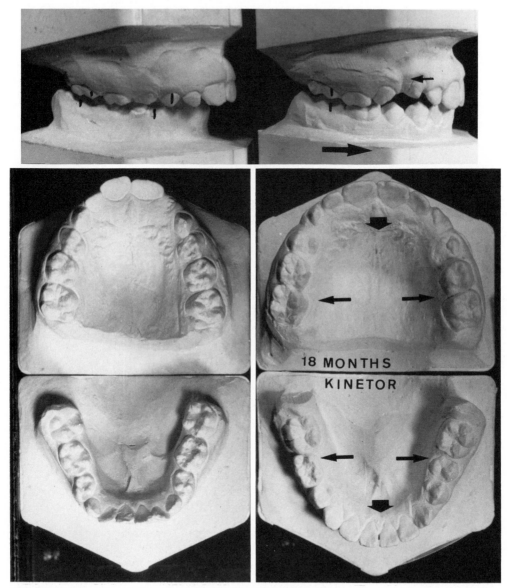

Figure 14–27. Case 8. Result of a year and a half of treatment with the Kinetor. Lingual inclination and crowding of lower incisors (large interincisor angle) were corrected by lip bumper and protrusion springs. The bumper as well as the Kinetor exert a favorable influence on the muscles of the lips, cheek, and tongue.

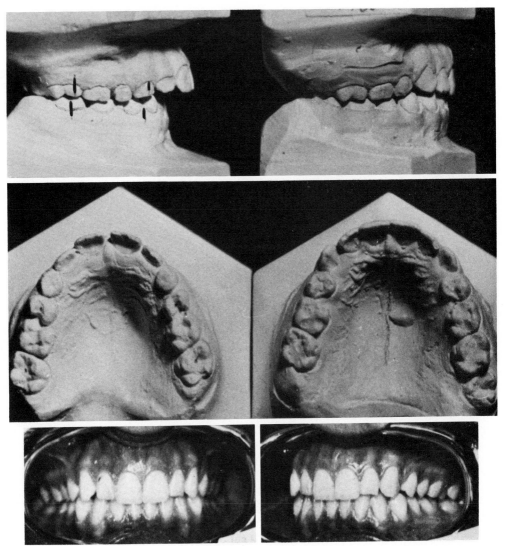

Figure 14–28. Case 9. Treatment with Kinetor from the ninth to the eleventh year of age. Oral photographs taken 10 years later.

ing fluid are added. The orthodontist may provide additional cleaning with an ultrasonic cleaner when he sees the patient.

The Kinetor is no orthodontic cure-all. A constricted maxilla with bilateral crossbite, combined with a deviation of the nasal septum, mouth breathing, etc., may require rapid splitting of the palatal suture. Other contraindications, according to Stockfisch, are severe Class III conditions and skeletal open bite. Other appliances have to be used for extremely rotated or markedly tipped incisors, or if extraction in the permanent dentition is necessary.

As stressed repeatedly, treatment with the Kinetor has to be undertaken in the mixed dentition. With some limitations, it should be successful also during the first two years of the permanent dentition. Stockfisch is positive that, used at the proper age and for the right kind of malocclusion, the Kinetor will correct two thirds of all malocclusions.

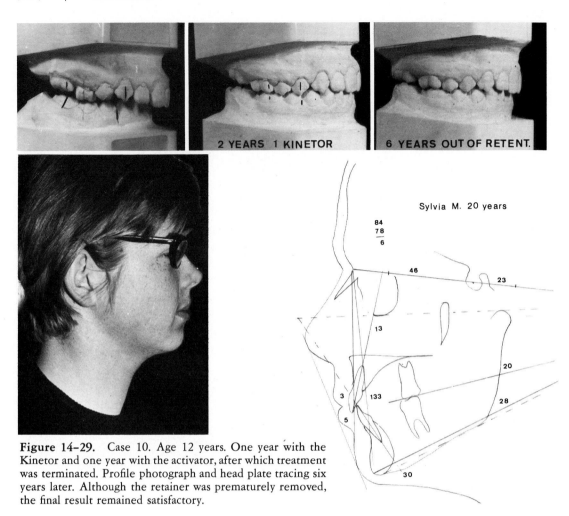

Figure 14-29. Case 10. Age 12 years. One year with the Kinetor and one year with the activator, after which treatment was terminated. Profile photograph and head plate tracing six years later. Although the retainer was prematurely removed, the final result remained satisfactory.

The clear basic design, the construction facilitated by the extensive use of prefabricated parts for two thirds of the appliances, simple manipulation and easy repairs (generally only the replacement of a broken vestibular loop), and last but not least, the speed with which correction is generally achieved, seem to justify the claim of Stockfisch that the Kinetor will enable the orthodontist to treat more patients than with any other appliance.

References

1. Graber, T. M.: Post mortems in posttreatment adjustment, Am. J. Orthod., 1966, p. 331.
2. Howland, J. P., and Brodie, A. G.: Pressures exerted by the Buccinator. Angle Orthod., *36*: 1–12, 1966.
3. Herren, R.: Form und Funktion in der kieferorthopädischen Therapie. Fortschr. Kieferorthop., 1963 Band 24, Heft 3 und 4.
4. Meroni-A. Meroni-Spinedi-Traverso-Bacigalupo: La gimnasia respiratoria y la aparatologia en el respirador bucal disgnásico. Rev. Circulo Argentino Odontol., *28*:1, 1964.
5. Meach, C. L.: A cephalometric comparison of bony profile changes in Class II/1 patients treated with extraoral force and functional jaw orthopedics. Am. J. Orthod., 1966, p. 353.
6. Schmuth: Über die Indikation einiger modifizierter FKO-Geräte. Fortschr. Kieferorthop., 1963, Band 24, Heft 3 und 4.

7. Schwarz, A. M.: Zahn-Mund-Kieferheilkunde, V. Band: *In* Anlehnung an die Funktionskiefer-orthopädie entwickelte Geräte, Seite 431 bis 433.
8. Sheppe, J.: Orthodontics, 1965.
9. Stockfisch, H.: Fernröntgen-Diagnose, Fernröntgen-Prognose für die kieferorthopädische Allgemein und Fachpraxis. Dr. Hüthig Verlag, Heidelberg, 1975.
10. Stockfisch, H.: Die neuzeitliche kieferorthopädische Praxis, 4. Auflage. Dr. Hüthig Verlag, Heidelberg, 1969.
11. Stockfisch, H.: Orthopedia de los maxilares, practica moderna, 1962 Editorial mundi, Buenos Aires.
12. Stockfisch, H.: Erfahrungen über die aktive und funktionelle Plattenbehandlung und über die Ausnutzung der kinetischen Muskelenergie bei kieferorthopädischen Massnahmen. Studienwoche 1960, Nederlandsche Vereeniging voor Orthodontische Studie.
13. Stockfisch, H.: Activateurs, les étapes de l'évolution des appareils a plaques. Société Francaise d'Orthopédie Dento-Faciale Congress Lyon, 1962.
14. Stockfisch, H.: Experience in active and functional plate treatment and the utilization of kinetic muscle energy in jaw-orthopedic methods. Int. J. Orthod., 2:3, 1974.
15. Stockfish, H.: Der Kinetor in der Kieferorthopädie. Dr. Hüthig Verlag. Heidelberg, 1966.
16. Stockfisch, H.: La distoclusion molaire inférieure (Classe II) et les problèmes d'appareillage. Orthop. Dento-Faciale, *1*:1, 1967.
17. Stockfisch, H.: Die rationelle Kinetortechnik mit Plastik-Fertigteilen und vorgetertigten Drahtteilen. Die Zahntechnik/Schweiz 2, 1967.
18. Stockfisch, H.: Successful treatment and avoidance of relapse in optimally timed and late treatment of Class II/1 Cases. Eur. Orthod. Soc., 1968, p. 295.
19. Stockfisch, H.: Rapid expansion of the maxilla. Success and relapse. Eur. Orthod. Soc., 1969.
20. Stockfisch, H.: Class III treatment with the elastic oral adaptor, the function corrector, the Kinetor, palatal expansion (splitting of the mid-palatal suture), light wire, and surgical shortening of the tongue. Eur. Orthod. Soc. 1970, p. 279.
21. Stockfisch, H.: Possibilities and limitations of the Kinetor bimaxillary appliance. Eur. Orthod. Soc., 1971, p. 317.
22. Stockfisch, H.: Posibilidades y limites de la terapeutica bimaxilar con el Kinetor en la oclusión cubierta y mordida abierta. Actas Soc. española Ortod., *17*:97, 1971.

CHAPTER 15

The Fränkel Appliance (The Function Corrector)*

The Andresen-Häupl appliance, the activator, which opened a new chapter in the history of removable orthodontic appliances, was followed by devices of a similar kind, but designed to make it possible to wear them also during the day. These appliance modifications were first introduced by Bimler and Balters. The function corrector, constructed by Rolf Fränkel of Zwickau, GDR, marks another stage in that development. The remarkable results achieved with this appliance have aroused considerable interest. Fränkel has conducted large-scale investigations on the measurable effects of therapy using the function corrector. These investigations, and his explanations of the theoretical background, making full use of our present orthodontic knowledge, are valuable additions to the clinical experience gained and should broaden our concepts in diagnosis and therapy. Charles Nord, one of the leaders of European orthodontics of this century, may prove to have been right when he called the Fränkel method "a revolution in orthodontic appliances."

THE CONSTRUCTION AND USE OF THE FUNCTION CORRECTOR (FR)†

The function corrector is constructed differently for different types of malocclusion. Fränkel describes four basic types of function correctors. The FR I is designed for correction of Class I and Class II, Division 1 malocclusions; the FR II for Class II, Division 2 malocclusions; the FR III for the treatment of Class III malocclusions; and the FR IV for open bites and bimaxillary protrusions.

In this chapter, primarily the FR I and FR III will be discussed. Although the appliance is intended mainly for the treatment of nonextraction cases, with slight modifications it can be used successfully for the treatment of extraction

---

*The authors are particularly grateful to Dr. Rolf Fränkel for his major text and illustration contributions to the chapter, and to Dr. Kaija Virolainen for her significant editorial assistance.

†The appliance was named by Fränkel "Funktionsregler" (FR)—function regulator. Although in the text the more idiomatic term "function corrector" is used, to maintain a unified terminology the abbreviation FR is retained.

cases as well. The description of these and other more sophisticated procedures is, however, beyond the scope of this book.

At first glance, the appliance looks rather complicated, and it must be emphasized that the directions for the construction of the appliance have to be followed with the greatest precision in every detail. Although it will take some time to become familiar with all the parts of the appliance, once correctly fashioned and used as advised, the appliance will need only a few subsequent adjustments.

The Function Corrector I (FR I)

There are three modifications of the FR I: FR Ia, FR Ib, and FR Ic.

FR Ia

The FR Ia (Fig. 15–1) is the original construction, which is still used for the treatment of Class I malocclusions in which there are minor or moderate crowding and concomitant arrested development of basal arches. It is especially well suited for the correction of deep bite Class I malocclusions where the maxillary incisors are protruded and mandibular incisors are retruded. It is also used for the correction of Class I deep overbites and for the treatment of mild Class II, Division 1 malocclusions in which the overjet does not exceed 5 mm.

The most conspicuous things about all function correctors are the two large buccal shields which have several important tasks to perform. In addition, the FR Ia has two lip pads with connecting wires, a labial bow, and two canine loops on the labial side.

On the lingual side, there is a palatal bow with occlusal supports on the maxillary molars (Fig. 15–2), and on the mandible, a lingual bow with U loops (Fig. 15–3).

When the function corrector is used for the correction of a distoclusion, the mandible is moved to a forward position. To hold this new position, the mandible is stabilized against the maxillary teeth (first molars and first premolars) with the aid of the palatal bow and the canine loops (see Fig. 15–2).

The palatal bow runs between the upper second premolar and the first

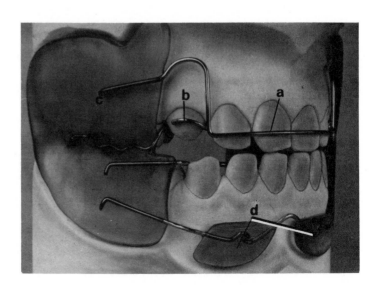

Figure 15–1. FR Ia: (a) labial bow, (b) canine loop, (c) buccal shield, and (d) lip pads.

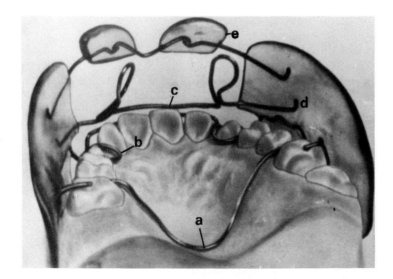

Figure 15-2. FR Ia on the maxillary cast: (a) palatal bow, (b) canine loop, (c) lingual bow, (d) buccal shield, and (e) lip pads.

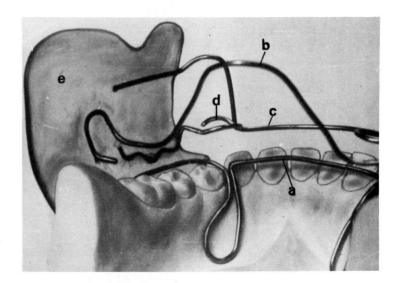

Figure 15-3. FR Ia on the mandibular cast: (a) lingual bow, (b) palatal bow, (c) labial bow, (d) canine loop, and (e) buccal shield.

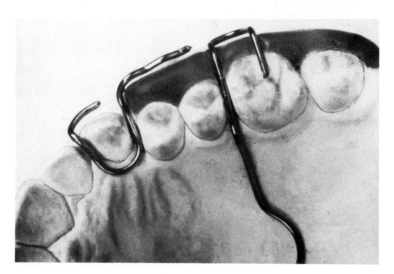

Figure 15-4. FR I: wax padding, the canine loop, and the palatal bow with the occlusal rest on the maxillary first molar.

molar and rests against the mesial surface of the first molar (Fig. 15–4). Besides buttressing the appliance against the first molars, the palatal bow helps to keep the appliance together. Its extensions, the occlusal supports between the mesiobuccal and distobuccal cusps of the maxillary first molars, prevent the appliance from sinking into the vestibular fold (Fig. 15–4). The canine loops buttress the appliance against the mesial aspects of the upper first premolars (Fig. 15–4). These loops can also be used to guide erupting canines into a proper position.

The main purpose of the lingual bow (Fig. 15–3) is to guide the mandible forward into its new position with the U loops; it also gives the appliance general support. The lingual bow is allowed to be in contact with the mandibular incisors only in those instances in which labial tipping of these teeth is desired.

The buccal shields (see Fig. 15–1) cover the buccal surfaces of the premolars and molars and the corresponding alveolar structures. The shields are designed to protect the growing alveolar bones from the harmful pressure of the buccinator mechanism. Therefore, they are constructed so as not to impinge on areas in which dentoalveolar development is desired. Furthermore, the shields must extend deep into the sulci to cause tension in the connective tissue fibers. This continuous stretching of the connective tissue fibers in the same direction stimulates new bone formation in the apical base.

Similar to the action of the buccal shields at the lateral aspects, the lip pads (see Fig. 15–1) eliminate the pressure exerted by an overactive mentalis muscle. The pads give mechanical support to the lower lip and prevent it from curling outward under the protruded maxillary incisors. Together with the U loops, the lip pads also have a function in positioning the mandible in the constructed mesial position.

Construction

The construction of the FR Ia, the original appliance, will be described in detail, since its construction is basic for all FR I's and also for the FR II.

The first step is the impression taking. The impressions should reproduce the whole expanse of the alveolar process up to the sulci and including maxillary tuberosities. However, to avoid distorting the soft tissues, impression trays should not reach too far into the sulci. The casts are mounted with the construction bite on a simple articulator.

The second step is the taking of a working or a construction bite. The treatment decision with regard to mandibular forward positioning is made by studying the patient's profile. The patient is asked to push the mandible forward; if the profile is then satisfactory, mandibular forward positioning with the function corrector is indicated (Fig. 15–5). In taking the construction bite, care is taken not to strain the facial musculature or the muscle balance between the protractor and retractor muscles.

If, however, the profile becomes worse when the mandible is positioned forward, extractions may have to be considered to reduce the procumbency.

For the FR Ia, the construction bite is taken with the teeth in an incisal edge-to-edge relationship (Fig. 15–6), except in Class I cases with shallow or normal overbite (these are taken with the teeth in habitual occlusion).

The bite registration is made with the aid of a base plate which conforms to the contour of the palate and to which lateral wax bite blocks have been added.

The next step in the fabrication of the FR I is the trimming of the plaster

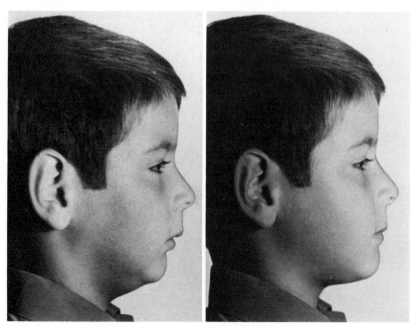

Figure 15-5. Profile analysis of a distoclusion: *left,* in habitual occlusion; *right,* mandible positioned forward.

casts for the buccal shields and the lip pads. This is one of the most difficult technical aspects in the construction of the function corrector and has to be done with meticulous care. To produce the tissue tension necessary for the appositional development of the apical bases, the buccal shields must extend high into the sulci in the areas where this development is desired. If the vestibular areas are not trimmed enough and the buccal shields are too short, the soft tissue attachments will fold inside the shield, counteracting the therapeutic effect of the appliance (Fig. 15–7). If the shields are too long, they will irritate the mucosa, and the patient cannot wear the appliance. The plaster casts, therefore, are trimmed back in the area of the maxillary tuberosities and the max-

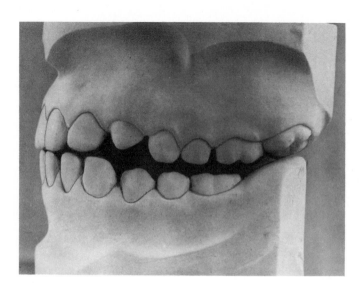

Figure 15-6. Construction bite for FR Ia in an incisal edge-to-edge position.

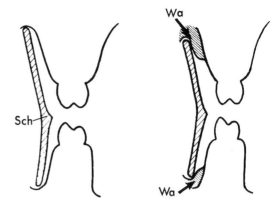

Figure 15-7. The buccal shields are extended to the vestibular fold (left); if they are too short (right), the soft tissues will invaginate between the shields and the alveolar process. If they are too long, they will irritate. Fitting must be precise to exert tension on the periosteal fibers.

illary first premolars (Fig. 15–8, arrow 2). Trimming of the lower lateral sulci is not necessary. All trimming has to be done with the patient present, taking great care and inspecting the anatomic conditions of the particular region. It is likewise important to trim in the anterior region of the mandibular sulci (Fig. 15–8, arrow 3). When the impression is taken, the depth of the sulcus usually is distorted and somewhat diminished. Hence, the sulcus is carefully trimmed about 5 mm. from the greatest curvature of the alveolar base so that the soft tissues do not get beneath the pads. In Figure 15–9, the solid line marks the real depth of the sulcus, and the interrupted line points out the distortion by the impression. Figure 15–9*B* shows the correct trimming of the sulcus. Seen from the side, the external surface of the alveolus should be nearly vertical after the trimming. In addition to the trimming of the sulci, the contacts between the maxillary first molars and second premolars and between the maxillary canines and first premolars are carved away. On the cast this is done by sawing a 1 mm. wide groove between the teeth (Figs. 15–2, 15–4, and 15–10). The grooves accommodate the palatal bow and the canine loops. It is better to carve the grooves too deep than too shallow to insure a firm seating of the appliance on the maxilla, a precondition for the forward placement of the mandible

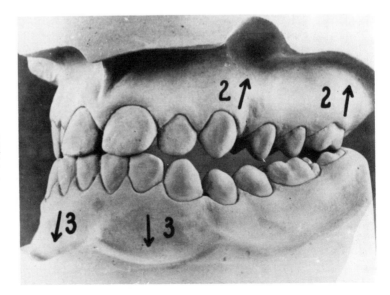

Figure 15-8. Areas of trimming of sulci for the buccal shields and the lip pads in FR I and FR II. *2,* Buccal shields. *3,* Lip pads.

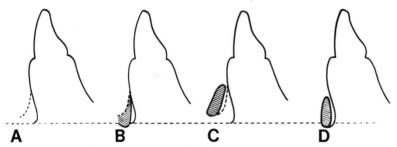

Figure 15–9. Position of the mandibular lip pads: (a) solid line, actual depth of the sulcus; interrupted line, distortion by impression taking; (b) correct trimming; (c) wrong position of the pad, caused by inadequate trimming; and (d) correct position of pad.

in the construction bite position. When first inserted, the wires will ride on the contact points, but subsequently they will lodge themselves between the teeth.

To achieve the desired expansion of the dental arches and the alveolar processes up to the apical base, the buccal shields have to be an appropriate distance from the lateral aspects of the teeth and the alveolus. Therefore, the next step after the trimming is to cover the buccal aspects of the models with a layer of wax. The thickness of this layer is determined individually according to the desired transverse development, but it must not exceed 3 mm. in the tooth area and 2.5 mm. at the alveolar area (Fig. 15–11). Otherwise the appliance will be too bulky and difficult to wear. The wax cover is especially important in the apical region of the maxillary first premolars, because in this area, in the majority of Class II, Division 1 malocclusions, the maxilla is narrowed transversely to the greatest degree. In the mandibular region, the wax cover is limited mainly to the teeth and a small part of the tissue below the gingival margin. Only a very thin layer of wax is necessary to cover the mandibular apical base. As shown in Figure 15–11, the waxing is done separately on the maxillary and mandibular casts. No wax is applied in the mandibular frontal region.

After the wax layer has been applied, the wires are bent and placed on the models (Fig. 15–12). The stabilizing and connecting wires are of heavier wire, whereas the tooth-moving wires are thinner. The stabilizing and connecting wires should not be in contact with the soft tissues in order to avoid abrasions. The wires situated in the vestibule which are not covered by the acrylic should not be more than 1.5 mm. from the alveolar mucosa. On the lingual side of the alveolar bone and on the palate, the distance between the wires and the mucosa should not be more than 0.75 mm. On the vestibular side, the wires should be bent to follow the natural grooves of the labial alveolar bone in order to avoid irritation of the soft tissues.

The wire parts, which will be embedded in the acrylic, should not contact the wax, nor should they be a greater distance from the wax surface than 0.75 mm. (Figs. 15–4 and 15–13). Otherwise, the buccal shields will become too thick and bulky. The ends of the wires are bent at right angles to the wax layer.

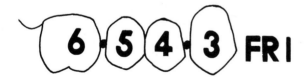

Figure 15–10. Position of wires between the buccal segment teeth in FR I and FR II after cast has been trimmed at contact points.

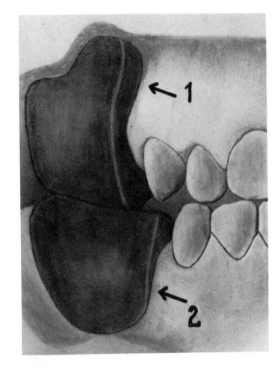

Figure 15–11. Wax padding under the buccal shield to establish space between tissue and the appliance in FR I and FR II. Note variable thickness between upper and lower arches.

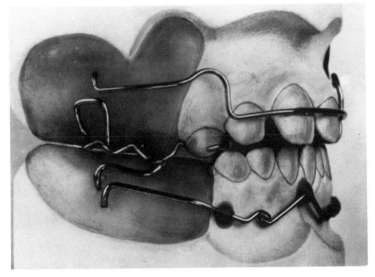

Figure 15–12. FR Ib with wires affixed by sticky wax and wax padding for shields before the application of cold-curing acrylic.

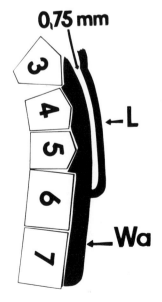

Figure 15–13. Wax padding (Wa) under the buccal shield. Correct distance between the labial arch (L) and the wax padding should be approximately 0.75 mm.

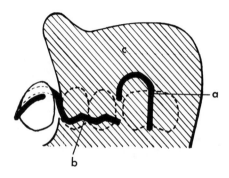

Figure 15-14. Side aspect of canine loop and occlusal rest: (a) canine loop, (b) occlusal rest, and (c) buccal shield.

The palatal bow (1.0 mm. in diameter) crosses the palate with a slight curve in a distal direction (see Figs. 15–2 and 15–4). This curve provides some extra length of wire to facilitate widening of the appliance, which is sometimes necessary as the apical bases develop laterally and begin to contact the buccal shields. The wire crosses the trimmed interdental space between the maxillary first molar and second premolar, makes a loop into the buccal shield, and emerges again to lie on the first molar between the buccal cusps (see Figs. 15–3, 15–4, and 15–12). If in the course of the treatment the wire in the interdental space between the second premolar and first molar impinges on the gingiva, the occlusal rest is bent toward the surface of the first molar to relieve the pressure.

The canine loop (0.9 mm. in diameter) is embedded in the buccal shield at the level of the occlusal plane (Figs. 15–1, 15–4, 15–12, 15–14, and 15–15). From there, the wire rises steeply to the gingival margin of the maxillary first premolar. The wire maintains contact with the mesial surface of the first premolar to secure the aforementioned intermaxillary stabilization of the appliance. If the canine loop is fashioned correctly, it can be bent occlusally to prevent the wire from impinging on the gingiva as the canine and premolar erupt further.

The shape and position of the labial bow (0.9 mm. in diameter) can be seen in Figures 15–1 and 15–12. The labial bow lies in the middle of the labial surfaces of the incisors and runs gingivally at right angles in the natural depression between the maxillary lateral incisor and the canine. It forms a gentle curve distally at the height of the middle of the canine root. This slight bend in the wire makes it possible to adjust the wire if necessary.

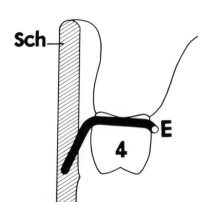

Figure 15-15. The canine loop (E) and the buccal shield (Sch). This shows the interproximal level of the canine loop when the appliance is fully seated.

The mandibular parts of the FR Ia are the lip pads and the lingual bow. The lip pads (see Fig. 15–1) are held in place by two wires (0.9 mm. in diameter) originating from the mandibular parts of the buccal shields. A third wire connects them; it is bent gingivally to allow for the movements of the frenum. It is preferable to use three wires instead of one in order to avoid adverse tension. The tags of all the wires are bent at right angles so that the pads will be prevented from rotating around the wires.

For the proper function of the FR Ia, the correct bending of the lingual bow with the U loops (0.9 mm. in diameter) is extremely important (see Fig. 15–3). Unless forward inclination of the mandibular incisors is desired, the wire should not be in contact with the teeth. The role of the U loops is to position the mandible forward. The loops are situated in the root area of the mandibular first premolars and are bent to follow the mandibular lingual contour as closely as possible. They should allow the mandible to slide easily into the appliance and should not impinge on or cause pain in the mucosa.

The lingual bow runs across the mandibular dentition between the canines and first premolars and enters the buccal shields at their frontal edge at the level of the occlusal plane. The wire should not lodge between the teeth; rather, it should stay slightly away from the teeth.

After the wires have been bent, they are secured on the model with modeling wax (see Fig. 15–12). The buccal shields and the lip pads are fabricated in cold-curing acrylic. The total thickness of the shields and the pads should not exceed 2.5 mm. All margins have to be well-rounded and perfectly polished.

The lip pads have the form of a parallelogram (see Fig. 15–1). The upper edge of the pads should be at least 5 mm. from the gingival border. The position of the lip is very important. Figure 15–9*D* shows the correct vertical position; Figure 15–9*C* shows a faulty position of the lip pads, which would produce abrasions on the inside of the lower lip.

Before the buccal shields are made, the maxillary and mandibular lateral wax coverings are joined by melting the contacting margins with a heated instrument.

FR Ib

The FR Ib is especially indicated for the treatment of Class II, Division 1 malocclusions with deep bite, where the overjet does not exceed 7 mm. and the distocclusion does not exceed an end-to-end relationship. Again, profile analysis is the decisive factor for the use of this appliance.

The FR Ib (Fig. 15–16) differs from the FR Ia in that it has a lingual plate instead of a lingual bow (Fig. 15–17). Because the lingual plate requires less alveolar height than the U loops, it is possible to use the FR Ib also in the treatment of mixed dentitions. The FR Ib is easier to construct, as the U loops of the lingual bow in the FR Ia are difficult to bend and can easily cause discomfort to the patient if not properly made.

The design and location of the lingual parts of the mandibular portion of the appliance are shown in Figures 15–17 and 15–18. The lingual plate is connected to the buccal shields with a wire 1 mm. in diameter and is bent over the contact points between the first and second premolars. The contact is not trimmed, as the connecting wire should not be allowed to wedge between the two premolars. If that occurred, an undesirable forward tipping of the first premolars would result. Embedded in the lingual plate is a wire (0.9 mm. in di-

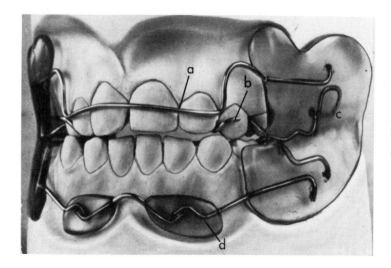

Figure 15-16. FR Ib: (a) labial bow, (b) canine loop, (c) buccal shield, and (d) lip pads.

Figure 15-17. FR Ib on the mandibular cast: (a) labial wire, (b) canine loop, (c) palatal bow, (d) lingual wires, (e) buccal shield, (f) lingual plate.

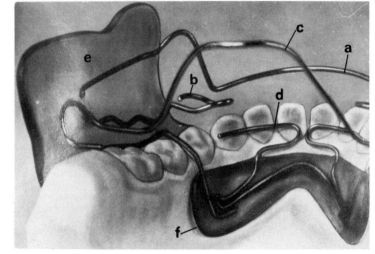

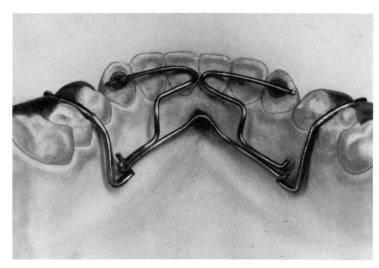

Figure 15-18. Lingual wires before application of acrylic (connecting wires to buccal shields should *not* be in contact with the mandibular teeth).

Figure 15-19. Slicing of the deciduous molars for FR I and FR II. Rad. E for canine loop; Rad. Pabü for palatal bow; E, canine loop; A, occlusal rest on maxillary second deciduous molar; Pabü, palatal bow.

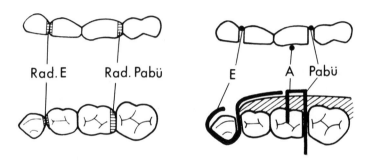

ameter) reinforcing the plate to prevent breakage at the midline where it is narrow because of the lingual frenum. The two lingual wires (0.8 mm. in diameter) emerge from the lingual plate in an occlusal direction and are then bent horizontally. They are kept from the incisors at a distance of 0.5 mm., about 3 mm. below their incisal edge. During the treatment, the lingual wires are brought into contact with the teeth if a retrusion of the mandibular incisors has to be corrected. Sometimes, toward the end of the treatment, the lingual wires are allowed to rest on the cingulum of the incisors to facilitate a leveling of the bite by their depressing action. According to the requirements of the case, lingual wires of 0.5 or 0.6 mm. diameter may be used to correct a strong lingual inclination of mandibular incisors, especially the central incisors, by active force. The wires may be fashioned differently to perform special tasks assigned to them.

When the FR Ib is used for treatment in the mixed dentition, the occlusal supports of the palatal bow are bent over the maxillary second deciduous molars (Fig. 15–19). The contacts between the deciduous canine and the first molar, and between the deciduous second molar and the first permanent molar, are carved away, but the mesial surface of the first permanent molar on the cast is not cut. In mixed dentition treatment, corresponding cuts will also be made on the teeth in the mouth before the appliance is inserted, because the occlusal surfaces of the deciduous molars are flat, and it would be difficult for the wires to lodge between the teeth. Construction bite for the FR Ib is taken in the same manner as for the FR Ia.

FR Ic

The FR Ic (Fig. 15–20) is indicated in the more severe Class II, Division 1 malocclusions, where the overjet is more than 7 mm. and the distocclusion exceeds an end-to-end cusp relationship. Immediate forward positioning of the mandible into a Class I relationship would not be tolerated by the patient because of the overjet; therefore, the construction bite is taken in an end-to-end molar relation (Fig. 15–21). After the mandible has become stabilized in this position, the FR Ic is adjusted by advancing the mandibular anterior part slightly forward so the mandible will again assume a more mesial position (Fig. 15–22). This forward adjustment is possible with the FR Ic because the buccal shields are split horizontally and vertically into two parts, so that the anterior part contains the wires for the lip pads and the lingual shield. The split buccal shields are held together by heavy horizontal wires, which are extensions of the connecting wires between the lingual plate and the buccal shield.

Cases treated with the FR I are shown in Figures 15–23 to 15–36.

Text continued on page 547

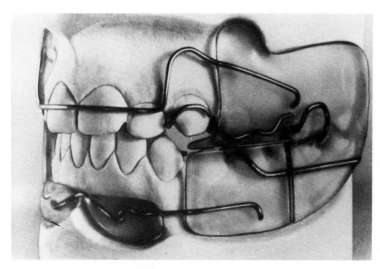

Figure 15–20. FR Ic. Note how the buccal shield may be split to pull the anterior part forward, moving lip pads anteriorly. Acrylic may then be added to stabilize the new relationship.

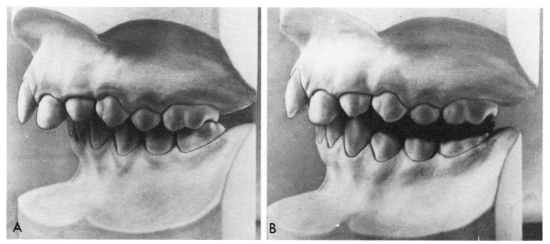

Figure 15–21. Construction bite for FR Ic is taken in an end-to-end molar relation. *A*, Habitual occlusion; *B*, construction bite relationship.

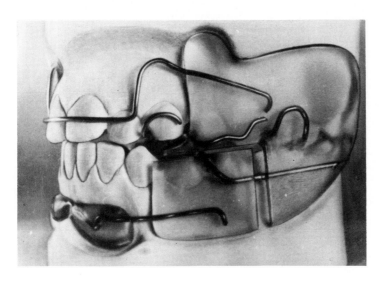

Figure 15–22. FR Ic advanced forward by pulling the mandibular anterior section of the appliance in a forward direction.

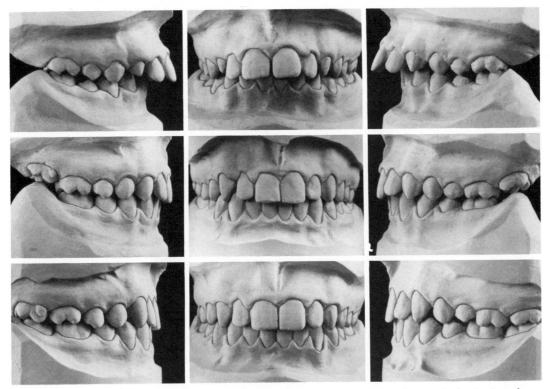

Figure 15–23.   Treatment with FR I. Patient B. P., male 12 years, 3 months of age at the beginning of treatment. Despite inadequate cooperation during the first year of treatment, a good result was obtained. Treatment time was nearly three years; retention lasted only half a year.

Casts and Measurements (mm.):	4|4	6|6	Maxillary Arch Length	4|4	6|6	Mandibular Arch Length
Top, beginning of treatment	37.0	48.5	24.5	37.0	49.0	18.5
Center, nearly 2 years later	40.5	51.0	19.5	38.5	51.0	18.0
Bottom, 3½ years later	42.5	53.5	19.0	39.5	54.0	14.0

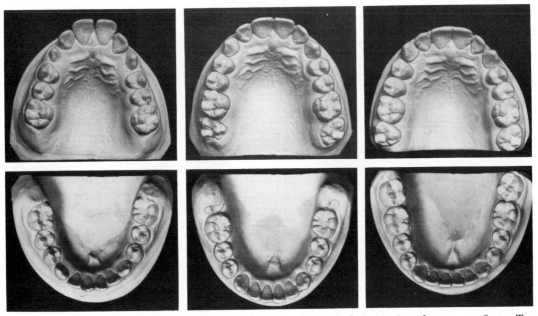

Figure 15–24.   Occlusal views of patient shown in Figure 15–23. *Left,* Beginning of treatment. *Center,* Two years later. *Right,* Three and one-half years later.

539

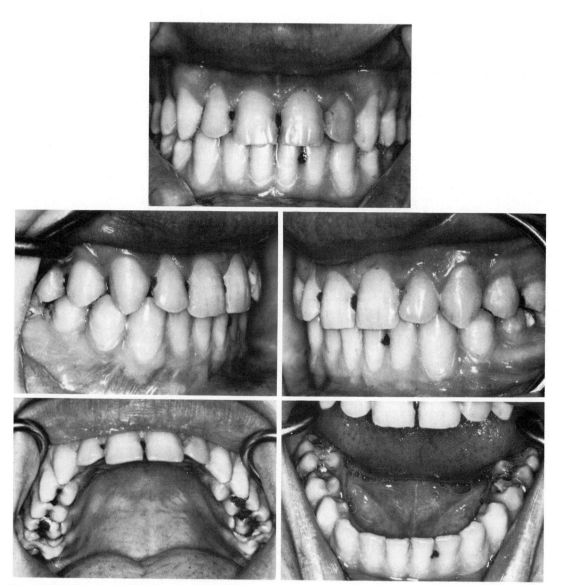

Figure 15–25. Dentition of patient B. P. (Figs. 15–23 and 15–24) three and a half years after wearing of appliance was discontinued. There is no relapse in arch width or in the region of the incisors. Dentoalveolar, palatal, and apical base expansion was well achieved.

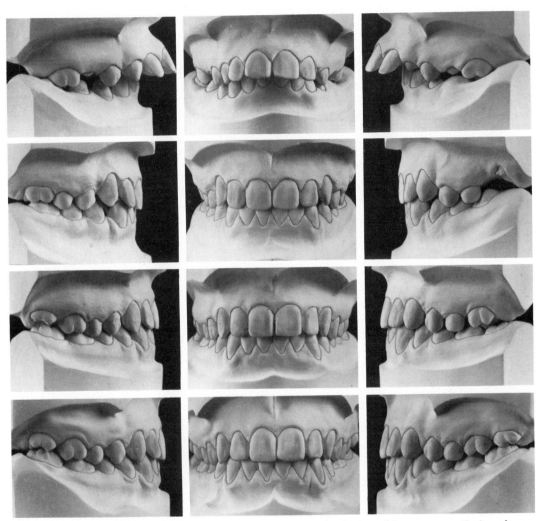

Figure 15–26. Patient J. N., male, age 9 years, 9 months at the beginning of the treatment. Carious destruction made extraction of all four first molars necessary. FR I was worn for a little over four years; retention lasted a little over two years.

Casts and Measurements (mm.):	4│4	Maxillary Arch Length
First row, beginning of treatment	35	26.5
Second row, 1½ years later	41	20.0
Third row, 6 years later	41.5	21.0
Fourth row, 8½ years later	41	21.0

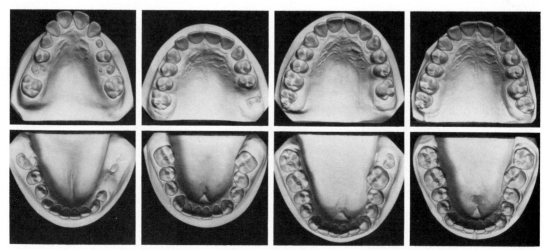

Figure 15-27. Occlusal views of patient shown in Figure 15-26. *Left,* Beginning of treatment. *Center left,* one and a half years later. *Center right,* six years later. *Right,* eight and a half years later.

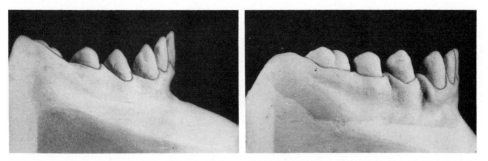

Figure 15-28. Lateral views of first and second mandibular casts of patient J. N. demonstrate the leveling of the bite as well as the uprighting of the tipped second molar. Time interval between the two casts was only one and a half years. This occurred without interference from any part of the appliance. Fränkel sees it as the consequence of keeping the cheeks away with the buccal shields. He assumes that molars are usually tipped lingually by the cheeks, inserting themselves between the maxillary and mandibular teeth.

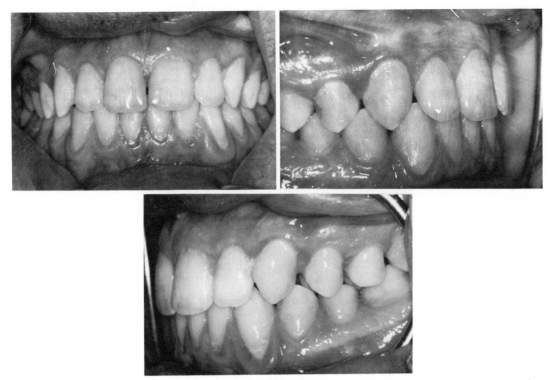

Figure 15–29. Patient J. N., three years out of retention. Six mm. expansion of the maxillary arch including apical base has been maintained, and the results were stable.

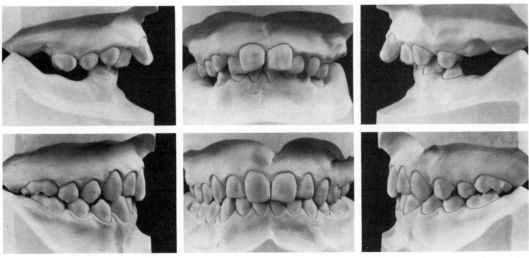

Figure 15–30. Patient S. K., girl, age 11 years, 2 months, at beginning of treatment. All four first molars were extracted prior to treatment. *Top row*, At beginning of treatment; bottom row, at end of treatment, three and a half years later.

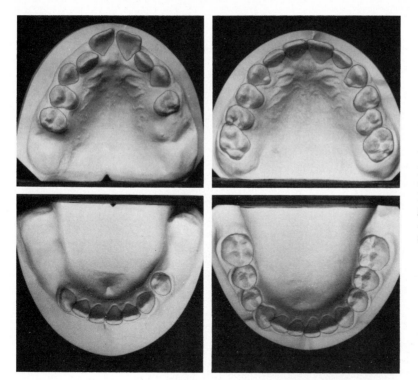

Figure 15-31. Occlusal views of patient shown in Figure 15-30. *Left,* At beginning of treatment. *Right,* At end of treatment, three and a half years later.

Figure 15-32. Cephalograms of patient S. K. demonstrate a typical development for this kind of treatment. Upper left cephalogram was taken at the beginning of treatment. Six months later (upper right) the mandible had moved forward and the patient was unable to occlude in a more posterior position, although only the incisors were in contact and there was a complete lateral open bite. Cephalogram taken one and a half years later (lower left) shows closing of bite. Last cephalogram (lower right) was taken three and a half years after the beginning of treatment.

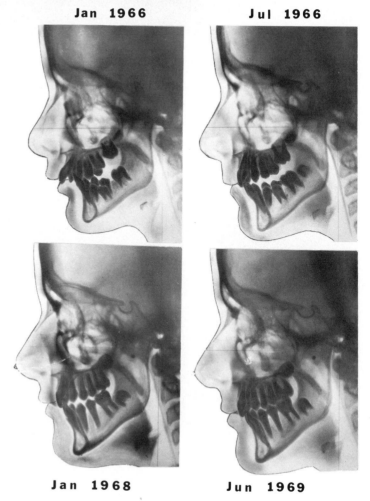

Jan 1966 **Jul 1966**

Jan 1968 **Jun 1969**

544

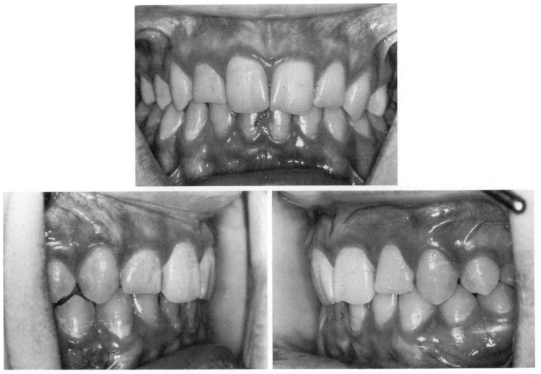

Figure 15–33. Post-treatment intraoral photographs of patient shown in Figure 15–32.

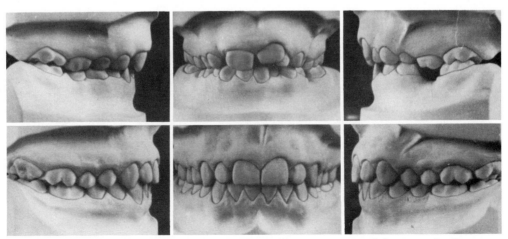

Figure 15–34. Patient T. T., age 8 years, male. Treatment in the mixed dentition. Appliance was worn day and night for two years; retention was done only at night for two years.

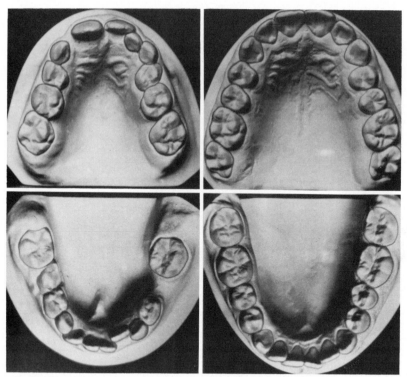

Figure 15–35.   Occlusal views of patient shown in Figure 15–34. *Left,* Before treatment. *Right,* After treatment.

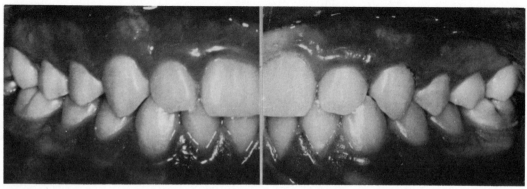

Figure 15–36.   Frontal view of patient shown in Figures 15–34 and 15–35, taken one and a half years out of retention.

FR II

The FR II (Fig. 15–37) is used for Class II, Division 2 malocclusions. If there is no strain in the facial musculature, the construction bite can be taken with the incisors in an edge-to-edge position; otherwise it is taken as for the FR Ic. If the maxillary incisors are retroclined, they should always first be tipped labially with an active plate.

The FR I is modified by adding a protrusion bow (0.8 mm. in diameter) behind the lingually inclined maxillary incisors (Fig. 15–38). The bow serves to maintain the protrusion of the maxillary incisors achieved before insertion of the FR II and eventually completes the labial tipping. The protrusion bow originates from the buccal shields and runs between the maxillary canines and the first premolar. Thus, it takes up the function of the canine loops in supporting the appliance against the maxilla. Therefore, the canine loops are bent differently in the FR II. They originate also from the buccal shield but embrace the canines buccally instead of lingually (Fig. 15–37).

Correction of the Class II, Division 2 malocclusion is achieved by changing the axial inclination of the maxillary incisors, by opening the vertical dimension, and by stimulating mandibular forward growth.

To avoid irritation on the inside of the lower lip in the vestibular fold, the lip pads in the FR II should be particularly well rounded because of the strong mentalis activity in Class II malocclusions. For the same reason, wearing of the FR II appliance should be started gradually, so that the patient's soft tissues become adjusted to the appliance.

As emphasized earlier, the firm seating of the appliance on the maxillary dentition is essential for the forward positioning of the mandible. The carving of the contacts between the first molar and the second premolar, and between the canine and the first premolar, is therefore a precondition for the effectiveness of the appliance. The mandibular movement, however, is not possible without removing the interference of the maxillary incisors first.

Cases treated with the FR II are shown in Figures 15–39 to 15–42.

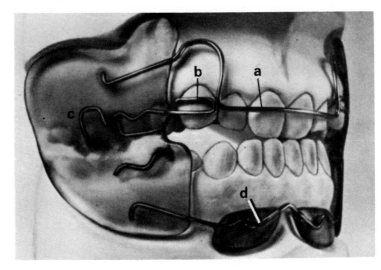

Figure 15–37. Function Corrector II. FR II in place on both maxillary and mandibular casts: (a) labial bow, (b) canine loop, (c) buccal shield, and (d) lip pads.

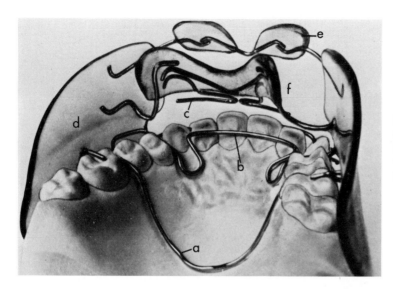

Figure 15-38. FR II on the maxillary cast: (a) palatal bow, (b) protrusion bow, (c) lingual wires, (d) buccal shield, (e) lip pads, and (f) lingual plate.

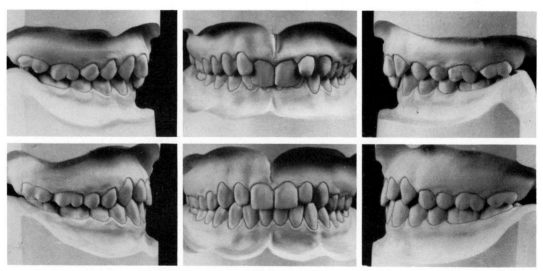

Figure 15-39.   Treatment with FR II. Girl, age 11 years, 7 months at beginning of treatment. *Top row,* At the beginning of treatment; *bottom row,* a little over two years later when active treatment was discontinued. Maxillary incisors were tipped forward by a plate prior to insertion of the function corrector. This procedure often makes it possible to complete treatment with one function corrector, because the construction bite can be taken immediately in a Class I relationship. In this case, two function correctors were needed, as it proved impossible to achieve Class I occlusion with the first.

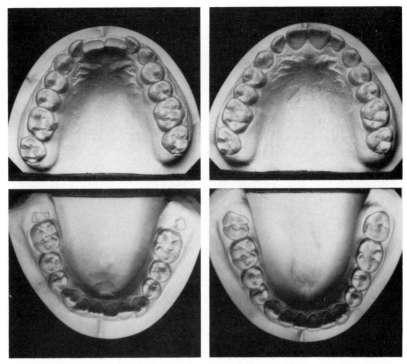

Figure 15–40. Occlusal views of patient shown in Figure 15–39. *Left*, Before treatment. *Right*, After two years of treatment.

Figure 15–41. Cephalograms of the patient shown in Figures 15–39 and 15–40 at beginning and end of treatment show the leveling of the bite and the resulting normal occlusion, as well as the correct relationship of the incisors.

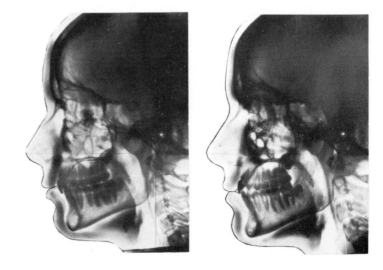

Mar 1967   Apr 1968

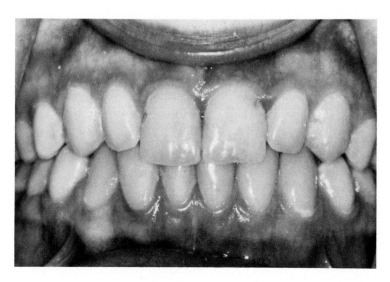

Figure 15-42. Intraoral view of patient in Figures 15-39 to 15-41 nearly three years after discontinuation of active treatment. Mandibular retention plate was still worn at this time.

FR III

The FR III (Fig. 15-43), which is used for the treatment of Class III malocclusions, also has buccal shields, but instead of lip pads in the mandibular anterior region, they are situated in the maxillary anterior region. The FR III has a palatal bow, a maxillary protrusion bow, a mandibular labial bow, and occlusal rests on the last mandibular molars.

The purpose of the lip pads is to eliminate the restricting pressure of the upper lip on the underdeveloped maxilla and to apply bone-stimulating tissue tension in the maxillary vestibular fold.

The pressure of the upper lip on the pads is transmitted by the appliance to the mandibular dentition with a distally directed force (Fig. 15-44). The mandible is held distally by a lower labial bow and by the buccal shields, which are in tight contact with the mandibular posterior teeth and the alveolar bone. In the FR III, the palatal bow has to run distally to the last maxillary molars to avoid a buttressing effect on the maxilla (Figs. 15-44 and 15-45). For the same

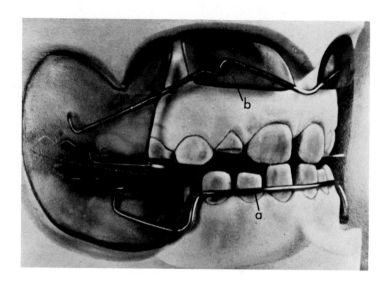

Figure 15-43. The FR III: (a) labial bow, (b) lip pads, and (c) buccal shields.

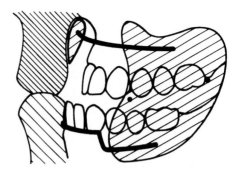

Figure 15–44. Schematic drawing of FR III. Maxillary lip pads are kept at a distance of about 3 mm. from the alveolar process. The pressure of the extended upper lip is transmitted by the lip pads on the buccal shields and on the mandibular dentition, which is gripped by the appliance. No acrylic part or wires impede the spontaneous development of the maxillary dentition and alveolar process.

reason, the protrusion bow crosses the alveolar crest well below the contact point between the canine and the first premolar.

Since the objective of the Class III treatment is to restrict mandibular growth and to stimulate maxillary growth, the buccal shields are constructed with this is mind. They are in contact with the mandibular teeth and the mandibular apical base; however, in the maxillary dentoalveolar area, they do not contact these structures. In this way, the buccinator mechanism is prevented from exerting pressure on the maxilla, and its development is stimulated. Likewise, the maxillary lip pads are kept about 2 to 3 mm. away from the alveolar process (see Figs. 15–44 and 15–50*B*). In addition, both the buccal shields and the lip pads are constructed to elicit bone-building stimulus by tension on the maxillary periosteum.

The construction bite is taken with the mandible in the most retruded position (Fig. 15–46). The bite is opened only enough to let the maxillary incisors move labially past the mandibular incisors. The amount of the bite opening is always kept at a minimum to make lip closure as easy as possible. The construction of the FR III varies slightly, depending on the amount of bite opening necessary to correct the anterior crossbite. If a deep bite is present, the bite is propped open with occlusal rests on the last maxillary molars (Fig. 15–47). These rests run between the occlusal surfaces of the maxillary molars and the palatal bow. If the overbite is very small, the occlusal rests on the last mandibular molars (Fig. 15–48), standard in all FR III's, are all that is needed to keep the bite open.

The maxillary cast has to be trimmed carefully. In the buccal shields this is done in the same way as for the FR I. In addition, the maxillary labial sulcus is trimmed for the lip pads. This trimming is done quite extensively after digital inspection. The pliable soft tissue under the upper lip will tolerate a deepening of the sulcus of about 5 mm. Proper trimming will position the lower margin of the lip pads at a distance of 7 to 8 mm. from the gingival border (see Fig. 15–43).

Figure 15–45. Relationship of maxillary protrusion bow (Probo) and palatal bow (Pabü) to the dentition.

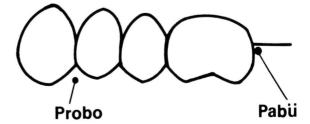

Probo　　　　　　　　**Pabü**

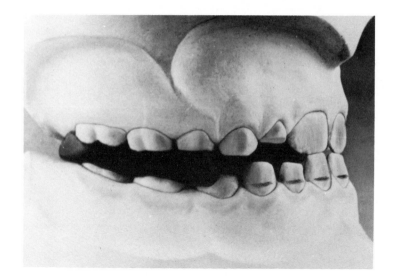

Figure 15–46. Construction bite for FR III. Note the marks on the incisors, which are scraped slightly to allow labial bow to fit tightly against teeth at this level on incisor and canine crowns.

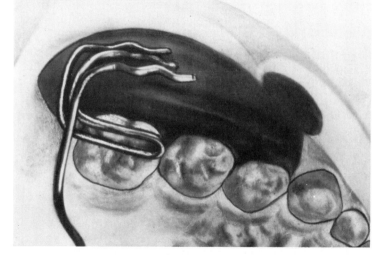

Figure 15–47. The occlusal rest on maxillary first molar in the FR III.

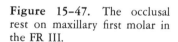

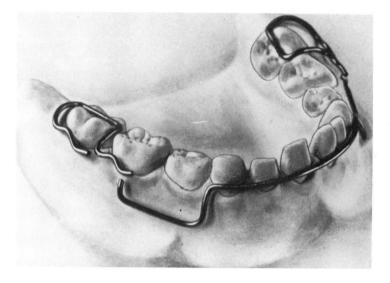

Figure 15–48. FR III: mandibular labial bow fitted into a groove carved across the labial surface of the six anterior teeth; occlusal rest on last mandibular molar. The low position of the labial bow prevents excessive lingual tipping of mandibular incisors.

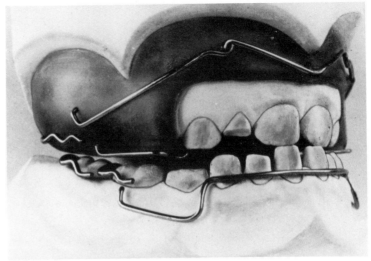

Figure 15-49. FR III with wires and wax padding before the application of cold-cure acrylic for the buccal shields and maxillary lip pads. Both shields and lip pads are 2 to 3 mm away from the vestibular mucosa. The periphery of these constructions, however, is at the fullest extension of the vestibule.

The buccal aspects of the maxillary teeth and alveolar process are again covered with wax, as in the construction of the FR I (Fig. 15–49). The wax layer under the lip pads should be 2 to 3 mm. thick, being thicker at the occlusal border. A 3 mm. thick wax padding will cover the buccal aspects of the maxillary lateral teeth.

The mandibular labial bow and the palatal bow are made of bent wire 1.0 to 1.1 mm. in diameter, the maxillary protrusion bow of 0.6 to 0.7 mm. diameter wire, and all the other wires of 0.9 mm. diameter wire. To ensure a close fit of the mandibular labial bow (see Figs. 15–43 and 15–48), a groove is carved on the plaster cast across the labial surface of the six anterior teeth, at the height of the papillae (see Fig. 15–46). If the labial bow is situated too high incisally, a pronounced retrusion of the mandibular incisors will occur. The occlusal rest for the last mandibular molar is bent to lie snugly in the occlusal fissure (see Fig. 15–48). The free ends are about 0.75 to 1 mm. away from the teeth and the mucosa.

The palatal bow originates in the buccal shields and has a shape similar to the palatal bow of the FR I and the FR II. It is kept about 0.5 mm. away from the palatal mucosa. As mentioned earlier, the bow has to run distally to the last maxillary molar to avoid buttressing against the maxilla (see Figs. 15–44, 15–45 and 15–47). For the same reason, the protrusion bow crosses the maxillary arch below the contact point between the canine and the first premolar. The bow contacts the maxillary incisors without pressure 2 mm. below the incisal edges. The wire must not contact the cinguli, as that would impede the eruption of the incisors.

With the wax padding in place and the wires fixed with modeling wax (Fig. 15–49), the acrylic can now be applied for the buccal shields and the lip pads. The shape of the buccal shields is illustrated in Figure 15–43. They are kept well away from the maxillary parts by the wax padding, but are in contact with the mandibular teeth and the alveolar process. The part of the shields that touches the gingival margins, however, has to be ground away to prevent irritation. The lip pads must be parallel to the slope of the alveolar process (Fig. 15–50*B*). When properly constructed, the lip pads will not touch the soft tissues and produce abrasions (Fig. 15–50*A*) when the patient opens his mouth and

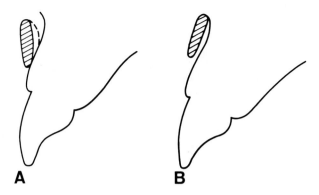

Figure 15–50. *A,* wrong, and *B,* correct position of maxillary lip pads.

the appliance is lowered with the mandible. As pointed out previously, the lip pads should extend well into the maxillary sulcus. The tension produced by the stretching of the soft tissues will also encourage maxillary development in an anterior direction. After the acrylic parts have been made, the margins of the buccal shields and lip pads are rounded and polished. The large surfaces of the appliance are also carefully polished.

In the course of treatment, the FR III is modified at certain times. A maxillary sagittal development is expected, and because of this, the mucosa may gradually contact the lip pads. If this happens, the tags of the wires holding the pads are freed by grinding away the acrylic around them (Fig. 15–51). The wires, which must be straight, are then pulled out of the buccal shields the necessary length to re-establish the right distance from the mucosa. When this has been accomplished, the holes are filled with cold-curing acrylic.

As treatment progresses, the maxillary and mandibular incisors will approach an edge-to-edge bite. At that time, the maxillary protrusion bow, until

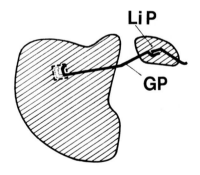

Figure 15–51. Forward adjustment of maxillary lip pads. Side and top view. Acrylic is set to permit wire to move forward in shield. New acrylic is then added.

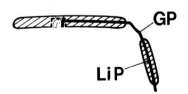

then only slightly in contact with the incisors, will be activated with a slight pressure against these teeth. It must be emphasized again that the wire must not press on the cinguli. The activation of the protrusion bow is meant to accelerate the labial movement of the maxillary incisors over the lower, to prevent "jiggling" of these teeth during the period when they alone contact the opposing mandibular teeth. As soon as the maxillary incisors are well over their mandibular counterparts, the maxillary stabilizing wires are removed. The occlusal rests on the mandibular molars are left intact. After that, the lateral open bite produced in the course of the treatment will gradually close.

Cases treated with the FR III are shown in Figures 15–52 to 15–55.

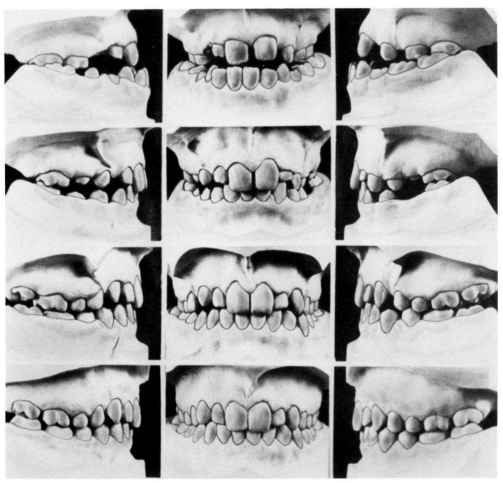

Figure 15–52. Patient R. Q. Male, age 10 years, 3 months at the beginning of treatment with FR III; dental age, however, was only about 8 years.

Top row, At the beginning of treatment; *second row,* after treatment with FR III for 20 months; *third row,* after retention of 2½ years (appliance only at night); appliance was removed after 2 more years of retention; *fourth row,* 1½ years after the appliance was entirely discarded.

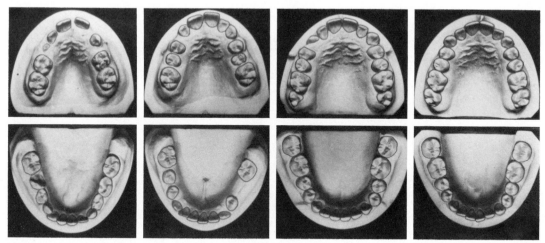

Figure 15-53.   Occlusal views of patient shown in Figure 15–52. *Left,* At beginning of treatment. *Center left,* After 20 months of treatment. *Center right,* After two and a half years in retention. *Right,* After one and a half years of retention.

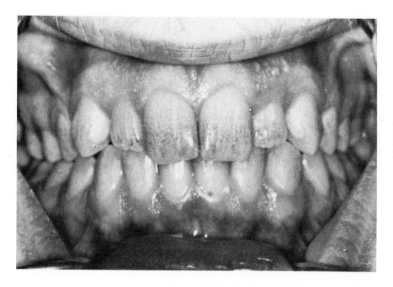

Figure 15-54.   Patient R. Q. (Figs. 15–52 and 15–53) at age 20 years.

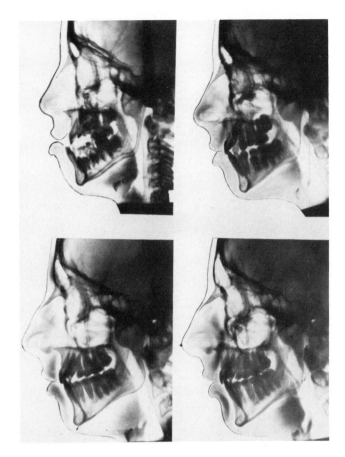

Figure 15–55. Cephalograms of patient R. Q. (Figs. 15–52 to 15–54). *Upper left,* At the beginning of treatment; *upper right,* 2 years later; *lower left,* after a period of retention of 2 years; *lower right,* after further retention for 10 months. Maxillary-mandibular plane angle decreased 9 degrees, gonial angle decreased 10 degrees, Na-ANS distance increased 9 mm., but Me-ANS distance increased only 3 mm.

FR IV

The last of the function correctors is the FR IV (Fig. 15–56), which is used for the correction of open bites and bimaxillary protrusions. It is used almost exclusively in the mixed dentition. In open bites of the permanent dentition, ei-

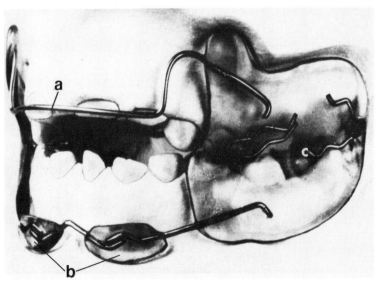
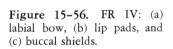

Figure 15–56. FR IV: (a) labial bow, (b) lip pads, and (c) buccal shields.

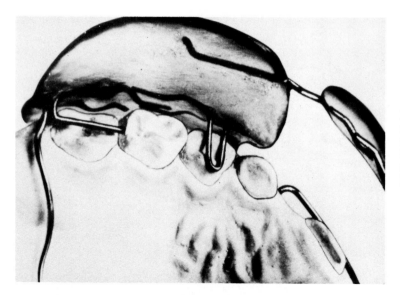

Figure 15-57. FR IV on maxillary cast. Note placement of occlusal rests and palatal bow, with canine loops being absent. There is no protrusion bow here, as in FR 2.

ther the FR I or the FR III is used, depending on jaw relationship. The FR IV has two buccal shields, two lower lip pads, a maxillary labial bow, a palatal bow, and four occlusal rests (on the maxillary first molars and deciduous first molars) to prevent tipping of the appliance (Fig. 15–57). The main objective of this appliance is to encourage normal muscle function and to establish a proper oral seal.

The construction of the FR IV is shown in Figures 15–56 and 15–57. The palatal bow is always placed behind the last molar. The occlusal rests may be adapted to the requirements of the particular case. They must not, however, impede the shifting of the appliance in a dorsal direction. Therefore, any trimming of interdental contacts or lodging occlusal rests between the teeth has to be avoided. For the treatment of bimaxillary protrusion, a mandibular labial bow (0.8 to 0.9 mm. diameter wire), similar to that of the FR III, may be added.

Mode of Action of the Function Corrector

It should be emphasized that the therapeutic effect of the function corrector is based on its interception of aberrations of the muscle function. The function corrector is not a tooth-moving orthodontic appliance. Neither is its mode of action the same as that of other (that is, activator type) functional appliances. The latter are in contact with the teeth and the alveolar bone and exert muscular pressure on these structures through the appliance, whereas the function corrector withholds muscle pressure from the developing jaw and dentoalveolar areas.

The function corrector, with its special biomechanical design, is capable of producing the following therapeutic changes in the orofacial complex:

1. Increase of transverse and sagittal intraoral space.
2. Increase of vertical intraoral space.
3. Forward positioning of the mandible.

4. Development of new patterns of motor function, improvement of muscle tonus, and establishment of proper oral seal.

1. *Increase of transverse and sagittal intraoral space* is achieved mainly through the buccal shields and the lip pads. Mechanical pressure on the perioral soft tissue band is regarded as an important factor in dentoalveolar crowding and arrested basal bone development. The buccal shields and lip pads eliminate the harmful mechanical pressure, thus favoring the forces acting on the inside of the oral cavity (tongue). According to Fränkel, when the forces of the cheeks are eliminated, the tooth tips laterally in the direction of least resistance. The alveolar walls in the coronal area are, likewise, deformed to the buccal. Although the root tip tends to deform the buccoapical area to the lingual, this movement is resisted by the thick lingual wall and the strong stretching effect of the buccal shield on the vestibular fold, with the resultant movement to the buccal (Fig. 15–58). Thus, the lateral movement of the teeth is not a tipping one, but a bodily tooth movement. The maxillary lip pads in the Class III treatment function in the same way, developing the maxillary base anteriorly without forward tipping of the maxillary incisors.

In addition to widening the dentoalveolar arches by deformation and transformation of the alveolar wall, the buccal shields and lip pads widen the arches by new bone formation in the apical base. Fränkel believes that the continuous stretching of the connective tissue fibers in the vestibular fold stimulates bone formation.

It is, however, important to note that the transverse and sagittal development of the apical base is possible only as long as there is still natural growth potential left. Possibilities for widening the mandibular base are over, therefore, around the age of nine, whereas the maxillary base can be widened for much longer. Accordingly, the optimal treatment time is the mixed dentition period.

2. *Increase of vertical intraoral space* is possible because the construction bite is taken so that, as the mandible is held forward, the bite is opened in the posterior segments. The elongation of the posterior teeth takes place according to the same principle that operates with anterior bite planes and activators, except

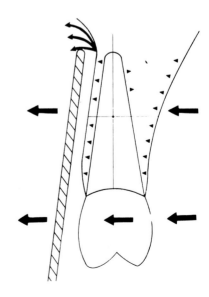

Figure 15–58. The effect of the buccal shield on the lateral expansion and bodily buccal movement of teeth. In the mixed dentition the buccal plate is very thin and quite active under the periosteum.

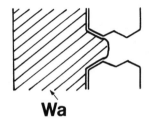

Wa

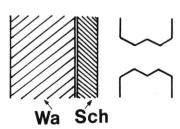

Wa Sch

Figure 15–59. Cheeks (Wa) interposed between maxillary and mandibular teeth without an appliance (above), and kept away by buccal shield (Sch) (below).

that in the treatment with the function corrector, buccal shields prevent the buccal soft tissue from invaginating between the teeth (Fig. 15–59). Fränkel believes that disturbance in vertical development is more often caused by the cheeks than by the effect of the tongue. According to Fränkel's experience, a spontaneous uprighting of mandibular teeth and leveling of the curve of Spee is always observed with the use of buccal shields, granting that there is space mesiodistally (see Fig. 15–28).

3. *Forward positioning of the mandible.* The proponents of the activator-type functional appliances claim that these appliances stimulate mandibular growth. However, there is evidence to show that sagittal improvement caused by these appliances is due to dentoalveolar changes and that these appliances tend to tip the mandibular incisors labially. The mode of action of the function corrector is different, and, therefore, it should not be grouped together with the activator-type appliances.

In the treatment with the function corrector, the position of the mandible is changed through gradual training of the protractor and retractor muscles, followed by condylar rebuilding. The lingual shield (or the U loops of the lingual bow) guide the mandible to a mesial position (Fig. 15–60). Whenever

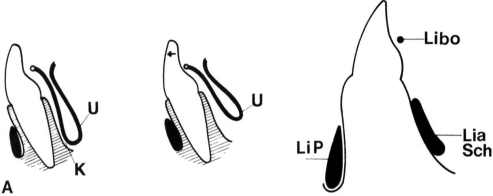

Figure 15–60. The effect of the U-loop and lingual plate on mandibular positioning through pressure sensation. The wires should not be in contact with the lingual surface of the incisors.

the mandible drops back, the pressure sensation on the lingual side of the alveolar process reactivates the protractor muscles, which are gradually conditioned to hold the mandible in the position determined by the construction bite. It is important not to overactivate these muscles. Therefore, the mandible is moved mesially in steps in the more severe Class II conditions (FR Ic). Fränkel is convinced that the stepwise mandibular forward positioning is each time followed by a renewed growth stimulation in the condylar process.

In order to change the position of the mandible without tipping the mandibular incisors forward, it is essential that the lingual bow or the lingual wires not be in contact with these teeth (Fig. 15–60). Also, to be successful, the patient should wear the appliance constantly.

4. *Development of new patterns of motor function, improvement of muscle tonus, and establishment of proper oral seal.* At the same time that the function corrector prevents the abnormal muscle forces from exerting their influence on the bony structures, it rehabilitates the muscles that have caused the deformity. The buccal shields and the lip pads massage the soft tissues, improving blood circulation. The shields loosen up tight muscles and improve tonicity where it is lacking. The buccal shields and the mandibular lip pads stretch the muscles of the buccinator mechanism in distoclusions (Fig. 15–61). The mandibular lip pads also prevent the action of an overactive mentalis muscle and, by supporting the lower lip, assist in establishing a proper oral seal.

After the insertion of the appliance, all movements—speaking, swallowing, and mimic movement—become muscle gymnastics. Therefore, conscious muscle exercises on the patient's part are not always necessary. However, if the perioral musculature is weak and flaccid and the patient habitually keeps the lips apart, it is essential to the success of the treatment that the patient make a special effort to keep his lips closed at all times. Because this is very difficult to

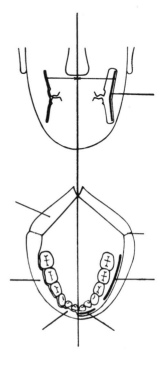

Figure 15–61. Effect of appliance on musculature. On the right side of the face, lateral soft tissues rest on dentition; on the left side, the buccal shield and lip pad take the pressure off the dental arches.

remember, the parent should give the child every morning a card with the letter "L" to remind him at school to keep the lips closed. The parents should control this by making a notation in a calendar every day. The patient is also asked to use certain lip exercises, such as holding a tongue blade or a slip of paper between the lips while watching television or reading.

In Class III malocclusions, where the tongue lies deep in the oral cavity, the patient is taught to improve the tongue position by lifting the tongue up against the narrowed maxilla and making clicking sounds with the tongue against the palate. The function corrector leaves the oral cavity free, which is a great advantage over the functional appliances. The movements of the tongue are not restricted by the bulk of the appliance, and the tongue can exert its molding effect on the palate and the maxillary apical base.

Clinical Handling of the Function Corrector

Before the appliance is inserted in the mouth, the margins of the acrylic parts are inspected for smoothness. The correct seating of the appliance on the maxilla and the mandible is examined separately. The shields should have the required distance from the alveolar parts to facilitate widening of the dental arches. The margins of the shields and pads should fit exactly in the sulci, but there should be no blanching of the mucosa. Blanching is most likely to occur in the region of the buccal frenula and the lower margin of the lip pads. The lip pads should be in a vertical position. If the lower margins tilt forward, the upper margins of the pads will rub against the mucosa as the patient opens and closes the mouth. A faulty position of the pads can be corrected by grinding a groove with a small fissure bur around the wire connecting the pads and then removing the wire. The position of the pads, now connected only with the buccal shields, is adjusted properly, and the connecting wire is inserted with cold-curing acrylic. Once the position of the lip pads is correct, there will never be any irritation at the depth of the sulcus. One has only to watch for irritation on the inside of the lower lip.

Although the function corrector is worn by the patient all the time (except while eating or brushing the teeth), the treatment with this appliance is started slowly and carefully, so that the patient's soft tissues, mucosa, and musculature can get used to the appliance gradually. The FR I and FR II should be used only one to two hours daily during the first two weeks. Then the patient's soft tissues are examined carefully, and if there is irritation, necessary grinding and adjustments are made.

During the next three weeks, the patient is allowed to wear the function corrector two to three hours during the day. If, after this time, the mucosa looks healthy, the patient is instructed to wear the appliance all day, but not at night. The patient should be completely adapted to wearing the FR I or FR II during the day before the appliance is worn at night. This usually takes two months. If the patient has not adapted to holding the constructed mesial position of the mandible, the jaw will drop back in sleep, and abrasions of the mucosa are likely to result. Patients become adjusted to wearing the FR III more readily; therefore, it can usually be worn at night after the first two weeks.

The appliance and treatment progress should be checked at four-week intervals. The mucosa of the vestibule is examined at every visit. Should abrasions exist, the shields and pads are polished and adjusted.

During the treatment, only a few changes are made with the appliance. In the FR I and FR II, the palatal bow and the canine loops (or the protrusion bow) should lodge well into the proximal spaces. As the teeth erupt, these wires will begin to impinge on the interdental papillae. When that happens, the canine loops (protrusion bow) should be bent occlusally and the molar supports on the maxillary first molars should be bent cervically to relieve the pressure. In the treatment of the Class II, Division 1 malocclusions with protruding maxillary incisors, the labial bow is activated slowly and carefully. The labial bow should contact the maxillary incisors with only minimal pressure. Too much pressure would cause the labial arch to slide gingivally and destabilize the appliance. To avoid this, a protrusion bow, similar to the one used in the FR II, can be added on the lingual side. The bow should rest on the cingula of the incisors in order to provide the necessary vertical support. Each time the labial bow is activated, the protrusion bow should be activated the same amount.

When the FR I or the FR II has been worn day and night for two months, improvement in transverse, sagittal, and vertical directions should be observed. After one more month, a lateral open bite should be apparent. This also is evidence of the proper cooperation of the patient. If cooperation has been adequate, an initial end-to-end molar relationship will be corrected in six months. With more severe cases necessitating the use of FR 1c, the distal relationship should be corrected in nine months. During the final phase of the treatment, the lateral open bite will close.

The adjustments for the FR III were discussed in connection with design of this appliance (see p. 554).

Treatment Timing

It is obvious that we can expect the best therapeutic effect from the function corrector during the time when the occlusion is forming and the soft and bony tissues are undergoing their most accelerated growth changes.

Optimum time to start the treatment is when the child is about $7\frac{1}{2}$ years old, or when the lower lateral incisors have erupted. However, Class III and open bite treatments should be begun as soon as the first molars have erupted. Treatment in the deciduous dentition is not advocated, because children at that age level are usually not mature enough to cooperate with the treatment. After the lower lateral incisors have erupted, the treatment plan is easier to make, and the lateral growth potential is still present. After the mandibular canines and premolars have erupted, stimulation of transverse development in the mandibular arch is limited. In the maxilla, however, possibilities for arch expansion are still good, even at a later age.

It is not recommended that treatment with the function corrector be started in the late mixed dentition, when the deciduous teeth already show advanced root resorption. It is better to wait until the maxillary premolars and the mandibular canines and first premolars have erupted. Only then is good intermaxillary stabilization possible.

Active treatment in the early period should last one and a half to two years, followed by a retention period of two years. If the treatment is started in the permanent dentition, a retention period of two to three years is needed. A long retention time is needed especially in Class II, Division 2 cases and in Class III cases.

The function corrector is of limited value in the treatment of difficult orthodontic problems in the permanent dentition. This is especially true of Class I malocclusion, the correction of which requires such controlled tooth movements as rotations and bodily movement. However, good results can be achieved in the permanent dentition in the treatment of deep bites and distoclusions. Sagittal change of mandibular position is still possible after puberty.

The function corrector is not an easy appliance to construct and to handle. Therefore, the inexperienced practitioner is advised to begin with the simpler malocclusions and not to treat the most severe neuromuscular skeletal problems immediately. The beginner is advised to start with Class III malocclusions, which usually can be treated successfully with the FR III, an appliance that is relatively easy to handle. With experience, it is then possible to treat the more difficult malocclusions with the more complex appliance construction.

Preconditions for the Success of Treatment

In addition to the proper appliance construction and handling, there are three important preconditions to achieving success in treatment with the function corrector:

1. The right indications for treatment.
2. The right psychological introduction of the appliance.
3. Cooperation of the patient and the parents.

These considerations are valid for any kind of orthodontic therapy, but are of significantly greater importance with the kind of treatment described here.

The cooperation of the patient, properly encouraged by the parents, is generally easier to obtain than one would expect, considering the size of the appliance and the necessity of wearing it continuously except during meals. There are only minor parts of the appliance inside the dental arches, so the speech impediment is minimal, even from the beginning. In fact, the children speak quite normally immediately after the appliance has been inserted.

An important factor in achieving a good cooperation from the patient is the right introduction of the appliance. The dramatic facial improvement brought about by the changed position of the mandible, the elimination of the mentolabial sulcus by the lower lip pads, the disappearance of the nasolabial fold, and support of the upper lip by the upper lip pads should be pointed out to children and parents. Therefore, it is essential that the appliance be made in such a way that after insertion the patient's facial contours are truly improved. Making the appliance too bulky would have the opposite effect on the child's face.

An important part of therapy with the function corrector is the patient's cooperation in carrying out the aforementioned lip exercises. These exercises are started as soon as the patient is accepted for treatment, before the insertion of an appliance. The patient must be reminded constantly to keep the lips closed.

Remarkable results achieved by the use of the FR have been reported by Fränkel and others. These results, and especially the demonstration of patients at the orthodontic clinic in Zwickau, GDR, are most impressive. Statistics on the widening of the dental arches, including the apical base and other dimensions, have been published. Fränkel has apparently been able to substantiate with cephalometric data his claim that the FR can bring about forward growth of the mandible.

The significant and stable expansion of the dental arches achieved as a result of treatment with the FR is contrary to the present generally skeptical attitude about the advantage and stability of such therapy. Lasting success should be dependent on how long the new form of the dentition is in harmony with the balance of lingual and labiobuccal muscular forces after treatment. A similar concern is valid for the forward positioning of the mandible, the maintenance of which needs a new dynamic equilibrium between the protractor and the retractor muscles.

This abbreviated account of Fränkel's explanations for the philosophy and operation of the function corrector omits most of the detailed and well-argued theoretical considerations in his writings, as well as the arguments in support of his concept which have appeared in publications on orthodontic research and related fields of knowledge. To learn more, the student of this novel and exciting method of therapy should turn to the original writings of Fränkel, which will add considerably to the practical and theoretical knowledge gained thus far.

References

1. Fränkel, R.: Funktionskieferorthopädie und der Mundvorhof als apparative Basis. Berlin, VEB Verlag Volk und Gesundheit, 1967.
2. Fränkel, R.: Technik und Handhabung der Funktionsregler. Berlin, VEB Verlag Volk und Gesundheit, 2nd ed., 1976.
3. Fränkel, R.: The theoretical concept underlying treatment with function correctors. Trans. Eur. Orthod. Soc., 1966, pp. 233–250.
4. Fränkel, R.: Treatment of Class II Division 1 malocclusion with functional correctors. Am. J. Orthod. 55:265–275, 1969.
5. Fränkel, R.: The functional matrix and its practical importance in orthodontics. Trans. Eur. Orthod. Soc., 1969, pp. 207–218.
6. Fränkel, R.: Maxillary retrusion in Class III and treatment with the function corrector III. Trans. Eur. Orthod. Soc., 1970, pp. 249–259.
7. Fränkel, R.: Decrowding during eruption under the screening influence of vestibular shields. Am. J. Orthod. 65:372, 406, 1974.
8. Fränkel, R., and Reiss, W.: Zur Problematik der Unterkiefer nachentwicklung der Distalbissfällen. Fortschr. Kieferorthop., 31:345–355, 1970.
9. Fränkel, R.: The guidance of eruption without extraction. Trans. Eur. Orthod. Soc., 1971, pp. 303–316.
10. Falck, F.: Vergleichende Untersuchungen uber die Entwicklung der apikalen Basis nach kieferorthopädischer Behandlung mit der aktiven Platten und dem Funktionsregler. Fortschr. Kieferorthop., 30:225, 1969.
11. Logan, W. R.: The vestibular appliance. Trans. Br. Soc. Study Orthod. Dent. Pract., 19:287, 1969.
12. Logan, W. R.: The clinical management of the Fränkel appliance Fr I. Trans. Br. Soc. Study Orthod. Dent. Pract., 21:205, 1971.
13. Eirew, H. L.: Dynamic functional appliances. Trans. Br. Soc. Study Orthod. Dent. Pract., 19: 287, 1969.
14. Adams, C. P.: An investigation into indications for and the effects of the function regulator. Trans. Eur. Orthod. Soc., 1969, p. 293.
15. Adams, C. P.: The design and construction of removable appliances, 4th ed. Bristol, John Wright & Sons, Ltd., 1970.
16. Renfroe, E. W.: The philosophy of extraction in orthodontic treatment. Trans. Eur. Orthod. Soc., 1966, p. 56.

17. Sather, A. H., and Nelson, D. H.: Effects of muscular anchorage appliances on deficient mandibular arch length. Am. J. Orthod., *60*:68, 1971.
18. Moss, M. L.: The primacy of functional matrices in orofacial growth. Dent. Pract., *19*:65, 1968.
19. Moss, M. L.: Differential roles of periosteal and capsular functional matrices in orofacial growth. Trans. Eur. Orthod. Soc., *45*:193, 1969.
20. Moss, M. L., and Salentijn, L.: The primary role of functional matrices in facial growth. Am. J. Orthod., *55*:566, 1969.
21. Moss, M. L., and Salentijn, L.: The capsular matrix. Am. J. Orthod., *56*:474, 1969.
22. Moss, M. L., and Salentijn, L.: Differences between the functional matrices in anterior open-bite and in deep over-bite. Am. J. Orthod., *60*:264, 1971.
23. Pac, J.: The early treatment of Class III malocclusion by the vestibule-plate. Trans. Eur. Orthod. Soc., *46*:239, 1970.
24. Leighton, B. G.: The value of prophecy in orthodontics. Dent. Pract., *21*:359, 1971.

CHAPTER 16

Removable Appliances with Extraoral Force

THE COMBINATION OF FIXED AND REMOVABLE APPLIANCES

In this world of either fixed or removable appliances, traditionally thought of as the American or European approach, there is an in-between approach which may combine some elements of both philosophies and produce treatment results that are attained more simply and successfully. Indeed, the combination or sequential use of removable and fixed appliances in certain categories of malocclusions and for certain specific treatment objectives may prove superior to either the fixed or the removable approach alone. We are all well aware of the criticisms leveled at removable appliances for trying to do too much with underpowered and limited tools with the persistent problems of partial correction and the need for compromise tooth extraction. And there is the equally valid concern for the overcomplexity of certain fixed appliance philosophies, which require a high level of technical training and competence, limiting both their use and the number of patients that can be served. In this era of expanding service under third-party payment plans and the proliferating demand for mixed dentition treatment, a rational approach to mechanotherapy is essential.

Since this book is devoted to removable appliances, the emphasis will be on the primary use of such devices, with minimal fixed appliances. For many years, American orthodontic specialists have been using bite plates, bite blocks, guide planes, palatal expansion appliances, removable canine retraction appliances, and the like to augment full-banded therapy. These will not be discussed in this chapter. Rather, the reader is referred to texts like *Current Orthodontic Concepts and Techniques* by the authors for a comprehensive handling of the subject.[1] Suffice it to say that removable appliances are quite valuable in the correction of overbite, crossbite, and impacted and malposed canines. Removable appliance texts, such as Schwarz's *Lehrgang der Gebissregelung*, also demonstrate the ingenious use of simple fixed appliance elements for correction of individual tooth malpositions, such as rotated or impacted teeth, in conjunction with active plates.[2] This chapter stresses fixed appliance augmentation in basal jaw malrelationship correction.

Class I malocclusions, with arch length problems, individual tooth irregularities, and crowding may make up the most frequent type of malocclusion in a broad population sample. But in the orthodontic practice, anteroposterior jaw malrelationships comprise the largest number of cases. In this group, Class II malocclusion is most frequent. The teeth are where they are because of the abnormal jaw malrelationship, aided and abetted by deforming and adaptive muscular activity. The correction of the anteroposterior dysplasia must be a prime treatment objective. With fixed appliances, great reliance has been placed on the use of intermaxillary elastics to achieve the correction. Depending on the particular technique, greater or lesser emphasis is placed on extraoral force to guide growth and to eliminate the apical base discrepancy. Then individual tooth malpositions are corrected by precise adjustments of arch wires and appurtenances.

Proponents of removable appliances are no less concerned with jaw malrelationships. The functional appliances, as exemplified by the Andresen activator, also attempt to correct the anteroposterior abnormality by moving the mandible forward with appliance guidance. The hope is to alleviate the apical base dysplasia, to reduce any discrepancies in the anteroposterior height ratios, and to retract maxillary anterior teeth and alveolar bone. If all Class II malocclusions were either mandibular retrusions or maxillary protrusions, the challenge would be clearer. The actual situations, however, are often combinations of both, creating the difficult task of assessing just how much mandibular underdevelopment is combined with maxillary anterior protrusion. The role of the lip musculature is significant, enhancing the discrepancy and probably having an effect on the anterior teeth in both the maxilla and mandible. Removable appliances seem effective in moving and holding the mandible forward (as the various chapters in this book tend to demonstrate). However, the retrusive effect on the maxillary complex is limited and often inadequate.

The perceptive diagnostician must first determine the area of greatest abnormality and then utilize the appliances that correct the malocclusion. In practice, he must compromise, with an arbitrary correction of the excessive overjet and basal dysplasia, concentrating on mechanotherapy that eliminates overjet but does not necessarily attack the primary area of abnormality. Many treatment procedures compromise by dragging lower teeth forward or tipping upper teeth excessively lingually, leaving the abnormal apical base relationship. Or therapy provides only a partial correction, requiring artificial tooth position goals, which are not likely to be stable in the face of dominant morphogenetic pattern and perioral muscle function.

Fixed mechanotherapy has also compromised, putting teeth in proper occlusion with normal overjet, but often at the expense of correct tooth to basal bone relationships within each jaw. Intermaxillary elastic traction has been the primary tool in this type of therapy. More effective is the use of extraoral appliances, as they attach to tooth-borne appliances, in an effort to eliminate maxillary protrusion and abnormal muscle activity. Even when it is possible to predict a probable downward or downward and backward growth of the mandible, extraoral force is directed against the maxilla to harmonize direction and increments of movement in this area with mandibular pattern. Orthopedics is a term that has been used by followers of both fixed and removable appliances. But true orthopedic guidance seems to be routinely possible only with extraoral force.

The ACCO of Margolis

Fixed appliances have no monopoly on utilization of extraoral force. Orthodontists started using facebows with modified Hawley retainers many years ago, when there was a dominant Class II pattern. Spengeman devised several varieties of removable appliances to hold back relapsing maxillary arches[3] (Fig. 16–1). Margolis started doing the same thing and realized that removable appliance–extraoral force combinations could not only serve as good retainers, but could actually be used as effective corrective mechanisms.[4] He called his appliance the ACCO (Figs. 16–2 to 16–5). Hundreds of orthodontists on the east coast of the United States have used this appliance in one form or another. Tennenbaum and Gabriel, of Argentina, have modified the appliance somewhat for treatment of both bilateral and unilateral Class II malocclusions and claim a high degree of success[5] (Figs. 16–6 and 16–7). The adaptation of acrylic over the labial wire of the Hawley type retainer gives added stability and better

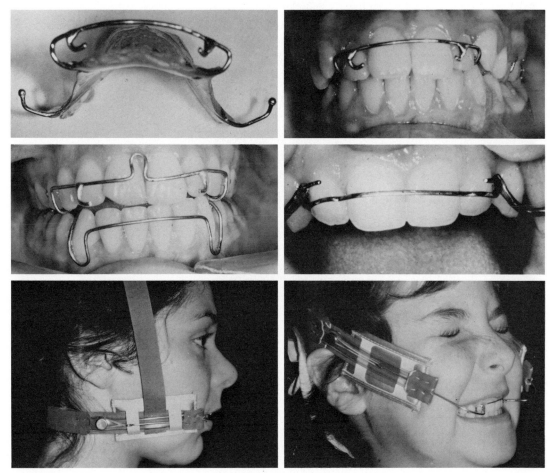

Figure 16–1. Modified Hawley-type maxillary retainer with spurs to receive extraoral force arms (J hooks). Labial bow may be plain (*top row*), or may have loops either in canine area or in incisor region (*middle, left*). Spurs may be below or above labial wire (*middle, right*). Conventional or high-pull headgear may be used (*lower row*). (Courtesy of Walter Spengeman.)

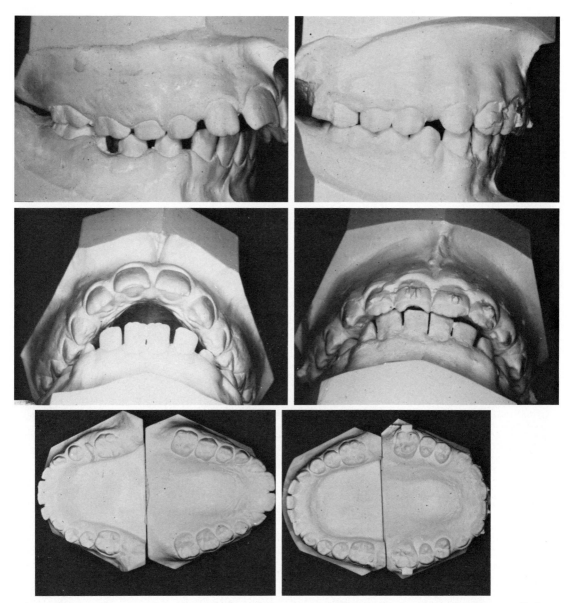

Figure 16-2. Plaster models of case demonstrating use of ACCO by Herbert Margolis. *Top row,* Before treatment with ACCO and nine months later, with bands placed to finish correction of incisor malpositions and to close spaces. *Middle row,* Frontal views showing change over same time interval. *Bottom row,* Occlusal views showing space reduction in both arches, but significant improvement in maxillary arch form in maxillary cast. (Courtesy of Herbert Margolis.)

retention to the appliance and reduces the tipping action that might occur, because of the reception of the extraoral force arms in the anterior region.

Margolis feels that the ACCO (AC for acrylic, CO for cervico-occipital anchorage) also prevents relapse of the torque adjustments that may have been achieved with fixed appliances. A conventional Hawley retainer neither holds the anteroposterior correction of the interdigitation nor the axial inclination of

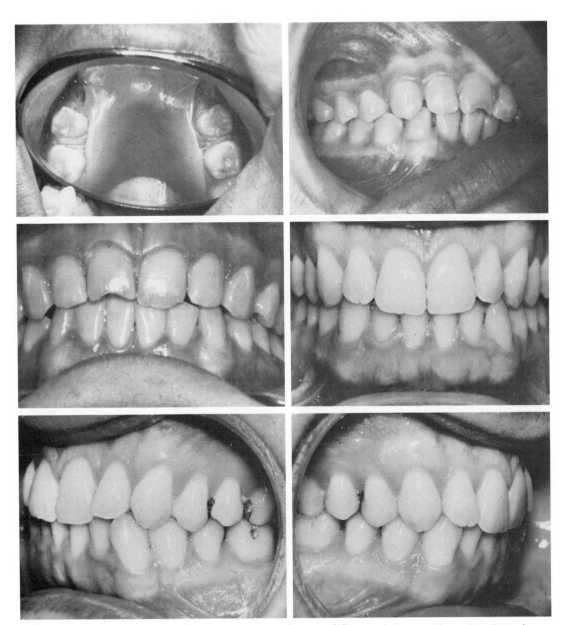

Figure 16-3. Intraoral views of patient in Figure 16-2. *Top left,* Palatal aspect with acrylic trimmed away from interproximal areas to allow distalization of buccal segments. Finger springs are against mesial surfaces of second deciduous molars. Usually only one side is activated at a time. *Top right,* Right side after 17 months' therapy with ACCO and "saddle arch." *Middle left,* Correction achieved by 17 months' therapy. *Middle right,* Frontal view 20 years later. *Bottom,* Side views of same patient, 20 years later, demonstrating stability of treated result. (Courtesy of Herbert Margolis and Harvey Peck.)

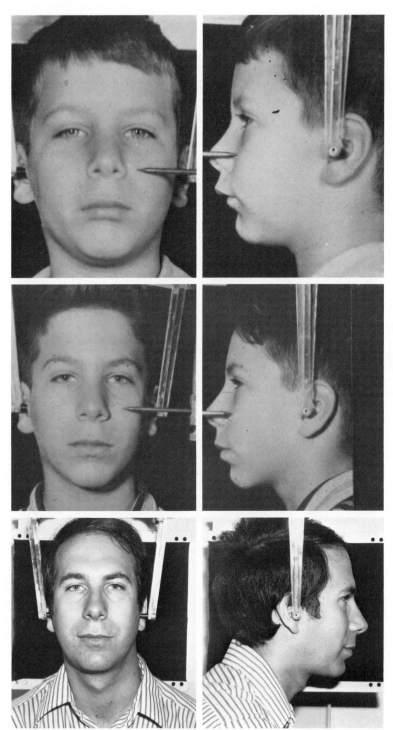

Figure 16–4. *Top,* Facial views, before treatment. *Middle,* Change after 17 months' therapy with ACCO. Bottom, 20 years later, with further autonomous improvement in facial balance. Same patient as Figures 16–2 and 16–3. (Courtesy of Herbert Margolis and Harvey Peck.)

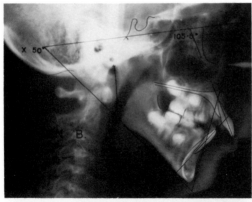
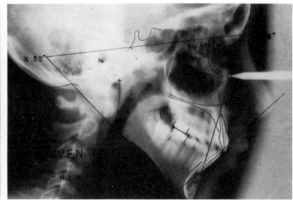
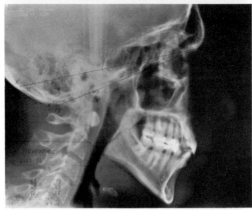

Figure 16-5. Cephalograms of patient in Figures 16-2 to 16-4 taken before treatment, after 17 months treatment, and after 20 years. Note increase in ramus height and stability of result. (Courtesy of Herbert Margolis and Harvey Peck.)

the incisors. With lingual pressure created by crimping the labial wire to close spaces, the teeth may actually be rocked on the lingual alveolar crest, actually tipping the apices labially. With the ACCO, this is reduced or eliminated. He also suggests soldering 0.040 inch tubes vertically to the labial wire between the maxillary lateral and canine teeth, instead of bending loops in the labial wire, as a possible alternative for reception of extraoral force arms. Also, an inclined plane is incorporated to free the mandible for all possible forward growth and elimination of functional retrusion. Keeping the opposing upper and lower posterior teeth apart stimulates eruption of the mandibular teeth, reducing the overbite and excessive curve of Spee. Acrylic is cut away from the lingual aspect of the maxillary posterior teeth, to permit finger springs to distalize premolar and molar teeth (see Figs. 16-3 and 16-6). One side at a time is distalized, with ball clasps or a passive finger spring on the opposite side to enhance retention of the appliance. After one side is moved back into a Class I relationship, a new ACCO is made, holding the completed side with ball clasps and putting finger springs on the remaining side to achieve the Class I correction.

Margolis instructs his patients to wear the ACCO 24 hours a day, plus extraoral force for at least 12 hours a day. He will usually use fixed appliances on the incisors for a short time to correct rotations, depress teeth, or close spaces and produce the required root torque in this area. Then he returns to the ACCO for any residual distalizing needed, plus retention. Figures 16-2 to 16-5 illustrate long-term results achieved with combined ACCO therapy to correct

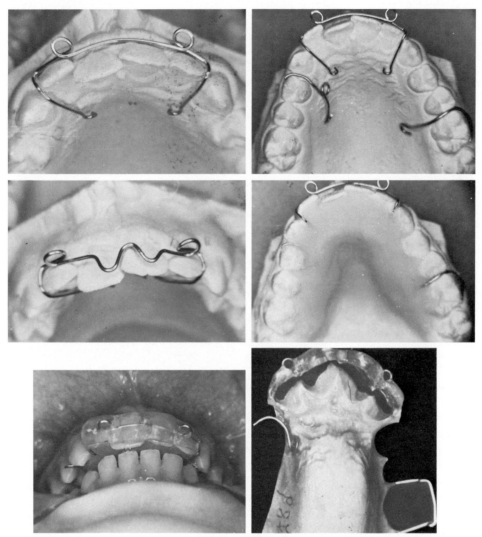

Figure 16-6. Fabrication of ACCO. Labial wire has loops bent in to receive extraoral force arms. It may be straight (*top left*) or undulated (*middle left*) to receive the labial acrylic augmentation. This part is done after palatal acrylic portion is completed (*middle right*). Labial acrylic may be added to the model or directly in the mouth (*lower left*). Various types of clasps or finger springs may be used to enhance stability and versatility (*lower right*). (Courtesy of Mario Tenenbaum.)

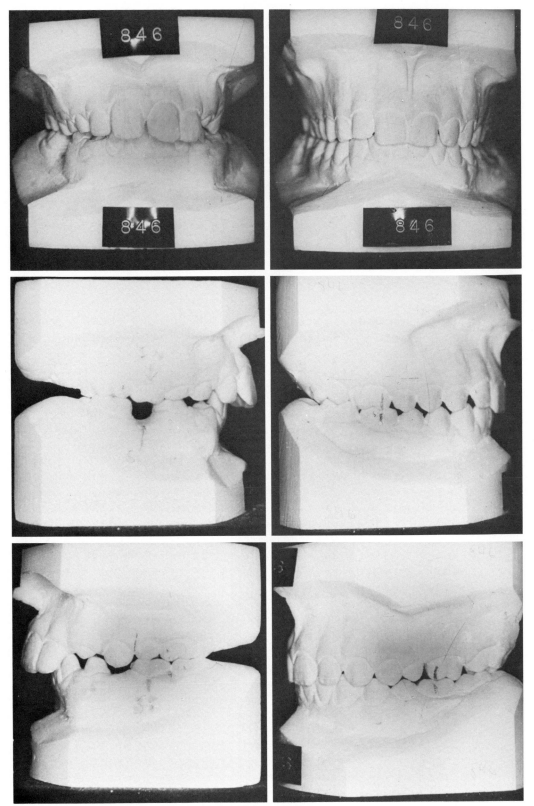

Figure 16–7

See following page for legend

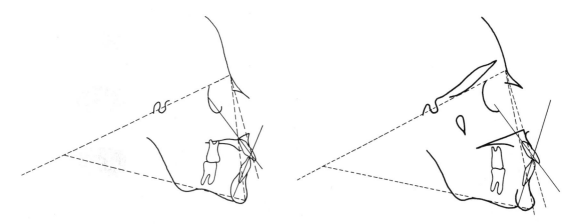

Figure 16–7. Study models and cephalometric tracings of patient with Class II malocclusion with excessive overjet and overbite. Only ACCO and extraoral force were used for the correction. (Courtesy of M. Tenenbaum and R. Gabriel.)

ACCO MODIFICATIONS

One of the authors (Graber) has used a modification of the ACCO for active retention for some years. The appliance is used in a manner similar to that recommended by Margolis and Tennenbaum. However, he achieves arch form and correction of anterior tooth malpositions first, along with space closure, with fixed appliances. Then he places the ACCO with or without a jackscrew to achieve expansion as needed (Fig. 16–8). The occlusal surfaces of the maxillary posterior teeth are covered to provide added retention and to free the possible interlocking effects of upper and lower buccal segments, as the Class II correction proceeds. A similar appliance, called the maxillary splint, employing extraoral parietal anchorage, has been used by Jacobson, with rather effective results.[6]

Force magnitude with the ACCO and similar appliances cannot be too great, since the appliance will become dislodged. This reduces the orthopedic potential. In the original use of such appliances, attempting to create orthopedic change in cleft palate cases, Graber used various configurations. The most successful appliances incorporated a labial bow and extraoral force arms directly in the palatal appliance, bending the arms to control direction of force and reduce dislodgement. The Graber appliance (Fig. 16–9) is a modification of the clear plastic palatal and occlusal coverage retainer designed by Ponitz,[7] similar to the Ortho-Tain retainer of Bergersen. This type of appliance works well as an active retainer for Class II cases, after arch form and contact relationship have been achieved by other appliances. Attempts have been made to use soft acrylic, covering the vestibular mucosa, to produce more basal bone change. Tissue irritation is a problem, however. Mills and Vig show a compara-

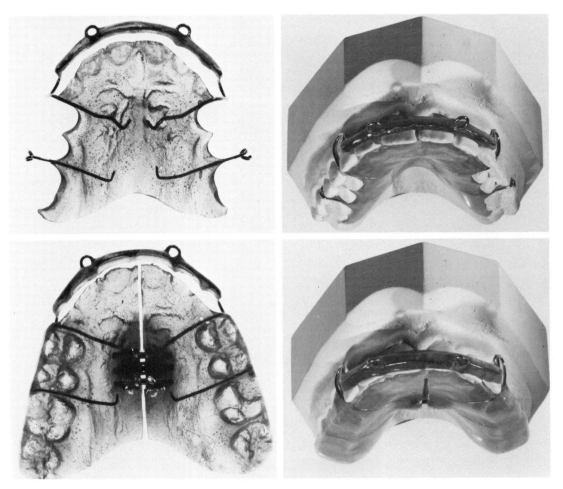

Figure 16–8. ACCO modifications. *Top,* Modified Hawley retainer, with loops bent in labial wire and acrylic added from canine to canine. Preformed arrow clasps are used at first molar embrasure. This appliance is used primarily for minor withholding of an incipient Class II malocclusion, or to prevent relapse of a corrected Class II malocclusion. *Bottom,* Jackscrew has been incorporated to provide increased buccal segment width. Acrylic is added over occlusal surfaces to enhance retention of appliance, to prevent buccal teeth from tipping excessively, and to free mandible from occlusal influence during downward and forward growth. Greater force magnitude is possible with this construction, producing a more orthopedic effect.

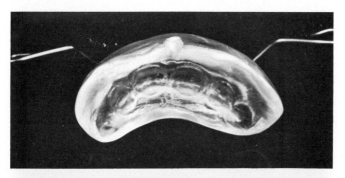

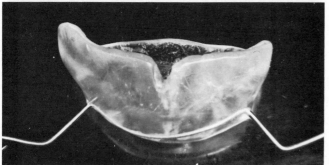

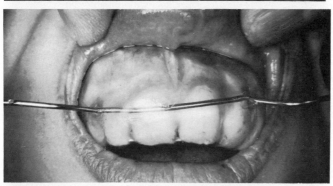

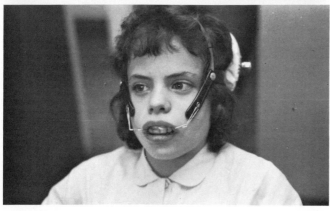

Figure 16–9. Soft plastic appliance, fabricated to fit maxillary arch in Class II, Division 1 malocclusion cases. Metal arms are incorporated in acrylic to receive motivating elastic or spring force from extraoral source. Appliance fits the teeth much like an elastoplastic positioner. Appliance must be relieved in area in contact with gingival mucosa on labial, to prevent irritation. Plastic in buccal vestibule stands away from tissue in premolar and canine areas to allow autonomous expansion. Action is similar to that of lateral shields of Fränkel function corrector. (From Graber, T. M., and Swain, B. F. (Eds.): Current Orthodontic Concepts and Techniques, 2nd ed. Philadelphia, W. B. Saunders Company, 1975.)

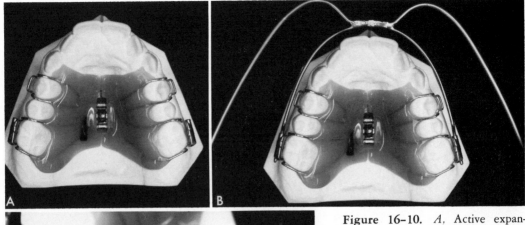

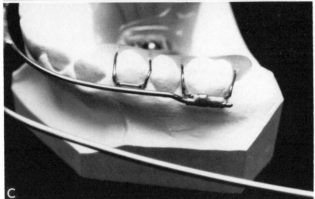

Figure 16–10. *A,* Active expansion plate, with jackscrew to maintain the posterior teeth in the alveolar trough as they are distalized, and to eliminate any maxillary arch narrowing. 0.040 inch buccal tubes are soldered to molar clasps to receive extraoral force facebow ends. *B,* Expansion plate with facebow inserted to show relationship to maxillary teeth from occlusal. *C,* Facebow arms inserted and illustrated from buccal to demonstrate occlusogingival relationship of facebow. (Courtesy of J. R. E. Mills.)

ble appliance, with the labial bow for extraoral force also incorporated in the acrylic.[8] Figure 16–10 shows how a cervical strap is used as the arrangement is fitted onto a mannikin. This type of appliance was described by McCallin in 1961.[9] Most recently, claiming to produce craniomaxillary orthopedic correction, Thurow also recommends the maxillary splint.[10] With minor fabrication and design variations, this appliance is the same one that has been used widely in England for some time.[8, 9]

Another modification suggested by Graber is first to align the maxillary teeth, achieve correct arch width and form, and then make a Vitallium casting to receive the extraoral force arms (Fig. 16–11). This makes an excellent retainer for Class II malocclusions where there is unfavorable growth direction or strong relapse tendencies. A bite plate can be incorporated on the lingual aspect if need be. Actually, if the mandibular incisors are not procumbent and some propulsive guidance is desired, the acrylic may be shaped on the lingual as a guide plane as well as a bite plate, analogous to the Vorbissplatte (forward biting plate) of Hotz (see Chapter 5). Care must be taken not to procline the lower incisors, however. Initial tooth inclination, direction of growth, guide plane angle, and amount of wear are factors that must be considered in such instances. Careful cephalometric records must be made periodically to assess treatment response. Such appliances are designed primarily for mild Class II problems.

Various modifications of removable appliances have been suggested to permit reception of extraoral force.[11-19] Hasund, in an excellent presentation

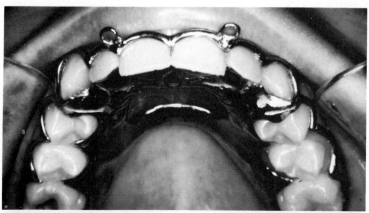

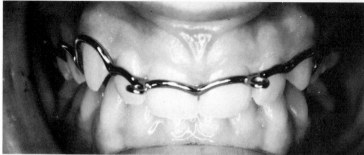

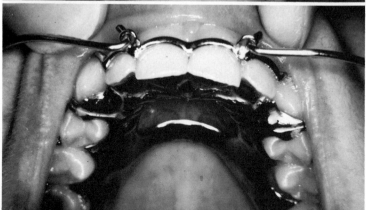

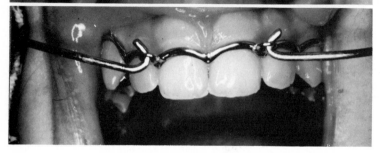

Figure 16–11. Cast Vitallium maxillary appliance. Arch form and width is first achieved by an active fixed or removable appliance. Then metal casting is made, similar to a cast partial denture, carefully surveyed to fit above greatest convexity of tooth surfaces, but not at gingival margin. Extraoral force arms insert in labial casting loops. Direction of pull best tolerated without dislodgement is in the horizontal. Precise fit on labial and lingual imparts primarily bodily force to incisors, as well as to other teeth. (From Graber, T. M., and Swain, B. F. (Eds.): Current Orthodontic Concepts and Techniques, 2nd ed. Philadelphia, W. B. Saunders Company, 1975.)

before the European Orthodontic Society in 1969, pointed out the importance of preparatory activator treatment in the mixed dentition, together with the use of extraoral force, in Class II, Division 1 malocclusions. Growth amounts and growth directions would affect the results of this first phase of treatment. Subsequent multibanded therapy and possible tooth sacrifice were usually considered necessary.[16]

Mills Fixed-Removable Combination

One very common modification of a removable appliance for reception of extraoral force is illustrated by Mills and Vig, where the round 0.036 or 0.040 inch buccal tube is soldered to the horizontal buccal members of the Adams clasps on the permanent maxillary first molars[8] (Figs. 16–10 to 16–15). The appliance of choice is usually a modified active plate. Magnitude of force is moderate at best for fear of dislodging the appliance.

If the operator desires to use only removable appliances to correct a conventional Class II, Division 1 malocclusion, then it usually requires two or three plates. It is necessary to eliminate the narrowness of the maxillary arch first. This may be done with an expansion plate (see Chapter 2). A jackscrew is an effective means of achieving the necessary force, although a Coffin type spring may be used (Figs. 16–12 to 16–15). Retraction of maxillary incisors to establish contact relationship and to correct arch form and tooth inclination is then necessary. A labial wire incorporated in the original expansion plate can be used. Or a new appliance may be constructed for just this purpose. Such an appliance (described in Chapter 2) would resemble a Hawley retainer. If there is a deep overbite, a bite plate may be incorporated to assist in the correction of the

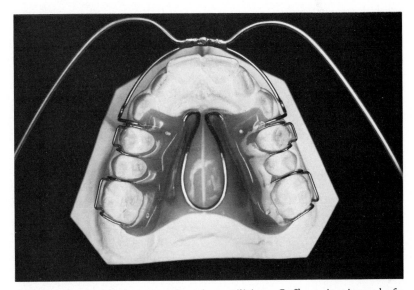

Figure 16–12. Active expansion plate, utilizing a Coffin spring, instead of a jackscrew. In this instance, the extraoral force facebow is soldered directly to the heavy labial bow of the appliance. In Figure 16–11, facebow may be removed. Direct soldering makes it somewhat easier for patient to insert, enhancing patient compliance. (Courtesy of J. R. E. Mills.)

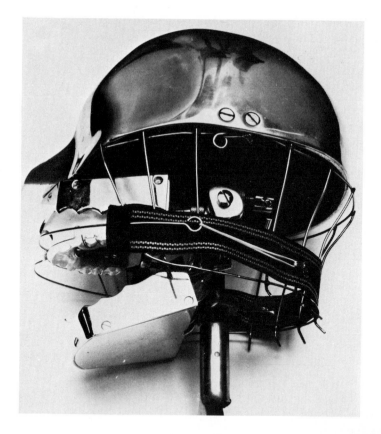

Figure 16-13. Coffin spring facebow combination (Figure 16-12) mounted on mannikin to show neck strap, elastic traction, direction of pull, etc. (Courtesy of J. R. E. Mills.)

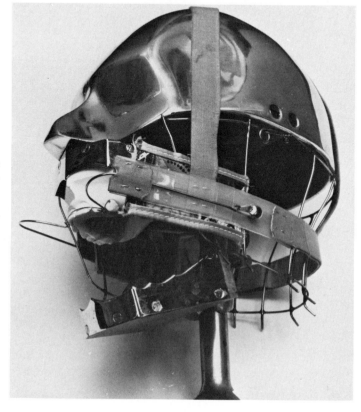

Figure 16-14. Active jackscrew expansion plate, illustrated in Figure 16-10, mounted on mannikin, showing use of a conventional headcap. Direction of force can be better controlled. (Courtesy of J. R. E. Mills.)

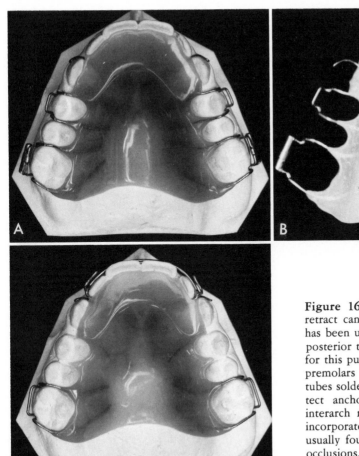

Figure 16–15. Removable appliance used to retract canines after initial expansion appliance has been used to correct arch form and distalize posterior teeth. *A,* Canine springs are illustrated for this purpose. Adams clasps are used on first premolars and first permanent molars. Buccal tubes soldered on first molar clasps serve to protect anchorage primarily, maintaining correct interarch relationship. The bite plate has been incorporated to decrease the excessive overbite usually found in most Class II, Division 1 malocclusions. *B,* Palatal view of appliance in *A.* Note retracting springs and spring guards, as well as soldered buccal tubes. *C,* Similar appliance, except that hooks or spurs are soldered to labial bow, to receive extraoral force arms, instead of conventional facebow inserting into buccal tubes on *A* and *B.* (See Figure 16–1 for similar design.) (Courtesy J. R. E. Mills.)

vertical discrepancy. After arch form has been achieved, a new appliance is made with acrylic coverage of the labial wire (like the ACCO), and, preferably, the posterior occlusal and buccal aspects. Loops for reception of the "J" hooks of the extraoral appliance may be placed in the anterior maxillary incisor region. A facebow may be incorporated directly, or buccal tubes may be soldered to the buccal of the first molar clasps, making sure that the tubes are sufficiently to the buccal to allow the facebow to be inserted and removed. Figures 16–10 to 16–17 demonstrate the different appliances used for one particular case, together with models and cephalometric tracings of the results obtained. Figure 16–18 shows a combined fixed and removable approach, which is discussed later.[8]

Again, a casting, as described previously (see Fig. 16–11) may be used at this stage, since tooth alignment, arch form, and contact relationship have been achieved. The maxillary arch now serves as the receptor (handle) for the extraoral force for growth guidance to harmonize maxillary growth direction and increments with mandibular basal and dentoalveolar growth and development.

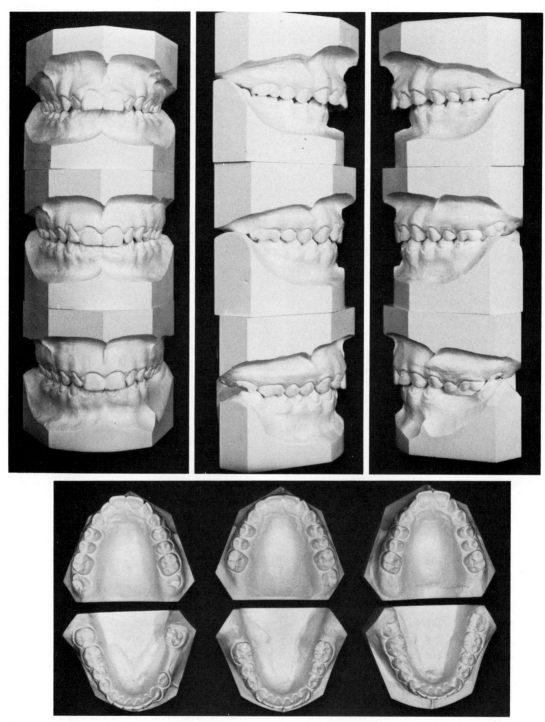

Figure 16–16. Study models of patient treated with a series of three appliances, adapted from Figures 16–10 to 16–15. Frontal, lateral, and occlusal views show results for a 13-year-old girl, with the usual sequelae of Class II, Division 1 treatment. All four second molars were removed, and the upper arch was distalized. This phase took 11 months. The canine retraction appliance was then fitted and worn for 5 months. The third appliance was worn for 4 months to retract and align the anterior segment. Models show malocclusion before treatment, at the end of active treatment, and 4 years out of retention. The lower left second premolar and first molar were lost because of caries in the period after appliance removal and the postretention casts. (Courtesy of J. R. E. Mills.)

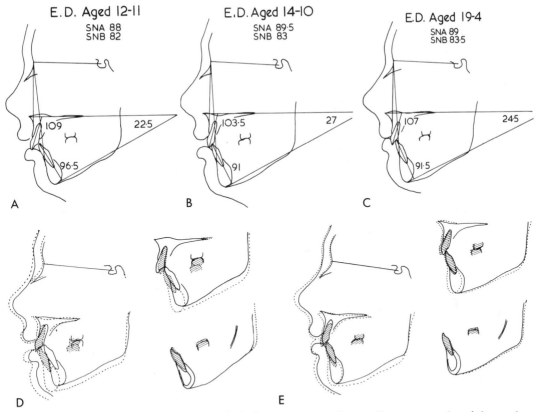

E.D. Aged 12-11
SNA 88
SNB 82

E.D. Aged 14-10
SNA 89·5
SNB 83

E.D. Aged 19·4
SNA 89
SNB 83·5

A   B   C

D   E

Figure 16–17. Cephalometric tracings made before treatment, after appliance removal, and 4 years later. *D* shows tracings of pretreatment and appliance removal time superimposed. *E* shows tracings made at end of treatment and 4 years later. Postretention changes are minimal. (Courtesy of J. R. E. Mills.)

Figure 16–18. Combination of fixed and removable appliances. Cemented molar bands, with double buccal tubes. Removable appliance fits with molar clasps, utilizing tubes for retention. Finger springs may retract canines, as in illustration, or achieve other objectives. Bite plane, guide plane, or occlusal blocks may be used, as indicated by specific malocclusion correction. (Courtesy of J. R. E. Mills.)

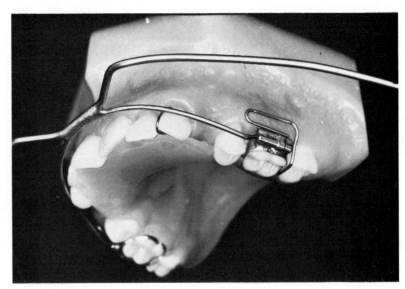

The greatest stability and resistance to displacement of the maxillary removable appliance are obtained if the appliance is kept completely passive, with no springs or screws for tooth movement. The only purpose should be reception of extraoral force. Since tooth movement should have been accomplished by this stage, the appliance should be fabricated so as to prevent further undesirable movement, such as lingual tipping of the maxillary incisors. For this reason, acrylic should cover as much as possible of both labial and lingual surfaces of the incisors. Or the casting should be accurately adapted into the interproximal areas, with broad labial coverage. The objective is to transmit the force to sutural areas and to stimulate directional growth changes primarily, not individual tooth movement.

If there is a unilateral Class II relationship, appliances may be diversified, as demonstrated by Margolis[4] and Tennenbaum and Gabriel.[5] After proper interdigitation has been achieved, the appliance should be modified to restore interdental retention on both sides. The "Achilles heel" of all these appliances is the danger of dislodgement. The tendency is for the neophyte to try to do too many things with the same appliance. By giving appliances specific duties, reciprocal disadvantageous forces are kept to a minimum.

An additional concern is that of prophylaxis. Broad acrylic or metal coverage of tooth surfaces may trap caries or decalcification-producing plaque. Assiduous brushing is a must. This has to be stressed and demonstrated before the appliance is placed. The need for patient compliance in wear also demands constant inspiration by the orthodontist and parents and vigilance at home. Indifferent cooperation and limited motivation will produce poor tissue response, just as with any conventional fixed or removable orthodontic appliance.

The most effective way of combining removable appliances with fixed appliance extraoral force is the use of cemented maxillary first permanent molar bands. Mills and Vig illustrate such a combination.[15] The round buccal tubes on the molar receive the facebow arms (Fig. 16–18). The edgewise tubes are there for any future fixed appliance therapy needed, such as alignment of maxillary incisors. The circumferential clasps fit above the double buccal tube assembly, enhancing retention of the removable appliance. An expansion screw may be incorporated in the removable appliance to provide the necessary arch width. If there is a habit problem, spurs may be incorporated in the palatal acrylic portion (Fig. 16–19). Tongue thrust may thus be intercepted, and tongue posture may be corrected.

The facebow is always inserted with a slight expansion, as the molars are to occlude with a wider part of the mandibular arch. The use of a bite plate helps guide the favorable eruption of the mandibular molars. Harvold has pointed out that by withholding the maxillary buccal segment eruption and stimulating the mandibular buccal segment eruption at the same time, full advantage is taken of the upward and forward eruption vector of the lower buccal teeth to provide a correction of the distocclusion by alveolodental adaptation.[20]

If the incisors have to be banded, this can be done as shown by Graber in his chapter on dentofacial orthopedics.[1] Mills and Vig show a similar approach.[15, 21] It cannot be stressed too strongly that the option of banding teeth is an essential of optimal therapy. Banding of incisors may be necessary, not only to align teeth but also to distribute the extraoral force, to depress the anterior teeth, and to elevate or tip down the anterior end of the palatal plane, as desired.

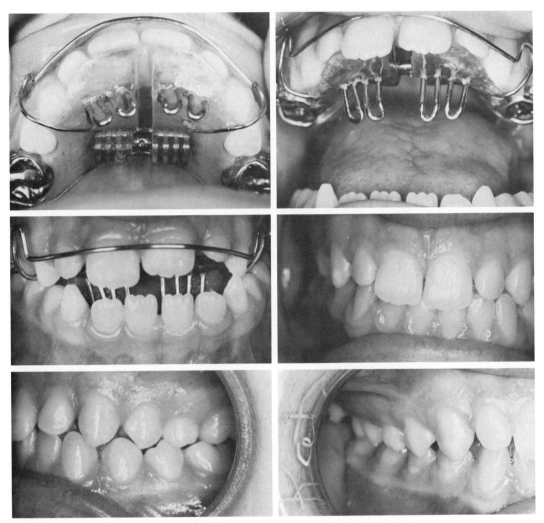

Figure 16–19. Fixed and removable appliance combination. Molar bands or full metal crowns have horizontal buccal tubes, which receive extraoral facebow. Jackscrew is used to correct crossbite with bilateral expansion, while anterior loops are embedded in acrylic to restrict abnormal finger and tongue activity. Acrylic may be carried over occlusal in open bite cases, or where necessary to correct anterior crossbite. Completed case is shown in middle right and lower figures.

Pfeiffer-Grobety Technique

Pfeiffer and Grobety strongly urge the melding of both fixed and removable appliances for the best possible result in Class II malocclusions.[18, 19] They make use of cemented maxillary first permanent molar bands. They write, "Since 1967, we have combined the action of these two appliances (activator and headgear), thinking that one would not be detrimental to the other. To our great surprise, we discovered that not only were their actions complementary but also that their respective effects increased so as to represent a highly efficient combination of therapies." Pfeiffer and Grobety have certain expectations from each element of their combined mechanotherapy for mixed dentition Class II, Division 1 cases. The activator (1) prevents, intercepts, and, if necessary, corrects pernicious habits (thumb sucking, lip sucking, reverse swallowing, mouth breathing); (2) acts as a space maintainer; (3) expands if necessary; (4) starts to correct the individual positions of teeth; (5) starts to correct the deep bite (within the freeway space limits); and (6) helps to correct the Class II relationship in three different ways: (a) The activator prevents vicious habits, reorients physiologic forces, and thus allows for the normal growth of the mandible. (b) The activator promotes, under the influence of the muscles of mandibular retraction, mesial movement of the lower teeth and distal movement of the upper teeth. (c) The activator possibly inhibits growth of the maxilla by means of the same muscles, which try to return to rest position.[18] In their opinion, the activator does not incite activation of mandibular growth, since they feel that this is a genetically defined potential that cannot be quantitatively altered.

That this is controversial is provable with experimental work, such as that of Petrovic, McNamara, Droschl, and Cederquist on mice and primates,[22-25] but still difficult to assess in humans. Yet the potential is undoubtedly there, and clinical evidence is strongly supportive of such possible influence on condylar growth and gonial angle change. The reader's attention is directed particularly to the chapters on the activator and its modifications and to the Fränkel appliance chapter (Chapter 15). This subject is also discussed in greater depth in Chapter 7.

Pfeiffer and Grobety's concern with mesial movement of the lower teeth as well as distal movement of the upper teeth will call attention to another controversial aspect of activator appliance effect.[18] One of the strongest criticisms of these appliances is their tendency to slide the mandibular teeth forward on the basal bone and to procline the mandibular incisors, all possible appliance defense against such movement notwithstanding. Certainly, it is hoped that forward movement of the mandibular teeth is minimal in most cases and that the effect of the various construction bites is to stimulate all possible forward mandibular growth, together with any changes in morphology that might assist in establishment of normal anteroposterior, maxillomandibular basal relationships.

In the combination of activator and cervical extraoral appliances used by Pfeiffer and Grobety, the authors list the following as the effects of the cervical appliance. (1) It slows down or interrupts growth of the maxilla. (2) It initiates a distal movement of the anchor molars, and, to some extent, the adjacent teeth. (3) It tips the anchor teeth either way, if desired. (4) It extrudes the molars, thereby opening the bite, but also rotating the mandible down and back. (5) It tips the palate down anteriorly.[18]

Here again, there is some question whether all these effects are desirable. Distalizing of molar teeth could impact second or third molars with mixed dentition therapy of this kind. Maxillary second molar crossbite may occur. In addition, the permanence of such distal driving is open to considerable question, as the movement is largely a tipping effect, with the molars uprighting later. Also, the extrusion of maxillary first molars is undesirable in certain Class II cases with steep mandibular planes and downward and backward growth vectors. Such action accentuates the basal discrepancy and increases facial convexity. Different types of extraoral force with a different direction of force application will depress or withhold maxillary molar extrusion, which is highly desirable in some instances. Alternatively, the extraoral force can be directed against the maxillary incisors with a high-pull vector, reducing the overbite while allowing the mandibular buccal segments to erupt upward and forward into a more normal anteroposterior relationship.

Text continued on page 594

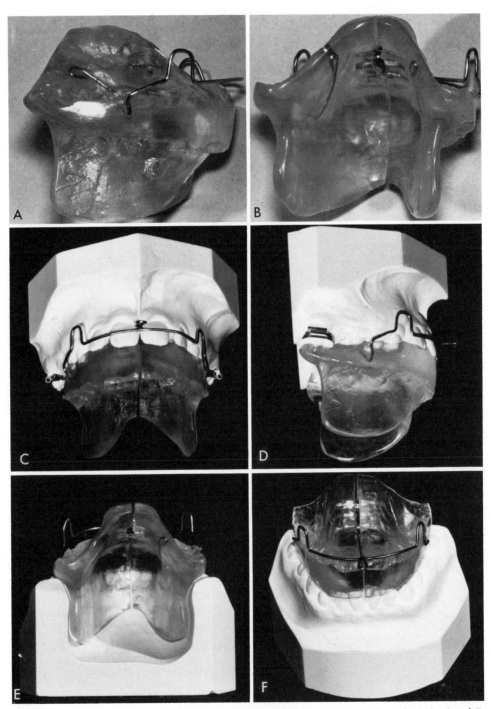

Figure 16–20. Six different aspects of the Pfeiffer-Grobety activator. Note clasps in *A* and *B*, which snap over buccal tubes on cemented molar bands in *C* and *D*. The lower wings are long and closely adapted. An expansion screw has also been incorporated. Acrylic covers the incisal third of the lower incisors to enhance bodily resistance. The spur on the labial bow serves as a restraining guide for the extraoral force facebow. (Courtesy of J. P. Pfeiffer and D. Grobety.)

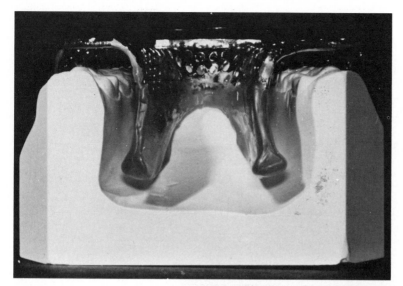

Figure 16–21. Lingual view of lower cast, with impression tray in place to illustrate method of obtaining maximum lingual extension and detail. The rims are extended 7 to 8 mm. by a rolled wax periphery that is coated with an adhesive. Space between tray and tissue allows adequate alginate bulk in the finished impression. Long flanges enhance appliance retention. (Courtesy of J. P. Pfeiffer and D. Grobety.)

Figure 16–22. Models in habitual occlusion, before treatment, with molar bands in place for extraoral force delivery, *left. Right,* Activator has been inserted between the models. The construction bite has brought the mandible 6 mm. anteriorly from postural rest position and has opened the bite 3 mm. beyond the postural rest vertical dimension. (Courtesy of J. P. Pfeiffer and D. Grobety.)

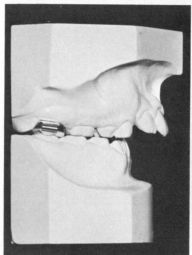
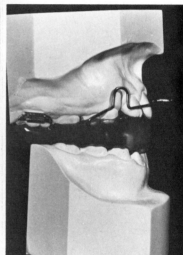

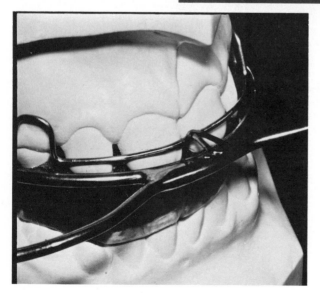

Figure 16–23. Both activator and extraoral force facebow are inserted on the models. Note the soldered spur that hooks over the activator labial bow to prevent possible loss of the removable appliance during sleeping hours. (Courtesy of J. P. Pfeiffer and D. Grobety.)

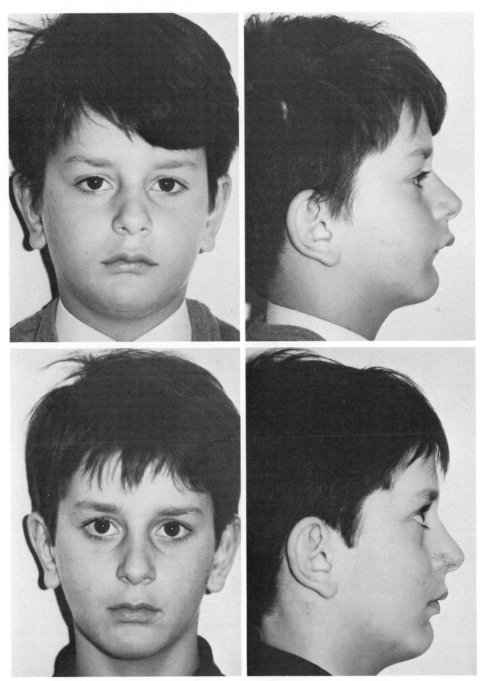

Figure 16–24. Frontal and profile views of severe Class II, Division 1 malocclusion, before and after 30 months of treatment. The improvement is primarily a distalizing effect on the maxillary arch, together with the elimination of abnormal perioral muscle function. (Courtesy of J. P. Pfeiffer and D. Grobety.)

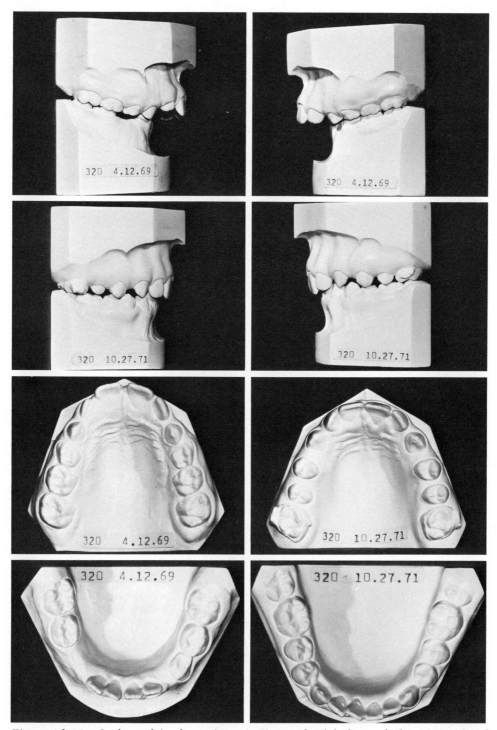

Figure 16–25. Study models of case shown in Figure 16–24, before and after 30 months of combined therapy. Excessive overjet has been eliminated, although some overbite and individual tooth irregularity remains. Subsequent multibanded therapy of less than one year completed the correction. (Courtesy of J. P. Pfeiffer and D. Grobety.)

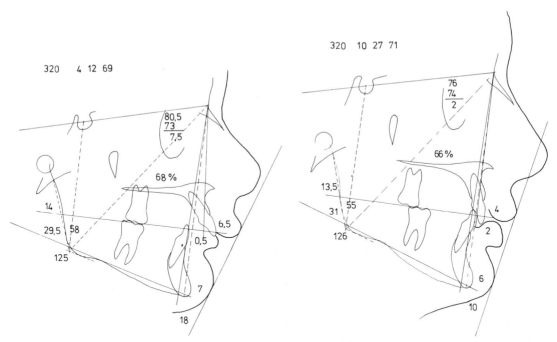

Figure 16-26. Cephalometric tracings of case shown in Figures 16–24 and 16–25, before and after combined treatment phase. Overjet and apical base discrepancy have been reduced. Facial esthetic improvement is seen in the improved Holdaway ratio. The mandibular plane has opened slightly, possibly owing to the distalizing effect on the maxillary teeth and to a primarily vertical growth direction. (Courtesy of J. P. Pfeiffer and D. Grobety.)

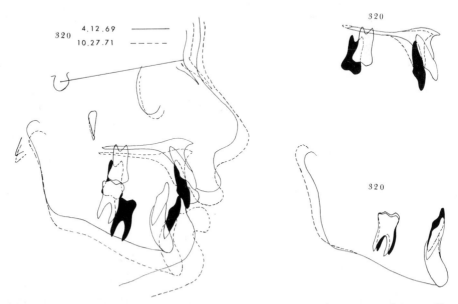

Figure 16-27. Superimpositions demonstrate change in total pattern, and in maxilla and mandible separately over the 30-month treatment period with extraoral force and activator for the case illustrated in Figures 16–24 to 16–26. The palatal plane has been tipped down anteriorly, and maxillary incisors have been retropositioned and uprighted. Maxillary molars have moved downward and backward, whereas lower molars show little change. Eruption of lower incisors, which tends to deepen the overbite, may be due to elimination of interposed lower lip. (Courtesy of J. P. Pfeiffer and F. Grobety.)

Nevertheless, with properly chosen cases and the ability to vary the choice and application of fixed and removable appliances to fit the treatment objectives, the combination of removable with extraoral force appliances is of great value in Class II, Division 1 malocclusions. Figure 16–20 shows six different aspects of the activator used by Pfeiffer and Grobety. The method of insuring long lingual flanges and maximum retention is shown in Figure 16–21. Figure 16–22 shows the models in occlusion before treatment, with molar bands in place, and then with the activator inserted between the models in the desired construction bite. The insertion of both activator and labial bow is illustrated in Figure 16–23. The dramatic facial changes achieved by combined activator–extraoral force therapy are shown in Figure 16–24. The models are shown in Figure 16–25 before and after 30 months of treatment. The cephalometric tracings in Figures 16–26 and 16–27 show the gratifying change that was accomplished.

Stockfisch Combination Therapy

Stockfisch (see Chapter 14) frequently uses extraoral force in conjunction with the Kinetor. He says, "In about 60-70% of all anomalies, full multi-banded therapy can be avoided by combination therapy—headgear and Kinetor." Even when further edgewise or straight wire treatment is necessary, the first period of combination therapy during the mixed dentition usually reduces fixed appliance treatment by one half. Figures 16–28 and 16–29 show the correction of a Class II malocclusion with deep overbite and an overjet of 10 mm., together with an arch constriction of about 10 mm. Molar bands with horizontal buccal tubes are placed first, and then the Kinetor is fabricated and placed, utilizing the buccal tubes for added appliance retention. Both can be worn together, with the Kinetor worn both day and night.

It is stressed here, as it has been in many places throughout the book, that the therapy described in this chapter is only one way to accomplish an objective. It may require simpler appliances, but it most certainly does not require less diagnostic study and acumen. For this reason, though it may seem paradoxical to some, the best qualified operators for removable appliances, or removable and fixed appliance combinations, must of necessity be the orthodontic specialists. Only they have sufficient training and experience and sufficient background to know what to do when, to know how to assess treatment results, and to know *when to change directions or appliances.* This book has been written for the orthodontic specialist, and it is hoped that those with lesser qualifications will realize the professional, ethical, and moral implications of embarking on a plan of treatment that will not serve the patient best. Providing less than optimum orthodontic guidance for a child simply because the dentist does not have the skill and training to do the job violates the Hippocratic oath. And weasel-wording and rationalizing about lesser fees and the supposed inability of orthodontic specialists to take care of all the patients will not make the situation any better. Only in those instances where orthodontic specialty guidance and consultation are not available, as in many small towns and rural areas, might the dentist feel justified to do his best in orthodontics, even though it would be of a lesser caliber than possible by an orthodontic specialist. For here, the alternative is nothing at all. Such a responsibility should not be taken lightly, because of the iatrogenic potential of some orthodontic mechanotherapy. The dentist should educate himself as completely as possible in the fields of

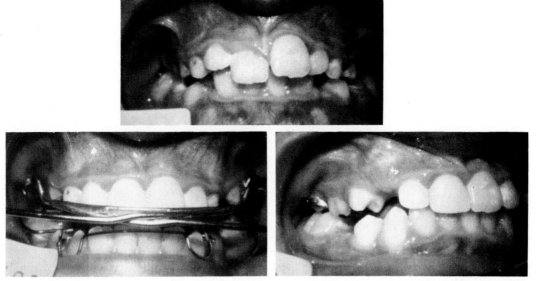

Figure 16–28. Combination therapy, with headgear and the Kinetor of Stockfisch. Molar bands with horizontal buccal tubes are cemented first, and then the Kinetor is fabricated to take advantage of added retention, with clasps over the buccal tubes. Top picture was taken at nine years. Bottom left is with both appliances in place. Kinetor is worn day and night, while headgear is used at night only. Lower right picture shows correction of 10 mm. overjet, deep bite, and 10 mm. maxillary arch constriction. Extraoral force can continue to be used after this first phase of treatment, as well as an anteriorly open activator, if desired, to guide the remaining teeth into place. Treatment time for the first phase of therapy was 20 months. (Courtesy of Dr. Hugo Stockfisch.)

craniofacial growth and development and in all aspects of orthodontic diagnosis. Continuing education courses are a must. If this reads like a sermon, such is the intent. Our ultimate responsibility is to the patient. It is our sacred moral duty always to do our best for society. If we cannot render the highest level of service, we should make sure the patient sees those who can. This is why medical and dental specialties exist.

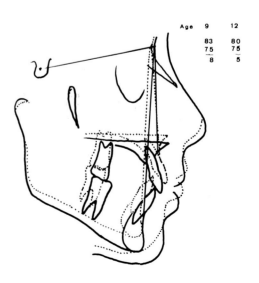

Figure 16–29. Same case as Figure 16–28. Tracings made at 9 and 12 years of age. SNaA angle has been reduced 3 degrees by the combination therapy. With SNaB staying at 75 degrees, the ANaB angle went from 8 to 5 degrees. (Courtesy of Dr. Hugo Stockfisch.)

References

1. Graber, T. M., and Swain, B. F. (Eds.): Current Orthodontic Concepts and Techniques, 2nd ed. Philadelphia, W. B. Saunders Company, 1975.
2. Schwarz, A. M.: Lehrgang der Gebissregelung. Vienna, Verlag Urban und Schwarzenberg. 1961, 2nd ed., vol. 2, 1956.
3. Spengeman, W. M.: Personal communication, August 24, 1967.
4. Margolis, H. I.: Personal communication, July 16, 1976.
5. Tennenbaum, M., and Gabriel, R.: Orthodontic treatment with removable plates and extraoral forces. Trans. Eur. Orthod. Soc., 1973, pp. 199–205.
6. Jacobson, A.: Personal communication, July 12, 1976.
7. Ponitz, R.: Invisible retainers. Am. J. Orthod., 59:266–272, 1971.
8. Mills, J. R. E., and Vig, K. W. L.: An approach to appliance therapy. Br. J. Orthod., 1:191–198, 1974.
9. McCallin, S. G.: Extraoral traction in orthodontics. Trans. Br. Soc. Study Orthod., 1961. pp. 1–14.
10. Thurow, R.: Craniomaxillary orthopedic correction with en masse dental control. Am. J. Orthod., 68:601–624, 1975.
11. Rosenmeyer, F., and Gil, R. A.: Distal movement of teeth with the removable Benac appliance, with or without extraoral force. Trans. Eur. Orthod. Soc., 1973, pp. 195–197.
12. Hill, C. V.: Controlled tooth movement. Dent. Pract., 52:13, 63, 1954.
13. Adams, C. P. The Design and Construction of Removable Orthodontic Appliances, 4th ed. Bristol, John Wright, 1970.
14. Usiskin, L. A., and Webb, W. G.: A comprehensive treatment of severe Class II, Division 1 malocclusion. Trans. Br. Soc. Study Orthod., 57:33–44, 1971.
15. Mills, J. R. E., and Vig, K. W. L.: An approach to appliance therapy, II. Br. J. Orthod., 2:29–36, 1975.
16. Hasund, A.: The use of activator in a system employing fixed appliances. Trans. Eur. Orthod. Soc., 1969, pp. 329–342.
17. Berg, R.: The selected use of different removable and fixed orthodontic appliances. Trans. Eur. Orthod. Soc., 1971, pp. 185–193.
18. Pfeiffer, J. P., and Grobety, D.: Simultaneous use of cervical appliance and activator: An orthopedic approach to fixed appliance therapy. Am. J. Orthod., 61:353–373, 1972.
19. Pfeiffer, J. P., and Grobety, D.: The Class II malocclusion: Differential diagnosis and clinical application of activators, extraoral traction and fixed appliances. Am. J. Orthod., 68:499–544, 1975.
20. Harvold, E. P., and Vargervik, K.: Morphogenetic response to activator treatment. Am. J. Orthod., 60:478–490, 1971.
21. Mills, J. R. E., and Vig, K. W. L.: An approach to appliance therapy, III. Br. J. Orthod., 2:93–101, 1975.
22. Charlier, J. P., and Petrovic, A.: Recherches sur la mandibule du rat en culture organes; le cartilage condylien a-t-il un potentiel de croissance independant? Orthod. Fr., 38:165–175, 1967.
23. McNamara, J. A., Jr.: Neuromuscular and skeletal adaptations to altered orofacial function. Ph.D. Dissertation, University of Michigan, 1972.
24. Droschl, H.: The effect of heavy orthopedic forces on the maxilla in the growing Saimiri Sciureus (Squirrel monkey). Am. J. Orthod., 63:449–461, 1973.
25. Cederquist, R., and Virolainen, K.: Craniofacial growth in the Squirrel monkey (Saimiri Sciureus). Am. J. Orthod., 69:592–593, 1976.

CHAPTER 17

Epilogue: A Philosophical Perspective

After some decades of rejection of fixed orthodontic appliances, in many countries in Europe, multibanded techniques are now used to a considerable and increasing extent. And there are signs that removable orthodontic appliances are finding more favor with orthodontists in North America. This certainly seems to be the trend for the future. The specific tasks assigned to these appliances are being clarified by practice. It is apparent that some experience is being gained where both types of appliances are in use in orthodontic practices, as indicated in Chapter 16.

One selective, logical, and economical approach, developed under the necessities of the British system of health care, is recommended by Mills and Vig. The objective is to fit the kind of treatment to the needs of each individual patient.[1] As they outline in their three-installment essay in the British Journal of Orthodontics, a few cases may be treated by judicious, guided extraction procedures alone. A large part of the average orthodontic practice may be treated with simple active plates. Extraoral traction may sometimes be added to the plates, either to reinforce anchorage or for distal movement of the posterior teeth. Such orthodontic treatment may often be supplemented or expedited by simple banded appliances. For a certain percentage of very difficult malocclusions, this combination technique would not be adequate. In another group of cases, an exceptionally high standard of achievement is required where much individual tooth movement is needed, such as torque, uprighting, paralleling, and rotational control. In these cases, fully banded techniques would and should be used. Since this arbitrary categorization of mechanotherapy demands is closely geared to the requirements of British orthodontics, it is questionable whether it will be used as a blueprint in other countries. Even in Britain, some change is foreseen, with continuing education in orthodontics likely to improve the caliber of service.[2] At present, extractions are anticipated in most cases,[3] with any subsequent movement by simple plates with springs. Myofunctional therapy finds little favor in Britain at present.[1, 4] Space closure is another sensitive and perhaps controversial subject. Provided the patient can be kept under close supervision, spontaneous closure of space is permitted. According to an investigation by Cookson,[5] 83 per cent of mandibular premolar extraction cases will demonstrate complete closure after four to six years. On the average, over 90 per cent of the change is due to forward movement of teeth in the buccal segments. Of course, whether the teeth are upright on either side of the extraction space is another question.

American orthodontists who have been trained in multibanded techniques, and who have become fully acquainted with removable appliances, insert them in a considerable number of cases, but usually only for relatively simple cases and for a short duration. For example, Col. C. L. Paul, an American orthodontist on duty in Heidelberg, recommended their use in the early mixed dentition in cases of anterior crossbite,[6] using acrylic bite blocks between the buccal segments and lingually placed springs to move the maxillary incisors labially. Plates with habit cribs are used to remedy abnormal tongue and finger habits, with a labial bow incorporated to retract and align protruded incisors, thus closing spaces.

Various spring designs can be used in conjunction with the labial bow to correct the malposition of individual teeth. Plates with spring appurtenances are also found useful in the late mixed or early permanent dentition to control and align palatally impacted or malposed canines and premolars. A rapidly growing field is the use of active plates in adults for minor correction. This is usually in conjunction with periodontal and prosthetic therapy. Despite the ample opportunity to observe treatment with removable appliances in Germany, most American orthodontists, at least in 1969 when the article was written, were not induced to go beyond the procedures recommended by Graber in his undergraduate orthodontic text.[7]

The orthodontist who uses removable appliances not only differs from his colleagues treating with fixed appliances by virtue of the mechanism he uses, but also diverges in his approach to diagnosis and treatment planning. As Stahl sees it,[8] the extended and correct three-dimensional analysis of the study models is the most important part of the diagnosis, especially for removable appliances, revealing even more than the cephalogram. The latter is regarded as indispensable, too, for it provides necessary information about the skeletal pattern. The orthodontist will depend to a great extent on precise measurements of existing space in the dental arch, together with the requirements of arch length for tooth alignment. With extraction of teeth contemplated, such information is of paramount importance. Those who use removable appliances exclusively are well aware of the limited efficiency of these devices for detailed tooth movement after extractions. Thus, there will be a certain reluctance to remove teeth, especially for patients who are 12 years old or older.

The risk of tipping teeth, the inability to parallel roots, the infraposition and rotation of teeth contiguous to the extraction site, as well as the uncontrolled or unsatisfactory space closure, will make the user of removable appliances more conservative than his fixed-appliance colleague. More cases will be started without extraction with removable appliances, awaiting the test of treatment response before tooth removal.

Where the potential of achieving optimal results from both fixed and removable appliances is equally feasible, it is possible to recognize the indications for removable appliances in a number of cases. Active plates as well as myofunctional appliances are recommended in the early mixed dentition, as indicated previously, for the correction of anterior crossbite, preferably immediately after the eruption of the incisors. Removable appliances, together with selective occlusal grinding in the buccal segments, work well in the correction of buccal crossbite and deviation of mandibular path of closure. Also handled well are the problems of space control and opening and maintaining spaces caused by premature loss of deciduous teeth. Rotation and alignment of single teeth are often amenable to correction by removable appliances. Finally, symmetric Class II malocclusions and not too severe Class III malocclusions are amenable to correction by myofunctional devices in both the mixed and permanent dentitions. The results shown by Fränkel in Chapter 15 provide dramatic proof of appliance-stimulated myofunctional potential. Such appliances also serve as retainers in mixed and permanent dentitions.

Another potential benefit of removable appliances is in treatment timing. The orthodontist trained to use removable appliances should be able to finish the treatment of a number of cases, or at least have them under retention, at a time when treatment with a multibanded appliance might not yet have been started. The younger patient often accepts appliances more readily than the teen-ager. The decisive factor here is the ability of the operator to correctly judge the indications for treatment with a particular removable appliance. This is of paramount importance. Protracted therapy that is started in the mixed and finished in the late permanent dentition will wear out the patient. Thus, unless there is a reasonable likelihood of correction by starting early, it may well be better to wait for the transitional dentition, taking advantage of the best growth potential, and completing therapy in one shorter time period.

Fixed and removable appliances can be used alternately or concurrently, as shown in Chapter 16. For example, in the early mixed dentition, Class II malocclusions may be first treated with conventional extraoral force, using a headgear. When a Class I occlusion is achieved, a myofunctional appliance or an active plate can be used for further orthodontic guidance. Another rational combination is to insert an active plate with springs to guide canines distally after the extraction of first premolars. Crowding is relieved, banding made easier, and treatment time reduced with fixed appliances. Simultaneous use of a headgear, with the face bow directed against the maxillary molars, and a removable appliance, worn during the day, work well. Sometimes, sectional banding is desirable, while a removable appliance is achieving other objectives. Again, after treatment with multibanded appliances is completed, active plates or myofunctional appliances are valuable as retainers, actively resisting relapse tendencies and dominance of the morphogenetic pattern. This wide-ranging application of removable appliances, as recommended by Stahl,[8] expresses the viewpoint of a new generation of German orthodontists who are making full and competent use of multibanded techniques, and yet do not forego the advantages of using removable appliances to obtain results in a simple and safe manner, often at an earlier age. Nevertheless, the need to use sophisticated and highly efficient multibanded appliances is recognized and no longer disputed in Germany.

There are, however, other good reasons why American orthodontists should devote more attention to removable appliances. There certainly has been a steady progress of orthodontic art and science, of know-how and technical refinement in America. Yet that is not all for the good. In this mechanistic and hurried world, we must also consider the iatrogenic potential. There may, perhaps, be a parallel betwen orthodontics and oncology. A delicate balance of chemotherapy is essential to insure the best tissue response and to prevent irreparable damage and possible demise for the cancer patient. Our challenge is less stringent, but root resorption, sheared alveolar crests, bone loss, tooth decalcification, and gingival damage are not likely to enhance dental health and longevity. As Graber pointed out a decade ago, "This headlong rush with efficient tooth-moving appliances and mass-extraction techniques to complete orthodontic correction in less and less time may be taking us in the wrong direction."[9] When Graber pleaded for a longer period of orthodontic management and responsibility, with two or three shorter periods of orthodontic mechanotherapy, he probably did not have the use of removable appliances in mind. Yet these could very well fill the bill.

Despite the increase in mixed dentition treatment, most multibanded techniques start therapy in the young permanent dentition. Only a relatively few have had routine observation to check the developing malocclusion and measures taken to break abnormal habits or orthopedically guide basal malrelationships with extraoral force. The case for interceptive and initial treatment at an earlier age has already been made by this book. In addition, in a recently published textbook devoted entirely to orthodontic treatment in the deciduous dentition, Taatz reported on a group of 300 orthodontically treated children.[10] Success was complete in 60 per cent and partial in 15 per cent. Nearly half the patients who were followed after therapy developed a normal permanent dentition without further treatment. Standards vary and treatment expectations could be less in this group. Nevertheless, the results are very impressive and carry a message for the average American orthodontist.

Gratifying results are often achieved by the very early use of small activator-like devices, worn around the clock for the treatment of Class II, Division 1 malocclusion. There could be a special advantage of beginning such treatment when the upper central incisors are erupting. These will thus be gently guided back from their dangerously protruded position. The forward positioning of the mandible and the facilitated lip closure should provide further protection and the frequent fractures of the upper incisors may be prevented. Certainly, quite a few cases could benefit by comparatively simple measures employed by the specialist. It is re-emphasized that there is the need for a proper diagnosis to discriminate between early or interceptive treatment and needless premature interference. There can be no shortcut or compromise in this critical area of orthodontic service.

The best and most efficient way to blend the use of fixed and removable appliances to fit the contemporary conditions and expectations of American orthodontists must yet be found. The importance of this question in satisfying

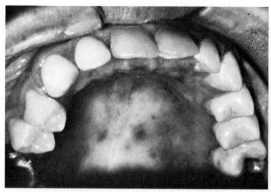 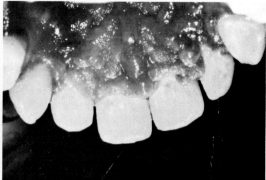

Figure 17–1. Twelve-year-old boy with hypertrophic gingivitis and decalcification and decay on lingual surfaces of maxillary teeth. The appliance was worn continuously, without proper hygiene and control of soft tissues. The patient was then referred by the general practitioner to the orthodontic specialist, after the damage had been done. Such examples of mismanagement and other cases of partial correction, improper appliance choice, extraction of the wrong teeth, and dissatisfied patients are being seen with increasing frequency in the United States today. (Courtesy of P. Herren.)

the expected future growing demand to expand treatment to cover larger segments of the population has been discussed in Chapter 1. It is to be stressed again that the possible damage by *removable appliances,* if not properly employed, should also be recognized. For example, an upper plate, worn continuously without proper hygiene and with irregular supervision by the operator, may cause gingivitis, caries, decalcification, and even bone loss (Fig. 17–1). Iatrogenic response is possible with any appliance, fixed or removable. Lost opportunity for the use of the most efficient appliance at the optimal growth and tissue response time, merely because the orthodontist wants to use a seemingly simple and less demanding removable appliance that can be fabricated by a technician and that takes less chair time, cannot be condoned. Nor can suspect economic motivation that rationalizes "early treatment" to save money for the patient, but produces an inferior result or wears the patient out in the process, be justified.

The removable appliances described in this book provide exciting possibilities not yet sufficiently appreciated by orthodontists in America. How they will use these tools cannot help but be a matter of historical interest and considerable importance to society in general and our children in particular.

References

1. Mills, J. R. E., and Vig, K. W. L.: An approach to appliance therapy. Br. J. Orthod., *1*:191–198, 1974; 2:29–36, 1975; 2:93–101, 1975.
2. Mills, J. R. E.: Continuing education for the orthodontist. Br. J. Orthod., *3*:35–38, 1976.
3. Mills, J. R. E.: Personal communication, 1975.
4. Mills, J. R. E.: Fixed and removable appliances in the treatment of Class II, Division 1 malocclusions. Transactions of the Third International Orthodontic Congress, J. T. Cook, ed. London, Crosby Lockwood Staples, 1975.
5. Cookson, A.: Space closure following loss of lower first premolars. Dent. Pract., *21*:411–416, 1971.
6. Paul, C. L., and Stahl, A.: Über die Indikation abnehmbarer Apparate im Rahmen der vorwiegend mit der Multibandtechnik durchgeführten kieferorthopädischen Behandlung. Osterr. Z. Stomatol., *66*:334–337, 1969.
7. Graber, T. M.: Orthodontics, Principles and Practice, 2nd ed. Philadelphia, W. B. Saunders Company, 1966 (3rd ed., 1972).
8. Stahl, A.: Personal communication, 1975.
9. Graber, T. M.: Postmortems in posttreatment adjustment. Am. J. Orthod., *52*:331–352, 1966.
10. Taatz, H.: Kieferorthopädische Prophylaxe und Frühbehandlung. Leipzig, J. A. Barth, 1976.

Index

Page numbers in *italics* indicate illustrations. Page numbers followed by (t) indicate tables.

ACCO appliance, 569–581
  fabrication of, *574*
  in Class II malocclusion, *576–577*
  modifications of, 576–581
  orthopedic changes and, 576–579
Acrylic, curing of, 335
  extension of, in Class II activator, 332–333
Activator, 133–336
  action of, theories of, 133–182
  advantages of, 308–309
  Andresen, 120–122, 133–135, 139, 152, 156, 183, *269*
  Andresen-Häupl, modifications of, 121–123, 203–206
  Bimler, *270*. See also *Bimler appliance*.
  bowtype, of Schwarz, 213–215
  clinical considerations in, 300–307
  condylar reaction to, 152–154
  construction bite in, 190–194, 291–300
  construction of, 194–206
    dislodging springs in, 329–330
    incisor protection and, 332–333
    labial arch in, 328–329
    labial arch wire in, 327, 333–334
    laboratory procedures in, 201–202
    lingual relief in, 327–328
    sequential treatment procedures in, 198–200
    technical directions for, 327–335
    treatment considerations in, 203–206
    trimming procedure and, 302–303, 331
  contraindications to, 326–327
  cutout, 247–252
  development of, 133–182
  disadvantages of, 308–309
  elastic open, 253–268. See also *Elastic open activator*.
  facial morphology and, 272, 282–287
  fitting of, 194–206
  fixed appliance combinations and, *149*, 168–169, 568–596
  functional occlusal plane changes and, 287–291
  Herren modification of, 209–213
  in Class II malocclusion, 133–152, 282–307, *310–321*, 326, 332–333
    advantages of, 163–164, 308–309
    applications of, 164–169
    bite registration in, 190–194, 291–300
    design of, 158–160
      clinical considerations in, 300–307
    Division 1, 184–194, *271*
    Division 2, *172–176*, 177, 206–207, *212*, 261–263, *270*, *314*, *315*

Activator (*Continued*)
  in Class II malocclusion, facial morphology and, 282–287
    fixed appliances and, 168–169
    hypothetical action of, 133–142
    limitations of, 160–163
    mandibular rotation in, 164–168
    occlusal plane changes in, 287–291
    possibilities of, 160–163
    post-treatment stability and, 169–178
    studies of, 142–152
    working bite of, *289*
  in Class III malocclusion, 207–209, *222*, 235, *244*, *245*, 263, *274*, 307–308, 322–325
    labial arch wire in, 333–334
  indications for, 309, 325–327
  Karwetsky U-bow, 216–227
  Klammt elastic open, 253–268. See also *Elastic open activator(s)*.
  labial arch in, 327–329, 333–334
  labial bow in, 197, *217*
  limitations of, 272–281
  management of, 169
  mandibular growth and, 154–156, 274, 278–282
  Metzelder modification of, 247–252
  midfacial growth and, 278–282
  modified, 139–148, 203–206
  muscle physiology and, *142–146*, 157–158, *293–296*, *300*
  occlusal changes and, 272–273, *273*
  original design of, 133–134, 142, 152–154
  orthopedic possibilities of, 278
  palate-free, 247–252
  Pfeiffer-Grobety, 587–594
  possibilities of, 160–163, 272–281
  Schmuth modification of, 215, *216*, *217*
  Schwarz modification of, 213–215
  skeletal dysplasia and, 273–274
  Slagsvold research in, 148, 169–178
  sleep and, 140–149
  soft-tissue changes and, *271*, 272
  technician, instructions for, 327–335
  tooth eruption and, 273–274
  trimming of, 302–303, 331
  use of, 183–229, 281
  vertical dimension and, 275–278
  Woodside technique in, 269–336
  Wunderer modification of, *208*

603

Active plate(s), applications of, 39–49
  components of, 12–13. See also names of
    specific components.
  construction of, 12–38
    elastics in, 35–37
    historical background of, 12–13
    labial wire in, 21–23
    of active elements, 21–36
    of baseplate, 13–15
    of clasps, 16–21
    screws in, 29–36
    springs in, 23–29
  fabrication of, 37–39
  in crossbite, 42–47
  maxillary, 68
  repair of, 37–39
  uses of, 39–49
  Y-plates, 44, 45, 47
Adams clasp, 19, 20–21, 110
Adaptability, physiological borderline of, 364
Adenoid tissue, reduction of, 76
Adolescent patients, 61
Ainsworth expansion arch, 376, 377
Allergic reactions, 110
Alveolar height, 351
Alveolar open bite, sucking and, 254
Andresen, Viggo, 120–123, 133–135, 139
    152, 156, 183, 269
Andresen appliance, 120–123, 269
Andresen-Häupl activator, 203–206
Angle(s), clivomaxillary, 341, 341
    facial, 340–342
Angle expansion arch, 376, 377
Anterior crossbite, 40, 263, 265, 367, 598
Anterior open bite, 510–512, 513
Anterior springs, in Bimler appliance,
    391–395, 451, 464, 465
Apertognathia. See Open bite.
Appliances, fixed, 567–596. See also Fixed
    appliances.
  functional, 118–132
  myodynamic, 124–125
  myotonic, 124
  removable. See Removable appliances.
Arch(es), bimaxillary, in Bimler appliance,
    483, 484
  dental. See Dental arch.
  expansion, of Ainsworth, 376, 377
    of Angle, 376, 377
    of Bimler, 401–402
    of Simon, 376, 377
  labial, in activator, 327–329, 333–334
    in Bimler appliance, 450, 541
  lingual, 376, 377
Arch wire(s), bimaxillary, 380
  development of, 377
  in Bimler appliance, 376–378, 380–381
  labial, 327, 333–334, 380
  lower, 380, 390–391
  stretching, 380
Arrow clasp, Schwarz, 16–17, 16, 17
Arrow pin clasps, 18, 19
Arrow-forming pliers of Schwarz, 16, 16
Ascher, Felix. See Bionator.
Autogenic inhibition, 296

Badcock plate, 12
Balters appliance. See Bionator.

Baseplate, of active plate, 13–15
Bilateral crossbite, 42, 46, 47, 49
Bimaxillary arch, in Bimler appliance, 483,
    484
Bimaxillary protrusion, 82, 372, 452–466
Bimler appliance, 270, 337–500
  action of, 400–402
  anterior springs in, 391–395, 451, 464, 465
  arch expansion and, 401–402
  arch wires in, 376–378, 423, 424
  arches for, 380–381
  as redoubled ellipse, 375–376, 375
  automatic effects of, 416–421
  bimaxillary arch in, 483, 484
  Bipro, 370, 372, 463–466
  "Blue Boy" case and, 421–442
  cephalometric analysis and, 338–347
  classification of, 366–367
  code letters for, 378
  color coding of, 372–376
  compensating manipulations of, 416–421
  Contra, 369, 462
  cuspid supports in, 446, 447, 452
  dental arch survey and, 356–365
  ellipse in, 388–389, 468–471
  evolution of, 373–374
  Extra, 369, 450
  extraction and, 448–462
  gnathic index formula and, 347–356
  "Green Girl" case in, 471–479
  Hypo, 369, 448
  in bimaxillary protrusion, 452–466
  in Class II malocclusion, 400
    Division 1, 368, 370, 402–416, 417, 418,
      421–442
    Division 2, 368, 370, 466–479
  in Class III malocclusion, 368, 370,
    479–498
  in cleft palate, 485
  in deep bite, 371
  in mandibular protrusion, 371
  in maxillary protrusion, 371
  in open bite, 463–466
  incisor classification and, 366–372
  interdental springs in, 443–448
  labial arch in, 450, 451
  lip bumper in, 425
  loop in, lower frontal, 397
  lower anterior section of, 395–399
  lower arch wire in, 390–391
  mandibular movement and, 400–402
  mandibular positioning and, 400
  mechanical stability of, 375–376
  molar supports in, 398, 426, 427, 466
  patient training and, 399
  practitioner position and, 499
  prefabricated parts of, 378–379
  presentation of, 399
  prestandard, 390–391, 396
  primary, 373, 373–374, 396
  problem grouping and, 372–376
  "Red Girl" case and, 452–462
  shape preservation in, 378–379
  Simplex, 392
  special, 369
  splint in, lower frontal, 397
  standard, 369, 398, 426, 427
  systematic handling program for, 379–384

Bimler appliance (*Continued*)
    tools for, 379–385
    training program for, 385–390
    type A, 367, *419*, 462–466
        labial arch adjustment in, *421, 422*
    type A₂, spécial, 444–445
    type B, 367, 466–471
    type B₂, *468*
    type C, 367, 479–485
    types of, 366–372, *370–371*
    U loop in, *374, 386–387*
    undulated connecting bar in, *486*
    upper portion of, 391–395
    variations in, 367–372
    "White Girl" case and, 402–416
    "Yellow Girl" case in, 488–498
Bimler ellipse, *388–389*
Bimler facial index, 339, *339*
Bimler two-dimensional caliper, *363*
Biomechanical orthodontics. See *Functional jaw orthopedics.*
Bionator of Balters, 229–246
    construction bite in, 236–240, *237, 238, 239*
    in Class II malocclusion, *241–243, 244, 246*
    in Class III malocclusion, *232*, 235–236, *245*
    in deep bite, *246*
    in open bite, *232*, 236, *244*
    maxillary cast of, *231*
    stabilization of, 233, 233(t)
    standard, *231*, 232–235
    vs. elastic open (Klammt) activator, 267–268
Bite. See also *Malocclusion; Overbite; Overjet; Protrusion; Retrusion.*
    closed. See *Closed bite.*
    construction. See *Construction bite.*
    crossed. See *Crossbite.*
    deep, 66, *246, 371*
    jumping of, *52*, 118–119
    open. See *Open bite.*
    raising, in Class III malocclusion, *494*
    registration of, in Class II malocclusion, 190–194, 291–307, 515–529
        neuromuscular concepts of, 292–296
    telescoped, 369, *462*
Bite plane(s), 15
"Blue Boy" case, 421–442
Bow, labial. See *Labial bow.*
Breathing, mouth. See *Mouth breathing.*
British health care system, orthodontics and, viii–ix, 597
Broad face, *339*
Bruxism, 230
Buccal crossbite, 82–83
Buccinator mechanism, *507*

Caliper, Bimler two-dimensional, *363*
Canine(s), alignment of, *43*, 47
    labial bow of, *23*
    rotation of, 29, *30*
Central maxillary incisor, crossbite of, *64*
Cephalometric analysis, Bimler, 338–347
Cheeks, pressure exerted by, 507

Chewing, Kinetor and, 505–507
Clasp(s), Adams, *19*, 20–21, *110*
    arrow, of Schwarz, 16–17, *16, 17*
    arrow pin, *18*, 19
    Duyzings, 21
    eyelet, *18*, 19
    in active plate, 16–21
    triangular, *17*, 18–19
Clasp knife reflex, *296*
Cleft palate, Bimler appliance in, *485*
Clivomaxillary angle, 341
Closed bite. See also *Malocclusion; Retrusion.*
    Bimler appliance in, 402–416, 421–422, 471–479
        appliance prescription in, 409
        construction of, 409–413
        long-term evaluation of, 413–416, 440–442
Coffin plate, 12
Coffin springs, 29, 391–395
Complete open bite, *285*
Condyle(s), activator therapy and, 152–154
Construction bite, in Bionator, 236–240, *237, 238, 239*
    in Class II malocclusion, *134*, 190–194
    in unilateral retro-occlusion, *58*
Contact sports, 68
Crossbite, *46*, 369
    active plate in, 42–47
    anterior, 40, 263, *265*, 367, 598
    bilateral, 42, *46, 47*, 49
    Bimler appliance and, *485*
    buccal, 82–83
    in Class II, Division 2 malocclusion, 206–207
    of central maxillary incisor, *64*
    unilateral, elastic open activator in, 265, *266*
    plate for, *43*
Crossbite springs, in Bimler appliance, *449*
Crouzon's disease, pseudo-, *354*
Crowding, *370*
    Bimler appliance in, *370*, 471–479
    elastic open activator and, 257–259
    with hypoplasia, Bimler appliance in, 452–462
Cuspid supports, in Bimler appliance, *446, 447*
Cutout activator, 247–252
Cybernator, 215, *216*

Deep bite, 66, *246, 371*
Deep face, *339–342*, 372
Deglutition, frequency of, 58–61
Denholtz muscle anchorage appliance, *91*
Dental arch, expansion of, 364–365
        Bimler appliance and, 401–402
        self-limitation of, 360–364
    height of, *263*, 358
    measurement of, 356–365, 407–409
        Pont index in, 357–358
    survey of, 356–365
    width of, 170(t), 171(t), 358, *362*
Dental arch analysis sheet, 358–360

Dentistry, third-party involvement in, 2–3
Dentition, deciduous, 70, 563
  Class II, Division 1 malocclusion in, *214*
  Fränkel appliance in, 563
  vestibular screen in, 70
 developing, active plates in, *48*
 early mixed, 598, 599
 mixed, Bimler appliance in, 36
  Fränkel appliance in, 563
  Kinetor and, 523
  overbite in, 230
 permanent, Fränkel appliance in, 564
Discomfort, with removable appliances, 55–57
Disharmony, facial, symptoms of, 349–351
Dolichoprosopy, *339–342*, 372
Double plate, 51–62, *54*, 56–57, *59, 60*
Double screen of Kraus, *81*
Duyzings clasps, 21
Dysplasia, leptoid, 355–356, *487*
 micro-rhinic, 352, *428, 487, 497*
 microtic, *487*
 skeletal, activator and, 273–274
 types of, 352–356
Dystosis craniofacialis, *354*

Eccentric screws, *34*
Eirew, Hans, on Bionator objectives, 229
 on functional appliances, viii
Elastic(s), in active plate, 35–37
 in Class II malocclusion, 99–103
 in Class III malocclusion, 37
 intermaxillary, 37, 109
 use of, *15*
Elastic bimaxillary wire appliance, 337–500.
  See also *Bimler appliance.*
Elastic open activator, 253–268
 action of, 257–268
 crowding and, 257–259
 in anterior crossbite, 263, *265*
 in Class II malocclusion, *264*
  Division 1, *258*, 259–261
  Division 2, 261–263
 in Class III malocclusion, 263–264
 in extraction cases, 266–267
 in open bite, 265, *267*
 in unilateral crossbite, 265, *266*
 modifications of, 257–259
 standard, 255–257, *255, 256, 257*
 vs. Bionator, 267–268
Encased screws, 33–34
Euryprosopy, *339*
Exerciser(s), rubber, 75, *75*
Expansion arch, Ainsworth, 376, *377*
 Angle, 376, *377*
 Simon, 376, *377*
Expansion plate(s), *43, 44*
Extraction, Bimler appliance and, 448–452
 feasibility of, 597–598
Extraction cases, elastic open activator in,
  266–267
Extraoral force, removable appliances with,
  567–596
  ACCO appliance in, 569–581
  Hawley appliance and, *569*
  Mills fixed-removable combination in,
   581–586
  Pfeiffer-Grobety technique in, 587–594

Extrinsic forces, 63–93. See also *Muscle forces.*
Eyelet clasps, *18*, 19

Face, angles of, 340–342
 broad, *339*
 deep, *339–342*, 372
 factor analysis and, 343–346
 long, *339–342*, 372, *498*
 lower, height of, 287(t)
 medium, *339–342*
 morphology of, activator and, 282–287
 structure of, disharmony in, 349–351
  formula for, 343–346
  harmony vs. norms in, 349–351
 types of, *339–342*
Facial formula, 342–343
Facial index, Bimler, 339
 Kollmann, 338–339
Facial polygon, 343–346
Farrar, John Nutting, 121n
Finger spring(s), *26*
Finger sucking, 73–74
Fixed appliances, activator and, in Class II
  malocclusions, *149*, 168–169
 removable appliances with, 567–596. See
  also under *Removable appliances.*
Force(s), extraoral. See *Extraoral force.*
 extrinsic, 63–93. See also *Muscle forces.*
Forward biting plate, 93–111. See also *Guide
 plane plate.*
Fossa, temporal, position of, *351*
Fränkel appliance (FR), 526–566
 action of, 558–562
 clinical handling of, 562–563
 construction of, 526–558
  of FR I, 527–547
   FR Ia and, 527–535
   FR Ib and, *533*, 535–537
   FR Ic and, 537–547
  of FR II, 547–549
  of FR III, 550–557
  of FR IV, 557–558
 in Class I malocclusion, 527–535
 in Class II malocclusions, 535–549
 in Class III malocclusion, 550–557
 in open bite, 557–558
 patient and, 562, 564
 success with, preconditions for, 564–565
 treatment timing and, 563–564
Function corrector, 526–566. See also
  Fränkel appliance.
Function regulator (FR), 526–566. See also
  Fränkel appliance.
Functional appliances, historical development
  of, 118–132
Functional jaw orthopedics, 118–132
 current concepts of, 123–132
 Fränkel appliance in, 126–129
 functional matrix concept in, 130–131
 future of, 123–132
 history of, 118–123
 indications and contraindications for, viii
 mandibular growth and, 129–130
 myodynamic appliances in, 124–125
 myotonic appliances in, 124
Functional matrix concept, 130–131
Functioning space, 127–128

Gebissformer, 337–500. See also *Bimler appliance*.
Gingivitis, hypertrophic, *600*
Gnathic index formula, 347–356
Graber appliance, 576–579, *578*
Great Britain, orthodontic practice in, 597
"Green Girl" case, 471–479
Growth, malocclusion and, Class II, 98
 Class III, *487*
 mandibular, activator therapy and, 129–130, 154–156, *282*
  functional jaw orthopedics and, 129–130
 Tanner chart of, *279, 280*
 vertical, activator and, 275–278
Growth disturbances, mechanism of, 352–356
 types of, *352*
Guide plane plate, 93–111
 complementary appliances with, 110–111
 construction of, *96*, 108–110
 contraindications against, 105
 forming of, in mouth, *95*
 in Class II malocclusion, 99–103
 morphologic factors and, 98–99
 reactivation of, *94, 96*
 structure of, 104–107
 treatment response and, 98

Harvold maxillary unit measurement, 286–287, 287(t)
Hasund, A. See *Fixed appliance, activator and.*
Häupl theory of orthodontic forces, 8–9
Hawley appliance, 65–66, *91*. See also *Active plate.*
 extraoral force with, *569*
 fabrication of, 37–38, *38*
 modifications of, *577*
Health insurance, 2–5
Helical coil spring(s), 25–29
Herren activator, 209–213
High labial bow, 25
Horizontal overbite, 171(t)
Hotz, Rudolf. See *Guide plane plate; Propulsor.*
Hyperflexion, mandibular, *487*
Hypoplasia, 369, 452–462

Iatrogenic damage, *600*
Incisor(s), central maxillary, crossbite of, *64*
 labial movement of, *46*
 lateral, alignment of, *43*
 occlusion of, *43*
 protection of, activator and, 332–333
 protrusive, *94*, 367, *368*
 retrusive, 367, *368*
 reversed, *368*
 sum of, 357–358
Inclined plane, 64–68
Inclined plane plate, removable, 93–111. See also *Guide plane.*
Inflammation, of palate, 110
Intermaxillary elastics, 109
Intermaxillary traction, in Class II malocclusion, 99–103
Intrusion, activator and, 275

Jaw orthopedics, functional, 118–132. See also *Functional jaw orthopedics.*

Karwetsky U-bow activator, 216–227
Kinetor, 501–524
 action of, 504–511
  chewing and, 505–507
 anterior, open bite and, *510, 511, 512, 513*
 construction of, 501–504, 514–520
 contraindications to, 523
 correction with, permanency of, 521–523, *524*
 design of, *514*
 in anterior open bite, 510–512, *513*
 in Class II malocclusion, Division 1, *519*, 520–521
  Division 2, *503, 504, 505, 506*
 in Class III malocclusion, *509, 510*
 in open bite, 521, *522*
 lip bumper and, 521, *522*
 maxillary expansion with, *508*
 modification of, 519
 open bite and, 521, *522*
 prefabricated parts for, *514, 515*
 rubber tubes in, 505–507
 stabilization of, 513–514
 tongue crib and, 521
 treatment timing and, 519–520
Kingsley plate, 12
Klammt elastic open activator, 253–268. See also *Elastic open activator(s).*
Kollmann facial index, 338–339, *339*
Kraus, Frantisek, 126–127
Kraus double oral screen, *80, 81*
Kraus vestibular screen, *79*

Labial arch, in activator, 327–329, 333–334
 in Bimler appliance, *450, 451*
Labial bow, activation of, *24*
 activator with, 197, *217*
 canine, *23*
 construction of, 108–110
 high, *25*
 in anterior alignment, *25*
 normal position of, 108–110
 of canine, *23*
Labial wire, in active plate, 21–23
Lateral incisors, alignment of, *43*
Leptoid dysplasia, *352*, 355–356, *487*
Leptoprosopy, *339–342*, 372, *498*
Lingual arch, 376, *377*
Lip(s), pressure exerted by, 507
 tonicity of, development of, 75, *76*
Lip bumper, Kinetor and, 521, *522*
 in Bimler appliance, *425*
 muscle forces and, 86–92
Lip habit, 70, 86–92
Lip molder. See *Vestibular screen.*
Lip shield, *90*
Long face, *339–342*, 372, *498*
Loop(s), frontal, in Bimler appliance, *382*
 U, in Bimler appliance, *386–387*
 vertical, form of, *108*
Loop spring, 27, *30*

Macrodontia, 369
Malocclusion, appliance indications in, ix
  Bimler classification of, 366–367
  Class I, 40–41
    activator and, 326
    Bimler appliance and, 452–462
    Fränkel appliance and, 527–535
  Class II, 40–41, 58, 59, 530
    ACCO appliance in, 575–578
    activator in, 133–152, 282–307, 310–321,
      326, 332–333
    Bimler appliance in, 400
    Bionator in, 241–243, 244, 246
    Division 1, 44, 51, 72, 73, 74, 98
      116–117, 276–277
      activator in, 110–111, 184–194, 271,
        272, 274, 275
      Bimler appliance in, 368, 370,
        402–416, 417–418, 421–442
      cutout activator in, 247, 248, 250–251
      double plate in, 60
      elastic open activator in, 258, 259–261
      fixed-removable combination treatment
        in, 581–586
      Fränkel appliance and, 535–549
      guide plane plate in, 93–111. See also
        Guide plane plate.
      in deciduous dentition, 214
      in nongrowing patient, 112–113
      Kinetor in, 519, 520–521
      propulsor in, 111–117
      treatment of, appliance structure in,
        104–107
        growth factors and, 98
        in late adolescence, 111
        morphologic factors in, 98–99
        response to, 98
    Class II, Division 2, 43, 247–250
      activator in, 206–207, 270
      Bimler appliance in, 368, 370, 466–471
      crossbite in, 206–207
      double plate in, 54, 57
      elastic open activator in, 261–263
      Fränkel appliance in, 270
      Kinetor in, 503, 504, 505, 506
      open bite in, 206
      elastic open activator in, 264
      elastics in, 99–103
      etiology of, 283
      guide plane in, 93–111
      intermaxillary traction in, 99–103
  Class III, 37, 40, 61
    activator in, 207–209, 274, 307–308,
      322–325, 333–334
    Bimler appliance in, 368, 370
    Bionator in, 232, 235–236, 245
    cutout activator in, 252
    double plate in, 60
    elastic open activator in, 263–264
    elastics in, 37
    Fränkel appliance in, 550–557
    Kinetor and, 509, 510
    prognosis in, 488, 497–498
    tongue thrust and, 510–512, 513
    types of, 485–498
  Class IV, Fränkel appliance in, 557–558
  oral screens in, 82–86, 83, 84, 85, 86
  pseudo Class III, 67

Mandible, closing of, 51
  growth of, activator and, 129–130, 154–
    156, 274, 278–282
    functional jaw orthopedics and, 129–130
  lateral deviation of, double plate in, 60
  movement of, Bimler appliance and,
    400, 402
  positioning of, 51
  rest position of, 136, 136–137
Mandibular hyperflexion, 487
Mandibular protrusion, Bimler appliance in,
  371
Mandibular unit, size of, 289(t)
Margolis appliance (ACCO), 569–581. See
  also ACCO appliance.
Masticator muscles, neural pathway of, 292
Maxillary arch, expansion of, 43
Maxillary incisor, central, crossbite of, 64
Maxillary plate, expansion of, Kinetor and,
  508
Maxillary protrusion, Bimler appliance for,
  371
Maxillary rotation, effect of, 354
Maxillary unit, Harvold measurement of,
  286–287, 287(t)
  size of, 289(t)
Maxillomandibular angle, 341–342
Medium face, 339–342
Mershon springs, 377
Mesoprosopy, 339–342
Metzelder activator, 247–252
Micro-rhinic dysplasia, 352–353, 428, 487,
  497
Microtic dysplasia, 353–355, 487
Midface, growth of, activator and, 278–282
Mills fixed-removable combination appliance,
  581–586
Mixed dentition. See Dentition, mixed.
Molar supports, Bimler appliance and, 398,
  426, 427, 466
Monobloc, 12, 119–120. See also Activator.
Mouth breathing, 56–57, 74–86
  masticator, neural pathway of, 292
Muscle forces, guide plane and, 64–68
  lip bumper and, 86–92
  oral screen and, 68–86
  Rogers exercises and, 120
  vestibular screen and, 68–86
Muscle(s), activator and, 156–158
Myodynamic appliances, 124–125
Myotonic appliances, 124

Nord plate, 12
Norwegian system. See Functional jaw
  orthopedics.

Occlusal plane, functional changes in,
  activator and, 287–291
Occlusion, changes in, activator treatment
  and, 272–273, 273. See also Malocclusion.
  of incisors, 43
Open bite, 51–62, 72, 77, 369
  alveolar, sucking habit and, 254

Open bite *(Continued)*
 anterior, 510–512, *513*
 Bimler appliance in, 463–466
 Bionator in, *232, 236, 244*
 complete, *285*
 cutout activator in, *249,* 250–251
 elastic open activator in, 265, *267*
 in Class II, Division 2 malocclusion
  Kinetor and, 521, *522*
 vestibular screen and, *82*
Oppenheim splint, 64–65, *65*
Oral adaptor, 337–500. See also *Bimler appliance.*
Oral screen(s). See also *Vestibular screen(s).*
 advantages of, 78–79
 breathing holes in, *75,* 76
 commercially available, *70*
 definition of, 76–77
 double, 77, *80*
 fabrication of, *71, 72*
 in malocclusions, 82–86, *83, 84, 85, 86*
 in mouth breathing, 74–86
 limitations of, 80–86
 muscle forces and, 68–86
 types of, *78*
Orthodontics, biomechanical. See *Functional jaw orthopedics.*
Orthodontic forces, Häupl theory of, 8–9
 Schwarz classification of, 7–8
Orthodontic screws, *31*
Orthodontic treatment, demand for, 2–5
 timing of, 599–600
Orthogonal reference system, *340, 345*
Orthopedics, ACCO appliance and, 576–579
 activator and, *278*
 functional jaw, 118–132. See also *Functional jaw orthopedics.*
Overbite, ACCO appliance in, *575–576*
 apparent, *285*
 horizontal, 171(t)
 in mixed dentition, 230
 vertical, activator and, 170(t)
Overclosure, activator and, *276–277*
Overjet, ACCO appliance in, *575–576*
 reduction of, *25*
 vestibular screen and, 77

Paddle spring, *27*
Palatal appliance, *15, 22*
Palate, cleft, Bimler appliance in, *485*
 inflammation of, 110
Palate-free activator, 247–252
Pan-dysplasia, *356, 487*
Patient, accommodation of, to appliances, 55–57
Periodontal disease, 230, *600*
Pfeiffer-Grobety technique, 587–594
Physiological borderline of adaptability, 364
Plate(s), active, 12–49. See also *Active plate.*
 Badcock, 12
 Coffin, 12
Plate, double, 51–62, *54, 56–57, 59, 60*
 expansion, *43, 44*
 for labial movement of incisor, *46*
 forward biting, 93–111. See also *Guide plane.*
 guide plane, 93–111. See also *Guide plane plate.*

Plate *(Continued)*
 Kingsley, 12
 Nord, 12
 removable inclined plane, 93–111. See also *Guide plane plate.*
 Robin, 12, 119–120. See also *Activator.*
Pliers, for Bimler appliance, 379, 383, *383*
Pont index, 357–358
Posteroclusion. See *Malocclusion, Class II.*
Profile, soft-tissue, activator and, *271,* 272
Propulsor, *114*
 in Class II, Division 1 malocclusion, 111–117
Protrusion, bimaxillary, 372
 Bimler appliance and, 452–466
 vestibular screen and, *82*
 mandibular, Bimler appliance in, *371*
 maxillary, Bimler appliance in, *371*
  dentoalveolar, 111
 of incisors, *94,* 367, *368*
Pseudo-Crouzon's disease, *354*
Pull screw, *36*

"Red Girl" case, 452–462
Reflex, clasp knife, *296*
Removable appliances. See also names of specific appliances.
 accommodation to, 55–57
 adolescent patients and, 61
 advantages of, 3–4
 biophysical development of, 5–10
 contact sports and, 68
 extraoral force with, 567–596. See also *Extraoral force.*
 extrinsic forces and, 63–92. See also *Muscle forces.*
 finger sucking and, 73–74
 fixed appliances with, 567–596
  ACCO appliance and, 569–581
  Graber appliance and, 576–579
  Margolis appliance and, 569–581
  Mills combination appliance and, 581–586
  Pfeiffer-Grobety technique in, 587–594
  Stockfisch combination therapy and, 594–595
 history of, 5–10
 iatrogenic damage and, *600*
 in Class II, Division 1 malocclusion, 93–117. See also *Malocclusion, Class II* and names of specific appliances.
 limitations of, 4, 597–601
 mouth breathing and, 56–57, 74–86
 muscle forces and, 63–92. See also *Muscle forces.*
 philosophical perspective on, 597–601
 simple, 63–92. See also names of specific appliances.
  guide plane, 64–68
  lip bumper, 86–92
  oral screen, 68–86
  vestibular screen, 68–86
 socioeconomic considerations and, 1–5
 swallowing and, 58–61
 young adults and, 61
Retro-occlusion, unilateral, *58,* 59
Retrusion, of incisors, 367, *368*
Reversal, of incisors, *368*
Robin, Pierre, 12, 119–120, 269

Rogers, Alfred P., 120
Rogers exercises, 120
Rubber exerciser, 75, *75*

Sagittal tooth movement, with Bimler
 appliance, 372
Schmuth activator, 215, *216, 217*
Schwarz, A. Martin. See *Active plate(s).*
Schwarz arrow-forming pliers, 16
Schwarz bow activator, 213–215
Schwarz classification, 7–8
Schwarz double plate, 51–62
Screen(s), double, *81*
 oral, 68–86
 vestibular, 68–86. See also *Vestibular screens.*
Screw(s), eccentric, *34*
 encased, *33*, 33–34
 in active plates, *36*
 orthodontic, *31*
 pull, *36*
 skeleton, *32*
 types of, *31–35*
 Weise jackscrew, *208, 209*
Separating medium, in activator construction,
 334
SI, 357–358
Simon expansion arch, 376, *377*
Skeletal dysplasia, activator and, 273–274
Skeleton screws, *32*
Slagsvold, Olaf, on activator, 133–152
 research of, 148, 169–178
Sleep, activator and, 140–147
Socioeconomic factors, removable appliances
 and, 1–5
Soft-tissue profile, activator and, *271, 272,
 275–277*
Spherical reference system, *347, 348*
Splint(s), frontal, for Bimler appliance, *382*
 Oppenheim, 64–65
Spring(s), anterior, in Bimler appliance,
 391–395, *451, 464–465*
 Coffin, 29
 in Bimler appliance, 391–395
 crossbite, in Bimler appliance, *449*
 dislodging, in activator, 329–330
 finger, *26*
 helical coil, 25–29
 in active plate, 23–29
 in Bimler appliance, 382, 391–395,
 443–448, *470*
 loop, *27, 30*
 Mershon, *377*
 paddle, *27*
Stockfisch combination therapy, 594–595
Stockfisch Kinetor, 501–524. See also
 Kinetor.
Stomatopedic records, *347, 349, 360, 361*
Sucking habit, 70, *254*
Sum of incisors (SI), 357–358
Swallowing, frequency of, 58–61

Tanner Growth and Development Chart,
 279, 280
Telescoped bite, 369, *462*
Temporal fossa, position of, *351*
Temporomandibular joint, disorders of, 230
Tenumbaum, Mario. See *ACCO appliance.*

Third-party involvement, in dentistry, 2–3
Tissue reaction, to orthodontic forces,
 theories of, 7–9
Tongue, action of, in Bionator therapy,
 229–230
 function of, in malocclusion, 230–231
Tongue crib, Kinetor and, 521
Tongue thrust, 70, 77
 anterior open bite and, 510–512, *513*
 Class III malocclusion and, 510–512, *513*
Tooth (teeth), anterior, alignment of, *25*
 as anchorage units, 100
 crowding of, Bimler appliance in, *370,*
 471–479
 elastic open activator and, 257–259
 with hypoplasia, 452–462
 eruption of, activator and, 273–274
 intrusion of, activator and, 275
 movement of, hazards of, 100
 sagittal, with Bimler appliance, 372
 rotation of, single, 29, *30*
Traction, intermaxillary, in Class II
 malocclusion, 99–103
Treatment timing, 599–600
Triangular clasps, *17*, 18–19
Trimming, of activator, 331

U-bow activator of Karwetsky, 216–227
U loop, in Bimler appliance, *386–387*
Unilateral crossbite, *43*, 265, *266*
Unilateral retro-occlusion, *58, 59*

Vertical overbite, activator therapy and, 170(t)
Vestibular screen(s), banded appliance and,
 87, 88
 definition of, 76–77
 function of, *69*
 in deciduous dentition, 70
 in finger sucking, 73–74
 in mouth breathing, 74–86
 limitations of, 80–86
 modification of, for banded appliance,
 87, 88
 muscle forces and, 68–86
 of Kraus, *79*
 open bite and, *82*
Vorbissplatte. See *Guide plane plate.*

Watry, F., 120
Weise jackscrew, *208, 209*
Whip appliance, 29, *30*
"White Girl" case, 402–416
Wire(s), arch, in activator, 327
 in Bimler appliance, 376–378, *423, 424*
 labial, in active plate, 21–23
 in Class III activator, 333–334

Woodside activator, 269–336. See also
 Activator.
Wunderer activator, *208*

Y-plates, *44, 45, 47*
"Yellow Girl" case, 488–498
Young adults, removable appliances in, 61